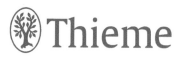

Medical Microbiology and Immunology Q&A

Melphine M. Harriott, PhD, D(ABMM), MT(ASCP)SM
Technical Director
Clinical Microbiology Laboratory
Ascension Michigan Laboratory Services
Detroit, Michigan, USA

Michelle Swanson-Mungerson, PhD
Associate Professor
Department of Microbiology and Immunology
Chicago College of Osteopathic Medicine
Midwestern University
Downers Grove, Illinois, USA

Samia Ragheb†, PhD
Formerly Assistant Professor
Department of Biomedical Sciences (Immunology)
William Beaumont School of Medicine
Oakland University
Rochester Hills, Michigan, USA

Matthew P. Jackson, PhD
Assistant Dean
Academic and Student Programs
Associate Professor
Microbiology, Immunology and Biochemistry
Wayne State University School of Medicine
Detroit, Michigan, USA

260 illustrations

Thieme
New York • Stuttgart • Delhi • Rio de Janeiro

Acquisitions Editor: Delia K. DeTurris
Managing Editor: Nidhi Chopra
Director, Editorial Services: Mary Jo Casey
Production Editor: Shivika
International Production Director: Andreas Schabert
Editorial Director: Sue Hodgson
International Marketing Director: Fiona Henderson
International Sales Director: Louisa Turrell
Director of Institutional Sales: Adam Bernacki
Senior Vice President and Chief Operating Officer: Sarah Vanderbilt
President: Brian D. Scanlan

Library of Congress Cataloging-in-Publication Data is available from the publisher

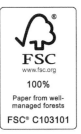

FSC
www.fsc.org
100%
Paper from well-managed forests
FSC® C103101

© 2019 Thieme Medical Publishers, Inc.
Thieme Publishers New York
333 Seventh Avenue, New York, NY 10001 USA
+1 800 782 3488, customerservice@thieme.com

Thieme Publishers Stuttgart
Rüdigerstrasse 14, 70469 Stuttgart, Germany
+49 [0]711 8931 421, customerservice@thieme.de

Thieme Publishers Delhi
A-12, Second Floor, Sector-2, Noida-201301
Uttar Pradesh, India
+91 120 45 566 00, customerservice@thieme.in

Thieme Publishers Rio de Janeiro,
Thieme Publicações Ltda.
Edifício Rodolpho de Paoli, 25º andar
Av. Nilo Peçanha, 50 – Sala 2508
Rio de Janeiro 20020-906, Brasil
+55 21 3172 2297

Cover design: Thieme Publishing Group
Typesetting by Thomson Digital

Printed in USA by King Printing Company, Inc.   5 4 3 2 1

ISBN 978-1-62623-382-9

Also available as an e-book:
eISBN 978-1-62623-383-6

Important note: Medicine is an ever-changing science undergoing continual development. Research and clinical experience are continually expanding our knowledge, in particular our knowledge of proper treatment and drug therapy. Insofar as this book mentions any dosage or application, readers may rest assured that the authors, editors, and publishers have made every effort to ensure that such references are in accordance with **the state of knowledge at the time of production of the book**.

Nevertheless, this does not involve, imply, or express any guarantee or responsibility on the part of the publishers in respect to any dosage instructions and forms of applications stated in the book. **Every user is requested to examine carefully** the manufacturers' leaflets accompanying each drug and to check, if necessary in consultation with a physician or specialist, whether the dosage schedules mentioned therein or the contraindications stated by the manufacturers differ from the statements made in the present book. Such examination is particularly important with drugs that are either rarely used or have been newly released on the market. Every dosage schedule or every form of application used is entirely at the user's own risk and responsibility. The authors and publishers request every user to report to the publishers any discrepancies or inaccuracies noticed. If errors in this work are found after publication, errata will be posted at www.thieme.com on the product description page.

Some of the product names, patents, and registered designs referred to in this book are in fact registered trademarks or proprietary names even though specific reference to this fact is not always made in the text. Therefore, the appearance of a name without designation as proprietary is not to be construed as a representation by the publisher that it is in the public domain. The knowledge base for medicine is always changing and expanding, especially regarding new methods for diagnosing diseases and proposed therapies or treatment regimens for those diseases. The author and publisher of this book have used reliable resources to provide the information in this book; however, given both the possibility for human error and the changing nature of medicine, neither the author nor the publisher warrants that the material contained in this book is completely accurate or complete in coverage and they disclaim all responsibility for any errors or omissions. Users of this book are encouraged to independently confirm any information contained herein believed to be in error. Although the contents of this book provide example patient vignettes and, through the explanations for the questions, offer diagnoses for medical conditions, the reader should not use the information contained herein for self-diagnosis, and should always seek the opinion of a health care provider if they suspect themselves to have an illness.

To my husband, Alwyn, and my parents, Melchizedek and Josephine, thank you for your unconditional love and support while I worked on this seemingly never-ending project. To my current and future students, thanks for pushing me to be better, dig deeper, and to know more. To my fellow authors, Matt, Michelle, and Sam, thank you for saying yes and for being part of this project.
Melphine M. Harriott

I want to thank my family for their support and understanding, since this project significantly added to our already hectic lives. I love you guys so much! I also want to thank my colleagues in the Department of Microbiology and Immunology in the Chicago College of Osteopathic Medicine (CCOM) for their guidance and mentorship during my time at CCOM. Furthermore, I want to thank the students that I work with at Midwestern University for always keeping me on my toes and making me think about immunology and infectious diseases from many different angles.
Michelle Swanson-Mungerson

To my fellow authors, without whom this project would not have been possible. Special thanks go to my family for their never-ending love and enduring support throughout the years.
Samia Ragheb[†]

To my fellow authors, Michelle, Sam, and Melphine whose boundless energy made this project happen. To my wife and daughter for their enduring love and support.
Matthew P. Jackson

[†]Prior to publication, our dear friend Samia Ragheb passed away. We are grateful for her dedication to her students, colleagues, and the field of immunology. She is greatly missed.—*Editors*

Contents

Preface

This book is a collection of multiple choice questions (MCQs) for the first- and second-year medical students to promote the learning of medical immunology and microbiology. The questions in this book reflect high yield information covered in a preclinical medical immunology/microbiology course and in the United States Medical Licensing Examination (USMLE) Step 1 and Comprehensive Osteopathic Medical Licensing Examination (COMLEX) Level 1.

This book contains 550 questions. It is divided into two sections, Immunology and Microbiology. For the Immunology section, where possible, the chapters are separated by subject matter. Some questions could not be categorized into one chapter; hence, these questions are included in a chapter titled "General Immunology." The Microbiology section is subdivided by organ system. Again, some questions could not be categorized under an organ system and were placed in the chapter on "General Microbiology."

The majority of the MCQs are similar to the type of questions that students may see on Step 1 medical board exams in the United States and are written using patient-centered vignettes. All questions are "one best answer"; in most cases, there are five answer choices.

Each MCQ is provided with the correct answer and an explanation. The explanation includes both the reasons why a given answer is correct and why the distractors are wrong. Some explanations include images to aid in the explanation.

In addition, each question is marked with a difficulty level. There are three levels of difficulty: easy (1), medium (2), and hard (3). Many questions are related to the highest levels of Bloom's taxonomy (e.g., interpretation of data and solution of problems) rather than being simple recall questions.

Both immunology and microbiology are fast-evolving disciplines. The authors have checked sources believed to be reliable, in order to provide information that is accurate and in accordance with the currently accepted evidence-based standards.

This book is not intended to be a substitute for immunology or microbiology textbooks. Students are strongly advised to consult their textbooks for more in-depth coverage of the subject matter.

Melphine M. Harriott, PhD, D(ABMM), MT(ASCP)SM
Michelle Swanson-Mungerson, PhD
Samia Ragheb†, PhD
Matthew P. Jackson, PhD

Acknowledgments

Several medical students played vital roles in the development of this book.

Thomas C. Bolig—Tom worked on this book while he was a fourth-year medical student at Wayne State University School of Medicine. He wrote several immunology and microbiology questions and provided feedback to the faculty authors. He is currently finishing a research fellowship at the National Institutes of Health and will pursue an Internal Medicine Residency after graduating from medical school.

Alexander S. Maris—Alex was a fourth-year medical student at Vanderbilt University School of Medicine while working on this project. He contributed several multiple choice questions to both the immunology and microbiology sections. He also reviewed and provided feedback for many of the chapters. He will be starting a Pathology Residency at Vanderbilt University Medical Center and plans to be a clinical microbiologist in the future.

Tom and Alex's contribution to this book is invaluable.

Other medical students who reviewed and provided feedback on the questions include:

Jocelyn Durlacher—third-year medical student at Vanderbilt University School of Medicine.

Lauren McNickle—third-year medical student at Frank H. Netter MD School of Medicine/Quinnipiac University.

Paige Peterson—fourth-year medical student at Frank H. Netter MD School of Medicine/Quinnipiac University.

Melphine M. Harriott, PhD, D(ABMM), MT(ASCP)SM
Michelle Swanson-Mungerson, PhD
Samia Ragheb†, PhD
Matthew P. Jackson, PhD

Contributors

Thomas C. Bolig, MS, MD
Resident Physician
Department of Internal Medicine
University of Michigan
Ann Arbor, Michigan, USA

Melphine M. Harriott, PhD, D(ABMM), MT(ASCP)SM
Technical Director
Clinical Microbiology Laboratory
Ascension Michigan Laboratory Services
Detroit, Michigan, USA

This work was completed in part while the author had the following affiliations:

Fellow, Clinical Microbiology
Department of Pathology, Microbiology and Immunology
Vanderbilt University Medical Center
Nashville, Tennessee, USA
Assistant Professor
Department of Microbiology and Immunology
Chicago College of Osteopathic Medicine
Midwestern University
Downers Grove, Illinois, USA

Matthew P. Jackson, PhD
Assistant Dean
Academic and Student Programs
Associate Professor
Microbiology, Immunology and Biochemistry
Wayne State University School of Medicine
Detroit, Michigan, USA

Alexander S. Maris, MD
Resident Physician
Department of Pathology, Microbiology and Immunology
Vanderbilt University Medical Center
Nashville, Tennessee, USA

Samia Ragheb†, PhD
Formerly Assistant Professor
Department of Biomedical Sciences (Immunology)
William Beaumont School of Medicine
Oakland University
Rochester Hills, Michigan, USA

Michelle Swanson-Mungerson, PhD
Associate Professor
Department of Microbiology and Immunology
Chicago College of Osteopathic Medicine
Midwestern University
Downers Grove, Illinois, USA

Abbreviations

ACh	acetylcholine		**ETEC**	enterotoxigenic *Escherichia coli*
ADP	adenosine diphosphate ribose		**GABA**	gamma aminobutyric acid
AFB	acid-fast bacilli		**GI**	gastrointestinal
AIDS	acquired immunodeficiency syndrome		**GNC**	gram-negative cocci
ALT	alanine amino transferase		**GNR**	gram-negative rod
AST	aspartate amino transferase		**GPC**	gram-positive cocci
ATP	adenosine triphosphate		**GPR**	gram-positive rod
cGMP	cyclic GMP		**HIV**	human immunodeficiency virus
CAMP	Christie, Atkins, Munch-Peterson		**IFN**	interferon
cAMP	cyclic adenosine monophosphate		**IL**	interleukin
CBC	complete blood count		**IV**	intravenous
CDC	Centers for Disease Control and Prevention		**IVDU**	intravenous drug use
CFU	colony forming unit		**KOH**	potassium hydroxide
cGMP	cyclic guanosine monophosphate		**LPS**	lipopolysaccharide
CO₂	carbon dioxide		**MAP**	mitogen-activated protein
COPD	chronic obstructive pulmonary disease		**MCV**	mean corpuscular volume
CSF	cerebrospinal fluid		**MHC**	major histocompatibility complex
CT	computed tomography		**MRI**	magnetic resonance imaging
DIC	disseminated intravascular coagulation		**O&P**	ova and parasite
DFA	direct fluorescent antibody		**PCR**	polymerase chain reaction
EAEC	enteroaggregative *Escherichia coli*		**PMNs**	polymorphonuclear cell
EAST	enteroaggregative heat stable toxin		**RBC**	red blood cell
EHEC	enterohemorrhagic *Escherichia coli*		**SNARE**	soluble attachment protein receptor
EPEC	enteropathogenic *Escherichia coli*		**STEC**	shiga-toxin producing *E. coli*
EIA	enzyme immunoassay		**TNF**	tumor necrosis factor
EIEC	enteroinvasive *Escherichia coli*		**UTIs**	urinary tract infections
ELISA	enzyme-linked immunosorbent assay		**WBC**	white blood cell

How to Use This Series

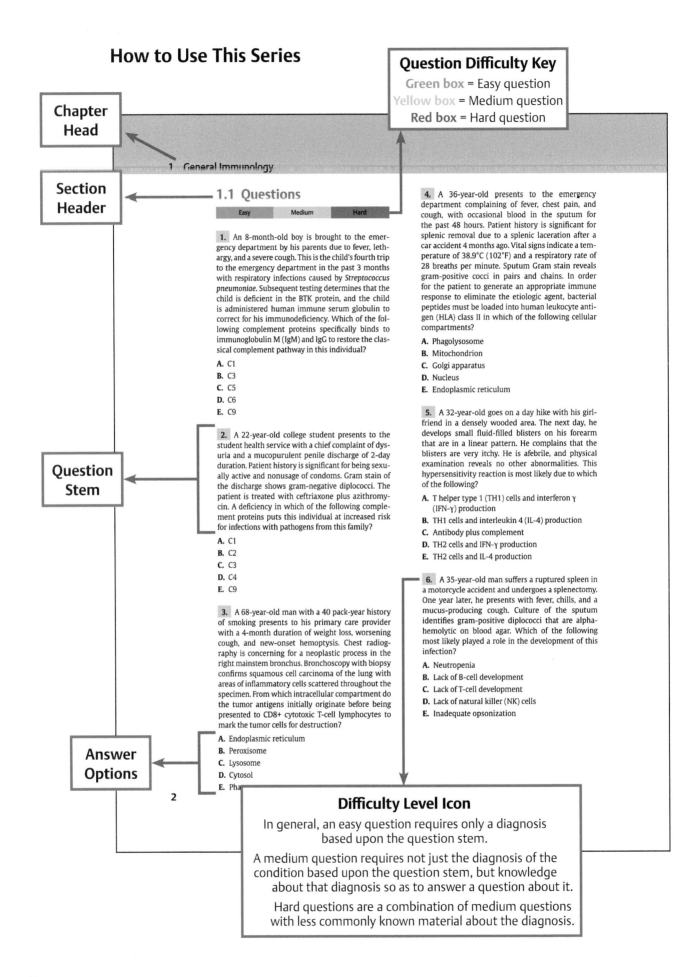

Chapter Head

Question Difficulty Key
Green box = Easy question
Yellow box = Medium question
Red box = Hard question

1 General Immunology

Section Header

1.1 Questions

Easy	Medium	Hard

Question Stem

1. An 8-month-old boy is brought to the emergency department by his parents due to fever, lethargy, and a severe cough. This is the child's fourth trip to the emergency department in the past 3 months with respiratory infections caused by *Streptococcus pneumoniae*. Subsequent testing determines that the child is deficient in the BTK protein, and the child is administered human immune serum globulin to correct for his immunodeficiency. Which of the following complement proteins specifically binds to immunoglobulin M (IgM) and IgG to restore the classical complement pathway in this individual?

A. C1
B. C3
C. C5
D. C6
E. C9

2. A 22-year-old college student presents to the student health service with a chief complaint of dysuria and a mucopurulent penile discharge of 2-day duration. Patient history is significant for being sexually active and nonusage of condoms. Gram stain of the discharge shows gram-negative diplococci. The patient is treated with ceftriaxone plus azithromycin. A deficiency in which of the following complement proteins puts this individual at increased risk for infections with pathogens from this family?

A. C1
B. C2
C. C3
D. C4
E. C9

3. A 68-year-old man with a 40 pack-year history of smoking presents to his primary care provider with a 4-month duration of weight loss, worsening cough, and new-onset hemoptysis. Chest radiography is concerning for a neoplastic process in the right mainstem bronchus. Bronchoscopy with biopsy confirms squamous cell carcinoma of the lung with areas of inflammatory cells scattered throughout the specimen. From which intracellular compartment do the tumor antigens initially originate before being presented to CD8+ cytotoxic T-cell lymphocytes to mark the tumor cells for destruction?

Answer Options

A. Endoplasmic reticulum
B. Peroxisome
C. Lysosome
D. Cytosol
E. Pha

2

4. A 36-year-old presents to the emergency department complaining of fever, chest pain, and cough, with occasional blood in the sputum for the past 48 hours. Patient history is significant for splenic removal due to a splenic laceration after a car accident 4 months ago. Vital signs indicate a temperature of 38.9°C (102°F) and a respiratory rate of 28 breaths per minute. Sputum Gram stain reveals gram-positive cocci in pairs and chains. In order for the patient to generate an appropriate immune response to eliminate the etiologic agent, bacterial peptides must be loaded into human leukocyte antigen (HLA) class II in which of the following cellular compartments?

A. Phagolysosome
B. Mitochondrion
C. Golgi apparatus
D. Nucleus
E. Endoplasmic reticulum

5. A 32-year-old goes on a day hike with his girlfriend in a densely wooded area. The next day, he develops small fluid-filled blisters on his forearm that are in a linear pattern. He complains that the blisters are very itchy. He is afebrile, and physical examination reveals no other abnormalities. This hypersensitivity reaction is most likely due to which of the following?

A. T helper type 1 (TH1) cells and interferon γ (IFN-γ) production
B. TH1 cells and interleukin 4 (IL-4) production
C. Antibody plus complement
D. TH2 cells and IFN-γ production
E. TH2 cells and IL-4 production

6. A 35-year-old man suffers a ruptured spleen in a motorcycle accident and undergoes a splenectomy. One year later, he presents with fever, chills, and a mucus-producing cough. Culture of the sputum identifies gram-positive diplococci that are alpha-hemolytic on blood agar. Which of the following most likely played a role in the development of this infection?

A. Neutropenia
B. Lack of B-cell development
C. Lack of T-cell development
D. Lack of natural killer (NK) cells
E. Inadequate opsonization

Difficulty Level Icon

In general, an easy question requires only a diagnosis based upon the question stem.

A medium question requires not just the diagnosis of the condition based upon the question stem, but knowledge about that diagnosis so as to answer a question about it.

Hard questions are a combination of medium questions with less commonly known material about the diagnosis.

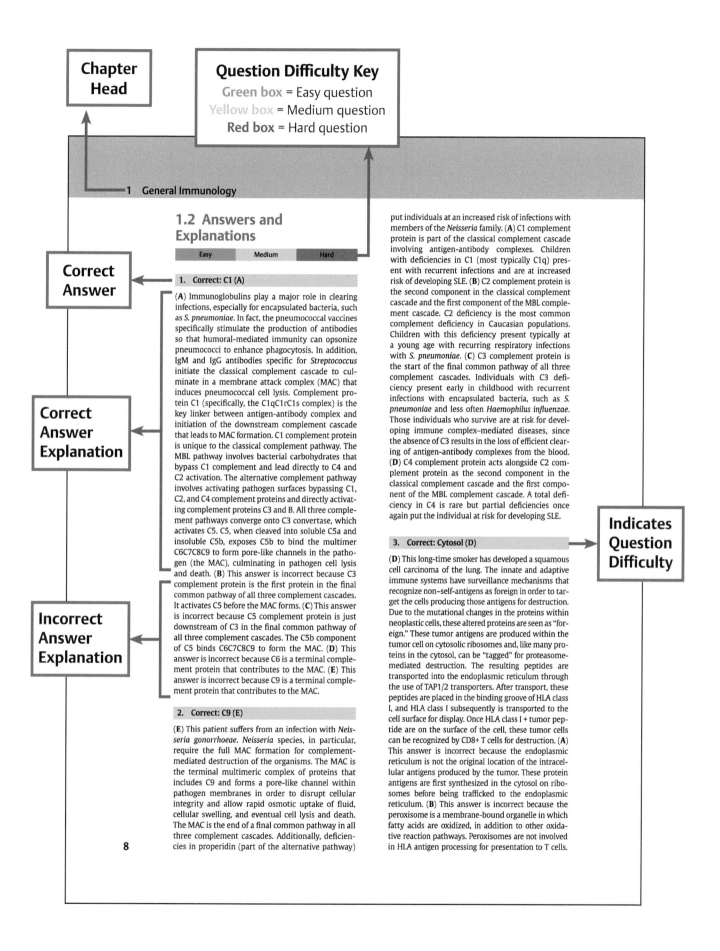

Chapter Head

Question Difficulty Key
Green box = Easy question
Yellow box = Medium question
Red box = Hard question

1 General Immunology

1.2 Answers and Explanations

| Easy | Medium | Hard |

Correct Answer

1. Correct: C1 (A)

(**A**) Immunoglobulins play a major role in clearing infections, especially for encapsulated bacteria, such as *S. pneumoniae*. In fact, the pneumococcal vaccines specifically stimulate the production of antibodies so that humoral-mediated immunity can opsonize pneumococci to enhance phagocytosis. In addition, IgM and IgG antibodies specific for *Streptococcus* initiate the classical complement cascade to culminate in a membrane attack complex (MAC) that induces pneumococcal cell lysis. Complement protein C1 (specifically, the C1qC1rC1s complex) is the key linker between antigen-antibody complex and initiation of the downstream complement cascade that leads to MAC formation. C1 complement protein is unique to the classical complement pathway. The MBL pathway involves bacterial carbohydrates that bypass C1 complement and lead directly to C4 and C2 activation. The alternative complement pathway involves activating pathogen surfaces bypassing C1, C2, and C4 complement proteins and directly activating complement proteins C3 and B. All three complement pathways converge onto C3 convertase, which activates C5. C5, when cleaved into soluble C5a and insoluble C5b, exposes C5b to bind the multimer C6C7C8C9 to form pore-like channels in the pathogen (the MAC), culminating in pathogen cell lysis and death. (**B**) This answer is incorrect because C3 complement protein is the first protein in the final common pathway of all three complement cascades. It activates C5 before the MAC forms. (**C**) This answer is incorrect because C5 complement protein is just downstream of C3 in the final common pathway of all three complement cascades. The C5b component of C5 binds C6C7C8C9 to form the MAC. (**D**) This answer is incorrect because C6 is a terminal complement protein that contributes to the MAC. (**E**) This answer is incorrect because C9 is a terminal complement protein that contributes to the MAC.

Correct Answer Explanation

Incorrect Answer Explanation

2. Correct: C9 (E)

(**E**) This patient suffers from an infection with *Neisseria gonorrhoeae*. *Neisseria* species, in particular, require the full MAC formation for complement-mediated destruction of the organisms. The MAC is the terminal multimeric complex of proteins that includes C9 and forms a pore-like channel within pathogen membranes in order to disrupt cellular integrity and allow rapid osmotic uptake of fluid, cellular swelling, and eventual cell lysis and death. The MAC is the end of a final common pathway in all three complement cascades. Additionally, deficiencies in properidin (part of the alternative pathway) put individuals at an increased risk of infections with members of the *Neisseria* family. (**A**) C1 complement protein is part of the classical complement cascade involving antigen-antibody complexes. Children with deficiencies in C1 (most typically C1q) present with recurrent infections and are at increased risk of developing SLE. (**B**) C2 complement protein is the second component in the classical complement cascade and the first component of the MBL complement cascade. C2 deficiency is the most common complement deficiency in Caucasian populations. Children with this deficiency present typically at a young age with recurring respiratory infections with *S. pneumoniae*. (**C**) C3 complement protein is the start of the final common pathway of all three complement cascades. Individuals with C3 deficiency present early in childhood with recurrent infections with encapsulated bacteria, such as *S. pneumoniae* and less often *Haemophilus influenzae*. Those individuals who survive are at risk for developing immune complex–mediated diseases, since the absence of C3 results in the loss of efficient clearing of antigen-antibody complexes from the blood. (**D**) C4 complement protein acts alongside C2 complement protein as the second component in the classical complement cascade and the first component of the MBL complement cascade. A total deficiency in C4 is rare but partial deficiencies once again put the individual at risk for developing SLE.

3. Correct: Cytosol (D)

(**D**) This long-time smoker has developed a squamous cell carcinoma of the lung. The innate and adaptive immune systems have surveillance mechanisms that recognize non–self-antigens as foreign in order to target the cells producing those antigens for destruction. Due to the mutational changes in the proteins within neoplastic cells, these altered proteins are seen as "foreign." These tumor antigens are produced within the tumor cell on cytosolic ribosomes and, like many proteins in the cytosol, can be "tagged" for proteasome-mediated destruction. The resulting peptides are transported into the endoplasmic reticulum through the use of TAP1/2 transporters. After transport, these peptides are placed in the binding groove of HLA class I, and HLA class I subsequently is transported to the cell surface for display. Once HLA class I + tumor peptide are on the surface of the cell, these tumor cells can be recognized by CD8+ T cells for destruction. (**A**) This answer is incorrect because the endoplasmic reticulum is not the original location of the intracellular antigens produced by the tumor. These protein antigens are first synthesized in the cytosol on ribosomes before being trafficked to the endoplasmic reticulum. (**B**) This answer is incorrect because the peroxisome is a membrane-bound organelle in which fatty acids are oxidized, in addition to other oxidative reaction pathways. Peroxisomes are not involved in HLA antigen processing for presentation to T cells.

Indicates Question Difficulty

8

Laboratory Values

	REFERENCE RANGE	SI REFERENCE INTERVALS
BLOOD, PLASMA, SERUM		
* Alanine aminotransferase (ALT), serum	8-20 U/L	8-20 U/L
Amylase, serum	25-125 U/L	25-125 U/L
* Aspartate aminotransferase (AST), serum	8-20 U/L	8-20 U/L
Bilirubin, serum (adult) Total // Direct	0.1-1.0 mg/dL // 0.0-0.3 mg/dL	2-17 µmol/L // 0-5 µmol/L
* Calcium, serum (Ca^{2+})	8.4-10.2 mg/dL	2.1-2.8 mmol/L
* Cholesterol, serum	Rec:<200 mg/dL	<5.2 mmol/L
Cortisol, serum	0800 h: 5-23 µg/dL // 1600 h: 3-15 µg/dL	138-635 nmol/L // 82-413 nmol/L
	2000 h: < 50% of 0800 h	Fraction of 0800 h: < 0.50
Creatine kinase, serum	Male: 25-90 U/L	25-90 U/L
	Female: 10-70 U/L	10-70 U/L
* Creatinine, serum	0.6-1.2 mg/dL	53-106 µmol/L
Electrolytes, serum		
Sodium (Na^+)	136-145 mEq/L	136-145 mmol/L
* Potassium (K^+)	3.5-5.0 mEq/L	3.5-5.0 mmol/L
Chloride (Cl^-)	95-105 mEq/L	95-105 mmol/L
Bicarbonate (HCO_3^-)	22-28 mEq/L	22-28 mmol/L
Magnesium (Mg^{2+})	1.5-2.0 mEq/L	0.75-1.0 mmol/L
Estriol, total, serum (in pregnancy)		
24-28 wks // 32-36 wks	30-170 ng/mL // 60-280 ng/mL	104-590 nmol/L // 208-970 nmol/L
28-32 wks // 36-40 wks	40-220 ng/mL // 80-350 ng/mL	140-760 nmol/L // 280-1210 nmol/L
Ferritin, serum	Male: 15-200 ng/mL	15-200 µg/L
	Female: 12-150 ng/mL	12-150 µg/L
Follicle-stimulating hormone, serum/plasma	Male: 4-25 mIU/mL	4-25 U/L
	Female: premenopause 4-30 mIU/mL	4-30 U/L
	midcycle peak 10-90 mIU/mL	10-90 U/L
	postmenopause 40-250 mIU/mL	40-250 U/L
Gases, arterial blood (room air)		
pH	7.35-7.45	[H^+] 36-44 nmol/L
PCO_2	33-45 mm Hg	4.4-5.9 kPa
PO_2	75-105 mm Hg	10.0-14.0 kPa
* Glucose, serum	Fasting: 70-110 mg/dL	3.8-6.1 mmol/L
	2-h postprandial: < 120 mg/dL	< 6.6 mmol/L
Growth hormone - arginine stimulation	Fasting: < 5 ng/mL	< 5 µg/L
	provocative stimuli: > 7 ng/mL	> 7 µg/L
Immunoglobulins, serum		
IgA	76-390 mg/dL	0.76-3.90 g/L
IgE	0-380 IU/mL	0-380 kIU/L
IgG	650-1500 mg/dL	6.5-15 g/L
IgM	40-345 mg/dL	0.4-3.45 g/L
Iron	50-170 µg/dL	9-30 µmol/L
Lactate dehydrogenase, serum	45-90 U/L	45-90 U/L
Luteinizing hormone, serum/plasma	Male: 6-23 mIU/mL	6-23 U/L
	Female: follicular phase 5-30 mIU/mL	5-30 U/L
	midcycle 75-150 mIU/mL	75-150 U/L
	postmenopause 30-200 mIU/mL	30-200 U/L
Osmolality, serum	275-295 mOsmol/kg H_2O	275-295 mOsmol/kg H_2O
Parathyroid hormone, serum, N-terminal	230-630 pg/mL	230-630 ng/L
* Phosphatase (alkaline), serum (p-NPP at 30°C)	20-70 U/L	20-70 U/L
* Phosphorus (inorganic), serum	3.0-4.5 mg/dL	1.0-1.5 mmol/L
Prolactin, serum (hPRL)	< 20 ng/mL	< 20 µg/L
* Proteins, serum		
Total (recumbent)	6.0-7.8 g/dL	60-78 g/L
Albumin	3.5-5.5 g/dL	35-55 g/L
Globulin	2.3-3.5 g/dL	23-35 g/L
Thyroid-stimulating hormone, serum or plasma	0.5-5.0 µU/mL	0.5-5.0 mU/L
Thyroidal iodine (^{123}I) uptake	8%-30% of administered dose/24 h	0.08-0.30/24 h
Thyroxine (T_4), serum	5-12 µg/dL	64-155 nmol/L
Triglycerides, serum	35-160 mg/dL	0.4-1.81 mmol/L
Triiodothyronine (T_3), serum (RIA)	115-190 ng/dL	1.8-2.9 nmol/L
Triiodothyronine (T_3) resin uptake	25%-35%	0.25-0.35
* Urea nitrogen, serum	7-18 mg/dL	1.2-3.0 mmol/L
* Uric acid, serum	3.0-8.2 mg/dL	0.18-0.48 mmol/L

* Included in the Biochemical Profile (SMA-12)

	REFERENCE RANGE	SI REFERENCE INTERVALS

BODY MASS INDEX (BMI)

Body mass index .... Adult: 19-25 kg/m²

CEREBROSPINAL FLUID

Cell count .... 0-5/mm³ .... $0\text{-}5 \times 10^6/L$

Chloride .... 118-132 mEq/L .... 118-132 mmol/L

Gamma globulin .... 3%-12% total proteins 0.03-0.12

Glucose .... 40-70 mg/dL .... 2.2-3.9 mmol/L

Pressure .... 70-180 mm H_2O .... 70-180 mm H_2O

Proteins, total .... 40 mg/dL .... 0.40 g/L

HEMATOLOGIC

Bleeding time (template) .... 2-7 minutes .... 2-7 minutes

Erythrocyte count.................................... Male: 4.3-5.9 million/mm³ .... $4.3\text{-}5.9 \times 10^{12}/L$

                                          Female: 3.5-5.5 million/mm³ .... $3.5\text{-}5.5 \times 10^{12}/L$

Erythrocyte sedimentation rate (Westergren) .... Male: 0-15 mm/h .... 0-15 mm/h

    Female: 0-20 mm/h....................................... 0-20 mm/h

Hematocrit .... Male: 41%-53% 0.41-0.53

    Female: 36%-46%............................. 0.36-0.46

Hemoglobin A_{1c} .... < 6% .... < 0.06

Hemoglobin, blood................................... Male: 13.5-17.5 g/dL .... 2.09-2.71 mmol/L

    Female: 12.0-16.0 g/dL .... 1.86-2.48 mmol/L

Hemoglobin, plasma .... 1-4 mg/dL .... 0.16-0.62 mmol/L

Leukocyte count and differential

    Leukocyte count .... 4500-11,000/mm³ .... $4.5\text{-}11.0 \times 10^9/L$

    Segmented neutrophils .... 54%-62% 0.54-0.62

    Bands .... 3%-5% 0.03-0.05

    Eosinophils .... 1%-3% 0.01-0.03

    Basophils.. 0%-0.75% 0-0.0075

    Lymphocytes .... 25%-33% 0.25-0.33

    Monocytes .... 3%-7% 0.03-0.07

Mean corpuscular hemoglobin .... 25.4-34.6 pg/cell .... 0.39-0.54 fmol/cell

Mean corpuscular hemoglobin concentration .... 31%-36% Hb/cell .... 4.81-5.58 mmol Hb/L

Mean corpuscular volume .... 80-100 μm³ .... 80-100 fL

Partial thromboplastin time (activated) .... 25-40 seconds .... 25-40 seconds

Platelet count .... 150,000-400,000/mm³ .... $150\text{-}400 \times 10^9/L$

Prothrombin time.................................... 11-15 seconds .... 11-15 seconds

Reticulocyte count .... 0.5%-1.5% 0.005-0.015

Thrombin time.. <2 seconds deviation from control .... <2 seconds deviation from control

Volume

    Plasma .... Male: 25-43 mL/kg .... 0.025-0.043 L/kg

    Female: 28-45 mL/kg .... 0.028-0.045 L/kg

    Red cell .... Male: 20-36 mL/kg .... 0.020-0.036 L/kg

    Female: 19-31 mL/kg .... 0.019-0.031 L/kg

SWEAT

Chloride.. 0-35 mmol/L .... 0-35 mmol/L

URINE

Calcium .... 100-300 mg/24 h .... 2.5-7.5 mmol/24 h

Chloride.. Varies with intake .... Varies with intake

Creatinine clearance .... Male: 97-137 mL/min

Female: 88-128 mL/min

Estriol, total (in pregnancy)

    30 wks .... 6-18 mg/24 h .... 21-62 μmol/24 h

    35 wks .... 9-28 mg/24 h .... 31-97 μmol/24 h

    40 wks .... 13-42 mg/24 h .... 45-146 μmol/24 h

17-Hydroxycorticosteroids .... Male: 3.0-10.0 mg/24 h .... 8.2-27.6 μmol/24 h

    Female: 2.0-8.0 mg/24 h .... 5.5-22.0 μmol/24 h

17-Ketosteroids, total .... Male: 8-20 mg/24 h .... 28-70 μmol/24 h

    Female: 6-15 mg/24 h .... 21-52 μmol/24 h

Osmolality .... 50-1400 mOsmol/kg H_2O

Oxalate .... 8-40 μg/mL .... 90-445 μmol/L

Potassium .... Varies with diet .... Varies with diet

Proteins, total .... 150 mg/24 h .... 0.15 g/24 h

Sodium .... Varies with diet .... Varies with diet

Uric acid .... Varies with diet .... Varies with diet

Additional Normal Laboratory Values

BLOOD	REFERENCE RANGE	SI REFERENCE INTERVALS
CD4:CD8 ratio	1–4	-------
CD4+ T-cell count	640–1175 cells/µL	$0.64–1.18 \times 10^9$/L
CD8+ T-cell count	335–875 cells/µL	$0.34–0.88 \times 10^9$/L

*Reference: Merck Manuals Professional Edition / Normal Laboratory Values

CSF	REFERENCE RANGE
Opening pressure	10-20 cm H_2O

URINE	REFERENCE RANGE	SI REFERENCE INTERVALS
Urinalysis, dipstick testing		
Bilirubin	Negative	-------
Blood	Negative	-------
Glucose	Negative	-------
Ketones	Negative	-------
Leukocyte esterase	Negative	-------
Nitrites	Negative	-------
pH	5-7	-------
Protein	Negative	-------
Specific gravity	1.002–1.030	-------
Urobilinogen	0.2-1.0 EU	-------
Urinalysis, microscopic		
Bacteria	Negative	-------
Casts	Occasional hyaline casts	-------
Red blood cells	0-2/high power field	-------
White blood cells	0-2/high power field	-------

*Reference: Merck Manuals Professional Edition/Normal Laboratory Values

Chapter 1

General Immunology

Alexander S. Maris, Samia Ragheb[†], and Thomas C. Bolig

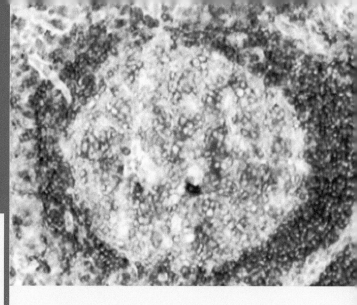

LEARNING OBJECTIVES

- Differentiate among the various proteins and mechanisms involved in the three major complement pathways.
- Understand the mechanisms by which complement proteins ultimately mediate microbial destruction.
- List the differences in intracellular pathways of antigen processing that ultimately result in antigen presentation to the appropriate T cell subsets.
- Discuss the major cellular and chemical actors in each hypersensitivity reaction.
- Describe the importance of splenic macrophages in the opsonization of encapsulated microbes.
- Compare active and passive immunity.
- Discuss the importance of interferon gamma and macrophage activation in the immune response.
- Describe the key chemical, enzyme, or immunoglobulin defects in the major congenital immunodeficiency disorders.
- Review the actions of the major cytokines and their associated key cellular effectors.
- Describe how the intracellular or extracellular nature of a pathogen determines what immune cell is most effective at combating that pathogen.
- Explain the critical role that apoptosis plays in central and peripheral immune tolerance.
- List key cytokines to their appropriate cellular effectors and actions.
- Discuss the increased incidence of infection in patients with hematopoietic malignancies.
- Describe the predominant mechanism of action for the major biologic immunotherapies.
- Recognize that foreign antigens may act as haptens that can lead to autoimmune disease.
- Describe how pathogen recognition receptors recognize various pathogen-associated molecular patterns.
- Describe the role of costimulatory receptors and ligands in the potent activation of T cells by antigen-presenting cells.
- Identify the major cellular markers of the various immune system cells.
- Recognize the hallmark malignant cells of the major hematopoietic malignancies.

- Recognize the clinical constellation of symptoms and laboratory findings associated with multiple myeloma.
- Recognize major cell-specific markers and match them to their corresponding cells.
- Describe how inappropriate adaptive immune system responses can lead to autoimmune disease.
- Recognize the clinical and laboratory findings associated with immune thrombocytopenic purpura.
- Recognize the characteristic clinical, laboratory, and immunofluorescent staining pattern of findings in Goodpasture's syndrome, an autoimmune disease.
- Recognize the characteristic clinical, laboratory, and histopathologic findings of gluten sensitive enteropathy (celiac disease).
- List which organs are immunoprivileged and relatively spared from autoimmunity.
- Recognize the importance of regulatory T cells and their effector molecules in host self-tolerance and protection from autoimmune disease.
- Discuss the immune response to viral infections.
- Differentiate between hypersensitivity reactions; describe the role of reticuloendothelial system in the clearance of immune complexes.
- Describe the immune response to mycobacteria.
- Discuss the susceptibility to pathogens for specific immunodeficiencies.

1.1 Questions

Easy	Medium	Hard

1. An 8-month-old boy is brought to the emergency department by his parents due to fever, lethargy, and a severe cough. This is the child's fourth trip to the emergency department in the past 3 months with respiratory infections caused by *Streptococcus pneumoniae*. Subsequent testing determines that the child is deficient in the BTK protein, and the child is administered human immune serum globulin to correct for his immunodeficiency. Which of the following complement proteins specifically binds to immunoglobulin M (IgM) and IgG to restore the classical complement pathway in this individual?

A. C1

B. C3

C. C5

D. C6

E. C9

2. A 22-year-old college student presents to the student health service with a chief complaint of dysuria and a mucopurulent penile discharge of 2-day duration. Patient history is significant for being sexually active and nonusage of condoms. Gram stain of the discharge shows gram-negative diplococci. The patient is treated with ceftriaxone plus azithromycin. A deficiency in which of the following complement proteins puts this individual at increased risk for infections with pathogens from this family?

A. C1

B. C2

C. C3

D. C4

E. C9

3. A 68-year-old man with a 40 pack-year history of smoking presents to his primary care provider with a 4-month duration of weight loss, worsening cough, and new-onset hemoptysis. Chest radiography is concerning for a neoplastic process in the right mainstem bronchus. Bronchoscopy with biopsy confirms squamous cell carcinoma of the lung with areas of inflammatory cells scattered throughout the specimen. From which intracellular compartment do the tumor antigens initially originate before being presented to CD8+ cytotoxic T-cell lymphocytes to mark the tumor cells for destruction?

A. Endoplasmic reticulum

B. Peroxisome

C. Lysosome

D. Cytosol

E. Phagosome

4. A 36-year-old presents to the emergency department complaining of fever, chest pain, and cough, with occasional blood in the sputum for the past 48 hours. Patient history is significant for splenic removal due to a splenic laceration after a car accident 4 months ago. Vital signs indicate a temperature of 38.9°C (102°F) and a respiratory rate of 28 breaths per minute. Sputum Gram stain reveals gram-positive cocci in pairs and chains. In order for the patient to generate an appropriate immune response to eliminate the etiologic agent, bacterial peptides must be loaded into human leukocyte antigen (HLA) class II in which of the following cellular compartments?

A. Phagolysosome

B. Mitochondrion

C. Golgi apparatus

D. Nucleus

E. Endoplasmic reticulum

5. A 32-year-old goes on a day hike with his girlfriend in a densely wooded area. The next day, he develops small fluid-filled blisters on his forearm that are in a linear pattern. He complains that the blisters are very itchy. He is afebrile, and physical examination reveals no other abnormalities. This hypersensitivity reaction is most likely due to which of the following?

A. T helper type 1 (TH1) cells and interferon γ (IFN-γ) production

B. TH1 cells and interleukin 4 (IL-4) production

C. Antibody plus complement

D. TH2 cells and IFN-γ production

E. TH2 cells and IL-4 production

6. A 35-year-old man suffers a ruptured spleen in a motorcycle accident and undergoes a splenectomy. One year later, he presents with fever, chills, and a mucus-producing cough. Culture of the sputum identifies gram-positive diplococci that are alpha-hemolytic on blood agar. Which of the following most likely played a role in the development of this infection?

A. Neutropenia

B. Lack of B-cell development

C. Lack of T-cell development

D. Lack of natural killer (NK) cells

E. Inadequate opsonization

7. A 24-year-old mother gives birth to a healthy 7-pound boy. She chooses to breastfeed her newborn. Which type of immunity is this baby receiving from his mother?

A. Passive innate immunity

B. Passive acquired immunity

C. Active innate immunity

D. Active acquired immunity

E. Innate adaptive immunity

8. A couple travels to South Africa and takes their 18-month-old daughter with them. Approximately 6 months later, the child develops a poor appetite, stops gaining weight, and develops a persistent cough. A chest X-ray shows multiple opacities of varying size. A tuberculin skin test is positive and a course of antibiotics is started. An immunological work-up revealed normal leukocyte counts. However, in vitro culture of white blood cells (WBCs) revealed a lack of tumor necrosis factor α (TNF-α) production. Which of the following conditions is most consistent with these clinical and laboratory findings?

A. Selective IgA deficiency

B. Common variable immunodeficiency

C. IFN-γ receptor 1 deficiency

D. Chronic granulomatous disease (CGD)

E. Autoimmune regulator (AIRE) deficiency

9. A 58-year-old woman undergoes a mastectomy and a course of chemotherapy. Monitoring of her absolute neutrophil count (ANC) shows that her ANC is 500 cells/μL (normal 1,500–8,000 cells/μL). Which of the following molecules would increase her ANC?

A. Granulocyte colony-stimulating factor (G-CSF)

B. IL-2

C. IFN-α

D. IFN-β

E. B cell activating factor (BAFF)

10. A 19-year-old college student develops a sore throat, fever, lymphadenopathy, and generalized malaise. He complains of feeling fatigued all the time. Physical examination shows an enlarged spleen. Pertinent laboratory findings are below:

- Complete blood count (CBC):
  - Red blood cells (RBCs): 5×10^6/μL
  - WBCs: 16,000/μL
  - Platelets: 130,000/μL
  - Monospot test: positive

Which of the following cell types is most likely to be involved in limiting this infection?

A. Neutrophil

B. B cell

C. CD4 T cell

D. CD8 T cell

E. Macrophage

11. Several mechanisms are important in maintaining central and peripheral immune tolerance. Apoptosis can maintain tolerance of the immune system in the periphery. Which of the following directly inhibits apoptosis?

A. IL-2

B. Fas ligand (FasL)

C. Caspase 3

D. TNF-α

E. B cell lymphoma 2 (Bcl-2)

12. A 13-year-old girl arrives in the emergency department in the middle of the night after experiencing vomiting and pain in the lower right abdomen. Appendicitis is suspected. Findings include a temperature of 38.3°C (101°F), pulse of 115 beats per minute, erythrocyte sedimentation rate (ESR) of 28 mm/h, and a WBC count of 12,000 per μL with 75% neutrophils. Which of the following molecules most likely triggered these physiological changes?

A. IL-1, IL-6, TNF-α

B. IL-12, IFN-γ

C. IL-4, IL-13

D. IFN-α, IFN-β

E. IL-10, transforming growth factor β (TGF-β)

13. A 67-year-old man develops severe painful shingles on the right side of his body. Physical examination shows a generalized lymphadenopathy with prominent cervical and axillary lymphadenopathy bilaterally and hepatosplenomegaly. A peripheral blood smear and a WBC count show lymphocytosis with normal appearing lymphocytes. Flow cytometry analysis is performed and demonstrates an unusually high percentage of CD5+CD19+ cells. Which of the following is the most likely diagnosis?

A. Acute lymphoblastic leukemia

B. Chronic lymphocytic leukemia (CLL)

C. Hairy cell leukemia

D. Adult T-cell leukemia

E. Hodgkin's lymphoma

14. A 60-year-old man suffers from uncontrolled hypertension for many years. He eventually develops end-stage renal failure and needs a kidney transplant. A first cousin has been identified as a suitable donor. Prior to surgery, induction therapy with daclizumab is initiated. What is the mechanism of action of this biologic immunotherapy?

A. Removal of passenger leukocytes in the graft

B. Blocking major histocompatibility complex (MHC) class I molecules

C. Blocking MHC class II molecules

D. Blocking IL-2R

E. Blocking T-cell co-stimulation

15. A 9-year-old boy is brought to the pediatrician with fever (38° [100.4°F]) and sore throat. During the physical examination, the pediatrician finds enlarged cervical lymph nodes, red swollen tonsils, and a tonsillar exudate. The pediatrician issues a prescription for penicillin as this patient had prior exposure to penicillin without incident. After 3 days, the boy complains of extreme fatigue. Laboratory analysis shows that his hemoglobin is 9 g/dL and bilirubin is 5 mg/dL. These later symptoms are most likely due to an immune response to:

A. Group A streptococcus antigen

B. Superantigen

C. Hapten

D. Pathogen-associated molecular patterns (PAMPs)

E. Damage-associated molecular patterns (DAMPs)

16. During spring break, a 20-year-old college student spent a week in Acapulco. After 4 days, he develops an abrupt onset of profuse watery diarrhea. He subsequently experiences five loose bowel movements each day. Within a few days, his symptoms resolve. Which of the following cell surface molecules allows immune recognition of the most likely organism causing this infection?

A. Cellular adhesion molecules

B. Toll-like receptors

C. Nucleotide-binding oligomerization domain (NOD)-like receptors

D. Retinoic acid-inducible gene I (RIG-I)

E. CD40

17. A 2-month-old boy is ready to begin his childhood vaccinations. At this stage, his antigen-specific T cells are naïve. For optimal activation and clonal expansion, naïve T cells are dependent on which of the following molecular interactions?

A. Binding of LFA-1 to ICAM-1

B. Binding of CD4 to MHC class II

C. Binding of CD8 to MHC class I

D. Binding of CD28 to B7-1 (CD80)

E. Binding of CTLA-4 to B7-1 (CD80)

18. A 62-year-old man who has previously enjoyed an active, healthy lifestyle is now suffering from frequent bacterial and viral infections. He now returns to his primary care physician because of an orbital infection and swollen hemorrhagic gums. On exam, he appears very pale. Pertinent laboratory results are below:

- CBC:
  - Hemoglobin: 8 g/dL
  - Platelets: 30,000/μL
  - WBCs: 20,000/μL
- Bone marrow analysis: 95% blasts
- Flow cytometry analysis of bone marrow aspirates shows a population of over 90% CD33+, CD117+ cells

Which of the following is the most likely diagnosis?

A. Acute myeloid leukemia (AML)

B. B cell acute lymphoblastic leukemia (B-ALL)

C. T cell acute lymphoblastic leukemia (T-ALL)

D. Severe combined immunodeficiency (SCID)

E. Acquired immunodeficiency syndrome (AIDS)

19. A 4-year-old boy has marked cervical lymph-adenopathy and splenomegaly. His mother states that he is always tired, has been less active, and seems to bruise quite easily. A blood work-up reveals anemia, neutropenia, and thrombocytopenia. Flow cytometry analysis shows a high percentage of CD10+, CD19+ cells and genetic analysis reveals hyperdiploidy. Which of the following is the most likely diagnosis?

A. Acute myeloid leukemia (AML)

B. B cell acute lymphoblastic leukemia (B-ALL)

C. T cell acute lymphoblastic leukemia (T-ALL)

D. Autoimmune lymphoproliferative syndrome

E. Hodgkin's lymphoma

20. A 55-year-old African American man presents with marked cervical lymphadenopathy. He has no other complaints. Histological examination of an excised lymph node shows histiocytes, eosinophils, lymphocytes, plasma cells, and some multinucleated Reed–Sternberg cells. Which of the following is the most likely diagnosis?

A. Hairy cell leukemia

B. Multiple myeloma

C. Hodgkin's lymphoma

D. Burkitt's lymphoma

E. Mantle cell lymphoma

21. A 70-year-old woman presents with a 3-month history of fatigue and backache. An X-ray of the lumbar spine shows severe demineralization, and magnetic resonance imaging (MRI) reveals lytic bone lesions and infiltration and destruction of L3 and L5. A CBC reveals anemia, and serum protein electrophoresis shows an abnormal paraprotein in the gamma globulin region. Serum creatinine is 2.7 mg/dL. Urine free light chain assay is pending. Which of the following is the most likely diagnosis?

A. Hodgkin's lymphoma

B. Marginal zone lymphoma

C. Mantle zone lymphoma

D. Follicular lymphoma

E. Multiple myeloma

22. A 26-year-old law intern complains of bruising easily and is experiencing menorrhagia. Palpation of the spleen reveals no abnormalities. Lab results are below:

- Prothrombin time: 12 seconds
- Partial thromboplastin time: 30 seconds
- Bleeding time: 11 minutes
- CBC:
  - RBCs: $5 \times 10^6/\mu L$
  - WBCs: $8,000/\mu L$
  - Platelets: $90,000/\mu L$
  - Hemoglobin: 13.5 g/dL

Which of the following autoantibodies is most likely responsible for her current condition?

A. Anti-Rh

B. Anti-penicillin

C. Anti-MHC class I

D. Antiglycoprotein IIb–IIIa

E. Anti–platelet endothelial cellular adhesion molecule (anti-PECAM-1)

23. A 26-year-old man presents with a 1-week history of coughing up blood. At the time of exam, he is afebrile and denies dyspnea. A chest X-ray shows bilateral infiltration. Urinalysis reveals proteinuria and hematuria and the presence of RBC casts. Immunofluorescent staining of a kidney biopsy shows smooth linear deposition of IgG and C3. Which of the following is the most likely diagnosis?

A. Tuberculosis (TB)

B. Systemic lupus erythematosus (SLE)

C. Goodpasture's syndrome

D. Bronchitis

E. Chronic obstructive pulmonary disease (COPD)

24. A mother brings her 2-year-old son to the pediatrician with a 2-week history of intermittent diarrhea. She also states that the boy does not seem to be growing over the past 3 months. Physical exam is unremarkable. When asked, the boy denies abdominal pain, but his mother states that his abdomen often becomes distended after meals and that his stools have a very unpleasant odor. An intestinal biopsy is ordered and shows villous atrophy, dense infiltration of lymphocytes in the lamina propria, and an increased number of intraepithelial lymphocytes. Which of the following is the most likely diagnosis?

A. Intestinal salmonellosis

B. Ulcerative colitis

C. Crohn's disease

D. Whipple's disease

E. Celiac disease

25. A 4-year-old girl presents with a 3-week history of twitching of the muscles around her mouth. Laboratory analysis reveals that her calcium levels are low and phosphorous levels are high. A subsequent biopsy of the parathyroid shows massive lymphocyte infiltration. Additionally, genetic testing demonstrates that the patient has two mutated copies of a gene that is inherited in an autosomal recessive pattern. This gene is found on chromosome 21q22.3 and is usually expressed by epithelial cells in the thymic medulla. The child is most likely deficient in which of the following?

A. MHC class I

B. MHC class II

C. Autoimmune regulator (AIRE)

D. CD28

E. CD80

26. Immunologically privileged sites contain sequestered self-antigens that are not usually the target of an autoimmune response. Injury to the tissue or organ may expose these sequestered antigens, and patients may subsequently develop autoimmune disease. Which of the following conditions is most likely to be caused by such an event?

A. Sympathetic ophthalmia

B. Psoriasis

C. Sjögren's syndrome

D. Graves' disease

E. Crohn's disease

27. Peripheral regulation of the immune system helps maintain tolerance against self-antigens. In several autoimmune diseases, defects of peripheral regulation have been shown to contribute to disease pathogenesis. Which of the following effector T-cell populations, if defective in number or function, contributes to defects in peripheral regulation?

A. T-bet expressing T cell

B. GATA-3 expressing T cell

C. RoRγt expressing T cell

D. Bcl-6 expressing T cell

E. FoxP3 expressing T cell

28. A 1-year-old girl is taken to a pediatrician's office by her father with a chief complaint that the girl has been fussy with a fever, infrequent loose stools, and mild nasal congestion over the last 4 days. Two days ago, she developed a rash around her trunk that has now migrated to her face and extremities. The pediatrician records a temperature of 36.7°C (98.7°F) and notes a blanching, maculopapular rash. Given the most likely diagnosis, which of the following binding interactions is needed to clear the infection?

A. IL-4 and IL-4 receptor

B. PD1 and PD-1 ligand

C. CD8 and MHC I

D. CTLA-4 and B7-2 (CD86)

E. CD40 and CD40 ligand

29. A 6-year-old boy is brought to the emergency department by his mother concerned over his fever, stiff neck, and headache. Vital signs reveal a temperature of 38.8°C (101.9°F). A lumbar puncture was performed and cerebrospinal fluid (CSF) was obtained. Gram stain of the CSF reveals gram-positive cocci in pairs and chains. Which of the following components is most critical for tagging this microorganism to enhance its engulfment by phagocytes?

A. C3b

B. C4a

C. C5a

D. C9

E. Mannose-binding lectin (MBL)

30. A 33-year-old woman with a past medical history significant for Raynaud's phenomenon presents to her physician's office for fatigue and unintended weight loss. She has been feeling very fatigued over the past few weeks, has lost 7 pounds, and feels feverish from time to time. She also notes that she has muscle aches and arthritis in her wrists and knees bilaterally. Her vital signs are: temperature 39°C (102.2°F), heart rate 89 beats per minute, and blood pressure 124/91. The woman has a malar rash and oral ulcer. Her cardiovascular exam is normal. Her lungs are clear to auscultation with no wheezes, rales, or rhonchi. Abdomen is nontender with mild splenomegaly. No joint erythema or deformities are present. Labs are pending. Given this woman's most likely diagnosis, what type of hypersensitivity reaction is responsible for the manifestations of her disease?

A. Type I hypersensitivity

B. Type II hypersensitivity

C. Type III hypersensitivity

D. Type IV hypersensitivity

31. A 59-year-old homeless man with past medical history of human immunodeficiency virus (HIV) is admitted for chest pain and dyspnea. The patient's vital signs are: temperature 40°C (104°F), heart rate 112 beats per minute, and blood pressure 101/70. Physical exam reveals that he appears cachectic and has bilateral cervical lymphadenopathy. He is aware and oriented to person, place, and time. His cardiovascular exam reveals tachycardia with regular rhythm. His lung exam is positive for rales throughout all lung fields and decreased fremitus in the posterior lower lung fields bilaterally. The trachea is midline. The abdomen is soft, nontender, and positive for hepatomegaly.

- CBC: pending
- Sputum Gram stain and culture: pending
- Blood cultures: pending
- Urine toxicology: negative
- Urine lipoarabinomannan: positive

Given the most likely diagnosis, which of the following ILs are necessary and specific for the clearance of the pathogen?

A. IL-1

B. IL-10

C. IL-12

D. IL-17

E. TGF-β

32. A 3-year-old boy with a history of recurrent infections has been diagnosed with X-linked agammaglobulinemia. To which of the following pathogens is he particularly susceptible?

A. Acid-fast bacilli

B. Encapsulated bacteria

C. Fungi

D. Intracellular parasite

E. Enveloped viruses

1.2 Answers and Explanations

Easy	Medium	Hard

1. Correct: C1 (A)

(**A**) Immunoglobulins play a major role in clearing infections, especially for encapsulated bacteria, such as *Streptococcus pneumoniae*. In fact, the pneumococcal vaccines specifically stimulate the production of antibodies so that humoral-mediated immunity can opsonize pneumococci to enhance phagocytosis. In addition, IgM and IgG antibodies specific for *Streptococcus* initiate the classical complement cascade to culminate in a membrane attack complex (MAC) that induces pneumococcal cell lysis. Complement protein

C1 (specifically, the C1qC1rC1s complex) is the key linker between antigen-antibody complex and initiation of the downstream complement cascade that leads to MAC formation. C1 complement protein is unique to the classical complement pathway. The mannose-binding lectin (MBL) pathway involves bacterial carbohydrates that bypass C1 complement and lead directly to C4 and C2 activation. The alternative complement pathway involves activating pathogen surfaces bypassing C1, C2, and C4 complement proteins and directly activating complement proteins C3 and B. All three complement pathways converge onto C3 convertase, which activates C5. C5, when cleaved into soluble C5a and insoluble C5b, exposes C5b to bind the multimer C6C7C8C9 to form pore-like channels in the pathogen (the MAC), culminating in pathogen cell lysis and death. (**B**) This answer is incorrect because C3 complement protein is the first protein in the final common pathway of all three complement cascades. It activates C5 before the MAC forms. (**C**) This answer is incorrect because C5 complement protein is just downstream of C3 in the final common pathway of all three complement cascades. The C5b component of C5 binds C6C7C8C9 to form the MAC. (**D**) This answer is incorrect because C6 is a terminal complement protein that contributes to the MAC. (**E**) This answer is incorrect because C9 is a terminal complement protein that contributes to the MAC.

2. Correct: C9 (E)

(**E**) This patient suffers from an infection with *Neisseria gonorrhoeae*. *Neisseria* species, in particular, require the full membrane attack complex (MAC) formation for complement-mediated destruction of the organisms. The MAC is the terminal multimeric complex of proteins that includes C9 and forms a pore-like channel within pathogen membranes in order to disrupt cellular integrity and allow rapid osmotic uptake of fluid, cellular swelling, and eventual cell lysis and death. The MAC is the end of a final common pathway in all three complement cascades. Additionally, deficiencies in properidin (part of the alternative pathway) put individuals at an increased risk of infections with members of the *Neisseria* family. (**A**) C1 complement protein is part of the classical complement cascade involving antigen-antibody complexes. Children with deficiencies in C1 (most typically C1q) present with recurrent infections and are at increased risk of developing systemic lupus erythematosus (SLE). (**B**) C2 complement protein is the second component in the classical complement cascade and the first component of the MBL complement cascade. C2 deficiency is the most common complement deficiency in Caucasian populations. Children with this deficiency present typically at a young age with recurring respiratory infections with *Streptococcus pneumoniae*. (**C**) C3 complement protein is the start of the final common pathway of all three complement cascades. Individuals with C3 deficiency present early in childhood with recurrent infections with encapsulated bacteria, such as *S. pneumoniae* and less often *Haemophilus influenzae.* Those individuals who survive are at risk for developing immune complex–mediated diseases, since the absence of C3 results in the loss of efficient clearing of antigen-antibody complexes from the blood. (**D**) C4 complement protein acts alongside C2 complement protein as the second component in the classical complement cascade and the first component of the MBL complement cascade. A total deficiency in C4 is rare but partial deficiencies once again put the individual at risk for developing SLE.

3. Correct: Cytosol (D)

(**D**) This long-time smoker has developed a squamous cell carcinoma of the lung. The innate and adaptive immune systems have surveillance mechanisms that recognize non–self-antigens as foreign in order to target the cells producing those antigens for destruction. Due to the mutational changes in the proteins within neoplastic cells, these altered proteins are seen as "foreign." These tumor antigens are produced within the tumor cell on cytosolic ribosomes and, like many proteins in the cytosol, can be "tagged" for proteasome-mediated destruction. The resulting peptides are transported into the endoplasmic reticulum through the use of TAP1/2 transporters. After transport, these peptides are placed in the binding groove of HLA class I, and HLA class I subsequently is transported to the cell surface for display. Once HLA class I + tumor peptide are on the surface of the cell, these tumor cells can be recognized by CD8+ T cells for destruction. (**A**) This answer is incorrect because the endoplasmic reticulum is not the original location of the intracellular antigens produced by the tumor. These protein antigens are first synthesized in the cytosol on ribosomes before being trafficked to the endoplasmic reticulum. (**B**) This answer is incorrect because the peroxisome is a membrane-bound organelle in which fatty acids are oxidized, in addition to other oxidative reaction pathways. Peroxisomes are not involved in HLA antigen processing for presentation to T cells. (**C**) This answer is incorrect because the lysosome is a membrane-bound acidified organelle that contains enzyme acid hydrolases that function at low pH to degrade sugars, proteins, and nucleic acids entering the cell in phagosomes from the extracellular environment. Lysosomes fuse with phagosomes to become phagolysosomes so that extracellular materials can be digested. The lysosome is implicated in processing extracellular antigens for presentation on HLA class II molecules to CD4+ T cells. (**E**) This answer is incorrect, because the phagosome is a membrane-enclosed vesicle containing large macromolecules entering the cell from the extracellular environment. Phagosomes fuse with lysosomes to become phagolysosomes so that extracellular materials can be digested. The phagosome is implicated in processing extracellular antigens for presentation on HLA class II molecules to CD4+ T cells.

4. Correct: Phagolysosome (A)

(**A**) This patient was splenectomized after suffering a splenic laceration following a motor vehicle collision with abdominal trauma. Asplenic patients are predisposed to infections with encapsulated microbes, including *Streptococcus pneumoniae.* Bacteria, including pneumococci, start out in the extracellular environment until they are phagocytosed by professional phagocytes (macrophages and dendritic cells). The bacteria are internalized into membrane-bound organelles called phagosomes that hold the undigested bacteria. These phagosomes fuse with lysosomes, which contain enzyme acid hydrolases to digest the materials into smaller components (monosaccharides, amino acids, nucleotides, etc.)—the fusion products are phagolysosomes. The endoplasmic reticulum then traffics membrane-bound vesicles containing HLA class II molecules studded in the membrane. These HLA class II–containing vesicles fuse with phagolysosomes, allowing the digested antigens access to HLA class II molecules in preparation for binding for antigen presentation. During this process, a peptide called class II–associated invariant chain (CLIP) is displaced from the antigen-binding site of the HLA class II molecules so that antigens can at last bind. These vesicles containing HLA class II:antigen complexes are then trafficked to the cell membrane surface where they are presented to CD4+ helper T cells. This antigen presentation event leads to the elaboration of proinflammatory and prokilling cytokines (e.g., IFN-γ) that signal to the macrophage and dendritic cell phagocytes to activate and kill their phagocytosed pathogens. (**B**) This answer is incorrect because the mitochondrion is the energy powerhouse of the cell, among other functions. Mitochondria are not the compartment in which HLA class II molecules are loaded for antigen presentation by macrophages and dendritic cells. (**C**) This answer is incorrect because Golgi apparatus is part of the exocytic pathway that HLA class II must utilize to reach the phagolysosome, but it is not the location in which it receives the bacterial-derived peptides. (**D**) This answer is incorrect, because the nucleus is a double membrane–bound organelle that houses the nucleic acid genome of the cell. Nuclei are not the location in which HLA class II molecules are loaded for antigen presentation by macrophages and dendritic cells. (**E**) This answer is incorrect, because the endoplasmic reticulum is the location in which HLA class II is loaded with invariant chain to prevent improper loading of self-peptides into the HLA class II molecules.

5. Correct: TH1 cells and IFN-γ production (A)

(**A**) This patient is suffering from a contact hypersensitivity due to poison ivy. The irritant from poison ivy is pentadecacatechol, which is an urushiol—a small lipid-like oily molecule. Pentadecacatechol penetrates the outer layers of the skin and binds to proteins on the surface of skin cells. In this form, it functions as a hapten and initiates an immune response that leads to blistering skin lesions. Haptenated self-proteins are taken up by Langerhans cells in the skin. Langerhans cells then migrate to a regional lymph node where they activate T cells. Hapten-specific effector TH1 cells then migrate to the skin where they initiate a delayed-type hypersensitivity response resulting in blistering. This response is mediated primarily by IFN-γ secretion by the TH1 cells that activated macrophages. Poison ivy is a classic case of contact dermatitis. Corticosteroids are the standard treatment. (**B**) IFN-γ is the "signature" cytokine that is produced by TH1 cells, while Th2 cells produce IL-4. (**C**) This is a case of poison ivy, which is due to a delayed-type hypersensitivity reaction. Thus, it is cell-mediated immune response, not an antibody-mediated response. (**D**) TH2 cells do not produce IFN-γ. IFN-γ is the "signature" cytokine that is produced by TH1 cells. IL-4 is the "signature" cytokine that is made by TH2 cells. (**E**) This is a case of poison ivy, which is due to a delayed-type hypersensitivity reaction. TH2 cells are responsible for immediate hypersensitivity reactions.

6. Correct: Inadequate opsonization (E)

(**E**) The spleen is an important organ for B-cell activation and differentiation. The production of pathogen-specific antibodies enhances opsonization and elimination of the organism by phagocytes. Macrophages and neutrophils express receptors for the Fc portion of IgG and are found in high abundance in the spleen. Opsonization is particularly important in eliminating encapsulated organisms such as *Streptococcus pneumoniae*. Asplenic patients are deficient in their ability to respond to polysaccharide antigens due to the lack of efficient opsonization. Individuals who lack a spleen are immunocompromised and are highly susceptible to infections and sepsis due to encapsulated organisms. It is highly recommended that asplenic individuals are vaccinated against these organisms. (**A**) Neutrophils develop in the bone marrow and not in the spleen. One side effect of splenectomy is neutrophilia. (**B**) B cells develop in the bone marrow. (**C**) T cells develop in the thymus. (**D**) NK cells develop in the bone marrow; they are an important defense mechanism against viral infections.

7. Correct: Passive acquired immunity (B)

(**B**) In this case, the infant is passively receiving IgA antibodies that were produced by his mother. Antibodies are made by plasma cells, which are the terminal state of differentiation of B cells that are part of the acquired/adaptive immune system. (**A**) Antibodies are not part of the innate immune system. (**C**) The infant is passively receiving antibodies in the breast milk. Antibodies are part of the acquired/adaptive

immune system. (**D**) The infant is passively receiving antibodies in the breast milk. The infant did not produce the antibodies; therefore, this does not represent active immunity. Active immunity is the result of a response to infection or vaccination. (**E**) Antibodies are part of the acquired/adaptive immune system. They are not part of the innate immune system.

8. Correct: IFN-γ receptor 1 deficiency (C)

(**C**) This child traveled to an area where tuberculosis (TB) is endemic. Children will exhibit symptoms of fever/chills, swollen lymph nodes, cough, sweating at night, and unintended weight loss, and are not as playful as before. Cellular immunity, and particularly activated macrophages, is required to combat the infection. IFN-γ is a potent activator of macrophages. A lack of IFN-γ production or a lack of expression of its receptor on the surface of macrophages will result in poor activation of the macrophages, deficient TNF-γ production, and difficulty killing intracellular pathogens such as *Mycobacterium tuberculosis*. (**A**) IgA does not play a significant role in neutralizing TB. TB is an intracellular infection; therefore, cellular immunity is required for protection. (**B**) Common variable immunodeficiency is one of the most frequently diagnosed primary immunodeficiencies. In these patients, B cells fail to differentiate into plasma cells. However, humoral immunity does not play a significant role in eliminating TB. (**D**) Chronic granulomatous disease (CGD) is caused by mutations in the NADPH (nicotinamide adenine dinucleotide phosphate) oxidase gene. This affects the capacity of phagocytes (neutrophils and macrophages) to kill organisms that they ingested. Patients with CGD are particularly susceptible to catalase positive bacterial infection. TNF-α production is not affected in individuals with CGD. (**E**) Autoimmune regulator (AIRE) deficiency affects the negative selection of T cells in the thymus and results in autoimmune disease. It does not affect IFN-γ production or TNF-α production.

9. Correct: Granulocyte colony-stimulating factor (G-CSF) (A)

(**A**) Granulocyte colony-stimulating factor (G-CSF) plays an important role in hematopoiesis. Recombinant G-CSF increases neutrophil production by the bone marrow and is used to treat neutropenia. G-CSF administration boosts production of neutrophils, thus protecting patients from life-threatening bacterial infections. The level of neutropenia post-chemotherapy may be mild, moderate, or severe. (**B**) IL-2 is a T-cell growth factor; following the activation of T cells, the expression of IL-2 and the high-affinity IL-2R "drives" T-cell proliferation. Lack of IL-2 production results in anergy of the T cell. (**C**) IFN-α is a type I IFN. Type I IFNs elicit an antiviral immune response from macrophages and NK cells and activate ribonucleases to inhibit viral protein synthesis in the infected cell. IFN-α is used to treat viral hepatitis. (**D**) IFN-β is another type I IFN. It is used to treat the autoimmune disease multiple sclerosis. (**E**) BAFF antagonists have been successfully used to treat some B cell–mediated autoimmune diseases in which high BAFF levels contribute to disease pathogenesis. BAFF itself has not been approved for the treatment of any human disease.

10. Correct: CD8 T cell (D)

(**D**) Epstein–Barr virus (EBV), the pathogen that causes infectious mononucleosis, is a DNA virus with tropism for B cells. Due to this tropism for B cells, EBV is also associated with cancers such as Hodgkin's and Burkitt's lymphoma. During an acute EBV infection, there is a significant increase in the number of CD8+ EBV-specific T cells. These help limit the infection by eliminating EBV-infected cells. After recognition of viral antigen in the context of MHC class I, CD8+ cytotoxic T-lymphocytes kill virally infected cells by two mechanisms: (1) they release the contents of their cytotoxic granules, which include perforin and granzyme, and (2) they kill the virally infected cells via Fas/FasL-mediated pathways. The CD8+ T cells have an abnormal appearance on peripheral smear as they react to the infected B cells. These reacting T cells are what are referred to as "atypical cells" on reports of blood smears. A robust T-cell response is necessary to mount an effective antiviral response. Patients can mount an antibody response to the infection; these may include antibodies to the viral capsid antigen, early antigen, and nuclear antigen. Seropositivity for these antibodies can confirm the diagnosis; however, the antibodies are not very effective at limiting the infection. (**A**) Neutrophils play an important role in the immune response to bacteria; they are not effective at eliminating virally infected cells. (**B**) B cells differentiate into plasma cells that produce antibodies. These virus-specific antibodies, if present in the patient, can only neutralize the virus while it is extracellular. Once the virus is intracellular, cellular immunity becomes the predominant mechanism of limiting this infection. (**C**) CD4 T cells play an important role within the immune system by helping to activate and coordinate other cell types. CD4 T cells play a role in the activation of CD8 T cells, but CD4 T cells do not directly kill the virus or virally infected cells. (**E**) Macrophages function as phagocytes and as antigen-presenting cells within the immune system. They are not effective at eliminating virally infected cells.

11. Correct: Bcl-2 (E)

(**E**) Apoptosis, or programmed cell death, is a form of controlled cellular destruction. Several genes have been identified that promote or inhibit the apoptotic pathway, such as Bcl-2. Increased expression of Bcl-2 has been implicated in several autoimmune diseases and cancers. (**A**) IL-2 is a T-cell growth factor; it "drives" the proliferation of activated T cells. (**B**) The

interaction of FasL with Fas on the surface of a cell triggers Fas trimerization and formation of the death-inducing signaling complex that promotes apoptosis. (**C**) Caspase 3 is one of several caspases that play a role in the execution phase of programmed cell death, which leads to chromatin condensation and DNA fragmentation. (**D**) TNF-α is a highly pleiotropic cytokine; it plays a role in the acute-phase response and in systemic inflammation. It can be expressed as a soluble trimeric molecule or as a membrane-bound molecule. The soluble trimeric form binds to TNF-receptor 1 (TNFRI). Signaling through the TNFR1 can lead to several outcomes; these include transcription of other cytokine genes or induction of apoptosis.

12. Correct: IL-1, IL-6, TNF-α (A)

(**A**) The high temperature, elevated WBC count with elevated neutrophils, and elevated ESR are all indicative of an acute-phase response. This is triggered by the release of proinflammatory cytokines (IL-1, IL-6, TNF-α) by tissue macrophages. These cytokines signal the bone marrow to increase WBC production, signal the hypothalamus to increase the body's temperature set point, and stimulate the liver to produce complement proteins and C-reactive protein. Increased acute-phase protein production affects plasma viscosity, thereby increasing the ESR. (**B**) IL-12, when produced by antigen-presenting cells during T-cell activation, will "drive" the differentiation of effector TH1 cells, which in turn produce IFN-γ. (**C**) IL-4 and IL-13 are cytokines that are made by effector TH2 cells. (**D**) IFN-α and IFN-β are both type I IFNs that play an essential role in limiting viral infection at epithelial barriers. (**E**) IL-10 and TGF-β are both immunoregulatory cytokines. They are produced by CD4+ Treg cells, as well as other cell types.

13. Correct: Chronic lymphocytic leukemia (B)

(**B**) As patients get older, immunosenescence increases their vulnerability to infection. Furthermore, patients with immune cell cancers are usually immunocompromised, as a secondary consequence of the malignancy. Chronic lymphocytic leukemia (CLL) usually occurs in older patients (>50 years old). It is more common in males, with a male-to-female ratio of 2:1. The most frequent clinical sign is enlargement of the cervical and axillary lymph nodes. The upper right quadrant of the flow cytometry histogram shows an unusually large percentage of B cells (CD19+) that express CD5. This is characteristic of CLL. (**A**) Acute lymphoblastic leukemia is characterized by an accumulation of lymphoblasts in the bone marrow. It is the most common immune malignancy in children. (**C**) Hairy cell leukemia is a relatively uncommon B-cell malignancy. Patients will usually present with infections and splenomegaly. They do not exhibit lymphadenopathy. A blood smear will show large lymphocytes with villous cytoplasmic projections. (**D**) Adult T-cell leukemia is associated with infection by the HTLV-1 virus. It is common in Japan and the Caribbean, but is rare in other populations. A blood smear would show lymphocytes with unusual morphology, having a "clover leaf" nucleus. (**E**) Hodgkin's lymphoma patients present with enlarged cervical lymph nodes. Histological examination of an excised lymph node would show characteristic multinucleated Reed–Sternberg cells. The presence of these cells is central to the diagnosis of Hodgkin's lymphoma.

14. Correct: Blocking IL-2R (D)

(**D**) Daclizumab is a monoclonal antibody against the IL-2R. Activated T cells produce IL-2 and express a high-affinity IL-2R. The autocrine interaction of IL-2 with its receptor "drives" T-cell proliferation. Interfering with the activation, proliferation, and clonal expansion of T cells that are targeting the graft will reduce the chances of graft rejection and extend the survival of the graft. Induction therapy involves treating prospective transplant recipients with anti-IL-2R antibodies prior to surgery. (**A**) Daclizumab is a humanized monoclonal antibody that targets the IL-2R and does not remove passenger leukocytes from the graft. (**B**) Daclizumab binds to CD25; it does not block MHC class I molecules. (**C**) Daclizumab binds to CD25; it does not block MHC class II molecules. (**E**) Daclizumab binds to CD25; it does not block the co-stimulation step of T-cell activation.

15. Correct: Hapten (C)

(**C**) This is a case of penicillin-induced hemolytic anemia. Penicillin can function as a hapten by binding to molecules on the surface of RBCs. This triggers production of IgG antibodies to penicillin. Upon subsequent exposure to penicillin, the antibodies will activate the classical complement pathway and lyse the RBCs. Alternatively, the Fc of the antibody molecule will bind to FcR on the surface of macrophages that are part of the reticuloendothelial system. Macrophages will clear and destroy the RBCs. (**A**) Group A streptococcus (*Streptococcus pyogenes*) is the most likely pathogen that is causing the sore throat. However, the new clinical signs and symptoms that include anemia are due to an immune response to penicillin that is bound to the surface of RBCs. (**B**) Superantigens induce the activation of large numbers of T cells. This results in a massive release of cytokines. Superantigens are not associated with hemolytic anemia. (**D**) Pathogen-associated molecular patterns (PAMPs) are common antigens found on many pathogens; they are recognized by pattern recognition receptors and activate the innate immune system. The new symptoms are due to an immune response to penicillin, not to the pathogen. (**E**) Damage-associated molecular patterns (DAMPs) are molecules that are released by diseased or dying cells, and they activate macrophages to initiate repair.

16. Correct: Toll-like receptors (B)

(**B**) This is a case of traveler's diarrhea, and enterotoxigenic *Escherichia coli* (ETEC) is responsible for most cases of traveler's diarrhea worldwide. This is usually a self-limiting infection with symptoms that last for a few days. Treatment involves drinking plenty of fluids and/or oral rehydration salts to avoid dehydration. Antibiotics are not usually required. Toll-like receptors are expressed on the cell surface of macrophages and epithelial cells. Some are expressed on the membranes of endosomes (intracellular vesicles). Toll-like receptors recognize common molecular patterns expressed by pathogens; these are called pathogen-associated molecular patterns (PAMPs). (**A**) Both leukocytes and epithelial cells express cellular adhesion molecules. These do not play a role in pathogen recognition by the innate immune system. Cellular adhesion molecules are necessary for allowing white cells to attach to endothelial or epithelial cells, which is necessary to recruit immune cells to the site of infection. (**C**) NOD-like receptors also recognize PAMPs. However, NOD-like receptors are expressed in the cell cytoplasm and not on the cell membrane. They respond to intracellular bacteria. ETEC is found on the surface of intestinal epithelium. (**D**) RIG-I is expressed in the cell cytoplasm and recognizes viral RNA. (**E**) CD40 is a transmembrane molecule that is expressed on the cell membrane of macrophages. It plays an important role in the interactions of macrophages and T cells. It does not play a role in pathogen recognition.

17. Correct: Binding of CD28 to B7-1 (D)

(**D**) During T-cell activation, adhesion molecules allow the T cells and the antigen-presenting cell to "stick" together so that the T cell can recognize the antigen that is presented in the context of MHC molecules. CD4 T cells recognize antigen in the context of MHC class II molecules, whereas CD8 T cells recognize antigen in the context of MHC class I molecules. A naïve T cell is defined as a T cell that has completed development in the thymus and has entered the periphery, but has yet to be stimulated. Naïve T cells are highly dependent on co-stimulation. This involves the interaction of CD28 on the T-cell surface with B7-1 or B7-2 molecules on the antigen-presenting cell. Ligation of CD28 by B7 molecules is necessary for clonal expansion. The co-stimulation step induces the expression of IL-2 (a T-cell growth factor) and the high-affinity IL-2R. The autocrine interaction of IL-2 with its receptor drives T-cell proliferation and clonal expansion. When a naïve T cell recognizes its antigen in the context of MHC but does not receive co-stimulation, it becomes anergic (nonresponsive). Unlike naïve T cells, T cells that have been previously stimulated are not dependent on co-stimulation. (**A**) LFA-1 and ICAM-1 are cellular adhesion molecules. The binding of LFA-1 on the T-cell surface with ICAM-1 on the antigen-presenting cell helps bring the two cells close together for adherence. (**B**) The CD4 molecule binds to MHC class II during T-cell activation and plays a role in signal transduction. (**C**) The CD8 molecule binds to MHC class I during T-cell activation and plays a role in signal transduction. (**E**) Binding of CTLA-4 to B7-1 delivers an inhibitory signal to the T cell.

18.   Correct: Acute myeloid leukemia (AML) (A)

(**A**) There are three main types of acute leukemia: myeloid origin, B-cell origin, and T-cell origin. Patients with leukemia also suffer from anemia, thrombocytopenia (hence the hemorrhagic gums), and immunodeficiency. The accumulation of malignant cells within the bone marrow prevents the development of other cell types and results in subsequent bone marrow failure. The flow cytometry analysis of the bone marrow shows that the malignant cells express CD33 (a myeloid marker) and CD117 (a receptor tyrosine kinase). The cells do not express B-cell markers (CD19, CD20) or T-cell markers (CD2, CD3). (**B**) The cells do not express any B-cell markers. (**C**) The cells do not express any T-cell markers. (**D**) Severe combined immunodeficiency (SCID) is a group of immunodeficiencies that are characterized by hypoplasia of lymphoid organs and decreased lymphocyte numbers (both B cells and T cells). RBC development and platelet development are normal. Patients with SCID will exhibit susceptibility to infection very early in life. (**E**) Acquired immunodeficiency syndrome (AIDS) is due to infection by the HIV virus. Hematopoiesis is normal in these patients. As the HIV virus wipes out the CD4+ T-cell population, patients become increasingly susceptible to infections, particularly opportunistic infections.

19.   Correct: B cell acute lymphoblastic leukemia (B-ALL) (B)

(**B**) Acute lymphoblastic leukemia is the most common malignancy of childhood; the majority of cases are diagnosed before the age of 6. Approximately 85% of cases are leukemias of B-cell origin, while the remaining 15% are leukemias of T-cell origin. Both CD10 and CD19 are B-cell markers. Patients suffer from bone marrow failure and present with symptoms of anemia, thrombocytopenia, and neutropenia. Patients will also present with lymphadenopathy, splenomegaly, and some organ infiltration. (**A**) Acute myeloid leukemias (AMLs) express CD33 and CD117. (**C**) The cells do not express any T-cell markers. (**D**) Autoimmune lymphoproliferative syndrome is a rare condition that affects approximately 500 people worldwide. Most cases are due to mutations in Fas, and a minority of cases are due to mutations in FasL. Defective apoptosis leads to lymphadenopathy, splenomegaly, autoimmune disease, and lymphomas. Patients have an increased percentage of CD4- CD8- T cells in the circulation. (**E**) Hodgkin's lymphoma

patients present with enlarged cervical lymph nodes. Histological examination of an excised lymph node would show characteristic multinucleated Reed–Sternberg cells. The presence of these cells is central to the diagnosis of Hodgkin's lymphoma.

20.   Correct: Hodgkin's lymphoma (C)

(**C**) Hodgkin's lymphoma patients present with enlarged cervical lymph nodes. Histological examination of an excised lymph node would show characteristic multinucleated Reed–Sternberg cells. The presence of these cells is central to the diagnosis of Hodgkin's lymphoma. (**A**) Hairy cell leukemia is a relatively uncommon B-cell malignancy. Patients will usually present with infections and with splenomegaly. They do not exhibit lymphadenopathy. A blood smear will show large lymphocytes with villous cytoplasmic projections. (**B**) Multiple myeloma patients usually present with complaints of back pain. The myeloma cells take over the bone marrow, resulting in lytic bone lesions. (**D**) Burkitt's lymphoma is associated with EBV infection. There is a translocation of the c-myc oncogene to the long arm of chromosome 14 in close proximity to the immunoglobulin heavy chain gene locus; this leads to B-cell transformation. (**E**) Mantle cell lymphoma is a B-cell malignancy of B cells in the mantle zone of the follicle. Like chronic lymphocytic leukemia (CLL), it has a characteristic phenotype of being CD19+ and CD5+; however, mantle cell lymphoma also expresses CD22 and CD23.

21.   Correct: Multiple myeloma (E)

(**E**) Cancerous plasma cells multiply in the bone marrow and crowd out other cell types. Patients with multiple myeloma will suffer from anemia. With more advanced disease, they will also suffer from neutropenia and become immunocompromised. Myeloma cells secrete copious amounts of immunoglobulin (monoclonal), resulting in a spike in the gamma globulin region of a serum protein electrophoresis. High levels of light chain are also found in the serum and urine. Because myeloma cells multiply in the bone marrow, lytic bone lesions develop, and patients will usually complain of back pain. (**A**) Hodgkin's lymphoma patients present with enlarged cervical lymph nodes. Histological examination of an excised lymph node would show characteristic multinucleated Reed–Sternberg cells. The presence of these cells is essential to the diagnosis of Hodgkin's lymphoma. (**B**) Marginal zone lymphoma is a cancer of B cells in the marginal zone of lymphoid follicles. (**C**) Mantle cell lymphoma is a B-cell malignancy of B cells in the mantle zone of the follicle. Like chronic lymphocytic leukemia (CLL), it has a characteristic phenotype of being CD19+ and CD5+; however, mantle cell lymphoma also expresses CD22 and CD23. (**D**) Follicular lymphoma is a cancer of B cells in the germinal center of lymphoid follicles. Constitutive over expression of bcl-2 leads to increased survival of B cells.

22. Correct: Antiglycoprotein IIb–IIIa (D)

(**D**) The patient is exhibiting symptoms of thrombocytopenia, in this case an autoimmune thrombocytopenia. In immune thrombocytopenic purpura (ITP), IgG autoantibodies against platelet antigens are responsible for removal of platelets from the circulation by the reticuloendothelial system. The normal lifespan of platelets is reduced from approximately 1 week to a few hours. Patients suffer from the typical symptoms of thrombocytopenia: deficiency of platelets in the blood, slow blood clotting, bleeding into tissues, and bruising. Patients do not exhibit signs of anemia or neutropenia. (**A**) This patient is not suffering from an autoimmune hemolytic anemia. Both the RBC count and hemoglobin level are normal. (**B**) This is not a case of penicillin-induced hemolytic anemia. The case history does not indicate exposure to penicillin, and the RBC and hemoglobin level are normal and do not suggest anemia. (**C**) In ITP, autoantibodies are directed against glycoprotein IIb–IIIa on the platelet membrane. They are not directed against MHC class I molecules. (**E**) PECAM-1 is also known as CD31. In ITP, autoantibodies are directed against glycoprotein IIb–IIIa on the platelet membrane. They are not directed against platelet endothelial cellular adhesion molecule (PECAM-1).

23. Correct: Goodpasture's syndrome (C)

(**C**) Patients with Goodpasture's syndrome have autoantibodies against type IV collagen, which is expressed in the basement membranes of alveoli and glomeruli. Therefore, patients will present with both pulmonary and renal symptoms. IgG anti-type IV collagen antibodies activate the classical complement pathway, thereby initiating an inflammatory response that damages alveoli and glomeruli. Alveolar hemorrhage will result in hemoptysis (coughing up blood). Damage to the glomerular basement membrane will affect the filtration unit; therefore, urinalysis will show proteinuria and hematuria. (**A**) Signs and symptoms of active tuberculosis (TB) include coughing with hemoptysis that lasts for several weeks along with fever, night sweats, and weight loss. The renal system is usually not affected. (**B**) The most commonly affected organs in systemic lupus erythematosus (SLE) are the vasculature, skin, joints, and kidneys. Damage to the glomerular basement membrane is due to the deposition of immune complexes that initiate an inflammatory response. Urinalysis will show evidence of proteinuria and hematuria. However, immunofluorescent staining of a kidney biopsy will not show a smooth pattern of staining; rather, the staining is often described as having a "lumpy bumpy" appearance. (**D**) Bronchitis

often develops from a respiratory infection, and is considered to be a very common acute condition. Patients may cough up blood, but the renal system is not involved. (**E**) Chronic obstructive pulmonary disease (COPD) is a chronic inflammatory lung disease, which is usually due to smoking or another irritant. Chronic bronchitis and emphysema are two common conditions that lead to COPD. Patients will complain of chest tightness, shortness of breath, and wheezing. The renal system is not involved.

24. Correct: Celiac disease (E)

(**E**) Patients with celiac disease develop a sensitivity to gluten. Both antibody-mediated and cell-mediated immune responses play a role in disease pathophysiology. The presence of the autoantibody IgA endomysial transglutaminase is pathognomonic for celiac disease. Additionally, large numbers of CD8+ T cells infiltrate the intestinal epithelium. The inflammatory process leads to the destruction of enterocytes. Villi that line the small intestine atrophy, resulting in lack of nutrient absorption and subsequent malnutrition. (**A**) The most common route of infection for salmonella is by contaminated water or food. Individuals will develop an acute diarrhea within 1 to 3 days after infection. Most individuals recover without medical intervention. (**B**) Ulcerative colitis is a chronic inflammatory disease, causing inflammation and ulcers in the digestive tract (particularly the colon and rectum). (**C**) Crohn's disease is a chronic inflammatory disease which can affect both the small intestine and the colon. However, the most commonly affected site is the terminal part of the ileum. In addition, the age of onset for most cases of inflammatory bowel disease (i.e., ulcerative colitis and Crohn's disease) is 15 to 40 years. (**D**) Whipple's disease is rare and is caused by the bacterium *Tropheryma whipplei*. The bacterium infects the lining of the small intestine, forming small lesions. Villi may be damaged in this disease, but there is no evidence of massive infiltration by CD8+ intraepithelial lymphocytes. Individuals at risk tend to be people 40 to 60 years of age who work outdoors and have frequent contact with sewage or wastewater.

25. Correct: Autoimmune regulator (AIRE) (C)

(**C**) Autoimmune regulator (AIRE) is expressed by thymic epithelial cells in the medulla and plays an important role in the negative selection of T cells. Defects in AIRE expression result in autoimmunity. The endocrine system is particularly vulnerable to autoimmune attack. If the parathyroid gland is affected, lack of production of parathyroid hormone results in dysregulation of calcium and phosphorous levels. Muscle twitching (tetany) is the result of low calcium levels. (**A**) MHC class I is expressed by all nucleated cells in the body. The HLA locus is on human chromosome 6. (**B**) MHC class II is expressed primarily by antigen-presenting cells. The HLA locus is on human chromosome 6. (D) CD28 is a transmembrane molecule that is expressed on T cells and plays an important role in the co-stimulation step during the activation of naïve T cells. (E) CD80, also known as B7-1, is a trans-membrane molecule that is expressed on the surface of antigen-presenting cells. The binding of CD80 to CD28 on the T-cell surface provides a co-stimulation signal during T-cell activation.

26. Correct: Sympathetic ophthalmia (A)

(A) The brain, eye, uterus, and testes are considered vital organs and restrict immune access; i.e., they are immunologically privileged sites. Sympathetic ophthalmia is a disease that occurs after trauma or surgery to one eye. The injury results in release of sequestered antigens, making them accessible to the immune system. Antigen-specific T cells become activated and mount an autoimmune attack, which can affect both eyes: the injured eye and the good eye. This is a granulomatous inflammation that causes much destruction and can lead to blindness. (B) Psoriasis is an inflammatory disease of the skin that results in scaly patches. The skin is not considered an immunoprivileged site. (C) Sjögren's syndrome is an autoimmune disease in which exocrine glands are the target of the immune response. Exocrine glands are not immunoprivileged. (D) Graves' disease is an autoimmune disease of the thyroid. The thyroid is not considered an immunoprivileged site. (E) Crohn's disease is a proinflammatory disease of the gut, which is not an immunoprivileged site.

27. Correct: FoxP3 expressing T cell (E)

(E) Of the CD4+ effector T-cell populations, Treg cells suppress the function of the other T-cell types (TH1, TH2, TH17, TfH). Treg cells express the FoxP3 transcription factor. They regulate other T cells through the production and secretion of regulatory cytokines, such as IL-10 and TGF-β. Phenotypically, Treg cells are characterized as expressing CD4 and CD25 on the cell surface. (A) The T-bet transcription factor is expressed by TH1 effector cells. (B) The Gata-3 transcription factor is expressed by TH2 effector cells. (C) The RoRγt transcription factor is expressed by TH17 effector cells. (D) The Bcl-6 transcription factor is expressed by TfH cells.

28. Correct: CD8 and MHC I (C)

(C) This patient most likely has roseola infantum or sixth disease. This syndrome is characterized by high fevers and a rash that originates around trunk and spreads to the face and extremities. Roseola is caused by human herpesvirus 6. For the body to clear a viral infection, CD8+ cytotoxic T cells must recognize viral antigen presented in the context of MHC I on the surface of virally infected cells. Once virus-infected cells are recognized via the CD8–MHC I interaction, cytotoxic T cells induce apoptosis in the infected cells, helping eliminate actively replicating virus. (A) This answer is incorrect, because IL-4 stimulating the IL-4 receptor is important for promoting Th2 responses that are not required for successful clearance of viral pathogens. (B) This answer is incorrect, because PD-1 and PD-1 ligand interaction is important for limiting (not promoting) T cell–mediated immune responses, including antitumor responses, autoimmune reactions, and chronic inflammatory conditions. (D) This answer is incorrect, because CTLA-4 interacting with CD86 limits T-cell activation. Binding of CD28 to CD86 sends an important co-stimulatory signal to T cells that is necessary for T-cell activation. (E) CD40 on B cells binds CD40 ligand on helper T cells to activate B cells. While B cells are not always critical in clearing viral infections (as in this case), antibody production by B cells can be neutralizing and provide long-term protection against re-infection against many viruses.

29. Correct: C3b (A)

(A) This child has meningitis with *Streptococcus pneumoniae*, an encapsulated gram-positive cocci that is difficult for macrophages, neutrophils, and dendritic cells to phagocytose. Therefore, one mechanism by which the immune system enhances the phagocytosis of these organisms is through opsonization. C3b of the complement pathway is a great opsonin that binds to C3b receptors on phagocytes to enhance the engulfment of these microorganisms and is critical for defense against bacterial infection. (B, C) These answers are incorrect, because C3a, C4a, and C5a are anaphylatoxins. They cause mast cells to degranulate and release histamine. C5a also attracts neutrophils to the endothelium. (D) This answer is incorrect, because C9 is a member of the membrane attack complex (MAC). C5b–C9 form the complex on the surface of bacterial and creates pores in cell walls. This process leads to lysis of the bacterium. The MAC is particularly critical in clearing *Neisseria* infections, since patients with deficiencies in C5–C9 are susceptible to *Neisseria* bacteremia. (E) Mannose-binding lectin (MBL) binds to bacteria and activates the complement pathway via proteases. It is not an opsonin.

30. Correct: Type III hypersensitivity (C)

(C) This patient most likely has systemic lupus erythematosus (SLE). In SLE, a large number of immune complexes are formed and are unable to be effectively cleared by the reticuloendothelial system. These immune complexes of antibodies against soluble self-antigens deposit in the vasculature activating complement and recruiting neutrophils, causing inflammation. Many patients with SLE have Raynaud's phenomenon, a small vessel vasculitis. Additional type III hypersensitivities include the Arthus reactions and serum sickness. (**A**) This answer is incorrect, because type I hypersensitivities are IgE-mediated and result in symptoms associated with season allergies and anaphylaxis. (**B**) This answer is incorrect, because type II hypersensitivities are when you produce antibodies of the IgM or IgG isotype that are specific for insoluble antigens (e.g., incompatible RBCs). Examples of type II hypersensitivities are Rh incompatibility and ABO blood incompatibility. (**D**) This answer is incorrect, because type IV hypersensitivities are mediated by T cells that result in reactions such as allergic contact dermatitis and graft versus host disease in transplants.

31. Correct: IL-12 (C)

(**C**) This man has miliary tuberculosis (TB) given his clinical presentation, X-ray findings, and positive urine antigen lipoarabinomannan. TB needs macrophages and the Th1 subset of T cells to clear the infection. IL-12 is secreted by macrophages and drives the development of the Th1 cells. Th1 cells stimulate macrophages and cell-mediated adaptive immunity, which are necessary to mount a protective response against *M. tuberculosis* infection. (**A**) This answer is incorrect, because IL-1 is a proinflammatory cytokines that induces fever and the secretion of acute-phase proteins. They are not specific to cell-mediated immunity that is required to clear *M. tuberculosis* infection. (**B**) IL-10 is an anti-inflammatory cytokine that inhibits Th1 cell development. This cytokine has an opposite effect of IL-12 and, therefore, would exacerbate, and not clear, infection with *M. tuberculosis*. (**D**) This answer is incorrect, because IL-17 recruits neutrophils to infection sites, which are not important in eradicating *M. tuberculosis*. (**E**) This answer is incorrect because TGF-β is important for promoting the formation of granulomas, not clearing *M. tuberculosis*.

32. Correct: Encapsulated bacteria (B)

(**B**) Individuals with X-linked agammaglobulinemia are primarily susceptible to recurrent bacterial sinopulmonary infections and enterovirus infections. This phenomenon is due to the lack of B-cell maturation. The humoral response is particularly important for the clearance of encapsulated bacteria due to the importance of opsonizing polysaccharide antigens. The large amount of secretory immunoglobulins is also important for gut mucosal immunity, which is why these patients also have recurrent enterovirus infections early in life. (**A**) This answer is incorrect, because acid-fast bacilli (e.g., mycobacteria) infections are seen in patients with cell-mediated immunity (i.e., T cell) deficiencies, which is not the case in this individual. (**C**) This answer is incorrect, because fungal infections are seen primarily in patients with T-cell deficiencies. Antibody responses are not absolutely necessary for the clearance of most fungal infections. (**D**) This answer is incorrect, because intracellular parasites require cell-mediated immunity. Antibodies cannot reach the parasites within the cell and therefore are not critical in the clearance of these pathogens. Only cell-mediated immunity can identify parasite-infected cells and eradicate them. (**E**) This answer is incorrect, because individuals with X-linked agammaglobulinemia are at increased risk of enterovirus infections, which are nonenveloped. Individuals with the loss of antibody protection still maintain T cell–mediated immunity to clear enveloped viruses.

Chapter 2

Inflammation

Samia Ragheb†

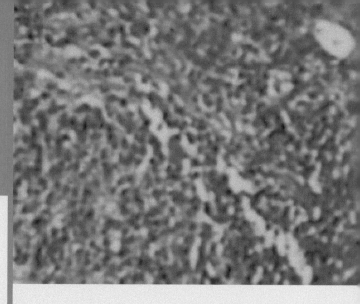

LEARNING OBJECTIVES

► Differentiate between innate immunity and acquired/adaptive immunity.

► Delineate each of the three complement pathways (classical, alternative, lectin), describe how each pathway is activated and regulated, and describe the biological consequences of complement activation.

► Delineate the cellular and molecular events that lead to acute or chronic inflammation.

► Delineate the function(s) of cytokines and chemokines in health and disease.

► Describe the use of immunotherapies (biologicals) in the management and treatment of immune-mediated disease; describe the mode of action of these immunotherapies.

► Describe the role of proinflammatory cytokines in the formation of an atheroma and delineate the immunopathogenesis of plaque development, progression, and rupture.

► Describe the structure of blood group antigens and the clinical consequences of blood type incompatibility.

► Describe central and peripheral regulatory mechanisms that prevent autoimmune reactions.

► Describe the immunopathogenesis, clinical presentation, histopathology, diagnosis, and therapy of inflammatory diseases that affect the endocrine system.

► Describe the cellular and molecular signals that influence T cell differentiation into effector T cell populations (TH1, TH2, TH9, TH17, TFH, Treg, CTL).

► Describe the histopathology, clinical presentation, diagnosis, and therapy of white blood cell malignancies.

► Explain how a diverse immunological repertoire is generated using limited genetic material and describe the role of allelic exclusion.

► Describe the process of T cell activation, co-stimulation, proliferation, anergy, and apoptosis.

► Delineate the cellular and molecular mechanisms that contribute to the immunopathology of systemic and organ-specific autoimmune diseases.

► Describe the structure, function, and anatomical distribution of human lymphoid organs.

► Differentiate between active and passive immunity.

► Describe the immunopathogenesis, clinical presentation, histopathology, diagnosis, and therapy of inflammatory diseases that affect the:

- respiratory tract.
- musculoskeletal system.

► Describe the structure of blood group antigens and the clinical consequences of blood type incompatibility.

2.1 Questions

Easy	Medium	Hard

1. The parents of a 2-week-old neonate brought their infant daughter to the pediatrician because of redness and swelling around the umbilical cord stump. At the time of exam, rectal measurement of body temperature is 39°C (102.2°F). White blood cell count is elevated with a predominance of polymorphonuclear cells. Which of the following peptide molecules most likely initiated the acute inflammatory response?

A. C5a

B. Intercellular adhesion molecule-1 (ICAM-1)

C. Immunoglobulin G (IgE)

D. Interleukin (IL)-2

E. Transforming growth factor β (TGF-β)

2. An intravenous drug user presents with a painful skin abscess, which is warm to the touch. Palpation of the infected site reveals fluctuance. Gram stain of the pus from the incision and drainage of the abscess shows many polymorphonuclear leukocytes (PMNs) and gram-positive cocci in clusters. Which of the following molecules is most likely responsible for the presence of the PMNs?

A. IL-1

B. IL-3

C. IL-8

D. IL-10

E. IL-12

3. Omalizumab is a humanized IgG1κ (immunoglobulin G, subclass 1, κ light chain) monoclonal antibody. It is potentially therapeutic in which of the following diseases?

A. Farmer's lung disease

B. Silicosis

C. Allergic asthma

D. Asbestosis

E. Sarcoidosis

4. A 50-year-old man, with a history of coronary artery disease, experiences chest pain while shoveling snow. Which of the following molecules most likely contributed to his condition?

A. IL-4, IL-13, TGF-β

B. Interferon γ (IFN-γ), myeloperoxidase, reactive oxygen species

C. IL-9, IL-10, TGF-β

D. IL-2, IL-13, vascular endothelial growth factor (VEGF)

E. IFN-β, IL-4, IL-10

5. A 36-year-old woman, who did not receive prenatal care, gives birth to her third child. The pregnancy and delivery were uncomplicated, and the neonate did not experience any trauma during childbirth. Twelve hours postpartum, the newborn is noted to be jaundiced. His bilirubin level at the time is 7 mg/dL (1.1 mg/dL direct bilirubin). Percentage of reticulocytes is 8% (normal = 2–5% in infants). Platelet and white blood cell counts are normal. The baby's blood type is A positive. Coombs test results are pending. What is the most likely cause of the baby's condition?

A. Blockage of the bile duct

B. Hemolytic anemia

C. Idiopathic thrombocytopenic purpura

D. Hemolytic-uremic syndrome

E. Hemorrhagic disease of the newborn

6. A 9-year-old girl has a history of tetany and complains of painful cramping and twitching of her hands and feet. Blood test results reveal the following: parathyroid hormone (PTH) is 100 pg/mL (normal = 230–630 pg/mL) and calcium is 6.0 mg/dL. Biopsy of the parathyroid gland shows infiltration by inflammatory cells. Which of the following is most likely to be defective in this patient?

A. Lymphocyte function-associated antigen 1 (LFA-1)

B. CD28

C. B7-1

D. Autoimmune regulator (AIRE)

E. GATA-3

7. A 7-year-old child is diagnosed with a mycobacterial infection. An immune work-up showed a homozygous deletion within the gene for the IL-12p40 subunit. The loss of this protein results in the inability of CD4+ T cells to become effector cells that produce high levels of which of the following?

A. IL-2

B. IL-4

C. IFN-β

D. IFN-γ

E. IL-10

8. A 70-year-old man presents with a 2-week history of back pain. He also reports that he has been feeling unusually tired. He has not had any significant lifestyle changes and has not recently engaged in any strenuous physical activity. Other than pallor, physical examination did not reveal abnormalities. X-ray showed several lytic lesions in the vertebrae and a bone marrow aspirate revealed 35% infiltration with plasma cells (normal: <5%). Pertinent laboratory findings are below.

- CBC:
    - RBCs: $3 \times 10^6/\mu L$ (normal = 4.3–$5.9 \times 10^6/\mu L$)
    - WBCs: $3,500/\mu L$ (normal = $4,500$–$11,000/\mu L$)
- IgG: 4,500 mg/dL (normal = 600–1,500 mg/dL)
- Urinalysis:
    - Dipstick: 0
    - Intratubular casts present
    - Positive Bence Jones proteins

Which of the following additional findings are most likely to be seen in this patient?

A. Serum IgG consists of equal proportions of IgG1, IgG2, IgG3, and IgG4

B. Both κ and λ light chains are in excessive quantities in the urine

C. High levels of IgA and IgM in the urine

D. Increased susceptibility to bacterial infections

9. Laboratory results from a serum protein electrophoresis show that there is a sharp spike in the gamma globulin peak. Further testing shows that the ratio of light chains is 1κ:6λ. Which of the following is most consistent with these findings?

A. IgG κ multiple myeloma

B. IgA λ multiple myeloma

C. IgM κ multiple myeloma

D. IgD κ multiple myeloma

E. IgE κ multiple myeloma

10. The germline DNA for the κ light chain in humans has 35 V-gene segments and 5 J-gene segments. If the recombination signal sequence next to J2 is defective, how many different variable regions can be generated, based on germline diversity only?

A. 0

B. 39

C. 40

D. 140

E. 175

11. A menstruating 16-year-old girl presents with fever up to 40°C (104°F), diarrhea, hypotension, malaise, and confusion. On exam, an erythematous rash is noted on her palms and soles. The most likely agent of this girl's condition is capable of crosslinking:

A. LFA-1 and ICAM-1

B. CD4 and major histocompatibility complex class II (MHC class II)

C. T cell receptor (TCR) and CD3

D. CD28 and B7

E. T cell receptor (TCR) Vβ and MHC class II

12. A 3-year-old boy with a history of recurrent respiratory infection is currently experiencing periodic diarrhea. A rectal thermometer recorded a temperature of 37.3°C (99.1°F). On physical examination, enlarged cervical lymph nodes and an enlarged spleen are noted. Blood tests show an elevated lymphocyte count and elevated polyclonal IgG levels. This boy is most likely to have a deficiency in:

A. Integrin β2

B. ZAP-70

C. CD28

D. CTLA-4

E. IL-2R γ chain

13. In one B cell, gene rearrangements create the variable region of the heavy chain and the light chain. Which of the following immunoglobulin gene rearrangements are not possible due to allelic exclusion?

A. Maternal H: maternal κ

B. Maternal H: maternal λ

C. Maternal κ: paternal λ

D. Paternal H: maternal κ

E. Paternal H: maternal λ

14. A 19-year-old woman is pregnant with her second child. Paternal identity is unknown. The woman's blood type is B negative. Which of the following would most likely complicate this pregnancy?

A. Biological father may be AB+

B. Biological father may be O-

C. Fetus has anti-B antibodies

D. Mother has anti-A antibodies

E. Mother has anti-B antibodies

15. A homebuilder in India steps on a rusty nail. Four days later, he experiences painful swelling of the foot around the injured site, muscle spasms, and stiffness in his neck. In which of the following anatomic sites is the immune system most likely to be stimulated first?

A. Adenoids and tonsils

B. Bone marrow

C. Thymus

D. Peyer's patches

E. Popliteal lymph nodes

16. On a hiking trip in southwestern Arizona, a 20-year-old man was bitten by a tiger rattlesnake whose venom is hemotoxic and neurotoxic. Symptoms included a burning pain at the puncture site, swelling, and weakness. He was rushed to the emergency department where he received IgG antivenom. The IgG antivenom provides the man with:

A. Natural and passive immunity

B. Natural and active immunity

C. Acquired and active immunity

D. Acquired and passive immunity

E. Natural and acquired immunity

17. A 19-year-old man is fatigued and presents with difficulty breathing. He works as a stable hand. A radiograph of the chest shows some loss of lung volume, and lung function tests show restrictive loss of lung function. A subsequent lung biopsy shows an inflammatory infiltrate with a few multinucleated giant cells. Which of the following most likely triggered this inflammatory response?

A. IgG

B. IgA

C. IgM

D. IgD

E. IgE

18. A 55-year-old woman presents with morning stiffness that lasts for several hours. She complains that the joints in her fingers and wrists are swollen and painful, but the symptoms seem to come and go. On exam, the pain, swelling, and stiffness are noted to be symmetrical. Radiography shows soft-tissue swelling and narrowing of the joint space. Pertinent laboratory findings are below:

- Erythrocyte sedimentation rate (ESR): 28 mm/h (normal < 20 mm/h)
- Antinuclear antibody (ANA): 1:320 (normal < 1:40)
- Rheumatoid factor: 1:128 (normal < 1:16)
- Anti–cyclic citrullinated peptide (anti-CCP): 42 EU/mL (normal < 20 EU/mL)
- Synovial fluid analysis:
  - Viscosity: low
  - Color: cloudy and yellow
  - WBCs: 3,500 μL

Which of the following is the most likely diagnosis?

A. Systemic lupus erythematosus

B. Rheumatoid arthritis (RA)

C. Osteoarthritis

D. Gout

E. Serum sickness

19. A 4-year-old girl has a history of multiple surgeries to correct a congenital heart defect. Her blood type is A positive and both parents have donated blood for her surgeries. Which of the following is the most likely ABO blood type of her parents?

A. AA and AB

B. AA and AO

C. AB and AB

D. AB and AO

E. BO and AA

20. ABO blood type incompatibility between mother and fetus is frequent, yet this does not pose a significant risk for hemolytic anemia in the newborn. Which of the following represents the most likely reason for this phenomenon?

A. Isohemagglutinins are IgG

B. Isohemagglutinins are IgA

C. Isohemagglutinins are IgM

D. Isohemagglutinins are IgD

E. Isohemagglutinins are IgE

21. An injured soldier is in immediate need of a blood transfusion. An army medic types the soldier's blood. None of the blood-typing antibodies agglutinated the soldier's red blood cells (RBCs). The soldier's blood type is most likely:

A. AB positive

B. AB negative

C. O positive

D. O negative

2.2 Answers and Explanations

Easy	Medium	Hard

1. Correct: C5a (A)

(**A**) This neonate is suffering from an infected umbilical cord stump and is displaying some characteristic signs and symptoms of inflammation. These include fever (calor), redness (rubor), pain (dolor), and swelling (tumor). This is a 2-week-old infant who has an innate immune response and has yet to acquire her own adaptive immunity. She is protected by her mother's IgG, which she received through transplacental transfer. If the infant were breast-fed, she would also receive antibodies (mostly IgA) from her mother's milk. The infectious pathogen is not specified, nor is it stated whether the mother has pathogen-specific protective antibodies to pass on to the infant. Therefore, it is not known which complement pathway was activated. Regardless, all complement pathways generate a C5 convertase, which cleaves C5 into C5a and C5b. C5a is a potent mediator of inflammation. Some of its biological effects include: (1) vasodilation, (2) upregulation of the expression of adhesion molecules on vascular endothelial cells, (3) chemoattraction of circulating white blood cells (the majority of which are neutrophils), and (4) local degranulation of mast cells. At the site of infection, tissue macrophages, upon activation, will also secrete proinflammatory cytokines (IL-1, IL-6, and TNF-α) and chemokines (CXCL-8/IL-8), which will amplify the inflammatory response and induce fever. Proinflammatory cytokines also increase the production of white blood cells by the bone marrow. (**B**) Intercellular adhesion molecule-1 (ICAM-1) is a transmembrane molecule that is expressed by activated vascular endothelial cells. Its ligands include LFA-1 and Mac-1, integrins that are expressed on the cell surface of circulating leukocytes. (**C**) IgE is an immunoglobulin isotype associated with allergic responses. The Fc portion of IgE binds to FcεR on the cell surface of basophils and tissue mast cells. (**D**) IL-2 is a cytokine that plays an important role in T cell activation. Once CD4+ T cells are activated by their specific antigen (in the context of MHC class II) and have received appropriate co-stimulation (interaction of CD28 with B7), they produce and secrete IL-2. They also upregulate the expression of the α-chain of the IL-2R. The IL-2R on activated T cells binds IL-2 with high affinity; this binding triggers proliferation of the T cell to generate "daughter" cells of the same specificity. (**E**) TGF-β is an immunoregulatory cytokine. It is one of the cytokines produced by CD4+ Treg cells; TGF-β has many biological effects and can alter the function of many cell types.

2. Correct: IL-8 (C)

(**C**) IL-8, also known as CXCL-8, is a chemokine produced by several cell types at sites of infection; these include macrophages, endothelial cells, and epithelial cells. Two receptors can bind IL-8, CXCR-1 and CXCR-2; these receptors are expressed on the cell surface of circulating neutrophils. Once neutrophils transmigrate from blood to tissue, they follow the chemokine gradient to the site of infection. (**A**) IL-1 is one of several proinflammatory cytokines that are produced by activated macrophages. The biological effects of these cytokines include upregulation of adhesion molecule expression on endothelial cells and increased production of white blood cells by the bone marrow. IL-1 also plays a role in thermoregulation; it induces fever by binding to receptors in the hypothalamus. (**B**) IL-3 induces the differentiation of hematopoietic stem cells into myeloid and lymphoid cell lineages. (**D**) IL-10, also known as cytokine synthesis inhibitory factor (CSIF), is an anti-inflammatory cytokine. It exerts its biological function by downregulating the expression of MHC class II molecules, downregulating B7 expression, inhibiting the function of TH1 effector cells, and inhibiting production of IFN-γ. (**E**) IL-12 is a proinflammatory cytokine. It is produced by a "classically" activated M1 type of macrophage and promotes differentiation of naïve T cells into the TH1 effector cell type.

3. Correct: Allergic asthma (C)

(**C**) The early phase of an allergic asthma attack is dependent on IgE that is bound to mast cells. Omalizumab is a monoclonal antibody that targets human IgE. It binds to the Fc portion of IgE, thereby interfering with its ability to bind to the FcεR on the surface of basophils and mast cells. Immune complexes of IgE bound to omalizumab are then cleared from the circulation. Omalizumab therapy decreases the amount of free IgE that is available to bind to the FcεR; this would reduce the probability of future asthma attacks. Clinical trials with omalizumab have also shown that as the level of free IgE is reduced, the expression of FcεR on basophils and mast cells is also downregulated. These two mechanisms of action—(1) removing IgE from the circulation and (2) reduced cell-surface expression of FcεR—contribute to the success of omalizumab therapy in asthmatic patients. (**A**) Farmer's lung disease is a hypersensitivity pneumonitis initiated by an IgG response to an inhaled antigen. Anti-IgE would not be helpful. (**B**) Silicosis is an occupational lung disease associated with jobs such as sandblasting and quarrying. The pathogenesis of this disease relies on the generation of reactive oxygen species from alveolar macrophages. This predominantly fibrogenic process is due mostly to TGF-β. It is not dependent on IgE. Therefore, anti-IgE therapy would not be helpful. (**D**) Asbestosis results from an inflammatory response to trapped asbestos fibers in the lung. It is an occupational disease and is not dependent on IgE. (**E**) Sarcoidosis is an inflammatory granulomatous disease and is not dependent on IgE. Sarcoid patients would not benefit from anti-IgE therapy.

4. Correct: IFN-γ, myeloperoxidase, reactive oxygen species (B)

(**B**) Coronary artery disease is largely due to atherosclerosis. Several biological pathways are involved in the formation of an atheroma; these include oxidative, inflammatory, and clotting pathways. It is not entirely clear how vascular injury is initiated, but areas of vessel bifurcation, where blood flow is more turbulent, are particularly vulnerable. Activated vascular endothelial cells produce platelet activating factor, which initiates clot formation. Activated tissue macrophages secrete proinflammatory cytokines that upregulate the expression of adhesion molecules on vascular endothelial cells. Activated macrophages and endothelial cells also secrete the chemokine IL-8, thereby attracting neutrophils. In addition, low-density lipoproteins (LDLs) become trapped in the vessel wall (intima). Both activated macrophages and neutrophils produce the myeloperoxidase enzyme. Myeloperoxidase modifies LDL into oxLDL, which is taken up by macrophages (foam cells) via scavenger receptors. Foam cells are macrophages that are full of oxLDL. This process potentiates the inflammatory response and initiates atheroma formation. Chronic inflammation contributes to thickening of the vessel wall and narrowing of the lumen (stenosis), thereby limiting blood flow. Over time, production of matrix metalloproteinases by inflammatory cells weakens the vessel wall and contributes to plaque rupture. (**A**) IL-4 and IL-13 are anti-inflammatory cytokines and do not contribute to the formation of an atheroma. Alternatively activated M2 macrophages contribute to plaque stability by secreting IL-4 and IL-13. TGF-β is an immunoregulatory cytokine. (**C**) IL-9 plays a role in asthma; it has not been implicated in cardiovascular inflammation. Both IL-10 and TGF-β are anti-inflammatory immunoregulatory cytokines and would inhibit cardiovascular inflammation. (**D**) IL-2 is required for the proliferation of T cells, but does not play a direct role in the formation of an atheroma. IL-13 is an anti-inflammatory cytokine. Vascular endothelial growth factor (VEGF) is a growth factor involved in angiogenesis; it helps

stabilize the plaque, preventing plaque rupture. (**E**) IFN-β is a type I interferon, which can downregulate macrophage function. Both IL-4 and IL-10 are anti-inflammatory cytokines.

5. Correct: Hemolytic anemia (B)

(**B**) The infant's symptoms and lab results are indicative of a hemolytic anemia. Hemolysis of RBCs will lead to elevated bilirubin levels, which cause yellowing of the skin and eyes. A normal percentage of reticulocytes is 0.5 to 2% in adults and 2 to 5% in infants. Reticulocytes are immature RBCs. An elevated percentage of reticulocytes is a sign of anemia as the bone marrow is ramping up RBC production. This infant is Rh+. Although the mother's blood type is unknown, it can be deduced that she is Rh- and the father is Rh+. This is her third pregnancy, and she was likely previously exposed and sensitized to Rh+ RBCs. Anti-Rh antibodies are IgG and can cross the placenta. Anti-Rh antibodies activate complement, thereby harming fetal RBCs by hemolysis. Infants with mild symptoms have hemolytic disease of the newborn and are treated with phototherapy. Severe disease may lead to erythroblastosis fetalis and death of the fetus. (**A**) Bilirubin is made in the liver and is removed from the body along with bile. Bile ducts transport bile from the liver to the intestines. Any blockage in bile ducts would result in elevated bilirubin levels. However, the higher percentage of reticulocytes is indicative of anemia. (**C**) The infant's platelet counts are normal, which would exclude acute idiopathic thrombocytopenic purpura. (**D**) *Escherichia coli* infection with the O157:H7 strain is a major cause of hemolytic-uremic syndrome in young children. The most common sources of infection include contaminated meat or produce. Patients with hemolytic-uremic syndrome suffer from hemolytic anemia, thrombocytopenia, and acute renal failure. (**E**) Hemorrhagic disease of the newborn is due to vitamin K deficiency with subsequent impaired production of coagulation factors. Infants have an increased risk of bleeding, especially after experiencing trauma during a complicated childbirth. Sites of bleeding may include the umbilical cord.

6. Correct: Autoimmune regulator (AIRE) (D)

(**D**) This child is suffering from a polyglandular autoimmune syndrome. Autoimmune polyglandular syndrome type 1 is a condition that is inherited in an autosomal recessive pattern and is due to a mutation in *AIRE*; this gene codes for the autoimmune regulator (AIRE) protein, which is normally expressed in the thymic medulla and plays an important role in the negative selection of T cells as they develop in the thymus. Defects in AIRE result in defects in central immune tolerance and in subsequent autoimmunity. Hormone-producing endocrine glands are particularly susceptible to autoimmune attack (the reasons for this are not entirely clear). The adrenal, parathyroid, and thyroid glands are affected. Inflammatory cell infiltration adversely impacts their function. Children affected by this condition have low levels of PTH and a subsequent calcium deficiency. Hypocalcemia is a major cause of tetany (muscle spasms and cramping). (A) LFA-1 (CD11a/CD18) is an integrin expressed on the surface of many white blood cells. It binds to ICAM. Cellular adhesion molecules are expressed on the cell surface of white blood cells and vascular endothelial cells. They govern leukocyte interactions, cell circulation and extravasation from blood to tissue, and cellular interaction with the extracellular matrix. (B) CD28 is a transmembrane molecule that is expressed on the surface of T cells. During T cell activation, the interaction of CD28 on the T cell with B7 on the antigen-presenting cell provides a co-stimulatory signal; this is generally considered a second step in the process of T cell activation. A naïve T cell must recognize its specific antigen in the context of MHC molecules (first step of T cell activation) and receive co-stimulation (second step of T cell activation). Without the co-stimulation step, a naïve T cell will not reach the threshold to become fully activated and will become anergic (unresponsive). (C) B7-1 or B7-2, also known as CD80/CD86, molecules are transmembrane molecules on the surface of antigen-presenting cells. A naïve T cell must recognize its specific antigen in the context of MHC molecules (first step of T cell activation) and receive co-stimulation (second step of T cell activation). The interaction of B7 molecules with CD28 on the T cell provides the co-stimulatory signal. (E) GATA-3 is a transcription factor that is required for T cells to differentiate into the TH2 effector cell type.

7. Correct: IFN-γ (D)

(D) This child has an infection with mycobacteria, an intracellular pathogen. During activation of a naïve T cell, production of IL-12 by the antigen-presenting cell will drive the differentiation of the T cell into a TH1 effector cell. TH1 cells play a critical role in immune defense against intracellular pathogens and protozoa. The "signature" cytokine made by TH1 cells is IFN-γ; it is a potent activator of macrophages. Activated macrophages have enhanced microbicidal capacity. This is due to several biological functions that can mobilize components of innate and adaptive immunity in a coordinated inflammatory response. These functions include: secretion of proinflammatory cytokines (IL-1, IL-6, and TNF-α) and chemokines, upregulation of the expression of MHC class II and B7 molecules (enhancing their capacity to present antigen and activate CD4+ T cells), upregulation of Fc and C3 receptors (enhancing their capacity to opsonize pathogens), enhanced phagocytosis, and enhanced respiratory burst. A lack of IL-12, with a subsequent lack of TH1 cells and IFN-γ, would jeopardize these biological functions of macrophages. (A) IL-2, also known as T cell growth factor, is a

cytokine that is required for the proliferation of T cells. Once activated, T cells produce IL-2 and express a high-affinity receptor for IL-2 (IL-2R). The autocrine interaction of IL-2 with its receptor drives T cell proliferation. (B) IL-4 is a cytokine that is required for the differentiation of TH2 cells; it is also produced by TH2 cells. IL-4 is a B cell growth factor, and it promotes isotype switching to IgG4 and IgE in humans. (C) IFN-β is a type I interferon. Virally infected cells make type I interferons (IFN-α and IFN-β); interferons limit viral replication and viral spread to neighboring cells. In addition to their antiviral properties, type I interferons have various biological effects and have been used therapeutically. IFN-α is used to treat hairy cell leukemia, multiple myeloma, and malignant melanoma; IFN-β is used to treat multiple sclerosis. (E) IL-10, also known as cytokine synthesis inhibitory factor (CSIF), is an anti-inflammatory immunoregulatory cytokine.

8. Correct: Increased susceptibility to bacterial infections (D)

(D) The patient is suffering from an IgG multiple myeloma. The malignant IgG-producing plasma cells multiply in the bone marrow and crowd out other cell types. Hematopoiesis is adversely affected; patients suffer from anemia and neutropenia, as is seen in this patient. In adults, neutrophils represent approximately 65% of circulating leukocytes. They are phagocytes of the innate immune system and are a first line of defense against bacterial infections. Additionally, multiple myeloma patients produce large amounts of immunoglobulin (monoclonal). Light chains are synthesized at a slightly faster rate than the heavy chains. Excess light chains are secreted in the urine; these are called Bence Jones proteins, and are found in the urine of 50 to 70% of multiple myeloma patients. In the nephron, Bence Jones proteins can occlude renal tubules; "intratubular casts" can cause injury and adversely affect renal function. The presence of Bence Jones protein in the patient's urine is consistent with the diagnosis of IgG multiple myeloma. (A) There are four IgG subclasses in humans with the following serum prevalence: IgG1 = 65%, IgG2 = 20%, IgG3 = 10%, and IgG4 = 5%. Therefore, in healthy individuals, IgG1 is the most prevalent. Although there is not enough information to deduce the IgG subclass in this multiple myeloma case, the prevalence of the four IgGs would not be equal. (B) As described above, multiple myeloma patients produce and excrete high levels of light chains that can be detected in the urine. Because the myeloma cells are producing a monoclonal antibody, and because each antibody molecule will only have only one type of light chain (either κ or λ), the light chains in the urine would be either κ or λ, but not both. (C) The myeloma cells are crowding out other plasma cells. The patient would have low levels of serum IgA and IgM. There would not be a large amount of either isotype in the urine.

9. Correct: IgA λ multiple myeloma (B)

(**B**) The normal ratio of κ:λ light chains is approximately 2:1. Although the question does not provide a clue as to the isotype of the immunoglobulin, the spike pattern in the electrophoresis, along with the high ratio of κ:λ, indicates a multiple myeloma that contains κ light chains. (**A**) Ratio of κ:λ is not indicative of a myeloma that produces κ light chains. (**C**) Ratio of κ:λ is not indicative of a myeloma that produces κ light chains. (**D**) Ratio of κ:λ is not indicative of a myeloma that produces κ light chains. (**E**) Ratio of κ:λ is not indicative of a myeloma that produces κ light chains.

10. Correct: 140 (D)

(**D**) With 35 V-gene segments and 5 J-gene segments, there would be 175 possible combinations (35 × 5). However, the recombination signal sequence next to J2 is defective; this eliminates the J2 segment, leaving four other J segments that can undergo gene rearrangements: 35 × 4 = 140 possible combinations. (**A**) The J2 segment will not be able to undergo gene rearrangement, but the other four J segments can rearrange. (**B**) To calculate the possible combinations, multiply 35 by 4. (**C**) To calculate the possible combinations, multiply 35 by 4. (**E**) To calculate the possible combinations, multiply 35 by 4.

11. Correct: T cell receptor (TCR) Vβ and MHC class II (E)

(**E**) Some bacterial exotoxins function as "superantigens" and can activate many clones of T cells. A conventional antigen is bound by MHC class II and presented to T cells. The T cell clone with specificity to that antigen would "recognize" the antigen when the variable regions of both the α and β chains of the T cell receptor (TCR) bind to the antigen. Superantigens do not fit in the antigen-binding grooves of MHC class II molecules and the TCR. Instead, they bind on the outside and crosslink the Vβ portion of the TCR with the MHC class II. Because a conventional antigen binds both the Vα and Vβ to reach the threshold to activate a T cell, whereas a superantigen binds the Vβ only, superantigens can activate many more T cell clones. These activated T cells, and macrophages, produce large amounts of various cytokines (called a cytokine storm). Many proinflammatory cytokines such as IFN-γ, IL-1, IL-6, IL-12, and TNF-α are released and initiate an acute inflammatory response. Bacterial exotoxin superantigens cause a sudden acute illness; symptoms such as pyrexia, hypotension, diarrhea, and rash are largely due to the effects of proinflammatory cytokines. This is a case of toxic shock syndrome; this condition has been linked to the use of superabsorbent tampons. *Staphylococcus aureus* exotoxins are the disease-causing superantigens; however, exotoxins of group A streptococci (*Streptococcus pyogenes*) have also been linked to cases of toxic shock syndrome. (**A**) LFA-1 and ICAM-1 are cellular adhesion molecules. They help the T cell and antigen-presenting cell to come together during T cell activation. Superantigens do not crosslink LFA-1 and ICAM-1. Superantigens crosslink TCR Vβ and MHC class II. (**B**) On CD4+ T cells, the CD4 molecule binds to nonpolymorphic regions on the β chain of the MHC class II molecule. The CD4 molecule also functions as a co-receptor and helps initiate signal transduction during T cell activation. Superantigens do not crosslink CD4 and MHC class II. Superantigens crosslink TCR Vβ and MHC class II. (**C**) The TCR is a heterodimer, made up of an α and β chain. The CD3 complex is associated with the TCR and contains immunoreceptor tyrosine-based activation motifs (ITAMs). Through these ITAMs, the CD3 complex initiates signal transduction during T cell activation. Superantigens crosslink TCR Vβ and MHC class II. They do not crosslink the TCR with the CD3 complex. (**D**) The interaction of CD28 on the T cell surface with B7 on the surface of the antigen-presenting cell provides a co-stimulatory signal during the activation of T cells. Superantigens do not crosslink CD28 and B7. They crosslink TCR Vβ and MHC class II.

12. Correct: CTLA-4 (D)

(**D**) CTLA-4 is a transmembrane molecule that plays an important role in the regulation of the immune system. The activation of a naïve T cell requires two steps. The first step involves the recognition of antigen by the T cell receptor (TCR). The second step involves a process known as co-stimulation, which is dependent on the binding of B7 on the antigen-presenting cell with CD28 on the T cell. Once the T cell is activated, the expression of CTLA-4 is upregulated. Like CD28, CTLA-4 can bind to B7 molecules; CTLA-4 competes with CD28, and CTLA-4 has higher binding affinity to B7 than does CD28. The binding of CTLA-4 to B7 delivers an inhibitory signal to the T cell so that the cell can become quiescent and stop proliferating. This sequence of events is one of several mechanisms to ensure proper regulation of the immune system in secondary lymphoid organs. CTLA-4 is also expressed by FoxP3+ Treg cells and plays a role in their function. A defect in CTLA-4 would result in uncontrolled lymphocyte proliferation. Insufficient expression of CTLA-4 leads to infiltrative and autoimmune diseases. CTLA-4 polymorphisms have also been reported for several autoimmune diseases. CTLA-4 deficiency is a rare condition in humans. Uncontrolled lymphocyte proliferation and infiltration of several organs can lead to organ dysfunction. Patients experience lymphadenopathy; furthermore, proper function of the lungs, gut, and various other organs will be affected by massive lymphocyte infiltration. Patients are diagnosed based on clinical symptoms, laboratory results, and genetic testing. Heterozygous individuals who have one good copy and one defective copy of the CTLA-4 gene will still experience clinical signs and symptoms. (**A**) Integrins play a role in cell adhesion and leukocyte circulation. Both LFA-1 (αLβ2) and Mac-1 (αMβ2) use the β2 chain (CD18). Leukocyte adhesion deficiency (LAD) is a rare disease, which is due to a defect in the β2 chain. In patients with LAD, white blood cells (the majority of which are neutrophils) cannot transmigrate from blood to tissue. Patients with LAD suffer from recurrent bacterial infections. (**B**) ZAP-70 is a tyrosine kinase that is associated with the ζ chain of the CD3 complex. It plays a role in signal transduction during T cell activation. (**C**) CD28 is a transmembrane molecule that is expressed on the cell surface of T cells; during T cell activation, the binding of CD28 to B7 molecules on the antigen-presenting cell provides a co-stimulation signal. This signal is required to reach the threshold of activation for a naïve T cell. Memory cells are less dependent on co-stimulation. (**E**) IL-2R γ chain is one of three transmembrane molecules that make up the IL-2R. The γ chain is also used by the receptors for several other cytokines, including IL-4, IL-7, IL-9, and IL-15. A mutation in the γ chain gene affects signal transduction by the receptors for these cytokines. Patients with a mutation in the γ chain suffer from X-linked severe combined immunodeficiency.

13.   Correct: Maternal κ: paternal λ (C)

(**C**) Allelic exclusion ensures that a B cell can produce only one heavy chain variable region and one light chain variable region. This ensures that the B cell will produce an antibody molecule with one specificity; i.e., each "arm" of the antibody molecule will have the same variable region. The heavy chain gene locus is on human chromosome 14. If the immunoglobulin gene rearrangements on the maternal chromosome are successful, then the heavy chain gene locus on the paternal chromosome 14 will not rearrange. The same principle applies to the gene rearrangements for κ and λ light chains. Each antibody molecule has two identical heavy chains and two identical light chains (either κ or λ). Therefore, answer choice **C** is not possible. (**A, B, D, E**) These combinations are possible.

14.   Correct: Biological father may be AB+ (A)

(**A**) This pregnant woman is Rh⁻; there is a high probability that she is carrying a fetus who is Rh⁺. The question stem does not provide information on the blood type of the biological father of the first child, the blood type of the first child, or the blood type of the biological father of this second child. However, most of the population (>80%) is Rh⁺. If this woman were exposed to Rh⁺ cells in the past, she would have anti-Rh antibodies; these are of the IgG isotype and can cross the placenta and harm an Rh⁺ fetus. A Coombs test is used to determine whether the mother has anti-Rh antibodies. To reduce the risk of sensitization to the Rh antigen, expectant mothers who are Rh⁻ are given intramuscular injections

of MICRhoGAM (anti-Rh) (which is RhoGAM that has lower amounts of the antibody); antepartum administration of MICRhoGAM is usually given at 28 weeks of pregnancy, whereas postpartum administration of RhoGAM is given within 48 hours of delivery. At delivery, the mother is exposed to the fetal RBCs. RhoGAM antibodies would bind to the Rh on the fetal RBCs and help clear them from the circulation. This reduces the risk of sensitization. Without RhoGAM, the risk of sensitization is 15 to 20%; with RhoGAM, the risk is reduced to 1 to 2%. (**B**) If both the mother and the biological father are Rh⁻, then the fetus will also be Rh⁻. (**C**) The fetal immune system is not yet mature and the fetus will not produce isohemagglutinin antibodies. (**D**) The ABO blood type of the biological father and that of the fetus are not known. However, differences in the ABO blood group antigens do not pose a risk to the fetus during pregnancy. Anti-A and anti-B are IgM antibodies and do not cross the placenta. ABO blood group antigen differences between mother and fetus are common and do not complicate the pregnancy. (**E**) The mother's blood type is B⁻. She would not have anti-B antibodies.

15.   Correct: Popliteal lymph nodes (E)

(**E**) *Clostridium tetani*, the causative pathogen of tetanus, is a bacterium that is found in contaminated dust, soil, and animal feces and is the most likely agent of this infection. When introduced into the body through a deep wound, bacterial endospores produce a powerful toxin, which impairs the function of motor neurons. Tetanus vaccinations have dramatically reduced the incidence of tetanus in developed countries; cases of tetanus are still found in underdeveloped countries where vaccination rates are low. Signs and symptoms of tetanus are due to the toxin; once released, it travels throughout the body via the lymphatics and vascular circulation. This toxin is powerful; minute amounts will cause symptoms prior to inducing a primary immune response. In this case, the homebuilder was injured in the sole of his foot when he stepped on the contaminated nail. Of the answer choices provided, the closest secondary immune organ is the popliteal lymph node. (**A**) Adenoids and tonsils are found in the upper respiratory tract. (**B**) Bone marrow is a primary lymphoid organ and is the site of hematopoiesis in humans. (**C**) The thymus is a primary lymphoid organ and is the site of T cell development in humans. (**D**) Peyer's patches are aggregations of follicles that are found in the ileum; they are secondary lymphoid organs in the gut.

16.   Correct: Acquired and passive immunity (D)

(**D**) Rattlesnake bites are life-threatening because of the toxicity of the venom. Hospitals located in areas where venomous snakes are prevalent stock antivenom. This is usually IgG from a horse that has been immunized. Therefore, this is passive, acquired immunity. The therapeutic horse antibody will save the victim's life. However, recipients of the horse IgG will subsequently experience symptoms of serum sickness. These symptoms may include chills, fever, rash, vasculitis, arthritis, or glomerulonephritis. Differences between horse IgG and human IgG will trigger an immune response in the recipients of horse antivenom, and these individuals will subsequently produce human IgG directed against the horse IgG. Immune complexes that are made up of human and horse IgGs will peak in the circulation at approximately 1 week after injection of the foreign horse IgG. These immune complexes will become trapped in the basement membrane in various tissues, triggering an acute and transient type III hypersensitivity reaction. (**A**) Natural and passive immunity is best exemplified by the passage of immunity from a mother to a child through breastfeeding or transplacentally. Even though the question is an example of passive immunity, since it is being injected into the patient, it is not "natural." (**B**) Natural and active immunity is best exemplified by a patient that is exposed to an infectious agent and generates an immune response to the etiologic agent. It is natural, because it is how we normally induce immune responses and it is active because the individual has to actively mount an immune response. Since the patient is being given the immunoglobulin, it is not an active response and therefore this response is incorrect. (**C**) Acquired and active immunity is best exemplified by the vaccination of a patient. The injection of antigen into a patient is not "natural" and it is active, because the patient has to actively mount their own immune response to the antigen. Since the patient is being given immunoglobulin, it is an acquired immunity, but it is not active immunity because the individual is not making their own immunoglobulin against the toxin. (**E**) Immune responses can be either natural or acquired—they cannot be both, so this is not the correct answer.

17. Correct: IgG (A)

(**A**) This is a case of Farmer's lung disease. The hypersensitivity pneumonitis is due to the formation of IgG antibodies to inhaled antigen. Immune complexes are deposited in the alveoli, where they activate complement, with resultant tissue damage due to a type III hypersensitivity. The inflammatory response compromises lung function. This is an occupational disease. The patient is a stable hand who works with hay. *Saccharopolyspora rectivirgula* (gram-positive rod) is found in moldy hay. (**B**) IgA is an important molecule for providing immunity at mucosal sites, including the respiratory system. However, IgA is not associated with the development of hypersensitivity reactions in the lungs and, therefore, is not the correct answer. (**C**) IgM is important molecule that can induce type II and type III hypersensitivity reactions

through the activation of complement. However, IgG antibodies specific for *S. rectivirgula* are the predominant isotype that promotes pathology in Farmer's lung. (**D**) IgD is an antibody molecule that is found on the surface of mature, naïve B cells and can serve an antigen receptor for activation of B cells. It is not actively secreted, and therefore does not contribute to antibody-mediated pathology in individuals. (**E**) IgE is an important mediator of type I hypersensitivities and asthma. However, in this individual, the pathology is consistent with Farmer's lung, which is a type III hypersensitivity that uses IgG, not IgE.

18. Correct: Rheumatoid arthritis (RA) (B)

(**B**) The elevated ESR is a nonspecific marker of inflammation. In the inflamed synovium, macrophages and neutrophils express peptidyl arginine deaminases. In the presence of calcium ions, these enzymes catalyze the deamination of proteins in the extracellular matrix (vimentin, fibrin, collagen) by converting arginine into citrulline. Thus, citrullinated protein antigens are generated during chronic inflammation. Cyclic citrullinated peptide (CCP) is a synthetic peptide that is used in diagnostic assays for rheumatoid arthritis (RA), a chronic inflammatory disease. Anti-CCP has a sensitivity of approximately 60%, but it is highly specific for RA with a specificity greater than 90%. The ANA test is nonspecific for RA. Although 70% of patients with RA have rheumatoid factor in the circulation, it is not diagnostic or specific for RA because it is also found in some healthy individuals and in patients with other immune-mediated diseases. Immune complex deposition contributes to joint inflammation. However, joint destruction is largely due to a highly proinflammatory immune response that is mediated by TH1 and TH17 cells, with resultant activation of macrophages (osteoclasts), neutrophils, and synovial fibroblasts. Production of matrix metalloproteinases contributes to the destruction of cartilage and the extracellular matrix. Low viscosity of synovial fluid is due to degradation of the extracellular matrix. (**A**) Patients with systemic lupus erythematosus may experience joint inflammation when immune complexes are deposited in the joint. However, these patients typically do not experience joint-space narrowing, bone erosion, and joint destruction. (**C**) Osteoarthritis is a degenerative disease; its pathology is not inflammatory as is seen in this patient. (**D**) Gout is a crystalline arthropathy. Urate crystals were not noted on synovial fluid analysis. (**E**) Serum sickness is due to an inflammatory response that is initiated by immune complex deposition with subsequent complement activation. It is an acute and transient inflammatory response.

19. Correct: AA and AO (B)

(**B**) This child's blood type is A⁺. She is Rh⁺ and would not have anti-Rh antibodies. Therefore, the Rh "status" of the parents would not be an issue in this case.

Because the child's blood type is A, she would have anti-B antibodies. She would not be able to receive any blood from a type B or a type AB donor. Answer choice B is the only one in which neither parent has a B genotype. (**A, C–E**) Because the child's blood type is A, she would have anti-B antibodies and therefore would react against at least one of the parents in each of these options.

20.   Correct: Isohemagglutinins are IgM (C)

(**C**) Human RBCs have a glycoprotein called H-antigen on the cell surface. Glycosylation adds additional terminal sugar moieties to the H-antigen. The A allele codes for an enzyme that covalently attaches *N*-acetylgalactosamine to the H-antigen, whereas the B allele codes for an enzyme that covalently attaches galactose to the H-antigen. The O allele has a deletion and does not code for a glycosyl transferase; therefore, it does not add additional sugar moieties to the H-antigen. An individual who is type A has anti-B antibodies, type B individuals have anti-A antibodies, type O individuals have both anti-A and anti-B, and people who have blood type AB do not have these antibodies. Anti-A and anti-B antibodies are called isohemagglutinins and they are of the IgM isotype. Because sugars have repeating epitopes, they are quite effective at crosslinking the B cell receptor and activating the B cell. The response of the B cell to sugar antigens is "T-independent"; i.e., it does not require T cell help. Without T cell help, B cells do not undergo isotype switching. Being IgM, isohemagglutinins do not cross the placenta and do not pose a risk to the fetus when there is ABO blood type incompatibility between mother and fetus. By contrast, Rh incompatibility between mother and fetus can put the fetus at risk. The Rh antigen is a protein and anti-Rh is an IgG, which can cross the placenta. When a mother is Rh⁻ and the fetus is Rh⁺, transplacental transfer of IgG anti-Rh puts the fetus at risk for hemolytic anemia. (**A,B,D,E**) Isohemagglutinins are IgM.

21.   Correct: O negative (D)

(**D**) A commercial panel of blood-typing antibodies would include anti-A, anti-B, and anti-Rh/D antibodies. If none of these antibodies agglutinated the soldier's RBCs, then the soldier's blood type is O⁻. (**A**) If the soldier's blood type is AB⁺, then all of the commercial antibodies (anti-A, anti-B, and anti-Rh) would agglutinate the soldier's RBCs. (**B**) If the soldier's blood type is AB⁻, then both the anti-A and the anti-B would agglutinate the soldier's RBCs. (**C**) If the soldier's type is O⁺, the anti-Rh antibody would agglutinate the soldier's RBCs, but there would be no agglutination reaction with the anti-A or the anti-B antibodies.

Chapter 3

Autoimmune Disease

Samia Ragheb[†]

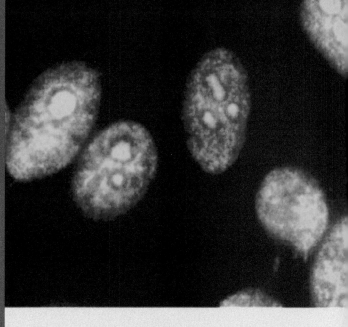

LEARNING OBJECTIVES

- ▶ Describe central and peripheral regulatory mechanisms that regulate autoimmune reactions.
- ▶ Describe the process of T cell activation, co-stimulation, proliferation, anergy, and apoptosis.
- ▶ Delineate the cellular and molecular mechanisms that contribute to the immunopathology of systemic and organ-specific autoimmune diseases.
- ▶ Describe the immunopathogenesis, clinical presentation, histopathology, diagnosis, and therapy of inflammatory diseases that:
  - – affect the nervous system and the neuromuscular junction.
  - – affect the musculoskeletal system.
  - – affect the skin and connective tissue.
  - – contribute to kidney pathology.
  - – affect the respiratory tract.
  - – affect the endocrine system.
  - – affect the gastrointestinal tract.
  - – affect the hematopoietic system.
- ▶ Describe leukocyte circulation and delineate the role of cytokines, chemokines, and cellular adhesion molecules in the extravasation of white blood cells during inflammation.
- ▶ Describe the use of immunotherapies (biologicals) in the management and treatment of immune-mediated disease; describe the mode of action of these immunotherapies.
- ▶ Describe the structure, function, and anatomical distribution of human lymphoid organs.
- ▶ Delineate the function(s) of cytokines and chemokines in health and disease.
- ▶ Distinguish between the role of CD4 and CD8 T cells within the immune system, including the role of effector T cell populations (TH1, TH2, TH9, TH17, TFH, Treg, CTL).

- ▶ Delineate the cellular and molecular events that lead to acute or chronic inflammation.
- ▶ Describe the protein structure and tissue distribution of the major histocompatibility complex class I and major histocompatibility complex class II molecules, and their function within the immune system.
- ▶ Define the structure and biological function of the five classes/isotypes of immunoglobulin.

3.1 Questions

Easy	Medium	Hard

1. A 24-month-old girl is brought to the pediatrician's office with cervical and axillary lymphadenopathy. She is afebrile. Physical exam reveals splenomegaly. The toddler has an elevated lymphocyte count and high immunoglobulin levels for all isotypes. Which of the following proteins is either absent or nonfunctional in this child?

A. CD95 (FAS)

B. Perforin

C. Granzyme

D. Interferon-γ (IFN-γ)

E. Interleukin 17 (IL-17)

2. A 36-year-old man presents to his primary care physician with diarrhea and severe abdominal cramps. He states that 2 days prior to the onset of symptoms, he was at a picnic where he consumed undercooked chicken. He is diagnosed with gastroenteritis and sent home with instruction to drink plenty of fluids. Within a few days, the symptoms subsided. Ten days later, the patient experiences ataxia and loss of cutaneous sensation, followed by ascending paralysis. Which of the following, if present, would best confirm his diagnosis?

A. Anti-acetylcholine (anti-ACh) antibodies

B. Anti-ACh receptor antibodies

C. Anti-voltage-gated calcium channel (anti-VGCC) antibodies

D. Anti-ganglioside antibodies

E. Anti-aquaporin 4 antibodies

3. A 37-year-old woman with multiple sclerosis (MS) is prescribed a humanized monoclonal antibody directed against the α4 integrin. The mechanism of action of this drug is to:

A. Inhibit the activation of microglia

B. Inhibit the activation of astrocytes

C. Inhibit oligodendrocyte cell death

D. Promote remyelination

E. Inhibit leukocyte transmigration into the central nervous system (CNS)

4. A computed tomography (CT) scan from a 28-year-old Caucasian woman with a history of myasthenia gravis (MG) reveals an enlarged thymus. Her neurologist recommends a thymectomy. Upon examination of the excised tissue, the pathologist identifies germinal centers in the thymic medulla, which resemble germinal centers that are found in lymph nodes. These germinal centers:

A. Act as a major repository of stem cells

B. Support the development of B cells and T cells

C. Support B-cell proliferation and differentiation

D. Support T-cell proliferation and differentiation

E. Are sites of negative selection of T cells

5. A 45-year-old man with a recent diagnosis of lung cancer presents for a routine visit to his primary care physician. He reports that he is having difficulty climbing stairs and his legs feel weak. A neurological exam shows poor muscle tone and decreased reflexes. An ocular exam is normal. A subsequent electromyography (EMG) study shows deficits in neuromuscular transmission. Within a few weeks, he starts radiation and 3,4-diaminopyridine is administered to increase acetylcholine (ACh) release. Analysis of the patient's serum will most likely show the presence of antibodies specific for:

A. Acetylcholine (ACh)

B. Acetylcholine receptors (AChRs)

C. Muscle-specific kinase (MuSK)

D. Voltage-gated calcium channel (VGCC)

E. Agrin

6. A 17-year-old girl practices the piano for hours each day while preparing for her Juilliard audition. Some pieces require sustained activity and are becoming increasingly difficult to play. She complains of becoming easily fatigued. An electromyogram (EMG) of the thenar eminence shows deficits. Which of the following laboratory findings would be most consistent with this condition?

A. Rheumatoid factor

B. Antinuclear antibodies (ANA)

C. Anti-acetylcholine receptor antibodies

D. Anti-myelin oligodendrocyte glycoprotein antibodies

E. Anti-neuronal antibodies

7. Which of the following is a characteristic of rheumatoid factor, which may be found in the synovial fluid of patients with rheumatoid arthritis (RA)?

A. Immunoglobulin M (IgM) reacting with the L chain of IgG
B. IgM reacting with the H chain of IgG
C. Antibody against collagen components
D. IgG reacting with the L chain of IgM
E. IgG reacting with the H chain of IgM

8. Therapy for rheumatoid arthritis (RA) involves the use of adalimumab, a human monoclonal antibody. Patients who receive this therapy are at a higher risk for infections, including tuberculosis. Which of the following is the target of adalimumab?

A. IFN-γ
B. IL-4
C. IL-17
D. Tumor necrosis factor α (TNF-α)
E. B cell activating factor (BAFF)

9. A 27-year-old African American woman presents to her primary care physician with general malaise, joint pain, and an erythematous rash on her face. She reports that her symptoms seem to flare with exposure to the sun. Except for the rash, the physical exam is normal. Routine blood work reveals a white blood cell (WBC) count of 6,500 cells/μL (normal range: 4,500–11,000/μL). Urinalysis reveals proteinuria with no evidence of red blood cells (RBCs), WBCs, or bacteria. Which of the following, if positive, would best confirm the diagnosis?

A. Antinuclear antibodies (ANA)
B. Anti-ribonucleoprotein antibodies (anti-Ro)
C. Anti-dsDNA antibodies
D. IgA in the urine
E. Rheumatoid factor

10. A 40-year-old man presents to his primary care physician with a 1-week history of fatigue and hemoptysis. Physical examination is unremarkable. Routine blood work is normal. Urinalysis reveals proteinuria and hematuria. A renal biopsy is performed and immunofluorescent staining for human IgG reveals a smooth, ribbon-like pattern of glomerular staining. Which of the following laboratory findings would best confirm this man's most likely diagnosis?

A. Antinuclear antibodies (ANA)
B. Anti-histone antibodies
C. Anti-dsDNA antibodies
D. Anti-collagen type IV antibodies
E. Bence Jones protein

11. A 36-year-old woman presents to the emergency department with a sudden loss of vision, paraparesis, and loss of bladder control. Magnetic resonance imaging (MRI) scan shows a large lesion in the spinal cord and increased signal from the optic nerve sheaths. Which of the following findings is most consistent with this patient's condition?

A. Anti-aquaporin 4 antibodies
B. Anti-myelin basic protein antibodies
C. Anti-proteolipid protein antibodies
D. Anti-myelin oligodendrocyte glycoprotein antibodies
E. Anti-LRP4 antibodies

12. A 30-year-old woman is experiencing facial numbness and blurry vision. One year earlier, she had experienced similar symptoms but did not seek medical attention because the symptoms subsided. She was pregnant at that time. Now, she is 3 months postpartum and the symptoms have returned. On examination, she shows signs of optic neuritis. A gadolinium-enhancing MRI shows two active lesions in the brain. The most likely mechanism mediating this disease is:

A. TH1-mediated response with IL-4 and IL-5 production
B. TH1-mediated response with IFN-γ and granulocyte-macrophage colony-stimulating factor (GM-CSF) production
C. TH2-mediated response with TNF-α production
D. TH2-mediated response with IL-10 and transforming growth factor β (TGF-β) production
E. TH2-mediated response with brain-derived neurotrophic factor (BDNF) production

13. During neuroinflammation in the central nervous system, the expression of MHC class I molecules on the cell surface of oligodendrocytes makes them susceptible to killing by:

A. Antibody plus complement
B. CD4+ T cells
C. CD8+ T cells
D. Activated astrocytes
E. Activated microglia

14. A 66-year-old retired policeman develops double vision and ptosis of one eyelid. Several months later, he has difficulty chewing and swallowing his food. Serologic tests reveal the presence of antibodies against molecules at the end plate of the neuromuscular junction. What is the most likely diagnosis?

A. Dermatomyositis

B. Inclusion body myopathy

C. Polymyositis

D. Lambert–Eaton myasthenic syndrome (LEMS)

E. Myasthenia gravis (MG)

15. A 24-year-old woman complains of general malaise and presents with an erythematous butterfly-shaped rash on her cheeks. She states that the rash flares up when she is outdoors. On exam, the physician notes that the nasolabial folds are spared. An immunological work-up shows that she is ANA positive in high titers and anti-dsDNA positive. Which of the following is the best first-choice treatment for her flare-ups?

A. Hydroxychloroquine

B. Azathioprine

C. Anti-CD3

D. Abatacept

E. Infliximab

16. A 25-year-old medical student has lost 10 pounds over the last 6 months. She complains of feeling tired most of the time, despite getting enough sleep. She recently spent a day at the beach and developed a rash on her face, which covered the bridge of her nose and her cheeks, but spared the nasolabial folds. Immunologic therapies that target which of the following molecules would best manage her condition?

A. α4 Integrin

B. CD80/86

C. IL-1 receptor

D. B cell activating factor (BAFF)

E. TNF-α

17. A 60-year-old woman complains of dry eyes, dry mouth, and dry, peeling lips. She has had several dental caries over the past 5 years. Physical examination reveals enlarged lacrimal and parotid salivary glands. Lymphocyte counts are normal and serological analysis indicates that immunoglobulin levels are normal. Further testing reveals the findings below:

- ANA: positive
- Rheumatoid factor: positive
- Anti-dsDNA: negative
- Anti-Ro: positive
- Anti-La: positive
- Anti-histone: negative

Which of the following is the most likely diagnosis?

A. Rheumatoid arthritis (RA)

B. Systemic lupus erythematosus (SLE)

C. Sjögren's syndrome

D. Scleroderma

E. Mixed connective tissue disease

18. In conditions of chronic inflammation, ectopic lymphoid follicles are found in inflamed tissues/organs. Which of the following chemokines plays an essential role in the recruitment of B cells into these follicles?

A. CCL2

B. CCL5

C. CXCL8

D. CXCL9

E. CXCL13

19. A 10-year-old girl is experiencing bouts of fever and chills and is feeling "achy." Her mother reports that she has generally experienced good health. Oral temperature is 40°C (104°F). Physical examination shows a child with normal height and weight for her age. Laboratory testing is pending. Which of the following receptors is expressed by hypothalamic thermoregulatory cells and most likely contribute to this child's fever?

A. IL-1R

B. IL-2R

C. IL-4R

D. IL-6R

E. IL-7R

20. A 4-year-old boy, who was previously healthy, complains of fatigue. He is of normal height and weight for his age. However, his mother states that he has recently lost weight, complains of thirst, needs to urinate frequently, and has started bed-wetting at night. Which of the following haplotypes is associated with this child's most likely condition?

A. HLA-B8

B. HLA-B27

C. HLA-DR2

D. HLA-DR3/DR4

E. HLA-DR15

21. A 35-year-old mother of two is experiencing joint swelling and pain in both hands. This affects her ability to get her children ready for school as it takes her at least 1 to 2 hours each morning to feel limber enough to function. Physical examination shows visible swelling of the interphalangeal joints and wrists. Which of the following shows a strong association with this women's most likely disease?

A. HLA-B8

B. HLA-B27

C. HLA-DR2

D. HLA-DR4

E. HLA-DR15

22. A 70-year-old woman with longstanding rheumatoid arthritis (RA) no longer responds to conventional immunosuppressants. Her physician considers prescribing an immunotherapeutic biologic agent. Which of the following immune molecules would be an appropriate target for this women's condition?

A. IFN-β

B. TNF-α

C. TGF-β

D. IL-3

E. IL-10

23. X-ray images of the hands of a patient with longstanding rheumatoid arthritis (RA) show narrowed joint spaces in the interphalangeal and metacarpophalangeal joints. Which of the following is directly responsible for the cartilage destruction?

A. IL-6

B. RANK ligand

C. Osteoblasts

D. Metalloproteinases

E. Prostaglandins

24. A 28-year-old man presents to his primary care physician with a 5-month history of low back pain. He also complains of morning stiffness in the lower back and hips, which appears to improve with exercise. He does not have a history of infection of the joints or bones. Physical examination reveals limitation of spinal mobility and radiologic imaging shows evidence of sacroiliitis. Arthrocentesis of the knee shows that synovial fluid is clear. Further testing reveals that he is HLA-B27 haplotype positive and rheumatoid factor negative. What is the most likely diagnosis?

A. Ankylosing spondylitis

B. Reactive arthritis

C. Rheumatoid arthritis (RA)

D. Psoriatic arthritis

E. Osteoarthritis

25. A 57-year-old woman is experiencing symmetrical painless weakness. Physical examination shows that the patient cannot easily rise from a seated position. Additionally, a purple rash around the eyelids and in the chest area is noted. Laboratory testing shows a creatine kinase level of 200 U/L (normal range: 10–70 U/L). A subsequent muscle biopsy reveals perifascicular inflammation and atrophy. Which of the following autoantibodies would best confirm the diagnosis?

A. Antinuclear antibodies (ANA)

B. Anti-dsDNA

C. Anti-tRNA synthetase

D. Anti-AChR

E. Anti-VGCC

26. A 35-year-old woman has been gaining weight and feeling lethargic over the past year. She is perplexed because her diet and level of physical activity have not changed. Physical examination reveals a goiter, which is firm to the touch and painless. A biopsy of the goiter is obtained. The pathology report indicates the presence of inflammatory cells. Which of the following laboratory results is most consistent with the most likely diagnosis?

A. Elevated T3

B. Elevated T4

C. Low thyroid-stimulating hormone (TSH)

D. Anti-TSH receptor agonist antibodies

E. Anti-thyroglobulin (anti-TG) antibodies

27. A 40-year-old woman was living in Ukraine at the time of the Chernobyl nuclear plant explosion in 1986. She was 10 years old at the time. This explosion released high levels of radioactive iodine. This woman is at increased risk of developing what autoimmune disease?

A. Hashimoto's thyroiditis

B. Graves' disease

C. Thyroid cancer

D. Hyperparathyroidism

E. Leukemia

28. A 42-year-old man is experiencing weight loss, despite no change in diet or physical activity. He appears to be quite irritable that he waited an additional 15 minutes for his appointment. Physical examination reveals a heart rate of 130 beats per min. Follow-up diagnostic testing shows that the patient suffers from Graves' disease. Which of the following most likely played a role in the development of his disease?

A. High levels of TSH

B. Presence of anti-thyroglobulin antibodies

C. Anti-TSH receptor agonist antibodies

D. Anti-TSH receptor blocking antibodies

E. Low levels of T3/T4

29. A 7-year-old girl is constantly thirsty and frequently urinates. Her mother states that she has lost weight despite a healthy appetite and healthy diet. Physical examination reveals that she is underweight for her age. Laboratory testing reveals a fasting blood glucose of 130 mg/dL (normal range: 70–110 mg/dL). Urinalysis shows the presence of glucose and ketones. Which of the following is most likely responsible for this child's condition?

A. Type I hypersensitivity

B. Type II hypersensitivity

C. Type III hypersensitivity

D. Type IV hypersensitivity

E. Type V hypersensitivity

30. A 56-year-old woman of Scandinavian descent is complaining of fatigue, shortness of breath, and a sore tongue. She appears pale, has dark circles around her eyes, and has dry cracked lips. Examination of the tongue reveals a "beefy" bright red tongue. A complete blood count (CBC) and vitamin B12 level are ordered and results are below:

- CBC:
  - Hemoglobin: 8.0 g/dL (normal range: 12–16 g/dL)
  - Reticulocytes: 3.0% (normal range: 0.5–1.5%)
  - RBCs: 2.2 million/μL (normal range: 3.5–5.5 million/μL)
  - WBCs: 6,500/μL (normal range: 4,500–11,000/μL)
  - Platelets: 250,000/μL (normal range: 150,000–400,000/μL)
- Vitamin B12: 75 pg/mL (normal range: 160–950 pg/mL)

Which of the following is the most likely diagnosis?

A. Autoimmune hemolytic anemia

B. Pernicious anemia

C. Iron deficiency anemia

D. Thalassemia

E. Sickle cell anemia

31. A 70-year-old woman presents to her primary care physician with fatigue and shortness of breath. She has enjoyed fairly good health throughout her life and there have been no changes in her diet or lifestyle. She continues to take a daily multivitamin and aspirin. On exam, her skin appears pale and there is noticeable pallor in the conjunctival mucosa and palmar creases. Which of the following would best confirm the most likely diagnosis?

A. Anti-AChR

B. Anti-VGCC

C. Anti-histidyl tRNA synthetase

D. Anti-intrinsic factor

E. Anti-thyroid peroxidase (anti-TPO) antibodies

32. An 18-year-old man is pale, fatigued, and has an enlarged spleen. He has a positive direct Coombs' test at 37°C and is diagnosed with a "warm"-type autoimmune hemolytic anemia. Which of the following immunopathologic mechanisms is most likely contributing to the anemia?

A. Type I hypersensitivity

B. Type II hypersensitivity

C. Type III hypersensitivity

D. Type IV hypersensitivity

E. Type V hypersensitivity

33. A 40-year-old woman presents to the emergency department with mucocutaneous bleeding from the nose and gums. She states that she bruises easily and experiences menorrhagia. She is currently not on any anticoagulant or antiplatelet therapy. Serological testing reveals the presence of IgG antibodies against platelet glycoproteins. Which of the following is most likely to play a role in the destruction of the platelets?

A. FcγR-mediated destruction by macrophages

B. Agglutination of platelets

C. Fibrin deposition

D. Thrombopoietin deficiency

E. Apoptosis

34. A 32-year-old woman presents to the emergency department with a sudden transient loss of vision in her left eye, which lasted for 30 minutes. She states that she also experienced some pain as she tried to move the affected eye. She states that she had a similar episode a few months prior to the current presentation. Upon consulting with an ophthalmologist, it was determined that she experienced an episode of optic neuritis. Testing reveals areas of demyelination of the optic nerve due to inflammation. Cerebrospinal fluid (CSF) was obtained for further analysis. Which of the following CSF findings would best confirm that this inflammatory process is due to an autoimmune mechanism?

A. Increased number of inflammatory cells

B. Increased glucose level

C. Increased protein level

D. Increased cytokine and chemokine levels

E. Presence of oligoclonal bands on electrophoresis

35. A 22-year-old law student develops a heliotrope-colored rash on her eyelids. She also experiences myalgias in her proximal muscles and complains that she has difficulty combing her hair and climbing stairs. On exam, the myalgias and proximal muscle weakness are found to be bilateral. A muscle biopsy reveals perimysium infiltration and perifascicular atrophy. Which of the following mechanisms is most likely involved in development of this disease?

A. An inflammatory polyneuropathy leading to paralysis

B. Antibodies that block neuromuscular transmission

C. Immune complex–mediated injury of small blood vessels

D. CD8+ T cell–mediated injury of myocytes

E. Antibodies against dystrophin

36. A 60-year-old man presents to his primary care physician with bilateral symmetrical muscle weakness. He also complains of weakness in his shoulders and thighs. No other abnormalities are observed during the physical examination. Laboratory results show an elevated erythrocyte sedimentation rate, elevated C-reactive protein (CRP), and elevated creatine phosphokinase. Which of the following is the most likely diagnosis?

A. Muscular dystrophy

B. Myasthenia gravis (MG)

C. Lambert–Eaton myasthenic syndrome (LEMS)

D. Dermatomyositis

E. Polymyositis

37. A 32-year-old woman with myasthenia gravis (MG) gives birth to a full-term 5-pound boy. Shortly after birth, the baby exhibits hypotonia and has difficulty breathing and suckling. He is transferred to the neonatal intensive care unit and is placed on a ventilator. Which of the following best explains why this baby is experiencing symptoms of MG?

A. HLA-DR3 and HLA-B8 haplotypes

B. IgG anti-AChR antibodies that crossed the placenta

C. IgM anti-AChR antibodies that crossed the placenta

D. Congenital myasthenic syndrome

E. X-linked myopathy

38. A 41-year-old woman has experienced several episodes of bilateral optic neuritis. Neuroimaging reveals lesions in the optic nerve and spinal cord, but not in the brain. Serologic testing shows the presence of anti-AQP4 (aquaporin 4) antibodies. What is the most likely diagnosis?

A. Encephalitis

B. Autoimmune polyneuropathy

C. Multiple sclerosis (MS)

D. Neuromyelitis optica (NMO)

E. Clinically isolated syndrome

39. A mother begins to introduce her baby daughter to solid foods at 8 months of age. Over the next few months, the baby exhibits abdominal distension, diarrhea, and failure to thrive. A biopsy of the small intestine shows an increase of intraepithelial lymphocytes, villus blunting, and increased numbers of WBCs in the lamina propria, which include T cells and plasma cells. Serologic testing would most likely reveal the presence of which of the following antibodies?

A. Anti-rotavirus antibodies

B. Anti-ganglioside antibodies

C. Anti-goblet cell antibodies

D. Anti-Paneth cell antibodies

E. Anti-gliadin antibodies

40. A 27-year-old man presents to his primary care physician with a 2-month history of nonbloody diarrhea and weight loss. A stool examination is negative for infectious pathogens. A colonoscopy reveals ulcers in the terminal ileum and areas of stenosis. The colon appears normal. Immunostaining of biopsy tissue from the terminal ileum would most likely show which of the following?

A. Eosinophils

B. TH1 and TH17 cells

C. TH2 cells

D. TH9 cells

E. CD8+ T cells

41. A 60-year-old man presents to urgent care with skin blisters. He states that a few months earlier he had experienced painful ulcerations in his oral mucosa for which he took over-the-counter benzocaine to alleviate the pain. Histological examination of the skin lesions shows epidermal separation with acantholysis and immunofluorescence shows IgG4 antibody binding to keratinocytes. Which of the following is the most likely diagnosis?

A. Urticaria

B. Psoriasis

C. Pemphigus vulgaris

D. Canker sores

E. Herpes

3.2 Answers and Explanations

Easy	Medium	Hard

1. Correct: CD95 (FAS) (A)

(**A**) FAS ligand/FAS death receptor–mediated apoptosis pathways play an important role in regulating the immune system. During both T cell and B cell

development, somatic recombination of TCR and BCR genes must result in a functional protein. Cells that undergo unsuccessful recombinations die by apoptosis. Negative selection of autoreactive T cells and B cells also involves apoptosis. In peripheral secondary lymphoid organs, FAS-mediated apoptosis plays a role in activation-induced death of T cells in order to prevent uncontrolled lymphocyte proliferation. A defect or lack of FAS ligand or FAS death receptor contributes to uncontrolled lymphoproliferation with subsequent lymphadenopathy and splenomegaly. Such is the case in patients with autoimmune lymphoproliferative syndrome (ALPS). Individuals with this disease present with enlarged lymph nodes, an enlarged spleen, hypergammaglobulinemia, and the presence of autoantibodies. The majority of cases are due to mutations in FAS receptor, while a minority of cases are due to mutations in FAS ligand. ALPS patients are predisposed to develop autoimmunity and lymphomas. (**B**) Perforin is found in the cytotoxic granules of CD8+ cytotoxic T cells and natural killer (NK) cells. Perforin is a pore-forming protein. It is similar in function to complement proteins that form the membrane attack complex; it punches holes in the target cell membrane, which allows granzymes to enter the target cell. (**C**) Granzymes are serine proteases that are found in the cytotoxic granules of CD8+ cytotoxic T cells and NK cells. Once delivered inside the target cell, they degrade proteins and activate the caspase enzyme system to trigger programmed cell death (apoptosis). (**D**) IFN-γ is a cytokine, which is primarily secreted by TH1 cells. It is a potent activator of macrophages; therefore, it plays an important role in type IV hypersensitivity reactions that are associated with many chronic inflammatory diseases (e.g., tuberculosis). (**E**) IL-17 is a proinflammatory cytokine, which is secreted by TH17 cells. It is involved in epithelial barrier protection and activation of neutrophils. It has also been implicated in several chronic inflammatory diseases, including Crohn's disease.

2. Correct: Anti-ganglioside antibodies (D)

(**D**) This is a case of Guillain–Barré syndrome (GBS), an acute inflammatory demyelinating peripheral neuropathy. There is evidence of molecular mimicry in GBS. Approximately two-thirds of cases are preceded by diarrhea due to *Campylobacter jejuni*. An immune response against *C. jejuni* results in IgG antibodies that cross-react with gangliosides in peripheral nerves. These antibodies activate the complement pathway, resulting in damage to the peripheral nerves. Both motor and sensory nerves can be affected. Patients experience loss of coordination (ataxia) and loss of sensation. They may also experience symptoms of ascending flaccid paralysis that starts in the hands or feet and move proximally. The paralysis is both acute and reversible. IgG antibodies have a half-life of approximately 3 to 4 weeks.

Once the infection is cleared and production of anti-ganglioside antibodies has stopped, symptoms will abate. Incidence of GBS is approximately 0.25 to 0.65 per 1,000 cases of *C. jejuni* infection. (**A**) The patient is presenting with motor and sensory issues, including lack of muscle coordination. This is not a description of someone with neuromuscular deficits; moreover, autoantibodies directed against the ACh neurotransmitter itself are not a common clinical entity. (**B**) The patient is presenting with motor and sensory issues, including lack of muscle coordination. This is not a description of someone with neuromuscular deficits; these patients (myasthenia gravis [MG]) usually complain of fatigue and weakness. (**C**) The patient is presenting with motor and sensory issues, including lack of muscle coordination. This is not a description of someone with neuromuscular deficits; these patients (LEMS) usually complain of fatigue and weakness. (**E**). Anti-AQP4 antibodies target a water channel found in the CNS; these autoantibodies are implicated in neuromyelitis optica (NMO). This patient is presenting with peripheral motor and sensory complaints.

3. Correct: Inhibit leukocyte transmigration into the central nervous system (CNS) (E)

(**E**) Integrins are cellular adhesion molecules on leukocytes; they bind to cellular adhesion molecules on the surface of endothelial cells. This allows leukocytes to transmigrate from the circulation into tissue. To transmigrate into the CNS, WBCs must cross a very tight blood–brain barrier. This involves interaction of VLA4 ($\alpha 4\beta 1$) on T cells with VCAM on the endothelial cell. Natalizumab is a monoclonal antibody that inhibits this binding by targeting the $\alpha 4$ integrin. (**A–D**) Since integrins are involved in leukocyte adhesion, circulation, and extravasation from blood to tissues, they are not involved in the activation of microglia (resident macrophages in the brain) or astrocytes, the protection of oligodendrocytes from injury or death, or the stimulation of oligodendrocytes to remyelinate the axon.

4. Correct: Support B-cell proliferation and differentiation (C)

(**C**) Germinal centers that are normally found in the cortex of lymph nodes are structures that support B cell activation, proliferation, and differentiation. The lack of germinal centers is usually suggestive of a B cell deficiency. In many patients with myasthenia gravis (MG) (~60–80%), germinal centers are found in the thymus; i.e., the pathology shows thymic follicular hyperplasia. Some patients with MG (~10–15%) have a thymoma. The remaining patients have a histologically normal thymus for their age. Thymectomy is usually recommended for those patients with follicular hyperplasia or thymoma. In patients with myasthenia, the presence of germinal centers in the thymus contributes to the disease by supporting the activation of autoreactive B cells

that produce autoantibodies against neuromuscular junction nicotinic AChRs (nAChR). (**A**) Stem cells are primarily found in the bone marrow and in fetal cord blood. Germinal centers are found in secondary lymphoid organs such as the lymph nodes, spleen, and mucosa-associated lymphoid tissue (MALT). They are sites of B cell activation, proliferation, and differentiation. (**B**) Prenatally, B cells develop in the liver and spleen; postnatally, they develop in the bone marrow. T cells develop in the thymus. (**D**) T cell proliferation and differentiation usually occur in the paracortical areas of the lymph node and in the perifollicular zone of the spleen. (**E**) Negative selection is a process that eliminates autoreactive T cells. This occurs in the thymic medulla as T cells develop.

5. Correct: Voltage-gated calcium channel (VGCC) (D)

(**D**) This is a case of Lambert–Eaton myasthenic syndrome (LEMS). There are two immune-mediated diseases that affect neuromuscular transmission. Myasthenia gravis (MG) is more common and affects the postsynaptic membrane of the neuromuscular junction. Patients with MG have autoantibodies to various skeletal muscle molecules; the most prevalent are anti-AChR antibodies. However, a minority of patients have anti-MuSK and anti-LRP4 antibodies. Patients with MG often present with ocular and bulbar symptoms first, followed by more generalized symptoms. LEMS affects the presynaptic motor nerve terminal. Antibodies to VGCCs will result in decreased vesicular ACh release, thereby inhibiting neuromuscular transmission. LEMS is also associated with small-cell carcinoma in the lung. Neuromuscular deficits in patients with LEMS are generalized. Unlike MG patients, LEMS patients do not present with ocular symptoms first. Another important distinction is that patients with MG will become more fatigued throughout the day, whereas patients with LEMS will get better with activity. (**A**) Patients with LEMS have decreased presynaptic ACh release. This is not due to the presence of antibodies to ACh itself; rather, it is due to antibodies that target the α subunit of voltage-gated Ca^{2+} channels (VGCCs). Ca^{2+} flow affects depolarization; therefore, there is reduction of vesicular ACh release, often to 10% or less of normal levels. Reduced ACh release leads to defects in neuromuscular transmission. (**B**) There are deficits in neuromuscular transmission in LEMS that are due to antibody-mediated damage to the presynaptic membrane of the neuromuscular junction. AChR is found on the postsynaptic membrane of the neuromuscular junction on the surface of skeletal muscle. (**C**) MuSK is a muscle-specific kinase found on the skeletal muscle membrane; it is the target of the immune response in a fraction of patients with MG. (**E**) Agrin is a component of skeletal muscle and plays an important role in the development of the neuromuscular junction; it is responsible for aggregation of postsynaptic ACh receptors during synaptogenesis.

6. Correct: Anti-acetylcholine receptor antibodies (C)

(**C**) This is a case of myasthenia gravis (MG). Patients with MG have antibodies against acetylcholine receptors (AChRs) on skeletal muscle. Anti-AChR antibodies interfere with neuromuscular transmission. They cause immune-mediated damage to the AChR by: (1) blocking binding of the ligand ACh to the receptor, (2) activating the classical complement pathway, and (3) increasing receptor turnover and internalization. This results in fewer functioning AChR on the postsynaptic muscle membrane. Sustained muscle activity while playing the piano would lead to fatigue. Patients with MG will usually feel fine in the morning, but feel increasingly weak and fatigued as the day progresses. (**A**) Rheumatoid factor is an antibody (usually IgM) directed against the Fc portion of IgG. It is usually found in patients with rheumatoid arthritis (RA), but can also be found in other autoimmune diseases. Sometimes, patients with MG may have rheumatoid factor in the circulation, but it is not diagnostic for MG. (**B**) Antinuclear antibodies (ANA) are found in several rheumatologic diseases, although they are not diagnostic for MG. (**D**) Anti-myelin oligodendrocyte glycoprotein antibodies are found in patients with multiple sclerosis (MS). (**E**) Anti-neuronal antibodies are found in patients with MS and in patients with neurodegenerative disease.

7. Correct: IgM reacting with the H chain of IgG (B)

(**B**) Rheumatoid factor is usually an IgM antibody directed against the Fc portion of an IgG antibody. It is frequently found in patients with rheumatoid arthritis (RA), but it is not diagnostic. Deposition of immune complexes in the joint will contribute to the inflammatory process that leads to joint destruction. (**A**) Rheumatoid factor is an IgM, which is directed against the Fc portion of IgG; therefore, it binds to the heavy H chain, not the light L chain. (**C**) Rheumatoid factor does not bind to collagen; it is an antibody against the Fc portion of IgG. (**D**) IgG is the target antigen for rheumatoid factor. (**E**) IgG is the target antigen for rheumatoid factor.

8. Correct: TNF-α (D)

(**D**) Adalimumab (Humira) is a fully human monoclonal antibody against TNF-α. It is used to treat chronic inflammatory diseases such as rheumatoid arthritis (RA) and Crohn's disease, where TH1 cells, TH17 cells, and macrophages contribute to disease pathophysiology. Because TNF-α plays an important role in macrophage biology, patients who receive TNF-α antagonist drugs are susceptible to many infections, particularly intracellular pathogens such as tuberculosis. (**A**) IFN-γ is a cytokine that is produced and secreted by TH1 effector cells. It is a potent activator of cells of the myeloid lineage. It also plays a role in isotype switching so that B cells may switch from IgM production to IgG production. (**B**) IL-4 is a cytokine that plays a role in the differentiation of a naïve T cell into a TH2 effector cell; it is also produced and secreted by TH2 cells. IL-4 plays a role in isotype switching so that B cells produce IgE. In atopic individuals (those predisposed to allergy), allergen crosslinking of IgE on the surface of mast cells leads to degranulation of mast cells. In turn, the mast cells themselves produce and secrete IL-4 and IL-13, which perpetuate the immune response in atopic individuals. (**C**) IL-17 is a proinflammatory cytokine, which is secreted by TH17 cells. It is involved in epithelial barrier protection and activation of neutrophils. It has also been implicated in several chronic inflammatory diseases. (**E**) B cell activating factor (BAFF) is a cytokine that is essential for survival and maturation of B cells in secondary lymphoid organs. At every stage of differentiation, B cells are dependent on BAFF (from naïve B cell to antibody-secreting plasma cell). Immunobiologicals that utilize antibodies against human BAFF are utilized in the treatment of systemic lupus erythematosus (SLE).

9. Correct: Anti-dsDNA antibodies (C)

(**C**) This is a fairly classic description of systemic lupus erythematosus (SLE). Patients with lupus have autoantibodies to many nuclear antigens. Lack of clearance of these antigen–antibody complexes results in immune complex deposition in the basement membrane in various tissues. SLE is a systemic disease with the potential to affect any organ system. The skin, joints, and kidneys are particularly vulnerable. Immune complexes activate the classical complement pathway; neutrophil infiltration and local mast cell activation result in damage to the basement membrane. Patients will generally experience joint pain and a photosensitive rash. In more advanced disease, the kidney glomeruli are damaged. Immune complex–mediated glomerulonephritis will affect glomerular filtration capacity; plasma proteins and/or RBCs will leak into the urine. Therefore, proteinuria and hematuria are common in patients with more advanced disease. Although SLE patients have antibodies to many nuclear components, anti-dsDNA and anti-Sm antibodies are specific and diagnostic for patients with lupus. (**A**) Although ANA are found in lupus patients, they are not diagnostic alone. ANA are also found in several other autoimmune diseases, including rheumatoid arthritis (RA) and Sjögren's syndrome. (**B**) Anti-Ro and anti-La antibodies are found in lupus patients and in Sjögren's syndrome patients. They are not diagnostic for lupus. Anti-dsDNA and anti-Sm antibodies are specific and diagnostic for SLE. (**D**) Immune complexes in patients with lupus consist of IgG antibodies that are bound to various nuclear antigens. In advanced disease, immune complex–mediated glomerulonephritis will adversely affect glomerular filtration. Leakage of plasma proteins in the urine results in proteinuria. Immunoglobulins in plasma will leak into the urine; however, the isotypes should reflect the isotype composition in the circulation (mostly IgG). IgA in the urine may be indicative of IgA nephropathy or an IgA multiple myeloma. (**E**) Rheumatoid factor is found in patients with RA and may be found in several other autoimmune diseases. It is an antibody (usually IgM) directed against the Fc portion of IgG.

10. Correct: Anti-collagen type IV antibodies (D)

(**D**) This is a case of Goodpasture's syndrome. The clues include: (1) a patient with both pulmonary and renal issues and (2) a smooth immunofluorescent staining pattern in the glomeruli, suggesting that the antibody is binding to antigen throughout the glomerular basement membrane (GBM). Patients with Goodpasture's syndrome have IgG antibodies against type IV collagen, which is found in the basement membrane in alveoli and glomeruli. These antibodies are generally referred to as anti-GBM. Because of damage to the basement membrane in these organs, patients will present with both pulmonary and renal disease. The coughing up of blood is a common finding due to alveolar hemorrhage. Urinalysis will show proteinuria and hematuria. Immunofluorescent staining shows a smooth staining pattern because the type IV collagen is found homogeneously throughout the GBM. In contrast, the staining pattern in lupus patients is "lumpy bumpy" because it depends on where the immune complexes get deposited in the glomeruli. Therefore, the staining pattern provides a clue to distinguish between these diseases. In Goodpasture's syndrome, there is a strong association with HLA-DR2. Treatment of patients with Goodpasture's syndrome includes plasmapheresis to remove the autoantibodies from the circulation and general immunosuppression. (**A–C, E**) This is a case of Goodpasture's syndrome. The clues include (1) a patient with both pulmonary and renal issues and (2) a smooth immunofluorescent staining pattern, suggesting that the antibody is binding to antigen throughout the GBM. Therefore, antinuclear antibodies (ANA), anti-histone antibodies, anti-dsDNA antibodies, and Bence Jones proteins are not diagnostic for Goodpasture's syndrome. Bence Jones proteins are light chains of antibody molecules; they are produced in excess and are found in the serum and urine of multiple myeloma patients.

11. Correct: Anti-aquaporin 4 antibodies (A)

(**A**) This is a case of neuromyelitis optica (NMO). Demyelination in NMO primarily affects the optic nerves and the spinal cord. By contrast, in multiple sclerosis (MS) there are demyelinating lesions in the brain, spinal cord, and optic nerves. Much of the damage in NMO is antibody-mediated, whereas much of the damage in MS is cell-mediated. Although the two diseases may be difficult to distinguish clinically, the question provides a clue that the disease is antibody-mediated. In NMO, patients have autoantibodies to aquaporin-4 (anti-AQP4). Aquaporins are transmembrane water channels that allow rapid water flux across cell membranes. AQP4 is the primary aquaporin in the CNS; it is found at the astrocyte end-foot processes that are found at the blood–brain barrier. In NMO, astrocytes are the primary target of the autoimmune response. However, the antibody-mediated inflammatory response also leads to demyelination. Oligodendrocytes and myelin appear to be secondary targets (due to collateral damage); the demyelination of NMO primarily affects the optic nerves and spinal cord. (**B–D**) Anti-MBP, anti-PLP, and anti-MOG antibodies are found in MS. This is a case of NMO. Although symptoms may be somewhat similar, demyelination in NMO is secondary to antibody-mediated inflammation. By contrast, CNS myelin is the target of the autoimmune response in MS and demyelination in MS is largely due to cell-mediated inflammation; lesions are found in the optic nerves, brain, and spinal cord. In NMO, lesions are in the optic nerves and spinal cord, but not usually found in the brain proper. (**E**) Anti-LRP4 antibodies are found in a fraction of myasthenia gravis (MG) patients.

12. Correct: TH1-mediated response with IFN-γ and GM-CSF production (B)

(**B**) Multiple sclerosis (MS) is an inflammatory demyelinating disease of the CNS. Lesions/plaques are usually found in CNS white matter in the brain and spinal cord. The optic nerve is part of the CNS and is usually one of the first areas affected. Gadolinium is used as a contrast agent in MRI and will "enhance" areas of active lesions where the blood–brain barrier is leaky from inflammatory disruption. The immune response in MS targets various myelin components, including myelin basic protein, proteolipid protein, and myelin oligodendrocyte glycoprotein. This immune response is highly proinflammatory and is due to a TH1-mediated inflammatory response with activation of microglia (CNS macrophages) and astrocytes. IFN-γ and GM-CSF are two cytokines that have been shown to activate these cells. Both macrophages and astrocytes contribute to injury and death of oligodendrocytes (myelin-forming cells in the CNS). This damage is mediated by secretion of TNF-α, reactive oxygen species, and nitric oxide, and matrix metalloproteinases (MMPs). Hormonal changes during pregnancy lead to immune deviation, shifting the immune response from TH1 to TH2. Disease remission due to pregnancy is frequent in MS patients. (**A**) Immune damage in the CNS in patients with MS is initiated and mediated by TH1 cells. However, these cells primarily secrete IFN-γ, not IL-4 and IL-5. (**C**) TH2 cells secrete many cytokines, including IL-4, IL-5, and IL-13; macrophages are a primary source for TNF-α. (**D**) The immune response in MS is mediated by TH1 cells, which secrete IFN-γ and GM-CSF. (**E**) BDNF is neuroprotective. Immune deviation therapies have been used in MS; they shift the immune response from a TH1 response to a TH2 response. Under these circumstances, TH2 cells have been shown to make BDNF.

13. Correct: CD8+ T cells (C)

(C) Myelin-specific CD8+ T cells are cytotoxic to oligodendrocytes, the myelin-forming cells of the CNS. CD8+ T cells recognize myelin antigens in the context of MHC class I, which is expressed by all nucleated cells in the human body, including oligodendrocytes. Multiple mechanisms lead to injury and death of oligodendrocytes. CD4+ TH1 cells produce proinflammatory cytokines such as IFN-γ and GM-CSF, which activate macrophages and astrocytes. In turn, both of these cell types contribute to neuroinflammation by secreting proinflammatory cytokines (IL-1, IL-6, TNF-α), reactive oxygen species, reactive nitrogen species, and matrix metalloproteinases (MMPs). Anti-myelin antibodies and anti-neuronal antibodies are also found in MS patients and these contribute to CNS damage by activating complement through the classical pathway. (A) Antibody plus complement can damage oligodendrocytes, but this is not dependent on the expression of MHC class I molecules. (B) CD4+ T cells recognize antigen in the context of MHC class II. (D) Activated astrocytes can damage oligodendrocytes by secreting TNF-α, reactive oxygen species, and nitric oxide. The expression of MHC class I by the oligodendrocyte is irrelevant to its susceptibility to these compounds. (E) Activated microglia can damage oligodendrocytes by secreting TNF-α, reactive oxygen species, nitric oxide, and MMPs. The expression of MHC class I by the oligodendrocyte is irrelevant to its susceptibility to these compounds.

14. Correct: Myasthenia gravis (MG) (E)

(E) Myasthenia gravis (MG) is an autoimmune disease in which the immune system targets the nicotinic acetylcholine receptor (nAChR) at the end plate of the neuromuscular junction. Damage to the nAChR leads to deficits in neuromuscular transmission. Patients experience muscle fatigability and weakness that peaks at the end of the day. Many patients will initially present with blurred vision and ptosis (drooping eyelids) prior to more generalized symptoms. Ocular symptoms and difficulty with chewing and swallowing food are some of the earliest symptoms of the disease. Symptoms tend to progress and worsen over time, affecting larger skeletal muscles and even muscles of respiration. Classically, MG affects young women (<40 years old) and old men (>60 years old). (A) Dermatomyositis is an inflammatory disease affecting skeletal muscle and skin. Patients will present with several distinctive rashes prior to developing weakness in proximal skeletal muscles. (B) Inclusion body myopathy is a hereditary autosomal genetic disorder, which causes progressive muscle weakness and wasting. It is not autoimmune-mediated. (C) Polymyositis is an inflammatory disease that affects proximal skeletal muscles. Histopathology shows inflammatory cells in the endomysium, with CD8+ T cells that surround and invade muscle fibers. This is evidence that CD8+ T cell-mediated cytotoxicity

plays a role in this disease. (D) Lambert–Eaton myasthenic syndrome (LEMS) is an autoimmune disease of the neuromuscular junction. The presynaptic membrane is the target of the autoimmune response, not the postsynaptic motor end plate. Patients with LEMS have antibodies directed against presynaptic voltage-gated calcium (Ca^{2+}) channels. Ca^{2+} flow affects the release of ACh from the motor nerve terminal.

15. Correct: Hydroxychloroquine (A)

(A) This is a fairly classic description of systemic lupus erythematosus (SLE). Although antinuclear antibodies (ANA) are found in lupus patients, they are neither diagnostic alone nor specific. ANA antibodies are also found in several other autoimmune diseases, including rheumatoid arthritis (RA) and Sjögren's syndrome. Anti-dsDNA and anti-Smith antibodies are specific and diagnostic for patients with lupus. SLE is due to a type III hypersensitivity. Immune complex deposition in the basement membrane in various tissues results in activation of complement with subsequent neutrophil recruitment, infiltration, and inflammation. Damage to the basement membrane will affect organ function. The most commonly affected tissues are the skin, joints, and glomeruli. For unknown reasons, anti-malarial drugs, such as hydroxychloroquine, are effective in controlling lupus flare-ups. (B) Azathioprine is an immunosuppressive drug that can be helpful in controlling advanced cases of lupus. (C) Anti-CD3 antibodies are used for depletion of T cells. They are not used to treat lupus, which is a systemic B cell–mediated autoimmune disease. (D) Abatacept is a fusion protein, which is made up of the extracellular portion of CTLA-4 and the Fc portion of IgG. It interferes with T cell co-stimulation and is not used to treat lupus. (E) Infliximab is an anti-TNF-α antibody and is not approved to treat lupus.

16. Correct: B cell activating factor (BAFF) (D)

(D) Patients with systemic lupus erythematosus (SLE) develop a classic "butterfly" rash across the face upon exposure to the sun. Lupus is a B cell–mediated systemic autoimmune disease. Overexpression of a cytokine called B cell activating factor (BAFF) has been shown to contribute to the survival and growth of autoreactive B cells. Studies have shown that SLE patients have high levels of BAFF in the circulation, which are elevated during periods of active disease (flare-ups). Belimumab is an anti-BAFF monoclonal antibody. Clinical trials of belimumab show improvement of symptoms in patients with SLE. (A) Natalizumab is a monoclonal antibody against an α4 integrin. It interferes with transmigration of leukocytes across the blood–brain barrier and is used to treat patients with multiple sclerosis (MS). (B) Abatacept is a fusion protein of the extracellular portion of CTLA-4 and the Fc portion of IgG. It interferes with the co-stimulation of T cells by interacting with CD80/CD86 since CTLA-4 has a higher affinity for cD80/86 than CD28. Abatacept is approved for the treatment of patients with rheumatoid arthritis (RA). (**C**) Anakinra is an IL-1R antagonist; it is used to treat RA. (**E**) Infliximab is a monoclonal antibody against TNF-α. It is used to treat patients with RA and patients with inflammatory bowel disease.

17. Correct: Sjögren's syndrome (C)

(**C**) This is a case of Sjögren's syndrome. In this disease, there is immune infiltration of the exocrine glands, resulting in tissue destruction and loss of function. Lacrimal and salivary glands are affected. Typically, the condition affects middle-aged women. The ratio of females to males is approximately 9:1 for Sjögren's syndrome patients. The female preponderance and disease onset around menopause support a strong role for hormones in the pathogenesis of this disease. Sjögren's syndrome may be a primary condition but can also be found in association with other autoimmune diseases (rheumatoid arthritis [RA], lupus, and systemic scleroderma). B cell hyperactivity is characteristic of Sjögren's syndrome. Patients have antibodies against ribonucleoprotein complexes (Ro/SSA and La/SSB); in advanced disease, they also exhibit hypergammaglobulinemia, and a small percentage of patients (5–10%) will develop non-Hodgkin's lymphoma. (**A**) The patient is not presenting with signs and symptoms of RA. These would include joint pain and swelling. Although the results indicate that the patient is rheumatoid factor positive, this is not specific for patients with RA. Rheumatoid factor can be found in other patients with rheumatological diseases and in healthy individuals as well. (**B**) The patient is not presenting with signs and symptoms of lupus. Furthermore, the anti-dsDNA test is negative. (**D**) Scleroderma is a chronic autoimmune disease whose hallmark is fibrosis of the skin and internal organs. In some patients, fibrosis is localized to the skin; they are classified as patients with scleroderma. In other patients, fibrosis involves the skin and various internal organs; they are classified as patients with systemic sclerosis. Systemic sclerosis can be potentially lethal. Its cause is still unknown but involves multiple factors, including genetic and environmental components. Patients with systemic sclerosis have antinuclear antibodies (ANA), antibodies to the enzyme DNA topoisomerase 1 (also called anti-Scl-70) and anti-centromere antibodies. (**E**). Mixed connective tissue disease is sometimes referred to as an overlap disease because its signs and symptoms overlap with several other diseases, including lupus, scleroderma, and polymyositis. Its etiology is unknown. Patients will usually present with swollen hands and joints and be positive for the anti-U1 ribonucleoprotein antibody.

18. Correct: CXCL13 (E)

(**E**) CXCL13, also known as B cell chemoattractant, is a chemokine that attracts B cells into the follicles of secondary lymphoid organs. It binds to the CXCR5 receptor on the surface of B cells. Normally, when B cells develop in the bone marrow, they then migrate to populate secondary lymphoid organs (lymph nodes, spleen, MALT, etc.). CXCL13 is one of several chemokines that are expressed by stromal cells; they "draw" B cells into the follicles by chemotaxis, where they undergo further maturation. In chronic inflammatory diseases, such as rheumatoid arthritis (RA), thyroiditis, and multiple sclerosis (MS), ectopic lymphoid follicles are found at sites of inflammation. CXCL13 is expressed in these follicles and serves to chemoattract B cells to inflamed tissues. (**A**) CCL2, also known as MCP-1, is a chemokine whose primary function is to recruit T cells, monocytes, and dendritic cells to sites of inflammation. Its receptor is CCR2, which is expressed on the cell surface of these cell types. (**B**) CCL5, also known as RANTES, binds to its receptor, CCR5. CCL5 chemoattracts T cells, monocytes, and dendritic cells to sites of inflammation. (**C**) CXCL8, also known as IL-8, recruits neutrophils, monocytes, and dendritic cells to sites of inflammation or infection. Two receptors have been identified that bind to IL-8; they are CXCR1 and CXCR2. (**D**) CXCL9 is a chemoattractant for effector TH1 cells; it binds to the receptor CXCR3.

19. Correct: IL-1R (A)

(**A**) The hypothalamus regulates body temperature. IL-1 is a proinflammatory acute phase cytokine with several functions. One of its important functions is to induce fever. Hypothalamic cells express receptors for IL-1 and respond by increasing body temperature. (**B**) IL-2R is expressed by T cells and other cell types. The interaction of IL-2 with its receptor induces the proliferation of T cells following activation. (**C**) IL-4R is expressed by various cell types, including T cells and B cells. The ligand IL-4 induces the differentiation of TH2 effector cells. IL-4 also functions as a B cell growth factor and promotes isotype switching to IgE production. (**D**) IL-6 is a pleiotropic cytokine with many functions. Receptors for IL-6 are expressed by various cells in the immune system (T cells, B cells, etc.) as well as cells that are not part of the immune system (endothelial cells, epithelial cells, and fibroblasts, for example). (**E**) IL-7 is a growth factor for both B cells and T cells, and it plays an important role in their development. It is secreted by stromal cells in the bone marrow and in the thymus. Other cell types, including dendritic cells and epithelial cells, also secrete IL-7.

20. Correct: HLA-DR3/DR4 (D)

(**D**) Type I diabetes affects approximately 30 million people worldwide. Patients mount an autoimmune response against pancreatic insulin-producing β-islet cells. A lack of insulin leads to hyperglycemia. In children, disease onset is usually between 3 and 10 years of age. Insulin replacement therapy is initiated within the first few years following diagnosis. As with all autoimmune diseases, pathogenesis of the disease is multifactorial and involves both genetic and environmental influences. HLA-DR3/DR4 haplotype shows a strong association with type I diabetes. (**A**) HLA-B8 does not confer an increased genetic risk for type I diabetes, but increases the risk for the development of Hashimoto's thyroiditis. (**B**) HLA-B27 does not confer an increased genetic risk for type I diabetes, but increases the risk for the development of ankylosing spondylitis. (**C**) HLA-DR2 does not confer an increased genetic risk for type I diabetes, but increases the risk for the development of systemic lupus erythematosus (SLE). (**E**) HLA-DR15 does not confer an increased genetic risk for type I diabetes, but increases the risk for the development of Goodpasture's syndrome.

21. Correct: HLA-DR4 (D)

(**D**) This patient is exhibiting classic signs and symptoms of early rheumatoid arthritis (RA). Inflammation will initially affect the smaller joints in the hand. In more established/advanced disease, larger joints may also be affected. Patients are usually very stiff in the mornings and it may take them several hours to feel functional. HLA-DR4 haplotype shows a strong association with RA; it is found in approximately 70% of RA patients. (**A**) HLA-B8 does not show a strong association with RA, but increases the risk for the development of Hashimoto's thyroiditis. (**B**) HLA-B27 does not show a strong association with RA, but increases the risk for the development of ankylosing spondylitis. (**C**) HLA-DR2 does not show a strong association with RA, but increases the risk for the development of systemic lupus erythematosus (SLE). (**E**) HLA-DR15 does not show a strong association with RA, but increases the risk for the development of Goodpasture's syndrome.

22. Correct: TNF-α (B)

(**B**) Rheumatoid arthritis (RA) is a highly proinflammatory disease. An influx of inflammatory cells into the synovial membrane ultimately leads to the destruction of cartilage and to bone erosion. TNF-α is a proinflammatory cytokine. Clinical trials of TNF-α antagonist drugs have demonstrated that targeting either TNF-α or its receptors is beneficial to patients with RA. Because TNF-α plays an important role in macrophage biology, patients who receive TNF-α antagonist drugs have a higher risk of infection; they are particularly susceptible to fungal infections and to tuberculosis. (**A**) IFN-β is a type I IFN. It does not play a significant role in the immunopathogenesis of RA. Recombinant IFN-β can be used to treat multiple sclerosis (MS). (**C**) TGF-β is an immunoregulatory cytokine. It is anti-inflammatory and, therefore, targeting this molecule would likely exacerbate this individual's symptoms. (**D**) IL-3 is a cytokine that functions as a colony-stimulating factor and plays a role in hematopoiesis. (**E**) IL-10 is an immunoregulatory cytokine. It is anti-inflammatory and, therefore, targeting this molecule would likely exacerbate this individual's symptoms.

23. Correct: Metalloproteinases (D)

(**D**) Rheumatoid arthritis (RA) is a complex autoimmune disease. Multiple mechanisms contribute to the immunopathology that leads to joint destruction. RA is a very debilitating disease; patients experience chronic pain, loss of function, and disability. Immune complexes that are made up of IgG and rheumatoid factor are deposited in the joint and initiate an inflammatory response. Furthermore, proinflammatory T cells (TH1 and TH17) secrete cytokines that activate macrophages and neutrophils. Proinflammatory cytokines affect several cell types: (1) macrophages and neutrophils release matrix metalloproteinases (MMPs). (2) synovial fibroblasts are also activated to release MMPs, and (3) chondrocytes switch from synthesizing matrix-building molecules to synthesizing MMPs that degrade the extracellular matrix. Proinflammatory cytokines also induce the expression of RANK ligand, which is a potent activator of osteoclasts. Osteoclasts are cells of the myeloid lineage. They are considered the tissue macrophages of bone and play an important role in the normal physiology of bone. Activated mature osteoclasts resorb bone. Destruction of cartilage and resorption/erosion of bone result in joint destruction. (**A**) IL-6 is a proinflammatory cytokine. It contributes to the immunopathogenesis of RA and blockade of IL-6 ameliorates RA. IL-6 itself does not destroy cartilage or bone directly. (**B**) RANK ligand plays an important role in the activation and differentiation of osteoclasts. It is not directly involved in the destruction of cartilage or bone. (**C**) Osteoblasts are bone-forming cells. The balance of osteoblasts and osteoclasts determines bone remodeling. (**E**) Prostaglandins are mediators of inflammation but do not directly contribute to joint destruction in patients with RA.

24. Correct: Ankylosing spondylitis (A)

(**A**) Ankylosing spondylitis is a disease that usually manifests in the second decade of life and affects males more than females. Male-to-female ratio is approximately 2:1. It has a strong association with HLA-B27 haplotype as studies have shown that approximately 90% of patients have HLA-B27. Initially, patients present with sacroiliitis, but the whole spine can be affected as the disease progresses. The target of the immune response in ankylosing spondylitis remains unknown. However, the affected joints show evidence of inflammatory infiltration, which is gradually replaced by cartilage and leads to bony fusions in the majority of patients. This affects the flexibility of the spine. Ankylosing spondylitis patients are negative for rheumatoid factor. The diagnosis is usually made based on clinical findings and radiological criteria. In more advanced disease, the spine has a "bamboo" appearance on X-ray. Biological agents that target TNF-α (a proinflammatory cytokine) have proven to be effective in ankylosing spondylitis. (**B**) Reactive arthritis is preceded by infection and will usually affect joints in the lower limbs. Approximately 50% of patients with reactive arthritis are HLA-B27 positive. Synovial fluid of patients with reactive arthritis will contain inflammatory cells and will appear cloudy. (**C**) Rheumatoid arthritis (RA) is associated with HLA-DR4. Patients will present with swelling, pain, and stiffness in the hands. (**D**) Some patients with psoriasis will also be affected by arthritis. Usually, the skin inflammation will manifest first followed by joint inflammation. The signs and symptoms of psoriatic arthritis resemble those of RA. (**E**) Osteoarthritis is a degenerative disease that is due to wear and tear of the joints. It is not an inflammatory disease and is classically seen in older patients or patients with history of joint injury.

25. Correct: Anti-tRNA synthetase (C)

(**C**) This patient is presenting with classic symptoms of dermatomyositis. These include symmetrical weakness of proximal muscles and skin manifestations. The classic rash around the eyelids is often described as a heliotrope rash because its shade is similar to the heliotrope plant. There is often a rash in the chest area, described as a "shawl" rash. Dermatomyositis is an inflammatory myopathy due to autoimmune damage to skeletal muscle. The immunopathology is due to a type III hypersensitivity. In patients with dermatomyositis, autoantibodies are directed against amino histidyl tRNA synthetases, which are involved in protein translation. The most common anti-tRNA synthetase is called anti-Jo-1. Antigen–antibody immune complexes are deposited and trapped in the basement membrane of vessels, thereby initiating a vasculitis, which is primarily manifested in skeletal muscle and skin. (**A**) Antinuclear antibodies (ANA) are elevated in the majority of patients with dermatomyositis. They are nonspecific and not diagnostic for the disease. (**B**) Anti-dsDNA antibodies are diagnostic for patients with systemic lupus erythematosus (SLE). (**D**) Anti-AChR antibodies are found in patients with myasthenia gravis (MG). Muscle fatigability and weakness are due to defects in postsynaptic neuromuscular transmission and not due to muscle inflammation. (**E**) Anti-VGCC antibodies are found in patients with Lambert–Eaton myasthenic syndrome (LEMS). Muscle weakness is due to defects in presynaptic neuromuscular transmission and not due to muscle inflammation.

26. Correct: Anti-thyroglobulin (anti-TG) antibodies (E)

(**E**) The patient is exhibiting signs of hypothyroidism due to thyroiditis. When inflammatory damage leads

to malfunction of the thyroid gland, constant pituitary stimulation of the gland to release hormones will lead to an enlarged thyroid (goiter). Women are more likely to be affected by autoimmune thyroiditis. In Hashimoto's thyroiditis, there is organ infiltration by macrophages and lymphocytes; in addition, the presence of germinal centers within the thyroid indicates that B cell activation and proliferation are playing a role in this disease. Antibodies include antithyroglobulin (anti-TG) antibodies and anti-thyroid peroxidase (anti-TPO) antibodies; they are positive in approximately 90% of patients with hypothyroidism. Both antibody-mediated and cell-mediated mechanisms contribute to the immunopathogenesis of thyroiditis. Thyroid follicles become destroyed and the inflammatory process eventually leads to fibrosis. Treatment of hypothyroidism comprises replacement of T4 (thyroxine), a key hormone in the regulation of metabolism. (**A**) T3 levels are decreased in hypothyroidism. (**B**) T4 levels are decreased in hypothyroidism. (**C**) Thyroid-stimulating hormone (TSH) levels are usually normal or elevated in hypothyroidism. (**D**) Anti-TSH receptor agonist antibodies (thyroid-stimulating immunoglobulin) are found in Graves' disease, a condition of hyperthyroidism. Some patients with Hashimoto's thyroiditis have antibodies that block or antagonize the TSH receptor.

27. Correct: Hashimoto's thyroiditis (A)

(**A**) Many children who were exposed to radioactive iodine from Chernobyl developed thyroid cancers. However, those who did not develop thyroid cancers have an increased prevalence of autoantibodies to thyroid antigens and an increased prevalence of autoimmune thyroiditis later in life. (**B**) Graves' disease is the most common cause of hyperthyroidism. Autoantibodies against the TSH receptor act as agonists and overstimulate the thyroid. Oral administration of radioactive iodine is sometimes used to treat hyperthyroidism. (**C**) Individuals who are exposed to high levels of radioactive iodine are likely to develop thyroid cancer. This is not an autoimmune condition. (**D**) Hyperparathyroidism is due to overactivity of one or more of the four parathyroid glands. It is not an autoimmune disease. (**E**) Individuals who are exposed to high levels of radioactive iodine may develop leukemias and lymphomas. These are not autoimmune conditions.

28. Correct: Anti-TSH receptor agonist antibodies (C)

(**C**) Graves' disease is an organ-specific autoimmune disease in which anti-TSH receptor antibodies mimic the ligand TSH and act as agonists to the TSH receptor. The consequence is overactivity of the thyroid gland (hyperthyroidism). The signs and symptoms of hyperthyroidism include an increased heart rate, increased metabolism that leads to unexplained

43

weight loss, and frequent irritability. In advanced disease, there are complications in which patients will also present with eye symptoms, such as periorbital edema. Graves' disease is the most common cause of hyperthyroidism. Anti-TG antibodies and anti-TPO antibodies are also found in patients with Graves' disease. However, the hallmark of this disease is the presence of anti-TSH-R stimulating antibodies; these are found in over 95% of patients. Patients with hyperthyroidism are treated with anti-thyroid drugs, radioactive iodine, or thyroidectomy. (**A**) TSH is produced by the pituitary. Graves' disease is not due to high levels of TSH. It is an autoimmune condition due to the presence of anti-TSH-R agonist antibodies. (**B**) Anti-TG antibodies are found in patients with Hashimoto's thyroiditis and in patients with Graves' disease. They are not diagnostic for Graves' disease. (**D**) Anti-TSH-R antibodies act as agonists, not as antagonists, of the TSH receptor in Graves' disease. As agonists, they stimulate the production of the thyroid hormones T3 and T4, whose levels are increased in patients who exhibit hyperthyroidism. (**E**) Levels of T3 and T4 are increased in Graves' disease.

29. Correct: Type IV hypersensitivity (D)

(**D**) This is a case of type I diabetes, also known as juvenile-onset diabetes, which is a type IV hypersensitivity. An autoimmune response against the pancreatic β-islet cells results in the CD8+ T cell–mediated destruction of the cells and decreased and/or complete loss of insulin production. While anti-insulin and anti-glutamic acid decarboxylase antibodies are positive in T1DM, they are markers of disease rather than the true agents of cytotoxicity against the pancreatic β-islet cells. Patients will have increased glucose levels in the blood; this glucose is not being utilized for energy and will be excreted in the urine because of the loss of insulin. The presence of ketones in urine indicates that the body is utilizing fat for energy instead of glucose. (**A**) A type I hypersensitivity is an immediate-type hypersensitivity that is IgE-mediated and involves degranulation of mast cells. (**B**) A type II hypersensitivity is an antibody-mediated cytotoxic hypersensitivity in which antibodies bind to and kill target cells. (**C**) A type III hypersensitivity is due to immune complex (antigen–antibody) deposition with subsequent complement activation, white cell recruitment, and inflammation. (**E**) A type V hypersensitivity is an antibody-mediated stimulatory hypersensitivity in which antibodies bind to and stimulate target cell receptors. The classic example is Graves' disease–mediated hyperthyroidism.

30. Correct: Pernicious anemia (B)

(**B**) Autoimmune atrophic gastritis is due to the production of autoantibodies against gastric parietal cells (specifically, gastric H^+/K^+ ATPase) and to their secreted product intrinsic factor. Absorption of vitamin B12 by enterocytes (epithelial cells in the ileum) is dependent on intrinsic factor. Approximately 10 to 15% of patients with gastritis will develop pernicious anemia. The anemia will manifest when stores of vitamin B12 are almost depleted. Antibodies to intrinsic factor are found in >95% of patients with pernicious anemia. Many patients with gastritis will be asymptomatic while the autoimmune destruction of gastric parietal cells is ongoing. Clinical symptoms will manifest when vitamin B12 levels are critically low. Vitamin B12 is necessary for the development of RBCs. Fatigue and pallor are a direct result of the anemia. Pernicious anemia is more common in females and in individuals of northern European (Scandinavian) descent. (**A**) Autoimmune hemolytic anemia is due to autoantibodies that are directed against various antigens on the surface of RBCs. The immunopathology involves direct destruction of RBCs. (**C**) Anemia due to iron deficiency is quite common. Iron is a component of heme, which is part of hemoglobin. (**D**) Thalassemia is a genetic inherited blood disorder. Mutations in hemoglobin genes result in low hemoglobin production. (**E**) Sickle cell anemia is an abnormality of RBCs. The sickle cell gene is inherited in an autosomal recessive pattern and results in a mutation in hemoglobin. This causes the RBCs to become rigid and sticky.

31. Correct: Anti-intrinsic factor (D)

(**D**) This is a vitamin-deficiency anemia due to lack of absorption of vitamin B12. Intrinsic factor plays a role in the absorption of vitamin B12 in the small intestine. Patients with pernicious anemia (autoimmune atrophic gastritis) have autoantibodies against intrinsic factor and are thus unable to absorb vitamin B12 from their diet. Because vitamin B12 is necessary for the development of RBCs, patients become anemic. Classically, B12 deficiency causes a macrocytic ("megaloblastic") anemia with hypersegmented neutrophils on peripheral blood smear. The clinical signs and symptoms of anemia are pallor, fatigue, and shortness of breath. Also, in contrast to B9 (folate) deficiency, which can also cause a megaloblastic anemia, B12 deficiency when chronic can lead to neurologic symptoms (weakness, sensory changes, gait difficulty). (**A**) Anti-AChR antibodies are found in patients with myasthenia gravis (MG). These patients experience fatigue due to deficits in postsynaptic neuromuscular transmission. They do not present with pallor. (**B**) Patients with Lambert–Eaton myasthenic syndrome (LEMS) experience deficits in neuromuscular transmission due to the presence of anti-VGCC antibodies directed against presynaptic voltage-gated calcium channels (VGCCs). They do not present with pallor. (**C**) Anti-histidyl tRNA synthetase antibodies are found in patients with inflammatory myopathies (dermatomyositis and polymyositis). They experience weakness in proximal muscles. (**E**) Anti-TPO antibodies are found in patients with hypothyroidism. These patients may experience constipation, delayed reflexes, bradycardia, fatigue, and weight gain, but they do not present with signs and symptoms of anemia.

32. Correct: Type II hypersensitivity (B)

(**B**) Autoimmune hemolytic anemia is equally prevalent in men and women. It can strike at any age but becomes more common with age, suggesting defects in immune regulation. Autoimmune hemolytic anemia that is due to "warm" antibodies (usually IgG) is more common than that due to "cold" antibodies (usually IgM). The terms warm and cold are based on the optimum temperature at which the antibodies bind to the RBCs. Autoantibodies cause destruction (hemolysis) of RBCs by two main mechanisms: (1) the antibodies can activate complement, which will lead to lysis of the RBCs, and (2) autoantibody-coated RBCs are cleared from the circulation via macrophages in the reticuloendothelial system (hence, the enlarged spleen). Several RBC autoantigens have been identified. In 70% of patients with autoimmune hemolytic anemia due to "warm" antibodies, the autoantigen is the Rh protein. In some patients, autoantibodies against glycophorin A have also been identified. Patients are usually treated with steroids, folate, IVIG, and sometimes rituximab (an anti-CD20 monoclonal antibody that targets antibody-secreting plasma cells. (**A**) A type I hypersensitivity is an immediate-type hypersensitivity that is IgE-mediated and involves degranulation of mast cells. (**C**) A type III hypersensitivity is due to immune complex (antigen–antibody) deposition with subsequent complement activation, white cell recruitment, and inflammation. (**D**) A type IV hypersensitivity is not antibody-mediated, but rather is mediated through T cells. Classic examples of type IV hypersensitivity reactions include allergic contact dermatitis and tuberculin reactions. (**E**) A type V hypersensitivity is an antibody-mediated stimulatory hypersensitivity in which antibodies bind to and stimulate target cell receptors. The classic example is Graves' disease–mediated hyperthyroidism.

33. Correct: FcγR-mediated destruction by macrophages (A)

(**A**) This woman is suffering from symptoms of thrombocytopenia, which is a fairly common disorder. Glycoprotein IIb/IIIa is the target antigen on the surface of platelets. The normal lifespan of platelets is approximately 7 to 10 days. In patients with thrombocytopenia, this is reduced to several hours. Reticuloendothelial system macrophages (liver and spleen) have FcγR to bind the Fc portion of IgG-bound platelets and cause their destruction. (**B**) Antibodies against platelet glycoproteins will cause agglutination of platelets. On its own, agglutination does not lead to platelet destruction. Rather, agglutination makes platelets highly susceptible to opsonization and phagocytosis by splenic macrophages and liver Kupffer's cells, which express Fc receptors for IgG. (**C**) Platelets are responsible for activation of the coagulation cascade with subsequent fibrin deposition. (**D**) Thrombopoietin is a hormone that regulates the production of platelets. (**E**) Platelets are not nucleated and thus cannot undergo apoptosis.

34. Correct: Presence of oligoclonal bands on electrophoresis (E)

(**E**) The blood–brain barrier provides a tight barrier that protects the CNS. This barrier may become "leaky" under several pathological conditions, which may include physical trauma, infection, or inflammation. When the barrier becomes leaky, components in plasma will enter the CNS. Therefore, the number of inflammatory cells, and the levels of glucose, proteins, cytokines, and chemokines may all change. This patient most likely has multiple sclerosis (MS), in which case changes in the above CSF parameters are not specific. The presence of oligoclonal bands on electrophoresis is strong evidence of intrathecal production of immunoglobulin, which is more specific for MS. Oligoclonal bands are found in the CSF in 85 to 95% of patients with MS; they aid in the diagnosis of MS. (**A**) An increased number of inflammatory cells in the CSF is a nonspecific finding. It may be due to autoimmune disease, infection, or physical trauma causing disruption of the blood–brain barrier. (**B**) Elevated CSF glucose may be seen in hyperglycemic patients (i.e., diabetics). Decreased CSF glucose (hypoglycorrhachia) is a nonspecific finding when there is an increased organism load in the CSF (bacteria, fungi, leukocytes, or even tumor cells). (**C**) Elevated CSF protein is a nonspecific finding that may occur in CNS/meningeal infection or inflammation. (**D**) Elevated CSF cytokines and chemokines are nonspecific findings of some kind of inflammatory CNS or meningeal process.

35. Correct: Immune complex–mediated injury of small blood vessels (C)

(**C**) Dermatomyositis is an inflammatory disorder of the skin and skeletal muscle. Patients will present with a distinctive skin rash and with muscle weakness. Many times the skin manifestations will precede the onset of muscle weakness. Skin manifestations include: (1) a purplish heliotrope rash on the eyelids, (2) scaly red plaques over the knuckles, elbows, and knees (called Gottron's papules), (3) dilated capillaries at the proximal nail fold, and (4) a "shawl" rash on the back, shoulders, and chest. The onset of muscle weakness is usually slow and progressive. Patients with dermatomyositis have anti-Jo-1 (antibody against the histidyl tRNA synthetase). Much of the immunopathology in dermatomyositis is due to complement-mediated inflammation and damage. Antigen–antibody immune complexes are deposited in small blood vessels where they activate the classical complement pathway. Anaphylatoxins (C3a and C5a) trigger the degranulation of mast cells, thereby increasing vessel permeability. C3a and

C5a also chemoattract neutrophils, which contribute to the vessel injury. This is a type III hypersensitivity vasculitis, resulting in damage to capillaries, hypoperfusion of muscle, and eventual muscle fiber ischemia and atrophy. (**A**) Chronic inflammatory polyneuropathy is a disease of peripheral nerves. Patients experience tingling, numbness, pain, and progressive muscle weakness—distal more so than proximal. Additionally, there are no skin manifestations in chronic inflammatory polyneuropathy. (**B**) Antibodies that block neuromuscular transmission can be directed against antigens at the motor nerve terminal (postsynaptic, as in myasthenia gravis [MG]) or antigens at the skeletal muscle surface (presynaptic, as in Lambert–Eaton myasthenic syndrome [LEMS]). They interfere with neuromuscular transmission. They do not play a role in the pathology of dermatomyositis. (**D**) CD8+ cytotoxic T cell–mediated damage to myocytes is an immunopathologic finding in polymyositis. Although similar to dermatomyositis in terms of signs and symptoms of muscle weakness, polymyositis is a milder disease without the skin manifestations that are found in patients with dermatomyositis. (**E**) Dystrophin is a protein found in muscle fiber sarcomeres. Mutations in the dystrophin gene lead to muscular dystrophy. Duchenne muscular dystrophy and the milder Becker muscular dystrophy are genetic conditions, not autoimmune.

36.   Correct: Polymyositis (E)

(**E**) Dermatomyositis is a vasculitis that is due to immune complex deposition. Polymyositis is an inflammatory autoimmune disease of skeletal muscle. Both polymyositis and dermatomyositis are inflammatory myopathies, but patients with dermatomyositis also have signs and symptoms affecting the skin. The immunopathogenesis of the two diseases is quite different. In polymyositis, CD8+ cytotoxic T cells invade muscle fibers that express MHC class I autoantigens. Perforin contained in the granules of cytotoxic T cells is primarily responsible for muscle pathology. Inflammatory cells are primarily found in the endomysium. Polymyositis affects adults and rarely affects children, whereas dermatomyositis affects both. (**A**) Muscular dystrophy is due to mutations in the dystrophin gene; its pathogenesis is not inflammatory. (**B**) Myasthenia gravis (MG) patients exhibit muscle weakness, which is due to deficits in postsynaptic neuromuscular transmission. Skeletal muscle is not inflamed in these patients. (**C**) Lambert–Eaton myasthenic syndrome (LEMS) is due to the presence of autoantibodies against voltage-gated calcium channels (VGCCs) at the presynaptic motor nerve terminal. These antibodies interfere with neuromuscular transmission, resulting in weakness. Skeletal muscle is not inflamed in these patients. (**D**) Dermatomyositis is an inflammatory myopathy. Patients present with proximal muscle weakness and with skin manifestations.

37.   Correct: IgG anti-AChR antibodies that crossed the placenta (B)

(**B**) In myasthenia gravis (MG), the pathogenic antibodies are primarily of the IgG isotype. If these antibodies cross the placenta, they can harm the fetus. For women with MG, up to 10% of patients will have newborns with signs and symptoms of MG. The muscle weakness is transient and will last as long as the mother's anti-AChR IgG is in the infant's circulation (the half-life of IgG is approximately 23 days). Anti-AChR antibodies can belong to any of the IgG subclasses, but the majority are of the IgG1 subclass. Newborns are treated with cholinesterase inhibitors to maximize the half-life of their released ACh neurotransmitters. (**A**) There is an increased association of HLA-DR3 and HLA-B8 with MG. However, even if the mother or newborn expressed these HLA haplotypes, the newborn would not exhibit signs and symptoms of myasthenia at birth. (**C**) IgM does not cross the placenta. In humans, the IgG antibody isotype can cross the placenta. (**D**) Congenital myasthenic syndrome is due to genetic defects that affect components of the neuromuscular junction. Symptoms may be similar to MG, but the pathogenesis is not autoimmune. (**E**) X-linked myopathy or muscular dystrophy is a rare condition in which patients exhibit muscle weakness in childhood. Its pathogenesis is genetic, not autoimmune.

38.   Correct: Neuromyelitis optica (NMO) (D)

(**D**) Neuromyelitis optica (NMO) is an inflammatory disease of the CNS. Patients have autoantibodies against a water channel protein called aquaporin 4 (AQP4). Anti-AQP4 autoantibodies target water channels at the astrocytic end feet that surround the blood–brain barrier. Immune-mediated damage is due to a type II hypersensitivity. Anti-AQP4 autoantibodies activate the classical complement pathway. Although the astrocyte is the primary target of the autoimmune response, oligodendrocytes suffer bystander/collateral injury resulting in demyelination. The activation of complement and the subsequent inflammatory response are responsible for massive demyelination that affects the optic nerves and the spinal cord. NMO has a high female:male ratio of 10:1. (**A**) Encephalitis is an acute inflammatory response. Its symptoms usually involve an acute onset of fever, headache, and confusion, which is not seen in this patient. (**B**) Autoimmune polyneuropathy is a disease of peripheral nerves, not the CNS. Autoimmune polyneuropathy may affect motor nerves, sensory nerves, or both. (**C**) Multiple sclerosis (MS) and NMO have similar signs and symptoms and can be difficult to differentiate clinically. Both are inflammatory demyelinating diseases of the CNS. Lesions in MS are found in the optic nerves, brain, and spinal cord. Lesions in NMO are restricted to the optic nerves and spinal cord. Serologic testing for anti-AQP4 antibodies can help distinguish between the two diseases.

(**E**) The term clinically isolated syndrome is used to refer to a patient's first neurological episode. It usually precedes a definite diagnosis of MS.

39. Correct: Anti-gliadin antibodies (E)

(**E**) Celiac disease (gluten-sensitive enteritis) primarily affects Caucasians. Its prevalence in the United States is approximately 1:150 to 1:300 people. Patients develop a sensitivity to gluten, which is found in wheat, barley, and rye. Gliadin (α,β,γ) is a protein in gluten-containing foods. Patients with celiac disease may have several autoantibodies that contribute to disease pathology. These include antibodies to gliadin proteins as well as anti-tissue transglutaminase 2 (anti-TTG2) antibodies. The relevance of anti-TTG2 antibodies is not entirely clear. Autoantibodies can be IgG and/or IgA. The presence of IgA antibodies is more strongly associated with the disease. Both antibody-mediated and cell-mediated immune responses play a role in disease pathophysiology. There are large numbers of CD8+ intraepithelial T cell lymphocytes in the intestinal epithelium. The inflammatory response leads to destruction of enterocytes and blunting of small bowel villi. These effects on the villi that line the small intestine lead to malabsorption of nutrients. Treatment involves exclusion of gluten-containing products from the diet; a gluten-free diet will usually lead to clinical improvement. (**A**) Rotavirus is a common cause of gastroenteritis in infants and children. Symptoms include fever, vomiting, and diarrhea. There is a risk of dehydration, but the illness is usually self-limiting. (**B**) Following infection with *Campylobacter*, pathogen-specific IgG antibodies cross-react with gangliosides in peripheral nerves. The resultant acute inflammatory demyelinating peripheral neuropathy is both acute and reversible. (**C**) Goblet cells are found at mucosal membranes; their role is to secrete mucus. (**D**) Paneth cells are found in the small intestine; they secrete antimicrobial peptides such as defensins.

40. Correct: TH1 and TH17 cells (B)

(**B**) Crohn's disease is an inflammatory bowel disease, which can affect any area of the gastrointestinal tract. The most common site for lesions is the ileum; the terminal ileum is affected in approximately two-thirds of patients. There are so-called "skip lesions" where areas of transmural inflammation are interspersed with areas of intestine that are not harmed; i.e., the inflammation is not continuous. Areas affected by inflammation will become ulcerated. Stools are typically not bloody, unless the colon and rectum are affected by disease. There is not a simple test for the diagnosis of Crohn's disease. Endoscopy can locate the areas of inflammation, which can differentiate between Crohn's disease and ulcerative colitis (a disease with similar signs and symptoms; however, the inflammation is mucosal and restricted to the colon and rectum). In Crohn's disease, TH1 and TH17 proinflammatory CD4+ T cells drive the inflammatory response. IFN-γ (made by TH1 cells) and IL-17 (made by TH17 cells) are expressed at high levels in the lamina propria; there is evidence that IFN-γ expression correlates with disease severity. Patients with active disease also have elevated C-reactive protein (CRP) levels. Therapy for patients with Crohn's disease may include glucocorticoids, azathioprine, and methotrexate. Increasingly, biologics are used; the anti-TNFα monoclonal antibodies infliximab and adalimumab can induce remission in patients with Crohn's disease. (**A**) Eosinophilic infiltrates are usually a hallmark of the immune response in allergy and in parasitic infections. (**C**) TH2 cells produce IL-4. Its functions include promoting isotype switching to IgE production and promoting IgE-mediated allergic responses. TH2 cells also produce IL-5, which activates eosinophils. (**D**) TH9 cells produce IL-9, which plays a role in allergic responses, asthma, and the immune response to parasitic helminth infections. (**E**) CD8+ T cell–mediated cytotoxicity does not play a major role in the pathogenesis of Crohn's disease.

41. Correct: Pemphigus vulgaris (C)

(**C**) The HLA haplotypes HLA-DR4 and HLA-DR6 show a strong association with pemphigus vulgaris, a rare blistering disease of the skin and oral mucosa. Keratinocytes are the predominant cell type in the epidermis. Junctional proteins, called desmosomes, hold the keratinocytes together, thus forming a tight epithelial barrier. Patients with pemphigus vulgaris have autoantibodies against desmoglein 3 (Dsg 3), a desmosomal cadherin. Anti-Dsg3 autoantibodies are responsible for disease pathology and are also critical for the diagnosis of pemphigus vulgaris. Antibody titers correlate with disease extent and severity. It is not clear how the antibodies trigger acantholysis (loss of intercellular connections within the epidermis). In humans, IgG4 antibodies do not activate complement and they do not bind well to Fcγ receptors on monocytes/macrophages. However, passive transfer experiments have shown that they are responsible for disease pathogenesis. These autoantibodies may play a role in keratinocyte cell detachment through steric hindrance or interference with function. (**A**) Urticaria, also known as hives, can be acute or chronic. Acute urticaria is due to an allergic response. In the majority of cases, chronic urticaria is considered idiopathic, of unknown cause. (**B**) Psoriasis is a chronic condition characterized by red plaques of inflamed skin that are covered with silvery-white scales. There is both a genetic and immune component to the pathogenesis of psoriasis, which involves excessive growth of the epidermis. (**D**) Canker sores are mouth ulcers that form in the oral mucosa. (**E**) Oral herpes is due to infection by the herpes simplex virus. Symptoms include groups of blisters that are commonly referred to as cold sores.

Chapter 4

Immunodeficiency Disorders

Michelle Swanson-Mungerson

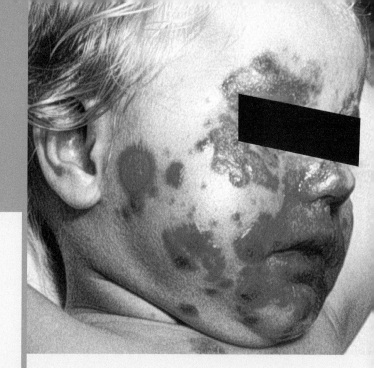

LEARNING OBJECTIVE

▶ Identify the symptoms, laboratory results, genetics, and treatments associated with immunodeficiencies.

4.1 Questions

Easy	Medium	Hard

1. A 6-month-old boy is brought to the emergency department by his parents with a chief complaint of fever, irritability, and cough. Vitals: temperature: 38.9°C (102°F), heart rate: 170 beats per minute, respiratory rate: 63 breaths per minute. Patient history is significant for two previous visits to the emergency department with similar symptoms in the past 2 months. Chest X-ray reveals consolidation in the left upper lobe. Gram stain of induced sputum demonstrates gram-positive lancet-shaped diplococci. Laboratory results reveal an elevated neutrophil count and the following:

Lymphocyte counts (×10^9/L)	Reported	Normal range
Total lymphocyte count	3.4	2.5–5.0
T lymphocytes (CD3)	2.9	1.5–3.0
B lymphocytes (CD19)	<0.01	0.3–1.0

Based on the most likely diagnosis, long-term management of this patient should include:

A. Recombinant human C5

B. Recombinant human granulocyte colony-stimulating factor (G-CSF)

C. Human immune serum globulin (HISG)

D. CTLA-4Ig fusion protein

E. Recombinant human interferon gamma (IFN-γ)

2. A 10-month-old boy presents to the emergency department with pneumonia. Since the age of 5 months, he has had recurrent pneumonia and sinusitis due to *Streptococcus pneumoniae*. Analysis of the peripheral blood indicates a lack of CD20+ cells, with normal numbers of CD4+, CD8+, and CD16+ cells. A defect is most likely to be present in which of the following genes?

A. *CD40L*

B. *Bruton's tyrosine kinase (BTK)*

C. *STAT3*

D. *ZAP-70*

E. *ATM (ataxia-telangiectasia mutated)*

3. An 8-month-old boy presents to urgent care with his parents with a chief complaint of fever, irritability, and cough. Vitals: temperature: 39.7°C (103.5°F), heart rate: 180 beats per minute, respiratory rate: 65 breaths per minute. Chest X-ray reveals consolidation in the right upper lobe. Bronchoalveolar lavage is positive for gram-positive lancet-shaped diplococci. Patient history is significant for three previous trips to the emergency department with similar symptoms and etiologic cause since his mother stopped breastfeeding 3 months ago. Laboratory blood tests reveal elevated numbers of neutrophils and normal T cell numbers, with an absence of B cells. Based on the information presented, which of the following assays would best confirm the immunological deficiency in the serum?

A. Immunoelectrophoresis

B. Polymerase chain reaction (PCR)

C. Western blot

D. Electrophoretic mobility shift assay (EMSA)

E. Direct immunofluorescence assay (DFA)

4. A 5-month-old boy is brought to the emergency department by his parents with a chief complaint of fever, irritability, and cough. Patient history is significant for two previous visits to the emergency department with lower respiratory infections; both were successfully treated with antibiotics. The boy had a brother who died from pneumonia before 1 year of age and has a 4-year-old sister who is healthy. Vitals: temperature: 38.9°C (102°F), heart rate: 170 beats per minute, respiratory rate: 63 breaths per minute. The child's chest X-ray reveals consolidation in the left upper lobe. Serum analysis reveals the following:

	Reported	Normal range
Total blood complement	56	41–90 hemolytic units
C1	22	16–33 mg/dL
C3	135	88–252 mg/dL
IgG	15 mg/dL	650–1,500 mg/dL
IgA	Not detected	76–390 mg/dL
IgM	5 mg/dL	40–345 mg/dL
Isohemagglutinins	Not detected	

Based on the information presented above, flow cytometric analysis of bone marrow from this child would most likely reveal

A. Decreased number of pre-B cells

B. Decreased number of pro-B cells

C. Increased number of immature B cells

D. Decreased number of hematopoietic stem cells

E. Increased number of plasma cells

5. Individuals with this Bruton's X-linked agammaglobulinemia (XLA) are highly resistant to infection with:

A. Cytomegalovirus (CMV)

B. Herpes simplex virus-2 (HSV-2)

C. Hepatitis B virus

D. Epstein–Barr virus (EBV)

E. Human immunodeficiency virus (HIV)

6. A 3-year-old boy is brought to the emergency department. His parents are concerned because their son initially complained of an earache, but now complains of his head hurting and he is vomiting and disoriented. Patient history is significant for frequent bouts of otitis media and lower respiratory tract infections. His mother and father are healthy, but the child's mother had a brother who was frequently ill and died of pneumonia at age 16. The boy's mother has a sister who is alive and healthy but also had a male cousin who died in infancy after multiple respiratory infections. Vitals: temperature: 38.9°C (102°F), heart rate: 185 beats per minute, respiratory rate: 67 breaths per minute. Physical examination reveals that the boy's left ear has an opacified tympanic membrane, while his right ear is normal. He has nuchal rigidity and is positive for both Kernig's and Brudzinski's signs. Based on the diagnosis of the child, if the patient's mother and father have another son together, what is the likelihood that the child will have the same disease?

A. 0%

B. 25%

C. 50%

D. 75%

E. 100%

7. A 3-month-old girl is brought to the emergency department by her parents with a chief complaint of fever, irritability, and dry cough. Vitals: temperature: 39.4°C (103°F), heart rate: 180 beats per minute, respiratory rate: 65 breaths per minute. Chest X-ray reveals diffuse bilateral infiltrates extending from the perihilar region without a thymic shadow. Gomori methenamine silver stain of the bronchoalveolar lavage sample reveals the presence of trophozoite and cyst forms. Analysis of peripheral blood mononuclear cells reveals normal numbers of CD20+ cells, CD18+ cells, and CD56+ cells, and an absence of CD3+ cells. Genetic analysis of this individual would most likely reveal a deletion in which of the following chromosomes?

A. Chromosome 2

B. Chromosome 11

C. Chromosome 17

D. Chromosome 21

E. Chromosome 22

8. A 7-month-old girl is brought to the emergency department by her parents due to the child's high fever, persistent coughing, and irritability. Patient history is significant for a congenital heart condition and recurrent respiratory infections. Vitals: temperature: 38.9°C (102°F), heart rate: 180 beats per minute, respiratory rate: 50 breaths per minute. Physical exam reveals cyanosis and labored breathing and laboratory values are significant for hypocalcemia. Based on the information given above, which of the following CD markers would most likely be absent or low when analyzing the blood cells of this patient by flow cytometry?

A. CD3

B. CD16

C. CD20

D. CD56

E. CD86

9. A 12-month-old girl presents with the following conditions: cleft palate, hypocalcemia, heart anomalies, and recurrent viral and fungal infections. Laboratory tests indicate the absence of CD3+ cells, with normal numbers of CD20+ cells. Based on this information, the most likely disorder is:

A. ZAP-70 deficiency

B. Bare lymphocyte syndrome (BLS)

C. DiGeorge's syndrome

D. AIDS

E. Adenosine deaminase severe combined immunodeficiency (ADA-SCID)

10. A 6-month-old boy is brought to the emergency department by his parents who are concerned that their son is extremely irritable and has a severe diaper rash that has now spread to the abdomen and back. Patient history is significant for repeated bacterial and viral infections that have led to multiple visits to the emergency department. Physical exam reveals large, red blisters on the abdomen, back, and buttocks. A KOH preparation demonstrates the presence of yeast, and blood work shows an increased neutrophil count, normal B cell, and CD4+ T cell numbers with an absence of CD8+ T cells. Additional tests indicate that the patient's lymphocytes do not proliferate in response to phytohemagglutinin. The most appropriate long-term management to treat this patient's underlying condition is

A. Bone marrow transplant

B. HISG injection

C. Thymus transplant

D. Granulocyte-macrophage colony-stimulating factor (GM-CSF) injection

E. Corticosteroids

11. An 8-month-old boy is brought to the emergency department by his parents with a chief complaint of diarrhea lasting more than 2 months. Parents deny any recent travel, and patient history is significant for recurrent respiratory infections that have resulted in numerous emergency department visits. On examination, the boy is significantly underweight and small for his age. Lymph nodes are palpable and tonsils are visible. Examination of peripheral blood by flow cytometry reveals the following:

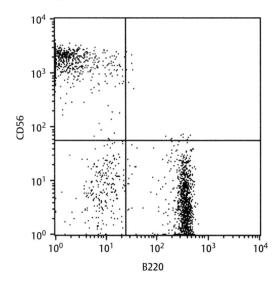

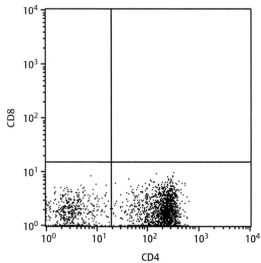

Based on the symptoms and the flow cytometry data, which of the following is deficient in this patient?

A. ZAP-70

B. Human leucocyte antigen (HLA) class II

C. STAT3

D. AIRE

E. BTK

12. A 3-month-old girl is brought to her pediatrician with concerns that the child has had diarrhea for 1 week. History is significant for multiple trips to the pediatrician's office for otitis media and pneumonia. Physical examination reveals that the child is in the 5th percentile for both height and weight, and upon examination of the oral cavity, tonsillar tissue is found to be present and the findings seen in the image below are noted.

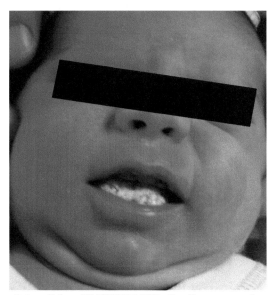

By James Heilman, MD [CC BY-SA 3.0 (https://creativecommons.org/licenses/by-sa/3.0)], from Wikimedia Commons

The child most likely lacks functioning:

A. Natural killer (NK) cells

B. Neutrophils

C. Macrophages

D. B cells

E. T cells

13. A mother brings her 5-month-old infant to the emergency department with concerns about her daughter's significant diarrhea, dehydration, and fever. Patient history is significant for a severe bout of pneumonia at 2 weeks of age. The child is up to date with her vaccines; the last vaccine that she received was the live oral rotavirus vaccine 1 week ago. Physical findings reveal a temperature of 38.9°C (102°F) and dry mucous membranes, and palpation reveals no rebound with guarding. Pertinent laboratory results are shown below:

Complete blood count (CBC)	Reported	Normal range
Total lymphocyte count	3.4	2.5–5.0
T lymphocytes (CD3)	1.5	1.5–3.0
CD4:CD8 ratio	100:1	2:1
B lymphocytes (CD20)	0.7	0.3–1.0

Enzyme immunoassay for rotavirus: positive

Based on the information provided, which of the following processes is most likely defective in this child?

A. Repair of double-stranded DNA breaks

B. Antigen presentation

C. Cytoskeletal reorganization

D. Isotype switch

E. T cell receptor signaling

14. A mother presents to the pediatrician's office with her 3-month-old baby girl, who has a diaper rash that will not go away and has white patches in her mouth. Patient history is significant for two visits to the emergency department, and she was diagnosed with pneumonia caused by *Pneumocystis jirovecii*. Chest X-rays from these visits denote the presence of a thymic shadow. Vital signs are normal. Physical findings reveal that she is small for her age, and lymph nodes are palpable, but not enlarged. Removal of her diaper reveals large, red blisters on the abdomen, back, and buttocks.

Which of the following test results, if negative, would be most consistent with the most likely diagnosis of the underlying cause of the current presentation?

A. Proliferation of white blood cells (WBCs) in response to concanavalin A

B. Sheep red blood cell (RBC) lysis by complement assay

C. CD18 expression on WBCs by flow cytometry

D. Total immunoglobulin by immunoelectrophoresis

E. ADA protein from peripheral blood by Western blot

15. Which of the following distinguishes between ZAP-70 deficiency and type I bare lymphocyte syndrome (BLS)? Only patients with ZAP-70 deficiency

A. Present before 2 years of age

B. Have decreased CD8+ T cells

C. Have normal levels of immunoglobulin M (IgM) and IgG

D. Have nonfunctional CD4+ T cells

E. Are deficient in HLA class I

16. A 6-year-old boy presents to the emergency department with a chief complaint of cough, fever, fatigue, and chest pain. Patient history is significant for recurrent respiratory and gastrointestinal (GI) infections, and asthma. At the time of the exam, the child's temperature is 39.4°C (103°F), heart rate is 150 beats per minute, and respiratory rate is 42 breaths per minute. Chest auscultation demonstrates significant bilateral crackles with expiratory wheezes, and a chest radiograph shows bilateral, diffuse pulmonary infiltrates with effusion. A complete blood count (CBC) reveals that neutrophil, eosinophil, lymphocyte, and platelet numbers are normal, with elevated IgE levels. Based on the patient's current presentation, patient history, and epidemiology, the most likely underlying immunodeficiency in this patient is

A. IgA deficiency syndrome

B. Wiskott–Aldrich syndrome

C. Hyper-IgE syndrome (HIES)

D. Bare lymphocyte syndrome (BLS)

E. Kostmann's syndrome

17. A mother brings her 6-year-old girl into the pediatrician's office because every time she eats scrambled eggs for breakfast, her daughter complains of stomach pain and breaks out into a rash. Based on the preliminary diagnosis, a total immunoglobulin panel and a radioallergosorbent test are ordered. The results are below:

Immunoglobulin panel	Reported
IgG	800 mg/dL
IgM	190 mg/dL
IgA	Undetectable
IgE	650 IU/mL
RAST score:	
Eggs	++++

This patient is at greatest increased risk for developing which of the following?

A. Systemic lupus erythematosus (SLE)

B. Scleroderma

C. Goodpasture's syndrome

D. Guillain–Barré syndrome

E. Hashimoto's thyroiditis

18. A mother brings her 12-month-old son into the pediatrician's office because every time he eats scrambled eggs for breakfast, her son gets fussy and breaks out into a rash. Based on the most likely preliminary diagnosis, a total immunoglobulin panel and a radioallergosorbent test are ordered. The results are below:

Immunoglobulin panel	Reported
IgG	950 mg/dL
IgM	225 mg/dL
IgA	Undetectable
IgE	685 IU/mL
RAST score:	
Eggs	++++

Which of the following vaccines would historically be contraindicated in this child?

A. Hepatitis B

B. Influenza

C. Human papillomavirus

D. Measles, mumps, and rubella

E. Varicella

19. A 34-year-old man presents to his physician complaining of fatigue, shortness of breath, and a tingling sensation in his feet. Patient history is significant for allergic asthma and celiac disease. Physical findings reveal a temperature that is normal, but the patient is pale. Laboratory analysis indicates that the patient is anemic and produces antibodies specific for intrinsic factor. An immunoglobulin panel of his blood also indicates the following:

Immunoglobulin panel	Reported
IgG	1,200 mg/dL
IgM	300 mg/dL
IgA	Undetectable
IgE	900 IU/mL

If this individual requires a transfusion of blood products, which of the following should not be administered to this patient?

A. Cryoprecipitate

B. Platelets

C. Type-matched RBCs

D. Type-matched whole blood

20. A 21-year-old man with a history of allergic asthma and severe eczema presents to the emergency department with a stab wound that lacerates the spleen. During surgery to repair the spleen, the patient receives 2 units of whole blood of the appropriate ABO and Rh type. As the surgery progresses over the next few hours, the patient's blood pressure drops to 80/55 mm Hg and he develops labored breathing (airway edema), consistent with anaphylaxis. Which of the following is the most likely to be absent in this patient?

A. IgA

B. Interleukin 13 (IL-13)

C. C9

D. Granzyme

E. IgE

21. A mother brings her 4-year-old child to the pediatrician concerned that her daughter is complaining of an ear ache. Patient history is significant for repeated cases of otitis media, sinusitis, and GI infections (at least four cases of sinusitis have occurred in the past year alone). Otoscope exam reveals an opaque, erythematous, tympanic membrane. Due to the recurrent infections, a CBC, T and B lymphocyte counts, and immunoglobulin testing are ordered. Results are below:

Complete blood count (CBC)	Reported	Normal
Erythrocyte count	4.3 million/mm^3	3.5–5.5 million/mm^3
Platelet count	185,000/mm^3	150,000–400,000/mm^3
Neutrophils	55%	54–62%
Eosinophils	2%	1–3%
Total lymphocytes	30%	25–33%
T lymphocytes (CD3)	2.0 × 10^3/µL	1.5–3.0 × 10^3/µL
CD4:CD8 ratio	2:1	2:1
B lymphocytes (CD20)	0.7 × 10^3/µL	0.3–1.0 × 10^3/µL
IgG	800 mg/dL	650–1,500 mg/dL
IgM	190 mg/dL	40–345 mg/dL
IgA	Undetectable	76–390 mg/dL
IgE	720 IU/mL	0–380 IU/mL

Based on this information, which of the following diseases is the child least likely to develop?

A. Common variable immunodeficiency (CVID)

B. Celiac disease

C. Pneumonia with encapsulated bacteria

D. Burkitt's lymphoma

E. Food allergies

22. A mother brings her 4-year-old daughter to the emergency department, as the child has a fever and is repeatedly coughing. Patient history is significant for repeated visits to the emergency department for severe allergy-induced asthma attacks and for pneumonia and severe sinusitis. Vital signs show a temperature of 38.9°C (102°F), a heart rate of 170 beats per minute, and a respiratory rate of 53 breaths per minute. Chest X-ray indicates consolidation in the right upper lobe. Laboratory results reveal the following:

Complete blood count (CBC)	Reported	Normal
Erythrocyte count	3.9 million/mm^3	3.5–5.5 million/mm^3
Platelet count	185,000/mm^3	150,000–400,000/mm^3
Neutrophils	60%	54–62%
Eosinophils	3%	1–3%
Total lymphocytes	29%	25–33%
T lymphocytes (CD3)	2.0 × 10^3/µL	1.5–3.0 × 10^3/µL
CD4:CD8 ratio	2:1	2:1
B lymphocytes (CD20)	0.7 × 10^3/µL	0.3–1.0 × 10^3/µL
IgG	1,400 mg/dL	650–1,500 mg/dL
IgM	220 mg/dL	40–345 mg/dL
IgA	Undetectable	76–390 mg/dL
IgE	380 IU/mL	0–380 IU/mL

Based on the presentation, lab results, and epidemiology, what is the most likely underlying disease that predisposes this child to the current illness?

A. IgA deficiency

B. Common variable immunodeficiency (CVID)

C. Wiskott–Aldrich syndrome

D. Omenn's syndrome

E. Job's syndrome (HIES)

23. A mother brings her 6-month-old girl to the pediatrician with a chief concern of a rash on her daughter's scalp. Patient history is significant for the repeated need for topical nystatin for diaper rash and fluconazole for recurrent bouts of white pseudomembranes on the tongue and oral mucosal surfaces. Vital signs are normal. Physical findings reveal an extensive red, flat rash with sharp scalloped edges that covers the majority of the child's scalp. Laboratory findings are shown below:

Complete blood count (CBC)	Reported	Normal range
Total lymphocyte count	3.4	2.5–5.0
T lymphocytes (CD3)	2	1.5–3.0
CD4:CD8 ratio	2:1	2:1
B lymphocytes (CD20)	0.7	0.3–1.0

Based on the patient's presentation and the laboratory data, a mutation in which of the following genes is most likely to be present?

A. *IL2RG* (IL-2 receptor gamma)
B. *STAT1* (signal transducer and activator of transcription 1)
C. *Properdin*
D. ZAP-70
E. *ATM* (ATM serine/threonine kinase)

24. An 8-month-old boy is brought to the pediatrician's office by his mother, due to his mother's concern over the fact that her son is irritable and is not eating well. Patient history is significant for recurrent diaper rash and folliculitis. Vital signs are normal. Physical findings reveal the presence of a white pseudomembrane on the tongue and oral mucosal surfaces. KOH preparation of skin scrapings reveals budding yeast. The most likely mechanism for this child's presentation is the insufficient production of:

A. IFN-γ, due to the loss of Th1 differentiation
B. IL-4, due to the loss of Th2 differentiation
C. Transforming growth factor beta (TGF-beta), due to the loss of Treg cell differentiation
D. IL-9, due to the loss of Th9 cell differentiation
E. IL-17, due to the loss of Th17 cell differentiation

25. A 3-year-old girl is brought to her pediatrician's office by her parents over their concern regarding the appearance of her nailbeds on her toes and fingers. Patient history is significant for hypoparathyroidism and multiple visits to her pediatrician's office for thrush and diaper rashes, which required fluconazole and nystatin to resolve. Physical exam reveals deformed, raised, yellowish-brown nails on 8 of the 10 toes and 6 of the 10 fingers. Neither the parents nor the girl's sister shares these similar symptoms. Colonies that grow from fingernail scrapings are white on Sabouraud agar with chloramphenicol and cycloheximide. Which of the following diseases can be *excluded* from the differential?

A. Autoimmune polyendocrinopathy-candidiasis-ectodermal dystrophy (APECED)
B. Type I bare lymphocyte syndrome (BLS)
C. Severe combined immunodeficiency (SCID)
D. Chronic mucocutaneous candidiasis (CMC)
E. HIV infection

26. A mother brings her 2-year-old son to the pediatrician's office complaining that her child has been coughing and wheezing, and is running a fever. Patient history is significant for recurrent eczema starting at 6 months of age, and repeated otitis media and respiratory infections. Previous laboratory results indicate that the child has repeatedly been thrombocytopenic at previous visits for respiratory infections, but the mother did not follow up regarding this concern. At the time of exam, the child has a temperature of 38.9°C (102°F), a heart rate of 170 beats per minute, and a respiratory rate of 45 breaths per minute. Chest X-ray reveals consolidation in the left upper lobe. Which of the following lab results is most consistent with the patient's most likely diagnosis?

A. Enhanced B cell responses to carbohydrate antigens
B. Unusually small platelets
C. Enhanced CTL-mediated lysis
D. Decreased macrophage numbers
E. Decreased von Willebrand factor

27. A newborn boy is born with a petechial rash and has prolonged bleeding from the umbilical stump. Syphilis, toxoplasmosis, HIV, CMV, and HSV-2 testing is negative. A peripheral blood smear indicates that the newborn is thrombocytopenic with small platelets. Over the course of the next 6 months, his mother takes him to the pediatrician with recurrent otitis media and pneumonia caused by *S. pneumoniae* and meningitis by *Haemophilus influenzae* type B, even though he was vaccinated shortly after birth. The defect in this patient leads to an inability of:

A. Macrophages to kill phagocytosed bacteria

B. Developing lymphocytes to repair double-stranded DNA breaks

C. Mature lymphocytes to reorganize actin cytoskeleton

D. CD4+ T cells to become Th17 cells

E. Nucleated cells to present peptide on HLA class I

28. A mother brings her 12-month-old son to the pediatrician for an itchy rash that will not go away. Patient history is significant for recurrent visits to the office over the last 4 months with sinusitis, otitis media, and pneumonia. Physical exam reveals multiple dry, red, scaly patches on the skin and multiple bruises that the mother says are due to her son learning to walk.

Lab values indicate:

Complete blood count (CBC)	Reported	Normal
Erythrocyte count	5.1 million/ mm^3	3.5–5.5 million/ mm^3
Platelet count	60 × 10^3/μL	150,000– 400,000/ mm^3
Platelet size	0.4 mm	2–4 mm
Neutrophils	58%	54–62%
Eosinophils	3%	1–3%
Total lymphocytes	31%	25–33%
T lymphocytes (CD3)	1.5 × 10^3/μL	1.5–3.0 × 10^3/μL
CD4:CD8 ratio	2:1	2:1
B lymphocytes (CD20)	0.7 × 10^3/μL	0.3–1.0 × 10^3/μL

Based on the patient's presentation and lab values, the most likely diagnosis is:

A. Ataxia-telangiectasia

B. Severe combined immunodeficiency (SCID)

C. Wiskott–Aldrich syndrome

D. AIDS

E. Omenn's syndrome

29. A 65-year-old woman presents to her primary care physician to ensure that her vaccinations are up to date. Patient history is significant for ongoing chemotherapy treatment for breast cancer. The vaccine for which of the following pathogens is contraindicated in this patient?

A. Influenza

B. *Streptococcus pneumoniae*

C. Varicella zoster virus

D. *Bordetella pertussis*

E. *Haemophilus influenzae*, type b

30. A mother brings her 2-month-old daughter to the emergency department, as the child has a fever and is repeatedly coughing. Patient history is significant for four visits to the emergency department with respiratory infections. Additionally, the mother and father of the child have no health issues, but the patient's paternal grandma had a brother who died in infancy after repeated bouts of bacterial pneumonia. At the time of exam, the child has a temperature of 38.9°C (102°F), a heart rate of 145 beats per minute, and a respiratory rate of 45 breaths per minute. Chest X-ray indicates consolidation in the left upper lobe and expectorated sputum demonstrates gram-positive cocci in pairs and chains. CBC results are below:

Complete blood count (CBC)	Reported	Normal
Erythrocyte count	4.2 million/ mm^3	3.5–5.5 million/mm^3
Platelet count	200,000/mm^3	150,000– 400,000/ mm^3
Neutrophils	4%	54–62%
Eosinophils	2%	1–3%
Total lymphocytes	31%	25–33%

Based on the patient's presentation and the information given, a mutation in which of the following genes is most likely to be present?

A. *WASP* (Wiskott–Aldrich syndrome protein)

B. *ADA*

C. *HAX-1* (HCLS-associated protein X-1)

D. *ITGB2* (beta-chain of CD18)

E. *ATM* (ATM serine/threonine kinase)

31. A mother brings her 5-day-old newborn to the emergency department complaining that her child has a fever and the umbilical cord stump is extremely red. The baby was born at 39-week gestation and all initial indications were that the baby was normal. Vital signs indicate a temperature of 38.9°C (102°F). Physical exam reveals that the abdomen is tender, swollen, and red. The umbilical stump is without pus and has a foul odor. Laboratory results reveal the following:

Complete blood count (CBC)	Reported	Normal
Erythrocyte count	5.2 million/mm³	3.5–5.5 million/mm³
Platelet count	235,000/mm³	150,000–400,000/mm³
Neutrophils	4%	54–62%
Eosinophils	3%	1–3%
Total lymphocytes	27%	25–33%

After immediate treatment for the child's current symptoms, what is the most appropriate long-term treatment for this patient?

A. Human immune serum globulin (HISG)
B. Granulocyte colonystimulating factor (G-CSF)
C. Recombinant interferon gamma (rIFN-γ)
D. Gene therapy with the *ELANE* (elastase, neutrophil expressed) gene
E. Recombinant IL-7

32. A mother brings her 7-week-old boy to an immunology specialist after a referral from his pediatrician. Patient history is significant for recurrent bacterial respiratory infections and laboratory results indicate a significant neutropenia, but no other abnormalities were reported. Analysis of a subsequent bone marrow aspiration reveals slightly decreased cellularity with an early myeloid "arrest" at the promyelocyte to myelocyte stage with atypical nuclei and cytoplasmic vacuolization. Based on the patient's medical history and laboratory results, the most likely diagnosis is

A. Wiskott–Aldrich syndrome
B. Autoimmune neutropenia
C. Cohen's syndrome
D. Kostmann's syndrome
E. Congenital amegakaryocytic thrombocytopenia

33. A couple presents to a genetics counselor to discuss the possibility of having a child with an inherited genetic disease. While the parents at the meeting have no significant medical history, the husband reveals that he had a sister that died early in life due to overwhelming infections and was diagnosed with severe congenital neutropenia. The husband said that his parents also both had no significant medical history. Based on this information, the husband has a high probability of carrying a mutated version of which of the following genes?

A. *HAX-1* (HCLS-associated protein X-1)
B. *CYBA* (cytochrome b)
C. *ELANE* (elastase, neutrophil expressed)
D. *LYST* (lysosomal trafficking regulator)
E. *CD40L* (CD40 ligand)

34. Which of the following vaccines could be life threatening to a child that has SCID?

A. *Haemophilus influenzae*, type b (ActHIB)
B. Hepatitis A/B (Twin Rix)
C. Measles, mumps, rubella (MMR)
D. Pneumococcal (Prevnar)
E. Influenza (Fluzone)

35. A 4-month-old boy is brought to the emergency department with a fever, cough, and rapid breathing. Patient history is significant for repeated, severe oral thrush and two episodes of pneumonia with *P. jirovecii*. At the time of the exam the child has a temperature of 38.9°C (102°F), a respiratory rate of 45 breaths per minute, and a heart rate of 110 beats per minute, and the absence of adenoids and any lymphadenopathy. Significant bilateral crackles with expiratory wheezes are observed upon auscultation and chest X-ray reveals bimodal consolidation and a lack of thymic shadow. Laboratory results are significant for the absence of B and T lymphocytes. After treatment for the immediate presentation, the most appropriate long-term management for this patient to treat the underlying condition is:

A. Bone marrow transplant
B. Human immune serum globulin (HISG) injection
C. Thymus transplant
D. GM-CSF injection
E. Corticosteroids

36. A 4-month-old boy is brought to the pediatrician's office with recurrent diarrhea. Patient history is significant for persistent oral candidal thrush, otitis media with *Streptococcus pneumoniae*, and pneumonia with *Pneumocystis jirovecii*. The mother says that the child has had diarrhea for over 3 weeks. Vital signs currently are normal. However, physical exam reveals a child that is under the 5th percentile for height and weight.

Complete blood count (CBC)	Reported	Normal
Erythrocyte count	4.3 million/mm^3	3.5–5.5 million/mm^3
Platelet count	200,000/mm^3	150,000–400,000/mm^3
Neutrophils	60%	54–62%
Eosinophils	2%	1–3%
Total lymphocytes	2%	25–33%
T lymphocytes (CD3)	0.1 × 10^3/μL	1.5–3.0 × 10^3/μL
B lymphocytes (CD20)	0.01 × 10^3/μL	0.3–1.0 × 10^3/μL
IgG	600 mg/dL	650–1,500 mg/dL
IgM	Undetectable	40–345 mg/dL

Which of the following clinical findings is most likely to be observed?

A. Silver hair and light-colored eyes

B. Hypercellularity of the bone marrow

C. Lack of pus at site of infection

D. Clefting of the palate

E. Lack of a thymic shadow

37. A 5-month-old girl is brought to the emergency department with a fever and severe cough. Patient history is significant for two previous trips to the emergency department with pneumonia and two previous visits for severe dehydration due to rotavirus-induced diarrhea. Family history is significant for having a sister who died at 2 months from a respiratory syncytial virus infection, despite treatment with monoclonal Ab treatment. The results of laboratory results are as follows:

Complete blood count (CBC)	Reported	Normal
Erythrocyte count	5.0 million/mm^3	3.5–5.5 million/mm^3
Platelet count	225,000/mm^3	150,000–400,000/mm^3
Neutrophils	61%	54–62%
Eosinophils	3%	1–3%
Total lymphocytes	1%	25–33%
T lymphocytes (CD3)	0.4 × 10^3/μL	1.5–3.0 × 10^3/μL
B lymphocytes (CD20)	0.04 × 10^3/μL	0.3–1.0 × 10^3/μL
IgG	300 mg/dL	650–1,500 mg/dL
IgM	Undetectable	40–345 mg/dL

Which of the following genes are most likely mutated in this child?

A. *WASP*

B. *ZAP-70*

C. *BTK*

D. *ADA*

E. *LYST*

38. A 4-month-old girl is analyzed for genetic mutations due to a failure to thrive, chronic diarrhea, recurrent fever, and a life-threatening infection after receiving the rotavirus vaccine. Family history is significant that her 2-year-old sister is healthy. Genetic analysis identifies a mutation in the *ADA* gene. The loss of lymphocytes in this individual is most likely due to the inability to:

A. Undergo V(D)J rearrangement

B. Convert toxic metabolites to nontoxic byproducts

C. Signal through cytokine receptors

D. Fix dsDNA breaks

E. Form an immunological synapse

39. A 3-month-old boy is brought to the emergency department with persistent diarrhea and dehydration. Patient history is significant for repeated oral candidiasis, otitis media with nontypeable *Haemophilus influenzae*, and pneumonia with *Pneumocystis jirovecii*. Physical exam reveals that the child is under the 5th percentile for height and weight. This child likely lacks:

A. Pro-B cells

B. Double-positive thymocytes

C. Promyelocytes

D. Megakaryocytes

E. NK cell precursor

40. A 3-month-old boy is brought to the emergency department with a fever, cough, and wheezing. Patient history is significant for repeated, severe oral *Candida* infections and two previous episodes of pneumonia. Family history is significant for a brother who had repeated respiratory infections and died from pneumonia at less than 1 year of age, but his sister is healthy. At the time of exam, the child has a temperature of 39.2°C (102.5°F), a respiratory rate of 35 breaths per minute, and a heart rate of 115 beats per minute. Significant bilateral crackles with expiratory wheezes are observed upon auscultation and chest X-ray reveals bimodal consolidation.

Complete blood count (CBC)	Reported	Normal
Erythrocyte count	5.1 million/mm^3	3.5–5.5 million/mm^3
Platelet count	200,000/mm^3	150,000–400,000/mm^3
Neutrophils	62%	54–62%
Eosinophils	2%	1–3%
Total lymphocytes	1%	25–33%
T lymphocytes (CD3)	0.05 × 10^3/μL	1.5–3.0 × 10^3/μL
B lymphocytes (CD20)	0.3 × 10^3/μL	0.3–1.0 × 10^3/μL
IgG	300 mg/dL	650–1,500 mg/dL
IgM	Undetectable	40–345 mg/dL

Which of the following proteins is most likely absent/nonfunctional in this patient?

A. ADA

B. Interleukin common gamma chain

C. Wiskott–Aldrich protein

D. Janus kinase 3

E. Recombinase activating gene 1

41. A 38-year-old man presents to his primary care physician with a chief complaint of fever, sore throat, and a rash. During his evaluation, the man indicates that he has been sexually active with multiple partners in the last 6 months and has not used any precautions. At the time of exam, the man has a temperature of 38.9°C (102°F). Enlarged tonsils without exudate, generalized lymphadenopathy, and a flat, red, rash on his chest and shoulders are noted on physical exam. Relevant laboratory results reveal the findings below:

Complete blood count (CBC)	Reported	Normal
Neutrophils	60%	54–62%
Eosinophils	2%	1–3%
Total lymphocytes	12%	25–33%
T lymphocytes (CD3)	0.6 × 10^3/μL	1.5–3.0 × 10^3/μL
CD4:CD8 ratio	0.7:1	2:1
B lymphocytes (CD20)	0.75 × 10^3/μL	0.3–1.0 × 10^3/μL

Antigen/antibody	Tests
HCV IgG	Negative
HAV IgG	Positive
HBcAg	Negative
HBsAg IgG	Negative
p24 Ag	Positive

Which of the following viral proteins is responsible for the rapid evolution of this virus over the course of infection?

A. Reverse transcriptase

B. gp40/gp120

C. Protease

D. p24 capsid antigen

E. Integrase

42. A 27-year-old woman presents to a community health clinic with nausea, fever, and a rash. Patient history is significant for intravenous drug abuse. At the time of exam, the woman has a temperature of 39.2°C (102.5°F). Physical exam reveals generalized lymphadenopathy, and a flat, red, rash on her chest. Relevant laboratory values are below:

Complete blood count (CBC)	Reported	Normal
Neutrophils	58%	54–62%
Eosinophils	1%	1–3%
Total lymphocytes	11%	25–33%
T lymphocytes (CD3)	$0.5 \times 10^3/\mu L$	$1.5–3.0 \times 10^3/\mu L$
CD4:CD8 ratio	0.5:1	2:1
B lymphocytes (CD20)	$0.75 \times 10^3/\mu L$	$0.3–1.0 \times 10^3/\mu L$

Antigen/antibody	Tests
HCV IgG	Negative
HAV IgG	Positive
HBcAg	Negative
HBsAg IgG	Negative
p24 Ag	Positive

Which of the following treatment options for this patient blocks the ability of the pathogen to mature into an infectious particle?

A. Nucleoside reverse transcriptase inhibitor

B. Integrase inhibitor

C. Protease inhibitor

D. Fusion inhibitor

E. Nonnucleoside reverse transcriptase inhibitor

43. A 48-year-old woman presents to a free health clinic for a follow-up after a 2-year absence. Patient history is significant for previous treatment with dolutegravir, tenofovir disoproxil fumarate, and emtricitabine. She has a longstanding history of drug abuse and homelessness. Physical exam is normal, but CD4 count is 380 cells/mm^3 and RNA viral load is 27,000 copies/mm^3. One month of the same treatment regimen is prescribed. When the patient returns for her follow-up 2 weeks later, the CD4+ T cell count has decreased further and the viral load has increased. A genotype resistance test is ordered. The most likely cause for this change in lab values is:

A. Evolution to a CCR5 strain of HIV

B. Mutations in the pol gene of HIV

C. Infection with a second strain of drug-resistant HIV

D. Thymic involution

E. Chromosomal translocation of the proviral genome

44. A 23-year-old woman presents to the clinic at her university complaining of nausea, fever, and a rash that has lasted a week. At the time of exam, the woman has a temperature of 39.2°C (102.5°F). Physical exam demonstrates generalized lymphadenopathy, and a flat, red, rash on her back and chest. Relevant laboratory values reveal:

Complete blood count (CBC)	Reported	Normal
Neutrophils	56%	54–62%
Eosinophils	3%	1–3%
Total lymphocytes	8%	25–33%
T lymphocytes (CD3)	$0.4 \times 10^3/\mu L$	$1.5–3.0 \times 10^3/\mu L$
CD4:CD8 ratio	0.6:1	2:1
B lymphocytes (CD20)	$0.75 \times 10^3/\mu L$	$0.3–1.0 \times 10^3/\mu L$
Alanine aminotransferase	18 U/L	8–20 U/L
Aspartate aminotransferase	20 U/L	8–20 U/L
Bilirubin	0.6 mg/dL	0.1–1.0 mg/dL

Antigen/antibody	Tests
HCV IgG	Negative
HAV IgG	Positive
HBcAg	Negative
HBsAg IgG	Negative
p24 Ag	Positive

Epidemiologically, this individual most likely acquired this infection through:

A. Working at a daycare center

B. Multiple body piercings

C. Unprotected sex with multiple partners

D. In utero transmission from her mother

E. Casual contact

45. To determine if an individual is infected with HIV, which of the following tests should be performed first?

A. Western blot analysis

B. CD4 count by flow cytometry

C. Syncytial formation assay

D. HIV antigen/antibody combination enzyme immunoassay

E. PCR for HIV RNA

46. A 6-month-old girl is brought to the emergency department by her mother with a deep, infected cut on her right arm. Patient history is significant for two prior trips to the emergency department for pneumonia caused by *Streptococcus pneumoniae*. Additionally, this child had a sister who died at 6 weeks of age due to an overwhelming infection caused by the same pathogen. The parents have no significant medical history. Vital signs reveal a temperature of 101°C (38.3°C). Physical examination reveals a child with a cut on her right arm that expresses purulent discharge and is warm to the touch. Additionally, the child appears to have light eyes and her hair has a silver sheen to it. A Gram stain from the infected site indicates the presence of gram-positive cocci in chains. Based on the presentation above, which of the following genes is most likely to be mutated in this child?

A. *ELANE*

B. *LYST*

C. *WASP*

D. *NEMO*

E. *NADPH oxidase*

47. A 4-month-old boy is brought to the emergency department by his mother with a fever, irritability, and a deep cough of 2 days' duration. Patient history is significant for two visits to the emergency department with pneumonia caused by *Streptococcus pneumoniae*. Parents have no significant medical history, but the child has a female cousin with a similar propensity for respiratory infections who "looks just like our son." Vitals: temperature: 38.9°C (102°F), heart rate: 170 breaths per minute, respiratory rate: 63 beats per minute. Chest X-ray reveals consolidation in the left upper lobe. Physical exam notes that the child has light eyes and light hair, but otherwise appears normal. The results of a CBC are listed below and the lab results also comment that the granulocytes contain giant azurophilic granules.

Complete blood count (CBC)	Reported	Normal
Erythrocyte count	4.5 million/mm^3	3.5–5.5 million/mm^3
Platelet count	225,000/mm^3	150,000–400,000/mm^3
Neutrophils	30%	54–62%
Eosinophils	2%	1–3%
Total lymphocytes	25%	25–33%

Based on the information above, his patient most likely has

A. Wiskott–Aldrich syndrome

B. Chronic granulomatous disease (CGD)

C. Kostmann's syndrome

D. Chédiak–Higashi syndrome

E. Griscelli's syndrome

48. A 6-month-old girl is brought to the emergency department by her father with a fever and persistent cough of 5 days' duration. Patient history is significant for five visits to the emergency department with pneumonia and bronchitis. The parents and their other child have no significant medical history. Vitals: temperature: 39.0°C (102.2°F), heart rate: 180 beats per minute, respiratory rate: 66 breaths per minute. Chest X-ray reveals consolidation in the right upper lobe. Physical exam notes that the child has fair skin, grey eyes, and light hair, but otherwise appears normal. The results of a CBC reveal minor neutropenia. Based on the most likely diagnosis, which of the following would most likely also be observed from a CBC in this patient?

A. Presence of Auer rods in a blast form

B. Small, dense hyperchromic RBCs

C. Elevated numbers of mononuclear cells with little cytoplasm

D. Abnormally small platelets

E. Giant azurophilic cytoplasmic granules in granulocytes

49. A 4-month-old boy is brought to a specialist due to recurrent and severe respiratory and skin infections, predominantly caused by *Staphylococcus* and *Streptococcus* species. His parents report that they have no significant medical issues and their other 4-year-old son has no medical problems. Physical exam reveals a relatively healthy looking child with fair skin and white hair with a metallic sheen. Based on the information above, what is the likelihood that their next son will have the same disease?

A. 0%

B. 25%

C. 50%

D. 75%

E. 100%

50. A 3-week-old boy is brought to the emergency department by his parents with a chief complaint of fever and fussiness of 2 days' duration. The boy was born at 39 weeks of gestation, weighed 3.2 kg, and seemed healthy. Vital signs reveal a temperature of 39°C (102.2°F). Physical exam shows abdominal distention, and omphalitis with no discharge. Gram stain of a biopsy specimen from the base of the umbilical stump reveals gram-negative bacilli. Which of the following cell types would be absent in an immunohistological analysis of a biopsy from the infected site?

A. NK cells

B. B cells

C. Neutrophils

D. T cells

E. Eosinophils

51. Individuals with leukocyte adhesion deficiency (LAD) are highly susceptible to which of the following pathogens?

A. Enveloped viruses

B. Helminths

C. Encapsulated organisms

D. Intracellular fungi

E. Protozoa

52. A 4-month-old girl presents to the immunology specialist's office with her parents with a chief concern of red ulcerative lesions. Patient history is significant in that she has been seen multiple times by her pediatrician for ulcers which started out as small erythematous papules that have now coalesced to form deep ulcerations with necrotic borders, despite topical antibiotic treatment. The child also had a delayed loss of her umbilical cord stump. A complete blood cell analysis reveals leukocytosis, with normal percentages of B cells and T cells and significantly elevated numbers of neutrophils. Which of the following is the most likely diagnosis?

A. Bare lymphocyte syndrome (BLS)

B. Chronic granulomatous disease (CGD)

C. Kostmann's syndrome

D. Myeloperoxidase deficiency

E. Leukocyte adhesion deficiency (LAD)

53. A consanguineous couple present to a genetics counselor to discuss the possibility of having a child with an inherited genetic disease. While each of them have no significant medical history, they reveal that a common relative had died early in life due to overwhelming infections and was diagnosed with severe leukocyte adhesion deficiency (LAD). The couple eventually has a child and LAD is suspected. Flow cytometry of the baby's blood cells is ordered. The absence of cells expressing which of the following markers would best confirm the diagnosis of LAD?

A. CD3

B. CD18

C. CD20

D. CD56

E. CD95

54. A 7-month-old boy is brought to the emergency department by his parents due to a fever and persistent cough of 1-week duration. Patient history is significant for multiple trips to the emergency department for pneumonia and severe otitis media, with his first presentation being at 7 weeks of age with *Pneumocystis jirovecii* pneumonia. At the time of the exam, the boy has a temperature of 39.7°C (103.5°F), a heart rate of 180 beats per minute, and a respiratory rate of 65 breaths per minute. Chest X-ray reveals consolidation in the right upper lobe. Laboratory blood tests reveal low levels of neutrophils, with normal T and B cell numbers, and the following serological results shown below:

	Reported	Normal range
Total blood complement	56 hemolytic units	41–90 hemolytic units
C1	22 mg/dL	16–33 mg/dL
C3	135 mg/dL	88–252 mg/dL
IgG	100 mg/dL	650–1,500 mg/dL
IgM	525 mg/dL	40–345 mg/dL
IgA	0 mg/dL	76–390 mg/dL
IgE	0 IU/mL	0–380 IU/mL

Based on the information given, this child likely has a mutation in which of the following genes?

A. *CD40L*

B. *ATM*

C. *TACI*

D. *BTK*

E. *STAT3*

55. A 9-month-old boy is brought to the emergency department by his parents due to a fever and a cough that has progressively gotten worse over the last 2 weeks. Patient history is significant for multiple trips to the emergency department for pneumonia and severe sinusitis. At the time of the exam, the boy has a temperature of 38.9°C (102.0°F), a heart rate of 175 beats per minute, and a respiratory rate of 70 breaths per minute. Chest auscultation demonstrates significant bilateral crackles with expiratory wheezes and rhonchi. A chest radiograph shows bilateral, symmetrical hilar interstitial shadowing. Laboratory blood tests reveal low levels of neutrophils, with normal T and B cell numbers, and the following serological results shown below.

	Reported	Normal range
Total blood complement	56 hemolytic units	41–90 hemolytic units
C1	22 mg/dL	16–33 mg/dL
C3	135 mg/dL	88–252 mg/dL
IgG	25 mg/dL	650–1,500 mg/dL
IgM	725 mg/dL	40–345 mg/dL
IgA	0 mg/dL	76–390 mg/dL
IgE	0 IU/mL	0–380 IU/mL

Based on the most likely diagnosis, this individual is at the highest risk for infections with which of the following?

A. *Mycobacterium tuberculosis*

B. *Candida albicans*

C. Human papillomavirus

D. *Streptococcus pneumoniae*

E. *Aspergillus fumigatus*

56. A 9-month-old boy is brought to an immunology specialist due to his repeated respiratory infections, which have resulted in multiple admissions to the hospital. Physical exam reveals a child that is small for his age with both lymphadenopathy and hepatosplenomegaly. However, the child appears normal without any additional motor or physical abnormality. Significant laboratory findings are below:

Lymphocyte counts	Reported	Normal range
Total lympho-cyte count	3.41×10^9/L	$2.5–5.0 \times 10^9$ c/L
T lymphocytes (CD3)	2.7×10^3/μL	$1.5–3.0 \times 10^3$/μL
B lymphocytes (CD20)	0.6×10^3/μL	$0.3–1.0 \times 10^3$/μL
Immunoglobulin panel		
IgG	48 mg/dL	650–1,500 mg/dL
IgM	625 mg/dL	40–345 mg/dL
IgA	5 mg/dL	76–390 mg/dL
IgE	0 IU/mL	0–380 IU/mL

Based on the most likely diagnosis, which of the following lab results is most likely to be seen in this patient?

A. Decreased memory B cells

B. Antigen-presenting cells lacking HLA class I

C. High levels of alpha-fetoprotein (AFP)

D. Antibodies specific for IgA

E. Presence of p24 antigen

57. An 11-month-old boy is brought to the emergency department with a low-grade fever with a significant cough of 3 days' duration. Patient history is significant for five previous visits to the emergency department with pneumonia, an abscess, sepsis, cellulitis, and abnormal wound healing. Physical exam reveals a normal-looking child with a temperature of 37.8°C (100°F), mild chest retraction, and rales in both lungs. Results from a bronchial lavage examination indicate the presence of *A. fumigatus*. CBC is normal, with lymphocyte and immunoglobulin levels in the normal range for his age. Examination of peripheral blood neutrophils by nitroblue tetrazolium (NBT) reduction test is negative. Based on this information, this patient most likely has

A. Leukocyte adhesion deficiency (LAD)

B. Job's syndrome

C. Chronic granulomatous disease (CGD)

D. Chédiak–Higashi syndrome

E. Toll-like receptor (TLR) deficiency

58. A 5-month-old boy was brought to the emergency department by his mother with a chief complaint of a scaly and dry rash of 6 weeks' duration and a huge "blister" on the child's leg. Patient history is significant for a previous abscess that required hospitalization, which grew *Staphylococcus aureus* upon culture. Additionally, the child was hospitalized with pneumonia at 4 months of age, which was also caused by *S. aureus*. Vital signs are normal, but physical exam reveals eczematic lesions, generalized lymphadenopathy, facial dysmorphism, and a 3-cm abscess, which lacks redness and warmth. CBC reveals no significant abnormalities, except for eosinophilia (40% of total WBC count). Based on the information given, what is the most likely diagnosis for the underlying cause of this child's presentation?

A. Severe atopic dermatitis

B. Wiskott–Aldrich syndrome

C. Job's syndrome

D. Severe combined immunodeficiency (SCID) syndrome

E. Omenn's syndrome

59. A 12-month-old boy is brought to the emergency department by his parents with a chief concern of numerous lesions on his neck, face, and upper chest of 5 days' duration. Patient history is significant for multiple admissions to the hospital for abscesses or respiratory infections caused by *Staphylococcus aureus*. Also, the patient's father has had similar issues with recurrent abscesses that are controlled by the constant treatment with antibiotics. Vital signs are normal and physical exam reveals multiple abscesses with mild cervical lymphadenopathy. Additionally, the child had facial abnormalities that included deep-set eyes, a protruding forehead, and a broad nasal base. Laboratory values indicate normal cellular distribution, except for eosinophilia, and an immunoglobulin panel reveals elevated levels of IgE. Based on the most likely diagnosis, this patient most likely has an inherent deficit in the ability to generate

A. Th1 cells

B. Th2 cells

C. Th9 cells

D. Th17 cells

E. Treg cells

60. A 7-month-old girl is brought to her pediatrician's office by her mother with a chief concern that her daughter has bumps on her face, neck, and scalp. Patient history is significant for multiple trips to the pediatrician's office for abscesses that culture out gram-positive cocci in clusters. Additionally, she has a brother who also is consistently in the pediatrician's office with similar symptoms. Vital signs are normal. Physical exam reveals cervical lymphadenopathy, and multiple abscesses on the face, neck, and scalp. Based on the most likely diagnosis of the underlying disease in this child, which of the following lab results is most likely to be seen in this patient?

A. Decreased IgE levels

B. Elevated B cell numbers

C. Increased glucose-6-phosphate dehydrogenase levels

D. Decreased complement levels

E. Elevated eosinophil numbers

61. A 3-month-old boy is brought to the emergency department by his father with a fever, cough, and a rash covering the majority of his body of 5 days' duration. Patient history is significant for two other respiratory infections, chronic diarrhea, and no significant weight gain since birth. At the time of exam, the boy has a temperature of 38.9°C (102°F), a respiratory rate of 45 breaths per minute, and a heart rate of 110 beats per minute. Physical exam shows lymphadenopathy and hepatosplenomegaly. Significant bilateral crackles with expiratory wheezes are observed upon auscultation, and chest X-ray reveals bimodal consolidation and the presence of a thymic shadow. Additionally, over half of the child's skin has erythroderma and desquamation. The child's lab values are as follows:

Complete blood count (CBC)	Reported	Normal
Erythrocyte count	4.8 million/mm^3	4.3–5.9 million/mm^3
Platelet count	300,000/mm^3	150,000–400,000/mm^3
Neutrophils	61%	54–62%
Eosinophils	5%	1–3%
Total lymphocytes	5%	25–33%
T lymphocytes (CD3)	0.4 × 10^3/μL	1.5–3.0 × 10^3/μL
CD4:CD8 ratio	100:1	2:1
B lymphocytes (CD20)	0.01 × 10^3/μL	0.3–1.0 × 10^3/μL

Based on the most likely diagnosis, which of the following genes is most likely mutated in this child?

A. *ADA*

B. *RAG1/2*

C. *STAT3*

D. *WASP*

E. *ZAP-70*

62. A 3-month-old boy is brought to an immunology specialist with a history of failure to thrive, chronic diarrhea, repeated respiratory infections, erythroderma, and desquamation. Based solely on this information, which of the following lab results would be most consistent with the most likely preliminary diagnosis?

A. Loss of all lymphocytes

B. Thrombocytopenia

C. Presence of polyclonal self-reactive T cells

D. Eosinophilia

E. Neutropenia

63. A 32-day-old baby is brought to the emergency department by her parents with a chief complaint of fever, wheezing, and a rash. The child was born at full term after an uncomplicated pregnancy. Patient history includes a previous hospitalization at 16 days in which the child was treated for seborrheic dermatitis with a secondary bacterial infection. He was treated with systemic antibiotics and a cortisone treatment and then released from the hospital. At the time of exam, the child has a temperature of 39.4°C (103°F), a respiratory rate of 45 breaths per minute, and a heart rate of 110 beats per minute. Physical exam shows lymphadenopathy and hepatosplenomegaly. Expiratory wheezes are observed upon auscultation and chest X-ray indicates consolidation in the right upper lobe. Additionally, over half of the child's skin has erythroderma and desquamation. After initial treatment for the immediate condition, what is the most appropriate long-term management for this patient to treat the underlying condition?

A. A bone marrow transplant

B. Regular human immune serum globulin (HISG) injections

C. A thymus transplant

D. Regular GM-CSF injections

E. Systemic corticosteroid treatments

64. A 3-year-old girl presents to her pediatrician's office with her mother for her annual checkup. Patient history is significant for recurrent pneumonia and bronchitis. Vital signs are normal, but physical exam reveals red capillaries that are spidery in appearance on the side of the face and neck. Additional observations note that the child is delayed in speech and has difficulty standing without wobbling. Based on the information given, this child is at the greatest risk for developing

A. Lymphoma

B. A skin infection with *Staphylococcus aureus*

C. An autoimmune disease

D. Anemia

E. A granuloma

65. A 10-year-old boy is brought to the emergency department with a fever and significant cough. Patient history is significant for repeated bouts with pneumonia that have resulted in hospital admissions. The patient is wheelchair bound, due to a progressive difficulty in walking. His parents have no significant medical history, but they have another child that is 5 years of age with recurrent respiratory infections, convulsions, and difficulty walking. The child's temperature is 38.9°C (102°F), heart rate is 145 beats per minute, and respiratory rate is 45 breaths per minute. The physician also notices dilated blood vessels on the bulbar conjunctivae and the left side of the child's face. Chest X-ray indicates consolidation in the left upper lobe. Complete blood cell count is significant for markedly decreased numbers of both B and T lymphocytes and a slight neutropenia. Based on the information given, what is the most likely underlying cause of this child's presentation?

A. ZAP-70 deficiency

B. Omenn's syndrome

C. Bare lymphocyte syndrome (BLS)

D. Ataxia-telangiectasia

E. Wiskott–Aldrich syndrome

66. A 19-month-old girl presents to the pediatrician's office with her mother with the chief complaint that the child has been severely irritable and has been tugging at her left ear. Patient history is significant for recurrent respiratory infections. The mother points out that the child is still not walking and is wobbly when standing, and postulates that this could be due to the ear infection. Vital signs are normal and physical examination reveals dilated blood vessels on the bulbar conjunctivae. Otoscope exam reveals an opaque, erythematous, tympanic membrane. Lab values are listed below:

Complete blood count (CBC)	Reported	Normal
Total lymphocyte count	1.0	2.5–5.0
T lymphocytes (CD3)	0.4	1.5–3.0
CD4:CD8 ratio	1:10	2:1
B lymphocytes (CD20)	0.1	0.3–1.0

Based on the information provided, which of the following processes in this patient is most likely defective?

A. Repair of double-stranded DNA breaks

B. Antigen presentation

C. Cytoskeletal reorganization

D. Isotype switch

E. T cell receptor signaling

67. An 8-week-old boy is brought to the emergency department by his parents with a chief complaint of fever and chronic bloody diarrhea. Patient history is significant for diabetic ketoacidosis, chronic diarrhea, and failure to thrive at 5 weeks of age. Vital signs indicate a temperature of 38.3°C (101°F) and physical exam reveals eczematic patches on his face. Biopsies taken during an endoscopy demonstrate villous atrophy and inflammation. Laboratory results reveal:

Complete blood count (CBC)	Reported	Normal
Erythrocyte count	5.2 million/mm^3	4.3–5.9 million/mm^3
Platelet count	180,000/mm^3	150,000–400,000/mm^3
Neutrophils	57%	54–62%
Eosinophils	6%	1–3%
Total lymphocytes	32%	25–33%
T lymphocytes (CD3)	1.7 × 10^3/μL	1.5–3.0 × 10^3/μL
B lymphocytes (CD20)	0.9 × 10^3/μL	0.3–1.0 × 10^3/μL
IgG	1,000 mg/dL	650–1,500 mg/dL
IgM	80 mg/dL	40–345 mg/dL
IgA	90 mg/dL	76–390 mg/dL
IgE	720 IU/mL	0–380 IU/mL

Based on the information presented, which of the following genes is most likely mutated in this child?

A. *RAG1/2*

B. *FASL*

C. *AIRE*

D. *NOD2*

E. *FOXP3*

68. A 12-week-old boy is brought back to the pediatrician's office with chronic diarrhea, a rash on his stomach, and a generalized malaise. Patient history is significant for repeated visits for refractive diarrhea and two hospitalizations for pneumonia. Vital signs are normal and physical exam reveals an infant with an eczematic rash on his abdomen, poor muscle tone, brittle hair, and a puffy face. Laboratory results demonstrate the following:

Complete blood count (CBC)	Reported	Normal
Erythrocyte count	4.3 million/mm^3	4.3–5.9 million/mm^3
Platelet count	285,000/mm^3	150,000–400,000/mm^3
Neutrophils	57%	54–62%
Eosinophils	7%	1–3%
Total lymphocytes	28%	25–33%
T lymphocytes (CD3)	1.7 × 10^3/μL	1.5–3.0 × 10^3/μL
B lymphocytes (CD20)	0.9 × 10^3/μL	0.3–1.0 × 10^3/μL
IgG	900 mg/dL	650–1,500 mg/dL
IgM	72 mg/dL	40–345 mg/dL
IgA	95 mg/dL	76–390 mg/dL
IgE	575 IU/mL	0–380 IU/mL
TSH	8 mU/mL	0.5–5.0 mU/mL
Free T4	2.5 mg/mL	5–12 mg/mL

Based on the most likely diagnosis, which of the following cell types is significantly decreased in this patient?

A. Th1 cells

B. Th2 cells

C. Th17 cells

D. Treg cells

E. Tfh cells

69. A 4-month-old boy is brought to the emergency department by his parents concerned with the child's vomiting and difficulty keeping the child awake. Patient history is significant for recurrent diarrhea, impaired weight gain, eczema, and two previous trips to the emergency department with pneumonia. Physical exam reveals a child that is small for his age, sunken eyes, dry mucous membranes, impaired consciousness, and breath that smells of ketones. Laboratory findings identify high levels of eosinophils, IgE, and the presence of anti-islet antibodies. Which of the following cell types is most likely to be decreased in this patient?

A. CD4+CD25+

B. CD16+CD56+

C. CD20+CD138+

D. CD8+CD95+

E. CD4+CD154+

70. A 14-week-old boy is diagnosed with early-onset thyroiditis and refractory diarrhea. A complete blood cell count and serum analysis reveals eosinophilia and high levels of IgE with a normal distribution of all other cell types. Based on the information given, which of the following findings would be most consistent with the most likely diagnosis?

A. Silver hair and light colored-eyes

B. Hypercellularity of the bone marrow

C. Eczematic lesions on the skin

D. Clefting of the palate

E. Lack of a thymic shadow

71. A 24-month-old boy is brought to his pediatrician by his mother for his annual physical. His mother claims that he has been less active lately and bruises easily. Patient history is significant for a year-long history of lymphadenopathy and splenomegaly. Vital signs are normal, but physical exam reveals a child that has multiple bruises and poor pallor. Laboratory results indicate the following:

Complete blood count (CBC)	Reported	Normal
Erythrocyte count	3.1 million/mm^3	4.3–5.9 million/mm^3
Platelet count	90,000/mm^3	150,000–400,000/mm^3
Neutrophils	60%	54–62%
Eosinophils	5%	1–3%
Total lymphocytes	50%	25–33%
T lymphocytes (CD3)	3.8×10^3/µL	1.5–3.0×10^3/µL
B lymphocytes (CD20)	1.8×10^3/µL	0.3–1.0×10^3/µL
IgG	2,200 mg/dL	650–1,500 mg/dL
IgM	185 mg/dL	40–345 mg/dL
IgA	500 mg/dL	76–390 mg/dL
IgE	495 IU/mL	0–380 IU/mL
Coombs' test	3+	

Based on the most likely diagnosis, analysis of the T cell repertoire would most likely reveal the presence of a high percentage of T cells with which of the following phenotypes?

A. CD4−CD8-

B. CD4−CD8+

C. CD4+CD25+

D. CD4+CD154-

E. CD4+BTLA+

72. A 12-month-old boy is admitted to the hospital with pneumonia. Patient history is significant for splenomegaly and hepatomegaly since 2 months after birth. He has been brought to the emergency department twice for pneumonitis caused by cytomegalovirus (CMV) infection. Physical exam reveals general lymphadenopathy and eczema on his chest and arms. His lab results indicate that he has anemia, thrombocytopenia, and increased levels of IgG, IgA, and IgE isotypes, and is positive by Coombs' test. Based on the information given, this child most likely is defective in which of the following?

A. CD40 ligand

B. STAT3

C. FAS

D. WASP

E. Transmembrane activator and CAML interactor (TACI)

73. A 2-year-old girl is referred to a specialist after a mutation in FAS was identified upon genetic screening. Patient history is significant for anemia, thrombocytopenia, and generalized lymphadenopathy. This patient is at an increased risk for developing

A. Hodgkin's lymphoma

B. Type I diabetes

C. Crohn's disease

D. *Neisseria* infections

E. Ataxia

74. A 24-month-old girl is brought to the pediatrician's office by her parents due to a recurrent fever and a rash. Patient history is significant for recurrent thrush as an infant. At the time of exam, the child's temperature is 38.1°C (100.5°F). Physical exam reveals that the child has dry, puffy skin with an urticaria-like rash on her abdomen. Her hair is short and brittle, as are her nails, which are raised, yellow, and have transverse grooves. Laboratory results reveal the presence of antibodies against CaSR (calcium-sensing receptor). Based on her underlying condition, which of the following is this child most likely to develop?

A. Adrenal insufficiency

B. Eosinophilia

C. Silver hair

D. Cleft palate

E. Eczema

75. A 12-year-old girl presents to her pediatrician for her annual physical. Patient history is significant for chronic mucocutaneous candidiasis (CMC), hyperparathyroidism, and adrenal insufficiency. Her parents have no significant medical history. Based on this information alone, what is the most likely underlying mutation in this individual?

A. *STAT1*

B. *ZAP-70*

C. *AIRE*

D. *Myeloperoxidase*

E. *STAT3*

76. A 16-year-old boy presents to the emergency department with abdominal pain and stridor. Physical examination is significant for defined areas of subcutaneous edema on his arms. The patient denies any pruritus associated with the skin lesions. This patient has presented to the emergency department before with similar symptoms, as has his sister and mother. Results of a CBC are normal and immunoglobulin levels are within the normal range. Which of the following substances is most likely absent in this patient?

A. Properdin

B. Myeloperoxidase

C. STAT3

D. C1 inhibitor (C1INH)

E. NADPH oxidase

77. An 18-year-old woman presents to the emergency department due to significant swelling of her lips and tongue. Patient history is significant for having her wisdom tooth extracted earlier that day. The patient denies eating anything unusual and/or wearing new makeup. Vital signs are normal, and physical examination reveals subcutaneous edema of her tongue and lips, which are not itchy. There is no additional sign of a rash. The patient says that her lips and tongue "tingled" and felt full before she felt the sites swelling over the next 3 hours. Her mother and paternal grandfather also have similar issues when they had dental work done. Which of the following is the best treatment for this patient?

A. Epinephrine

B. Recombinant C1INH

C. Antihistamines

D. Bradykinin β2-receptor agonist

E. Leukotriene inhibitor

78. A 9-year-old girl is brought to her pediatrician's office because she has complained of being tired and "achy" and has had a low-grade fever on and off for 6 weeks. Patient history is significant for recurrent infections with *Streptococcus pneumoniae*. At the time of exam, the girl's temperature is 38.3°C (101°F) and physical exam demonstrates lymphadenopathy, swelling of the joints of her hands, and a malar rash on her face. Based on the most likely diagnosis, this child is most likely deficient in which of the following?

A. Complement 3 (C3)

B. IFN-α

C. CD40 ligand

D. Complement 9 (C9)

E. IL-17

79. A 12-year-old boy presents to the emergency department with meningitis that is determined to be caused by *Neisseria meningitides*. Due to the severity of his disease, it was determined that his CH50 was normal, indicating that his classical pathway of complement is fine. His AH50, analyzing the alternate pathway of complement, is low. The function of the protein that is most likely missing in this child is to:

A. Stabilize the C3 convertase of the alternative pathway

B. Destabilize the active C1 into C1q, C1r, and C1s

C. Act as an opsonin and form the C5 convertase

D. Compete with factor B for binding to surface-bound C3b

E. Prevent polymerization of C9 and formation of membrane attack complex (MAC)

80. A 12-month-old girl is brought to the emergency department by her parents with a 2-day history of cough and fever. Patient history is significant for repeated rhinitis and pneumonia. Vital signs reveal a temperature of 38.9°C (102°F), a heart rate of 170 beats per minute, and a respiratory rate of 63 breaths per minute. Chest X-ray reveals consolidation in the left upper lobe. Peripheral blood analysis reveals only a severe reduction in the number of T cells in the blood, with a complete loss of CD8+ T cells and normal numbers of CD4+ T cells. Further analysis reveals that the CD4+ T cells proliferate in response to stimuli. Based on the information given, which of the following laboratory results are most consistent with the most likely diagnosis of this patient's underlying condition?

A. Hypogammaglobulinemia by enzyme immunoassay

B. Decreased HLA class I expression by flow cytometry

C. Giant azurophilic granules in neutrophils

D. Positive for HIV RNA genomes by reverse transcription PCR (RT-PCR)

E. Decreased CH50 by complement assay

81. A 6-month-old girl is brought to the emergency department by her parents with a fever and cough of 1-day duration. Patient history is significant for four visits to the emergency department with pneumonia and chronic diarrhea. Vital signs reveal a temperature of 38.9°C (102°F), a heart rate of 177 beats per minute, and a respiratory rate of 68 breaths per minute. Chest X-ray reveals bilateral consolidation. Peripheral blood analysis reveals only a severe reduction in the number of CD4+ T cells in the blood, with no deficiency in the number of CD8+ T cells and B cells. Immunoglobulin levels of all isotypes are below normal levels. Which of the following is most likely the underlying cause of this child's presentation?

A. ZAP-70 deficiency

B. Bruton's XLA

C. Wiskott–Aldrich syndrome

D. HLA class II deficiency

E. Common variable immunodeficiency (CVID)

4.2 Answers and Explanations

Easy	Medium	Hard

1. Correct: Human immune serum globulin (HISG) (C)

(**C**) The patient has Bruton's XLA and the treatment for these individuals is monthly injections with human immune serum globulin (HISG). (**A**) is incorrect since the patient's deficiency is in the production of B cells and therefore antibodies (serum immunoglobulins). Providing additional complement will not help this patient due to the loss of the classical complement pathway. (**B**) This answer is incorrect, because recombinant G-CSF is used to treat neutropenia, and since the lab indicates that the patient's neutrophil numbers are elevated (due to the infection), this treatment would not be helpful. (**D**) This answer is incorrect, because CTLA-4Ig fusion protein (such as abatacept and belatacept) inhibits T cell activation by blocking the interaction of CD28 on T cells with CD80 or CD86 on antigen-presenting cells. This is ineffective in treating this patient as it is not a T cell defect. CTLA4Ig is FDA-approved for use in severe-to-moderate adult rheumatoid arthritis and juvenile idiopathic arthritis, and is in clinical trials to treat other conditions. (**E**) This answer is incorrect, because recombinant human IFN-γ is used to treat patients who have deficiencies in intracellular killing of pathogens, such as chronic granulomatous disease (CGD). The rIFN-γ increases the activation state of macrophages and other phagocytes to help patients with phagocytic immunodeficiencies, not B cell deficiencies.

2. Correct: *Bruton's tyrosine kinase (BTK)* (B)

(**B**) Many genetic mutations responsible for the loss of immune function are now being identified. BTK is a critical protein in the pre-B cell receptor signaling pathway that is required for the differentiation of pre-B cells into immature B cells. With an absent or nonfunctional *BTK* gene, there is no signal generated by the μ heavy chain complexed with the surrogate light chain (pre-BCR), so developing B cells are arrested at the pre-B cell stage. (**A**) This answer is incorrect, because mutations in *CD40L* lead to hyper-IgM syndrome, which result in serum levels containing high levels of IgM, but little to no other isotypes. This is because CD40L (CD154) on the T cell must interact with CD40 on B cells to induce isotype switch. (**C**) This answer is incorrect, because mutations in *STAT3* are associated with Job's syndrome or HIES . This patient does not have B cells and therefore are unable to produce IgE. (**D**) This answer is incorrect because the lab values are not consistent with an individual with ZAP-70 deficiency. ZAP-70 is an important molecule in the T cell receptor signaling pathway. Individuals with two mutated copies of *ZAP-70* will have a loss of CD8+ T cells, with the presence of nonfunctional CD4+ T cells. Since the patient has normal levels of CD8+ T cells, this is not consistent with the lab results. (**E**) This answer is incorrect, because mutations in *ATM* are associated with ataxia-telangiectasia. These patients have low numbers of both B and T cell numbers, which is inconsistent with the lab results. In addition, individuals with mutations in ATM also have neurological and other organ system involvement.

3. Correct: Immunoelectrophoresis (A)

(**A**) The patient's diagnosis is consistent with hypogammaglobulinemia due to the recurrent infections with encapsulated gram-positive bacteria, *Streptococcus pneumoniae*, and due to the fact that the infections began after the loss of maternal Ig protection from breastfeeding. Additional information demonstrating the lack of B cells also suggests that the individual will be deficient in serum immunoglobulins (antibodies). Immunoelectrophoresis, which separates serum proteins based on size and charge, followed by immunoprecipitation with antihuman sera (human antiglobulin) would result in the absence of a precipitation band in the gamma globulin fraction, thereby confirming the lack of immunoglobulins in this patient. (**B**) This answer is incorrect, because PCR only amplifies cellular DNA. Incidentally, an XLA patient is likely PCR positive for the immunoglobulin gene (i.e., normal). (**C**) The Western blot is a highly specific test: it can measure antigen-specific antibodies, but not general immunoglobulins. Western blot is sometimes used to test for the presence of the BTK protein in XLA, but is not the best answer. (**D**) This answer is incorrect, because the electrophoretic mobility shift assay (EMSA) looks for the ability of transcription factors to bind to DNA. (E) This answer is incorrect because a direct immunofluorescence assay (DFA) is used to assess the presence of an antigen bound to cells or tissues. It is used to detect the presence of immune complexes bound to kidney tissue in systemic lupus erythematosus (SLE).

4. Correct: Decreased number of pre-B cells (A)

(**A**) The individual suffers from Bruton's XLA due to a mutation in the *BTK* gene. *BTK* encodes for BTK, which is an important signaling molecule through the pre-B cell receptor. During the pro-B cell stage, the rearranged μ heavy chain assembles with the surrogate light chain to form the pre-BCR. Expression of the pre-BCR on the cell surface indicates the cells transition to a pre-B cell. The pre-BCR induces a signaling cascade that utilizes BTK to promote proliferation and differentiation of the pre-B cell to an immature B cell. Therefore, in boys with a BTK deficiency, the pre-BCR signal is not generated so the pre-B cells cannot proliferate, resulting in decreased numbers of pre-B cells. (**B**) This answer is incorrect, since the block in development occurs *after* the pre-B cell stage so the number of upstream hematopoietic stem cells and pro-B cells are normal. (**C**) This answer is incorrect, because as stated above, the pre-B cells cannot become immature B cells. (**D**) This answer is incorrect, since the block in development occurs *after* the pre-B cell stage so the number of upstream hematopoietic stem cells and pro-B cells are normal. (**E**) This answer is incorrect; one would expect no plasma cells in the bone marrow since their precursors, the mature B cell, are not being produced. Interestingly, Bruton's XLA is considered a "leaky" defect since almost all patients have some serum immunoglobulin (particularly IgM) and a few (<1%) circulating mature B cells (primarily IgM+). This is thought to result from pre-BCR signals from other tyrosine kinases that compensate for the absence of BTK.

5. Correct: Epstein–Barr virus (EBV) (D)

(**D**) Individuals with Bruton's XLA are deficient in mature B cells due to an inability to develop past the pre-B cell stage. EBV infects mature, peripheral B cells and ultimately remains latent in this cell type. In the absence of B cells, individuals with this immunodeficiency are highly resistant to infection with EBV. (**A**) This answer is incorrect, because cytomegalovirus (CMV) can infect numerous cell types, including epithelial and endothelial cells, fibroblasts, and lymphocytes. Therefore, a deficiency in B cells does not provide resistance to infection with CMV. (**B**) This answer is incorrect, because HSV-2 infects epithelial and neuronal cells, not B cells. (**C**) This answer is incorrect, because hepatitis B has a high tropism for hepatocytes, not B cells. There is some indication that chronic hepatitis B can contribute to the development of B cell lymphomas, but there is no indication that B cell immunodeficiency prevents individuals from hepatitis B infection. (**E**) This answer is incorrect because HIV infects CD4+ T lymphocytes, not B cells.

6. Correct: 50% (C)

Inheritance pattern for X-linked inherited diseases

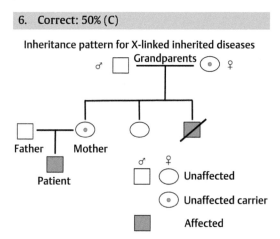

(**C**) The child suffers from Bruton's XLA, which is an X-linked recessive disease. Based on mendelian genetics, the child has a 50% chance of receiving the X chromosome that contains the BTK mutant from the mother. (**A**) This answer is incorrect, because the mother is a carrier and therefore there is a statistical chance of passing on the mutated BTK gene. (**B, D**) These answers are incorrect, because X-linked recessive diseases cannot be inherited in that pattern. (**E**) This answer is incorrect, because for the likelihood to be 100%, the mother would have to carry two BTK mutated X chromosomes. If she did have two mutated X chromosomes at the BTK locus, she would demonstrate symptoms. Since she is healthy, she is a carrier.

7. Correct: Chromosome 22 (E)

(**E**) The infant has pneumonia caused by *Pneumocystis jirovecii* and ultimately suffers from DiGeorge's syndrome. DiGeorge's syndrome is caused by a deletion in chromosome 22 (22q11.2 region). This deletion causes a defect in the development of the third and fourth pharyngeal pouches during development and results in abnormal thymus development, as well as hypoparathyroidism, and cardiovascular and facial anomalies. (**A**) This answer is incorrect in that chromosome 2 is associated with mutations in *ZAP-70*. Individuals with ZAP-70 deficiency have an immunodeficiency that results in the loss of CD8+ T cells, with the production of nonfunctional CD4+ T cells. The size of the thymus may be decreased in ZAP-70 individuals, but is not typically absent. (**B**) This answer is incorrect, since chromosome 11 is the location of the genes encoding the RAG proteins. A mutation and/or deletion in the genes encoding the RAG proteins results in the loss of both B and T cells, and can be associated with the development of Omenn's syndrome. (**C**) This answer is incorrect, since chromosome 17 is the location of the *STAT3* gene, and mutations/deletions in this gene on chromosome 17 are associated with the development Job's syndrome (HIES), which

is not consistent with the current presentation. (**D**) This answer is incorrect, because chromosome 21 harbors the *AIRE* gene, which can cause the recessive form of chronic mucocutaneous candidiasis (CMC) when an individual inherits two mutated and/or deleted copies of this gene. These individuals harbor both B and T cells, but the T cells are unable to respond to *Candida*. In this case, the individual is not making any T cells, so the lab results are not consistent with this mutation.

8. Correct: CD3 (A)

(**A**) The patient has DiGeorge's syndrome, which manifests with abnormal thymus development, as well as hypoparathyroidism, cardiovascular, and facial anomalies. Due to the thymus being absent or hypoplastic in this individual (depending on the chromosome 22 deletion), T cells are unable to undergo T cell development and thus they will have no or low numbers of CD3+ T cells in the blood. (**B, D**) These answers are incorrect, because both CD16 and CD56 are found on NK cells that do not require the thymus for development. (**C**) This answer is incorrect, since CD20 is a B cell marker and B cell development occurs normally in patients with DiGeorge's syndrome. However, antibody responses are poor due to a lack of T cell help. (**E**) This answer is incorrect, as CD86 is a co-stimulatory molecule predominantly found on activated B cells and antigen-presenting cells.

9. Correct: DiGeorge's syndrome (C)

(**C**) The patient presents with classical symptoms of DiGeorge's syndrome: hypoparathyroidism, cardiovascular effects, a cleft palate, and low to no T cells due to no thymus or thymic hypoplasia. Individuals with DiGeorge's syndrome have a deletion in chromosome 22 (22q11.2 region), which results in a defect in the development of the third and fourth pharyngeal pouches during fetal development, which ultimately effects the development of facial structures, heart, thyroid, parathyroid, and thymic tissues. (**A**) This answer is incorrect, since ZAP-70 deficiency leads to an absence of CD8+ T cells, but normal numbers of nonfunctional CD4+ T cells. Additionally, ZAP-70 deficiency is not associated with the other symptoms presented. (**B**) This answer is not the best answer because, even though bare lymphocyte syndrome (BLS) can lead to the loss of T cells, the other symptoms are not consistent with BLS. (**D**) This answer is incorrect, since HIV infection leads to the specific loss of CD4+ T cells, not both CD4+ and CD8+ T cells. (**E**) This answer is incorrect, since ADA-SCID leads to the loss of both B and T cells. ADA deficiency results in the accumulation of toxic metabolites that kill developing B and T cells.

10. Correct: Bone marrow transplant (A)

(**A**) This individual suffers from ZAP-70 deficiency, which results in defective T cell receptor signaling.

73

T cell development is affected because the developing T cells are unable to undergo appropriate positive/negative selection. Individuals with ZAP-70 mutations have no to low numbers of CD8+ T cells, but generate normal to elevated numbers of CD4+ T cells that are nonfunctional. CD4+ T cells do not proliferate in response to mitogens, such as phytohemagglutinin. Since the genetic defect is inherent to the T cells, the only long-term cure for this child is a bone marrow transplant to introduce healthy precursor cells for normal T cell development. (**B**) This answer is incorrect, since HISG treatment is used as a treatment for B cell deficiencies and/or agammaglobulinemia. (**C**) This answer is incorrect, because as stated above, there is no overt problem with the thymus itself. Thymic transplant is an option for individuals with DiGeorge's syndrome, in which the defect is in development of the thymus. (**D**) This answer is incorrect, since GM-CSF is used to treat neutropenia to increase the number of circulating neutrophils, which is not the issue in this case. (**E**) This answer is incorrect, since corticosteroids are potent anti-inflammatories used to cause immunosuppression when the immune system is hyperactive and/or targeting self (autoimmunity). This individual is already immunosuppressed, so treating him with corticosteroids would dampen any remaining immune function and would not be appropriate.

11. Correct: ZAP-70 (A)

(**A**) The patient has a deficiency in ZAP-70, which causes an immunodeficiency that results in the absence of CD8+ T cells and the production of nonfunctional CD4+ T cells. ZAP-70 is a kinase that is required for signaling through the T cell receptor. In its absence, individuals are unable to develop CD8+ T cells, and the CD4+ T cells that are produced are nonfunctional in that they cannot adequately signal through the T cell receptor in response to antigen. (**B**) This answer is incorrect because the absence of HLA class II (as seen in some forms of bare lymphocyte syndrome [BLS]) results in the loss of CD4+ T cells. HLA class II is required for selection of developing CD4+ T cells in the thymus and the absence of HLA class II results in the inability to generate CD4+ T cells. Since this individual has CD4+ T cells in their peripheral blood, these lab results are not consistent with an HLA class II deficiency. (**C**) This answer is incorrect, because STAT3 deficiencies are associated with the development of Job's syndrome. This patient does not exhibit the symptoms associated with Job's syndrome, such as eczema and skin infections, and CD8+ T cells are present in patients with a STAT3 deficiency. (**D**) This answer is incorrect, because AIRE is associated with the recessive form of chronic mucocutaneous candidiasis (CMC). Patients with *AIRE* mutations present with normal numbers of T cells, but have issues with autoimmune responses and a propensity for recurrent candidal infections, which the patient does not exhibit. (**E**) This answer is

incorrect, because BTK is important in B cell development and its absence results in a block of B cell development at the pre-B cell stage. This individual has normal numbers of B cells by flow cytometry.

12. Correct: T cells (E)

(**E**) The child most likely has a T cell deficiency, including ZAP-70 deficiency. ZAP-70 deficiency generates inadequate signaling through the TCR during development in the thymus and results in the absence of CD8+ T cells and low numbers of nonfunctional CD4+ T cells. In the differential would also be DiGeorge's syndrome, but since the child does not exhibit additional characteristics associated with DiGeorge's syndrome (hypocalcemia, cleft palate, heart anomalies), ZAP-70 deficiency is more likely. (**A**) This answer is incorrect, because patients who have classic NK cell deficiency are characterized by severe, recurrent, or atypical herpes virus infection and papillomavirus infections. They have significant issues controlling infections with cytomegalovirus (CMV), varicella zoster virus, Herpes simplex virus (HSV), and Epstein–Barr virus (EBV). (**B**) This answer is incorrect, because individuals with deficiencies in neutrophils present with otitis media, oropharyngeal infections, respiratory infections, cellulitis, and skin infections, commonly due to gram-positive bacteria. While this child does have recurrent otitis media and pneumonia, this child is "failing to thrive," which is commonly seen in children with ZAP-70 deficiency and other children with T cell immunodeficiencies. (**C**) This answer is incorrect, because a lack of macrophages results in invasive fungal infections including histoplasmosis and aspergillosis and persistent human papillomavirus infections, as seen in the recently identified MonoMAC syndrome, which this patient does not have. Individuals with this syndrome additionally have a much later age of onset (mean > 30 years), whereas this patient is an infant. (**D**) This answer is not the best answer, because individuals with B cell deficiencies usually present beyond 4 to 6 months of age due the presence of maternal antibodies acquired during gestation and through breastfeeding. Additionally, while infants with B cell deficiencies may present with otitis media, sinusitis, and recurrent pneumonia, issues with fungal infections are uncommon.

13. Correct: T cell receptor signaling (E)

(**E**) This infant has ZAP-70 deficiency, which results in deficient signaling through the T cell receptor. ZAP-70 is a kinase that transmits signals after TCR engagement to induce normal T cell development and T cell activation. Individuals with this deficiency demonstrate an inability to control live attenuated vaccines and present with opportunistic infections. Furthermore, these patients do not produce CD8+ T cells and produce CD4+ T cells that are nonfunctional in response to antigen, due to the inability to transduce signals generated from the TCR. (**A**) This answer is incorrect, because individuals with the inability to repair double-stranded DNA breaks result in the loss of both B cells and T cells, as recombination of immunoglobulin and the T cell receptor requires repair of double-stranded DNA breaks. Since this individual has normal B cell numbers and a deficiency in only CD8+ T cells, this process is unlikely to be defective. (**B**) This answer is incorrect, because when antigen presentation is defective, T cell development is also affected since developing thymocytes are selected on HLA class I and II. Individuals with deficiencies in antigen presentation, such as bare lymphocyte syndrome (BLS), show overall decreases in T cell numbers, not just CD8+ T cells. (**C**) This answer is incorrect, because immunological deficiencies associated with cytoskeletal reorganization result in Wiskott–Aldrich syndrome. This X-linked immunodeficiency presents with normal numbers of B and T cells, but has eczema and opportunistic infections. Defective WASP is unlikely in this child, since the patient is female and there are deficiencies in T cells that would not be expected in Wiskott–Aldrich syndrome. (**D**) This answer is incorrect, because individuals with deficiencies in isotype switch (such as in X-linked hyper-IgM syndrome) have normal T cell numbers and present with recurrent bacterial infections with encapsulated bacteria. Defects in isotype switch are unlikely the overriding issue in this patient at this time, since IgM and IgA levels are normal in individuals with ZAP-70, and at 5 months, there is still residual maternal IgG to provide protection.

14. Correct: Proliferation of WBCs in response to concanavalin A (A)

(**A**) The patient has a T cell immunodeficiency caused by a mutation in *ZAP-70*. Individuals with this deficiency have difficulty controlling fungal infections, including pneumonia and diaper rash caused by *Candida*. Individuals with this immunodeficiency produce CD4+ T cells, but they do not respond to signals that require ZAP-70 for activation. Therefore, T cells from these patients are unable to respond to T cell mitogens, such as concanavalin A and phytohemagglutinin. However, T cells from these patients can proliferate to PMA + ionomycin, which bypass early T cell receptor signaling events, or IL-2, which induces T cell proliferation independent of ZAP-70. (**B**) This answer is incorrect, because individuals with ZAP-70 immunodeficiency have an intact complement system. Therefore, this diagnostic test with patient serum will result in the lysis of sheep RBC. (**C**) This answer is incorrect, because individuals with CD18 deficiency manifest with leukocyte adhesion deficiency (LAD). Common symptoms of LAD patients include delayed separation of the umbilical cord, recurrent bacterial infections on the skin and mucosal surfaces, and impaired wound healing. (**D**) This answer is incorrect, because the individuals with ZAP-70 deficiency generate B cells that are capable of producing immunoglobulin.

Immunoglobulin levels may vary between individuals with this disease, but they should have detectable immunoglobulin by immunoelectrophoresis. (**E**) This answer is incorrect, because ADA deficiency results in the loss of both B cells and T cells and presents with an SCID phenotype. While ZAP-70 deficiency has similar, but usually milder, features of SCID, this individual has a thymic shadow, which is not typically seen in SCID patients.

15. Correct: Have nonfunctional CD4+ T cells (D)

(**D**) Individuals with ZAP-70 deficiency produce CD4+ T cells, but they are nonfunctional since these T cells are unable to transmit signals through the TCR. In contrast, individuals with type I bare lymphocyte syndrome (BLS) have normal CD4+ T cell populations that are functional. Individuals with type I BLS have deficiencies in HLA class I presentation, so CD4+ T cells that recognize HLA class II are normal. (**A**) This answer is incorrect because patients with ZAP-70 deficiency and type I BLS typical both present before 2 years of age. (**B**) This answer is incorrect, because patients with both of these immunodeficiencies have decreased CD8+ T cell levels. In ZAP-70-deficient patients, the decrease in CD8+ T cells is due to the lack of TCR signaling by developing T cells that recognize HLA class I during development. In type I BLS, HLA class I is not expressed in these individuals and therefore CD8+ T cells do not develop during T cell development. (**C**) Individuals with ZAP-70 deficiency have nonfunctional CD4+ T cells and therefore these CD4+ T cells are ineffective in providing T cell help for isotype switch to IgG. Therefore, they have decreased levels of IgG. In contrast, individuals with type I BLS have normal levels of both IgM and IgG, because the only T cell subset that is absent/deficient in these individuals is CD8+ T cells, not CD4+ T cells. (**E**) This answer is incorrect, because individuals with mutations in ZAP-70 have normal HLA expression, since the defect is intrinsic to T cell signaling. Patients with type I BLS have a deficiency in HLA class I.

16. Correct: IgA deficiency syndrome (A)

(**A**) This patient has IgA deficiency, which is the most common genetic immunodeficiency. Patients with IgA deficiency have a loss of IgA at mucosal sites; therefore, they are highly susceptible to respiratory and mucosal infections. Additionally, they tend to have IgE-mediated symptoms, such as allergies and asthma, which are likely due to penetration of allergens across mucous membranes. (**B**) This answer is incorrect, because even though individuals with Wiskott–Aldrich syndrome manifest with recurrent respiratory infections, they typically exhibit with eczema and additional recurring opportunistic infections. Additionally, patients with Wiskott–Aldrich syndrome have thrombocytopenia with unusually small platelets. This patient has normal platelet numbers. (**C**) This answer is incorrect, because individuals with HIES (also known as Job's syndrome) present with eczema and recurrent infections with *Candida* and *Staphylococcus* and blood eosinophilia. As suggested by the syndrome name, these individuals have elevated levels of IgE in their serum. While elevations of IgE are seen in this patient, this patient does not demonstrate the eosinophilia found in HIES. (**D**) This answer is incorrect, because individuals with bare lymphocyte syndrome (BLS) present with all types of opportunistic infections, with no indication of allergies and/or asthma. Additionally, individuals with BLS have a decrease in T cell numbers, which is inconsistent with this individual's laboratory findings. (**E**) This answer is incorrect, because individuals with Kostmann's syndrome (also known as congenital agranulocytosis) have an almost complete lack of peripheral blood neutrophils, which is inconsistent with this patient's laboratory findings.

17. Correct: Systemic lupus erythematosus (A)

(**A**) Approximately 20 to 30% of individuals with IgA deficiency develop autoimmune disorders. Of the autoimmune diseases identified in IgA-deficient individuals, the most common are: systemic lupus erythematosus (SLE), Graves' disease, vitiligo, type I diabetes, immune thrombocytopenia, and both juvenile and adult-onset rheumatoid arthritis. (**B–E**) These answers are incorrect because they are not associated with individuals with IgA deficiency.

18. Correct: Influenza (B)

(**B**) The individual has an allergy to eggs. The influenza vaccine is produced in eggs and therefore the vaccine has residual egg products that could induce an allergic reaction. Newer formulations of the vaccine are made in cells, not eggs, and can be used in patients with egg allergies. (**A, C**) These answers are incorrect, because they are both recombinant vaccines in which limited viral proteins are produced in yeast. Therefore, the vaccine consists of viral proteins and some residual yeast proteins, which should not be harmful to this patient. (**D, E**) These answers are incorrect, because, even though they are live attenuated viruses, they are safe to administer to patients with IgA deficiency.

19. Correct: Type-matched whole blood (D)

(**D**) This patient has multiple clinical issues. First, he has pernicious anemia, which is causing the current symptoms. Pernicious anemia is associated with IgA deficiency, which is indicated by the lack of detectable IgA in the immunoglobulin panel and the history of severe allergic asthma and celiac disease (both of which are associated with IgA deficiency). Due to the lack of IgA, this patient sees IgA as "foreign" and may have antibodies specific for IgA. Therefore, the administration of whole blood (which contains plasma with IgA antibodies) may induce

an anaphylactic reaction. (**A, B**) These answers are incorrect because the cryoprecipitate that contains clotting factors or platelets would not be expected to have an adverse effect in this patient. (**C**) This answer is incorrect, because typed-matched RBCs for this patient would not have any additional blood components (e.g., donor antibodies) that would specifically induce a transfusion reaction.

20. Correct: IgA (A)

(**A**) This individual's underlying medical condition is selective IgA deficiency (sIgAD). Individuals with sIgAD can experience severe allergies, including asthma and eczema. Because the patient does not express IgA, this individual sees IgA as foreign and has made antibodies against IgA (probably from a previous transfusion or other exposure to blood from an IgA+ individual). Therefore, the preformed antibodies react with the transfused IgA, which sets off an anaphylactic reaction. (**B**) This answer is incorrect for multiple reasons. First, polymorphisms that increase IL-13 (not deficiencies) predispose an individual to asthma and eczema. Thus, the patient history is not consistent with an IL-13 deficiency. Second, a deficiency in IL-13 would not result in an anaphylactic response after a transfusion of ABO and Rh-matched whole blood. (**C**) This answer is incorrect because C9 deficiencies would not predispose individuals to anaphylaxis after transfusion with whole blood. While transfusion reactions against IgA are mediated by IgG complement activation, the activation of C9 is not a requirement for this reaction to have its effect. (**D**) This answer is incorrect because a granzyme deficiency would not predispose this individual to allergies, eczema, and/or transfusion reaction-induced anaphylaxis after whole blood transfusion. A deficiency in granzymes would affect the ability of NK and CTLs to kill target cells, including tumor cells and cells that have intracellular infections. (**E**) This answer is incorrect, because individuals with IgA deficiency have higher levels of circulating IgE, not an absence of IgE. Furthermore, IgE that is specific for IgA can also contribute the anaphylactic reaction against IgA if the patient has IgE specific for IgA.

21. Correct: Burkitt's lymphoma (D)

(**D**) The child has selective IgA deficiency (sIgAD). Individuals with sIgAD may have increased risk of cancer, but not for lymphoproliferative disorders such as Burkitt's lymphoma. (**A**) This answer is incorrect, because it has been shown that individuals with sIgAD have progressed to CVID. The likelihood to progress in CVID may be more likely in familial and MHC-associated sIgAD. (**B**) This answer is incorrect, because individuals with sIgAD have an increased risk of developing celiac disease, in addition to other autoimmune diseases such as systemic lupus erythematosus (SLE), Grave's diseases, and rheumatoid arthritis. (**C**) This answer is incorrect, because individuals with

IgA deficiency are at increased risk of developing respiratory infections, especially with *Streptococcus pneumoniae* and *Haemophilus influenzae*. (**E**) This answer is incorrect, because individuals with IgA deficiency are at an increased risk of developing food allergies. It is postulated that the absence of dimeric IgA may allow for the abnormal passage of food through the gut lining, allowing for the activation of B cells specific for food antigens and the development of food allergies.

22. Correct: IgA deficiency (A)

(**A**) IgA deficiency is the most common immunodeficiency, affecting anywhere from 1:500 to 1:700 individuals. Many individuals with IgA deficiency are asymptomatic, but those that manifest with symptoms tend to have significant issues with allergies and recurrent sinopulmonary infections. (**B**) This answer is incorrect, mainly because common variable immunodeficiency (CVID) is not as common as IgA deficiency and the age of presentation is inconsistent with CVID, which does not normally present until at least adolescence. (**C**) This answer is incorrect, because epidemiologically, Wiskott–Aldrich syndrome is less common than IgA deficiency. Individuals with Wiskott–Aldrich syndrome have normal numbers of B cells, eczema, thrombocytopenia, and overall defective antibody production, which is inconsistent with this patient's presentation. (**D**) This answer is incorrect, because these individuals with Omenn's syndrome have very few B cells, elevated IgE levels, and eosinophilia. Furthermore, individuals with Omenn's syndrome present with a severe phenotype early after birth. Therefore, the lab results and the age of presentation are inconsistent with this disease. (**E**) This answer is incorrect, because this is a very rare disease (1:1,000,000 people) and the patient's level of IgE is within the normal range (albeit at the high end). Individuals with HIES have recurrent infections, pneumonia, eczema, extremely high levels of IgE, and eosinophilia due to the predominant production of Th2 cells.

23. Correct: *STAT1* (signal transducer and activator of transcription 1) (B)

(**B**) The patient suffers from chronic mucocutaneous candidiasis (CMC) caused by gain of function mutations in the STAT1 gene. Due to the dominant STAT1 function, the ability of CD4+ T cells to become TH17 cells is impaired. The lack of IL-17 production by TH17 cells leads to chronic or persistent candidal infections of the mouth, esophagus, digestive and genital mucosae, nails, and/or skin. (**A**) This answer is incorrect, because mutations in the IL2RG results in severe combined immunodeficiency (SCID). Individuals with SCID can have recurrent fungal infections due to the absence of an adaptive immune cells, but the lab results indicate that the individual has normal numbers of B and T cells and therefore SCID is not likely. (**C**) This answer is incorrect, since properidin is part of the

alternative complement pathway that does not have a significant impact on fighting fungal infections. (**D**) This answer is incorrect, because the individual has normal T cell numbers, which is not the case in ZAP-70-deficient individuals who have no CD8+ T cells and nonfunctional CD4+ T cells. (**E**) This answer is incorrect, because mutations in ATM also lead to the loss of both B and T cells, since ATM is involved in the repair of double-stranded DNA breaks that occur during the rearrangement of the genes for immunoglobulin B cells and the T cell receptor in T cells.

24. Correct: IL-17, due to the loss of Th17 cell differentiation (E)

(**E**) This patient has chronic mucocutaneous candidiasis (CMC) with decreases in Th17 cells that produce IL-17 to control *Candida* infections. The loss of Th17 cells and/or their function can be due to the gain of function mutation in STAT1 that inhibits Th17 cell development or due to recessive mutations in AIRE that lead to the production of neutralizing autoantibodies against IL-17. (**A**) This answer is incorrect, because deficiencies in IFN-γ are not necessarily associated with *Candida* infections, but are associated with an increased frequency of mycobacteria infections. (**B**) This answer is incorrect, because the loss of IL-4 and Th2 cells does not result in enhanced fungal infections. IL-4 is important for promoting humoral immune responses and type I hypersensitivities, but has limited importance in fighting fungal infections. (**C**) This answer is incorrect, because the loss of Treg cells is associated with the development of autoimmune diseases—not the disease symptoms presented in this case. (**D**) This answer is incorrect, because Th9 cells that produce IL-9 are not relevant in protection against candidal infections, but do seem to be important for the expulsion of certain types of parasitic worms, including *Nippostrongylus brasiliensis*.

25. Correct: Type I bare lymphocyte syndrome (B)

(**B**) Patients with type I bare lymphocyte syndrome (BLS) do not express HLA class I and therefore have deficiencies in cytotoxic T cell responses, which are not critical in chronic *Candida* infections. Therefore, type I BLS can be excluded from the differential. (**A**) This answer is incorrect, since this patient likely has APECED, based on the recurrent candida infections and hypoparathyroidism. Therefore, it should be at the top of the differential. (**C**) This answer is incorrect, since individuals with SCID are highly susceptible to *Candida* infections. However, in SCID patients, candida infections can become invasive with systemic spread, which distinguishes it from CMC or APECED. (**D**) This answer is incorrect, since this patient is exhibiting signs of CMC. (**E**) This answer is incorrect, because HIV-positive patients are also at increased risk of *Candida* infections, such as thrush. While this answer is unlikely, due to the child's age and the parents not manifesting with similar symptoms (e.g., they do not appear to have HIV), it still cannot be excluded from the differential.

26.   Correct: Unusually small platelets (B)

(**B**) The patient has Wiskott–Aldrich syndrome, which results from a mutation in the WAS gene. These individuals have normal numbers of lymphocytes, but these cells are unable to form fixed conjugates and tightly bind other cells. In addition, these individuals have decreased numbers of platelets that are very small. Because of these factors, patients with Wiskott–Aldrich syndrome are immunodeficient and bruise easily, with trouble controlling bleeding after minor injuries. (**A**) This answer is incorrect, because B cells in these patients are unable to undergo the cytoskeletal reorganization that is required for the capping of the immunoglobulin to one pole of the B cell that is required for generating an activation signal in response to carbohydrate antigens. (**C**) This answer is incorrect, because CTL lysis is also decreased in these patients, since CTLs are unable to reorganize the cytoskeleton to tightly grab target cells and direct lysosomal contents at the target. (**D**) This answer is incorrect, because even though the ability of macrophages to phagocytose antigen and chemotaxis is negatively impacted in Wiskott–Aldrich syndrome, their total numbers are unaffected. (**E**) This answer is incorrect, because von Willebrand factor, which is important for blood clotting, is not impacted in Wiskott–Aldrich syndrome. Patients with mutations in either WASp or von Willebrand factor can both demonstrate trouble in controlling bleeding. However, the immune manifestations seen in Wiskott–Aldrich syndrome are not seen in individuals lacking or having reduced von Willebrand factor.

27.   Correct: Mature lymphocytes to reorganize actin cytoskeleton (C)

(**C**) This infant boy has Wiskott–Aldrich syndrome, which is an X-linked disease that harbors mutations in the WAS protein that is critical for actin cytoskeletal rearrangement in immune cells. This mutation leads to the loss of cytoskeletal reorganization to form the immunological synapse, which affects the activation of T cells and the ability of NK and CD8+ T cells to kill target cells. Because of these deficiencies, the child is immunosuppressed. The thrombocytopenia seen in this child is caused by increased clearance, reduced platelet survival, and immune-mediated mechanisms. (**A**) This answer is incorrect, because the ability of macrophages to kill phagocytosed bacteria is intact in Wiskott–Aldrich patients: the killing pathways are just fine. However, in Wiskott–Aldrich syndrome patients, their macrophages have a defect in phagocytosis and chemotaxis, since actin reorganization is important for these effects to occur. (**B**) This answer is incorrect, because if this patient had an inability to repair double-stranded DNA breaks, they would have an SCID phenotype. They would have more severe and

recurrent infections with all types of opportunistic pathogens, and they would have normal platelet numbers. (**D**) This answer is incorrect, because the inability of CD4+ T cells to become Th17 cells is associated with Job's syndrome (HIES), which does not exhibit significant thrombocytopenia with unusually small platelets. Individuals with HIES or Wiskott–Aldrich syndrome both develop eczema as part of the disease course, so HIES is within the differential of this patient, but the thrombocytopenia makes C the best answer. (**E**) This answer is incorrect, because individuals with the inability to present HLA class I have bare lymphocyte syndrome (BLS) and exhibit immunodeficiency, but have more trouble with a wider range of opportunistic pathogens. Furthermore, they do not exhibit thrombocytopenia with unusually small platelets.

28.   Correct: Wiskott–Aldrich syndrome (C)

(**C**) The patient is a male who presents with repeated opportunistic infections, despite normal numbers of B and T cells. As this child gets older, it is likely that his B cell and T cell numbers will drop below normal. Additional information demonstrates that the individual bruises easily and has microthrombocytopenia, which is the most consistent with Wiskott–Aldrich syndrome. (**A**) This answer is incorrect, because individuals with ataxia-telangiectasia present with decreased numbers of B and T cells due to the importance of the ATM gene in repairing double-stranded DNA breaks that occur during B and T cell development. (**B**) This answer is incorrect, because individuals with SCID present with decreased numbers of B and T cell numbers, which is not seen in this patient. (**D**) This answer is incorrect, because individuals who are at the AIDS stage of HIV infection would demonstrate significantly decreased CD4+ T cell numbers and a CD4:CD8 ratio less than 2:1. (**E**) This answer is incorrect, because this immunodeficiency results in the absence of B cells, but some autoreactive T cells persist. Individuals with Omenn's syndrome present with lymphadenopathy and splenomegaly due to the proliferation of self-reactive T cells and eosinophilia, which is not present in this patient.

29.   Correct: Varicella zoster virus (C)

(**C**) The patient is likely neutropenic due to chemotherapy treatment, which targets and kills rapidly dividing cells. Neutrophils have a short half-life, and therefore, the neutrophil progenitors continuously proliferate to restore the neutrophil numbers. When neutrophil counts drop, patients become immunocompromised, as they lose the first line of defense against pathogens. Because of this, neutropenic patients should not receive live vaccines. The varicella zoster virus vaccine is a live attenuated vaccine and therefore should not be given. (**A**) This answer is incorrect, because the influenza vaccine is not a live attenuated vaccine. Therefore, it is safe to give to someone who is neutropenic. (**B**) This answer is incorrect, because there are multiple pneumococcal vaccines that target the polysaccharides of *Streptococcus pneumoniae*. These vaccines are safe to give to immunocompromised individuals and may provide some protection against these bacteria. (**D**) This answer is incorrect, because the Tdap vaccine protects against tetanus, diphtheria, and pertussis and is comprised of toxoids from each of these pathogens. These toxoids are chemically inactivated and safe to give to the immunocompromised. (**E**) This answer is incorrect, because the vaccines that target *Haemophilus influenzae* type B are either polysaccharides or polysaccharides conjugated to proteins and are safe to give to immunocompromised individuals.

30. Correct: *HAX-1* (HCLS-associated protein X-1) (C)

(**C**) The patient suffers from Kostmann's syndrome, which results in severe neutropenia that makes the patient highly susceptible to bacterial and fungal infections. Autosomal recessive mutations in HAX-1 constitute approximately 15% of severe congenital neutropenia. It is possible that the patient's grandmother's brother died with a similar disease. However, since this disease was not seen in every generation (which would be an autosomal dominant trait), it must be inherited in a recessive manner, which is consistent with mutations in HAX-1 gene. (**A**) This answer is incorrect, because individuals with mutations in WASP have Wiskott–Aldrich syndrome, which can have neutropenia associated with the disease. However, these patients also have additional symptoms including significant thrombocytopenia and the platelets that they have are unusually small. Since this patient does not have any of these symptoms, this is not the best answer. (**B**) This answer is incorrect, because individuals with mutations in ADA have an SCID phenotype and lack B cells and T cells. This patient's lab values indicate that she is deficient in neutrophils with normal lymphocyte numbers. (**D**) This answer is incorrect, because a mutation in ITGB2 results in the loss of the functional CD18 molecule that is important for the adhesion of neutrophils to endothelial cells before they extravasate to the site of infection. Individuals with this mutation have "leukocyte adhesion deficiency (LAD)" and can manifest with the patient symptoms. However, their laboratory values tend to demonstrate neutrophilia, not neutropenia. (**E**) This answer is incorrect, because mutations in the ATM gene result in ataxia-telangiectasia. The ATM gene encodes a protein that is important for the repair of double-stranded DNA breaks. Mutations in this gene result in decreases in B and T cells, and the impairment of cells to undergo isotype switch, since all of these processes require dsDNA repair. Since this patient has normal numbers of B and T cells, this answer is unlikely.

31. Correct: Granulocyte colonystimulating factor (G-CSF) (B)

(**B**) The patient suffers from Kostmann's syndrome, which results in severe neutropenia that makes

the patient highly susceptible to oropharyngeal problems, otitis media, respiratory infections, cellulitis, and skin infections. The neutrophil precursors do not mature into neutrophils and results in a severe neutropenia as seen in this individual. Treatment with G-CSF has been successful in increasing the numbers of circulating neutrophils in these patients and is a standard treatment for these individuals. (**A**) This answer is incorrect, because individuals with Kostmann's syndrome have normal B cell development and antibody responses. Therefore, HISG treatment would not be beneficial, especially for respiratory infections, since the immunoglobulin in HISG does not readily reach mucosal sites. (**C**) This answer is incorrect, because rIFN-γ is used in the treatment of individuals who have normal numbers of neutrophils, but are deficient in intracellular killing (as seen in myeloperoxidase deficiency). rIFN-γ is used to treat individuals with killing deficiencies, not deficiencies in the cells themselves. (**D**) This answer is incorrect, for the following reason. While 50% of severe congenital neutropenia is caused by mutations in the *ELANE* gene, gene therapy with a "good" form of the *ELANE* gene would not be helpful, since the *ELANE* mutation is an autosomal dominant mutation. The introduction of this gene would not correct the neutropenia. (**E**) This answer is incorrect, because recombinant IL-7 can be used to treat T cell deficiencies, but has no effect on neutropenias. IL-7 is an important growth factor for developing lymphocytes (B and T cells), not granulocytes including neutrophils.

32. Correct: Kostmann's syndrome (D)

(**D**) This patient presents with Kostmann's syndrome, which results in a severe neutropenia. The analysis of the bone marrow is consistent with this presentation, because the developing neutrophils are stunted at the neutrophil precursor stage (promyelocyte/myelocyte). (**A**) This answer is incorrect, because individuals with Wiskott–Aldrich syndrome also have thrombocytopenia with unusually small platelets. This finding was not seen in this patient. (**B**) This answer is incorrect, because bone marrow aspirates of individuals with autoimmune neutropenia show normal bone marrow cellularity with a late myeloid arrest, which is inconsistent with the lab findings presented. Additionally, the age of onset is typically a bit older (7–9 months) and the symptoms are typically milder than are presented in this scenario. (**C**) This answer is incorrect, because individuals with Cohen's syndrome also present with hypotonia and other distinct features, which are not present in this patient. Furthermore, bone marrow aspirates from patients with this syndrome have neutropenia with normal or hypercellular marrow, while the patient who presents in this scenario has hypocellular bone marrow. (**E**) This answer is incorrect, because, even though it is associated with bone marrow failure and loss of platelets, there is a failure to make both megakaryocytes and platelets, which was not found in the analysis of the bone marrow aspirate.

33.   Correct: *HAX-1* (HCLS-associated protein X-1) (A)

(**A**) The husband in this situation had a sister with two mutations in the *HAX-1* gene. Severe congenital neutropenia occurs when an individual acquires two mutated copies of the *HAX-1* gene (and thus is a recessive mutation). Since the husband and his parents have no significant medical history, it is likely that both of his parents were heterozygous for a mutation in the *HAX-1* gene. Because both of his parents were heterozygous, there is a 50% chance that he carries a mutated form of the HAX-1 gene. (**B**) This answer is incorrect, because mutations associated with *CYBA* lead to loss of intracellular killing by neutrophils and other phagocytes, not a decrease in the number of neutrophils. (**C**) This answer is incorrect because, even though this mutation can lead to a severe congenital neutropenia, mutations in *ELANE* are dominant. Therefore, if the husband in this situation carried this mutation, he would also have severe congenital neutropenia. Since he has no significant medical history, this is unlikely. (**D**) This answer is incorrect, because mutations in the *LYST* gene (that are associated with Chédiak–Higashi syndrome) do not have a deficiency in the quantity of neutrophils. Patients with this mutation have a deficiency in neutrophil-dependent killing of pathogens. (**E**) This answer is incorrect, because mutations in *CD40*L, which can lead to hyper-IgM syndrome, are X-linked. Since the husband in this situation had a sister, not a brother, who had severe congenital neutropenia, it is unlikely that he carries a mutation in the *CD40L* gene.

34.   Correct: Measles, mumps, rubella (MMR) (C)

(**C**) A child with SCID does not have a functional adaptive immune response. The MMR vaccine is a live attenuated vaccine that can cause severe, even life-threatening, infections in immunocompromised. (**A**) This answer is incorrect, because the *Haemophilus influenzae*, type b vaccine (ActHIB) is a polysaccharide–protein conjugate vaccine that is safe to give to immunocompromised patients. (**B**) This answer is incorrect, because hepatitis A/B (TwinRix) is a recombinant protein vaccine that is safe to give to immunocompromised patients. (**D**) This answer is incorrect, because the pneumococcal vaccine (Prevnar) is polysaccharide-conjugate vaccine that is safe to give to immunocompromised patients. (**E**) This answer is incorrect, because the influenza (Fluzone) is a split-virus vaccine that is safe to administer to immunocompromised patients.

In contrast, FluMist is a live attenuated vaccine that could cause significant illness in this patient.

35.   Correct: Bone marrow transplant (A)

(**A**) This patient has severe combined immunodeficiency (SCID). The repeated infections with opportunistic pathogens and the absence of detectable lymphatic tissue and thymus are consistently found in patients with SCID. This is a congenital defect that can only be compensated for with a bone marrow transplant. (**B**) This answer is incorrect, because it will not repair the defect and cure this individual. HISG can be used as a prophylactic treatment to provide protection of this child until the bone marrow transplant is performed. (**C**) This answer is incorrect, because the thymus is not the problem—the inherent defect in this individual is the development of T cells. Even if the thymus were to be transplanted, there would be no developing thymocytes to populate this transplanted organ. (**D**) This answer is incorrect, because GM-CSF is used to correct neutrophil deficiencies, which is not the problem in SCID. The neutrophil numbers are fine in these patients, and GM-CSF will not correct the defect in T and B cell development. (**E**) This answer is incorrect, because corticosteroids are immunosuppressive, which would suppress any ability of the child to fight infections with the immunity that he has in the absence of B and T cells.

36.   Correct: Lack of a thymic shadow (E)

(**E**) This child has SCID. The IgG in this infant is from transplacental transfer from the mother during fetal development, so there are times that IgG levels can be misleading in infants. The lack of any IgM in this child in combination with the lack of CD20 cells indicates that there is a B cell deficiency. Additionally, the lack of detectable T cells indicates that there is a T cell deficiency as well. Children born with SCID consistently present with diarrhea, failure to thrive, candida infections, and respiratory infections. Many times, the chest X-ray performed during a respiratory infection will demonstrate the lack of a thymic shadow. (**A**) This answer is incorrect, because silver hair and light-colored eyes are associated with Chédiak–Higashi syndrome, which is a disease in which neutrophils are unable to kill phagocytosed pathogens and CTLs are unable to kill target cells. Furthermore, B and T cell numbers are relatively normal in these patients, which is inconsistent with the current patient. (**B**) This answer is incorrect, because hypercellularity of the bone marrow is associated with BTK deficiency. In this disease, B cell development is blocked at the pro-B cell stage, resulting in an accumulation of pro-B cells in the bone marrow, resulting in hypercellularity. In BTK deficiency, children will lack B cells, but have normal T cell numbers, which is inconsistent with this child's presentation. (**C**) This answer is incorrect, because the lack of pus at the site of infection is consistent with deficiencies in neutrophils, not lymphocytes as is seen in SCID. Individuals with lazy leukocyte syndrome or leukocyte adhesion deficiency (LAD) will present with recurrent infections with a lack of pus at the site of infection. (**D**) This answer is incorrect, because clefting of the palate is consistent with DiGeorge's syndrome, but not SCID.

37. Correct: *ADA* (D)

(**D**) This patient has SCID due to a mutation in ADA. ADA deficiency leads to an SCID phenotype due to the accumulation of toxic metabolites in developing B and T cells. (**A**) This answer is incorrect, because WASP is mutated in individuals with Wiskott–Aldrich syndrome. Patients with this syndrome have normal B and T cells; however, the cells do not function correctly. In addition, patients with this disease also demonstrate thrombocytopenia, with unusually small platelets, which was not evident in this patient. (**B**) This answer is incorrect, because ZAP-70 is mutated in individuals with ZAP-70 deficiency. Patients with ZAP-70 deficiency demonstrate an absence of CD8+ T cells and nonfunctional CD4+ T cells, due to a lack of normal T cell receptor signaling. B cell numbers are normal in these individuals, which is in contrast to this patient. (**C**) This answer is incorrect, because BTK is mutated in individuals with Bruton's X-linked hypogammaglobulinemia. BTK is required for normal B cell development, and these boys do not produce B cells, but have normal T cell numbers, which is in contrast to this patient. (**E**) This answer is incorrect, because LYST is mutated in Chédiak–Higashi syndrome. Patients with this disease have a mutation in the LYST gene that encodes a protein critical for microtubule polymerization, and thus lysozyme generation and function. Individuals with this disease have a normal distribution of immune cells, but have neutrophils that are deficient in intracellular killing and CTLs that are unable to release cytotoxic granules to kill target cells.

38. Correct: Convert toxic metabolites to nontoxic byproducts (B)

(**B**) This child has SCID due to a mutation in the *ADA* gene. ADA is responsible for converting toxic metabolites to nontoxic byproducts in developing lymphocytes. In the absence of ADA, the toxic metabolites induce the death of developing B and T lymphocytes. (**A**) This answer is incorrect, because the SCID phenotype induced by an inability of developing lymphocytes to undergo V(D)J rearrangement is due to mutations in the *RAG* gene. (**C**) This answer is incorrect, because the SCID phenotype induced by an inability of developing lymphocytes to signal through cytokine receptors is due to mutations in the *IL2RG* gene. (**D**) This answer

is incorrect, because one form of the SCID phenotype induced by an inability of developing lymphocytes to fix double-stranded DNA breaks that occur during V(D)J recombination is due to mutations in the *ATM* gene. Additional mutations in *Artemis* and *DNA ligase IV* can also cause an SCID phenotype due to the inability of developing lymphocytes to fix double-stranded DNA breaks. (**E**) This answer is incorrect, because the SCID phenotype induced by an inability of lymphocytes to form an immunological synapse is due to mutations in the *WASP* gene. Individuals with Wiskott–Aldrich syndrome that have mutations in the *WASP* gene have normal number of B and T cells but, since they do not function appropriately, can present with a milder form of SCID.

39. Correct: Double-positive thymocytes (B)

(**B**) This child likely has SCID, which results in the lack of mature T and B lymphocytes. Therefore, T cell development will not occur to the double-positive thymocyte stage in the thymus and patients with SCID will lack these T cell precursors. Even in forms of SCID that have mutations that allow for the development of B cells (e.g., T – B + SCID seen with mutations of the IL-2R common gamma chain, JAK3, and IL-7Ra chain), these individuals will not have double-positive thymocytes. (**A**) This answer is incorrect, because even though many forms of SCID are negative for mature B cells, they will develop to this early stage of B cell development. Pro-B cells are detectable by the expression of the B cell marker, CD19, which can be found in the bone marrow of human SCID patients. (**C**) This answer is incorrect, because promyelocytes are precursors of neutrophil development and are still seen in individuals with neutropenia. While neutropenic children can have many of the same clinical presentations as SCID (e.g., persistent bacterial and fungal infections), these children still have promyelocytes. It is just that the promyelocytes do not fully develop into neutrophils. (**D**) This answer is incorrect, because megakaryocytes are precursors for platelets, and this child shows no evidence of platelet deficiency. (**E**) This answer is incorrect, because NK cell immunodeficiency typically presents with severe, recurrent, or atypical herpes infections and papillomaviruses, which is inconsistent with this patient's presentation.

40. Correct: Interleukin common gamma chain (B)

(**B**) This patient presents with X-linked SCID, which is an X-linked disease associated with mutations in the interleukin common gamma chain. The fact that another brother died from repeated infections during the first year of life, but the sister is healthy, indicates an X-linked form of severe combined immunodeficiency (SCID). In X-linked SCID, the individuals develop B cells, but they are nonfunctional due to the fact that the common gamma chain is required for signaling through multiple cytokine receptors, including IL-2, IL-4, IL-7, IL-9, IL-15, and IL-21. Therefore, these patients will produce B cells, which are nonfunctional due to the need of T cell help and the lack of responsiveness to these cytokines. (**A**) This answer is incorrect, because ADA deficiency results in an autosomal recessive SCID in which no B cells and T cells develop. (**C**) This answer is incorrect, because even though Wiskott–Aldrich syndrome is an X-linked immunodeficiency, males with mutations in *WASP* develop B cells and T cells. However, these lymphocytes are nonfunctional due to the inability to form immunological synapses, since WASP is required for cytoskeletal reorganization. These patients also have thrombocytopenia, which is not indicated in this case. (**D**) This answer is incorrect, because JAK3 deficiency is an autosomal recessive pattern, and this patient's history indicates an X-linked SCID. JAK3 deficiency and IL-2RG are clinically and immunologically indistinguishable, except for their inheritance pattern. (**E**) This answer is incorrect, because nonfunctional RAG proteins are associated with the development of Omenn's syndrome in which there are no B cells produced, with the production of a few T cell clones that tend to be self-reactive and proliferate extensively in these patients.

41. Correct: Reverse transcriptase (A)

(**A**) This individual is undergoing a primary HIV infection. The reverse transcriptase of HIV does not have significant proofreading activity and therefore introduces many mutations into the viral genome as it reverse transcribes the viral RNA into the double-stranded DNA intermediate. These introduced mutations lead to the evolution of HIV over the course of infection of this individual. (**B**) This answer is incorrect, because even though mutations into the envelope gene that encode gp40/gp120 influence the ability of the virus to evade the immune system and change the co-receptor used for entry, this is not the *cause* of the evolution. The reverse transcriptase is responsible for introducing the mutations in the *env* gene that leads to changes into the envelope protein. (**C**) This answer is incorrect, because the protease only functions to cleave the polyproteins of HIV into their final form so that the HIV virus matures into infectious particles. (**D**) This answer is incorrect, because the p24 capsid antigen is not involved in the evolution of the virus, but rather is mainly an important protein for diagnosis. (**E**) This answer is incorrect, because integrase is important for introducing the HIV double-stranded DNA viral intermediate into the host chromosome and is absolutely required for the continuation of the viral life cycle within an individual cell. It does not, however, promote the evolution of the virus over the course of infection.

42. Correct: Protease inhibitor (C)

(**C**) This woman is demonstrating the signs of a primary infection with HIV. As part of the current recommendations, all individuals that are HIV-positive are to be treated with active antiretroviral therapy, which includes two reverse-transcriptase inhibitors and a second class of antiretroviral therapeutic drugs. Protease inhibitors block the ability of protease to cleave the HIV polyproteins into their final form, which is required for HIV maturation into an infectious viral particle. (**A, E**) These answers are incorrect, because these two HIV inhibitors inhibit the activities of HIV's reverse transcriptase, which is required for replication of the virus, but not maturation of the virus. (**B**) This answer is incorrect, because the integrase inhibitor blocks the ability of HIV integrase to incorporate the HIV double-stranded DNA intermediate into the host genome. While this enzyme is critical for propagating the virus, it is not critical for HIV maturation. (**D**) This answer is incorrect, because this inhibitor blocks the ability of HIV to enter the cell. It blocks the ability of HIV to use the CCR5 co-receptor that is required for viral entry, but does not affect HIV viral maturation.

43. Correct: Mutations in the pol gene of HIV (B)

(**B**) Noncompliance in HIV-infected patients puts these individuals at a significantly higher risk of developing a mutation that confers resistance to HIV antiretroviral drugs. Therefore, the lack of improvement in this individual after reinitiating antiretroviral treatment is most likely due to mutations in the HIV strain that make it resistance to drugs previously used in this patient. Since the *pol* gene encodes the enzymes that are targeted by antiretroviral therapy (reverse transcriptase, protease, integrase), mutations in this gene are likely responsible for the resistance to the antiretroviral therapy. (**A**) This answer is incorrect, because it is the evolution from a CCR5 to a CXCR4 strain of HIV that results in a dramatic drop in CD4+ T cell counts and an increase in viral load. Therefore, (**A**) could have been correct if it was written as "evolution to a CXCR4 strain of HIV," but not the other way around. (**C**) This answer is incorrect, because, even though infection with a second strain of drug-resistant HIV is possible, it is more likely that the patient's lack of adherence to antiretroviral therapy resulted in mutations that confer resistance to her previous drug regimen. (**D**) This answer is incorrect, because thymic evolution does not significantly contribute to worsening symptoms and lab results in HIV patients. Since the patient is 48 years old, the thymus has undergone substantial thymic involution, independent of HIV infection. (**E**) This answer is incorrect, because the proviral genome does not move within the host chromosome once it has been inserted.

44. Correct: Unprotected sex with multiple partners (C)

(**C**) This individual is undergoing a primary response to HIV infection. In the United States, the primary mode of transmission is through unprotected sex. (**A**) This answer is incorrect, because working at a daycare center is a risk factor for acquiring hepatitis A, not HIV. This individual is positive for IgG specific for Hepatitis A virus (HAV), meaning that she either was immunized against HAV or has previously had the disease. Either way, the presence of IgG against hepatitis A indicates that she is immune to hepatitis A. Additionally, she does not have any signs of liver malfunction, further supporting that this patient's signs are not from a hepatitis virus infection. (**B**) This answer is incorrect, because multiple body piercings increases the risk for hepatitis C, not necessarily HIV. Additionally, the patient does not show elevated liver enzymes, indicating that her symptoms are not from an infection with hepatitis C (with most HCV-infected patients presenting with symptoms after initial infection). (**D**) This answer is incorrect, because it is highly unlikely that a 23-year-old woman would just now show with symptoms of HIV infection that she acquired in utero. (**E**) This answer is incorrect, because HIV cannot be acquired through casual contact. HIV is transmitted through the sharing of bodily fluids.

45. Correct: HIV antigen/antibody combination enzyme immunoassay (D)

(**D**) A combination enzyme immunoassay (EIA) that tests for both p24 Ag and anti-HIV antibodies is the test that is first performed in HIV diagnosis. See Centers for Disease Control and Prevention (CDC) algorithm at the end of this answer. If the individual is positive by this combination EIA, a follow-up EIA is performed to distinguish between infection with HIV-1 and HIV-2. (**A**) This answer is incorrect, because the Western blot is the previous confirmatory test for HIV infection. Due to its low sensitivity, it has not been the primary screening test for HIV positivity. Due to the increased sensitivity and specificity of EIAs in recent years, the Western blot is not currently used in the algorithm for HIV diagnosis. (**B**) This answer is incorrect, because while CD4 count by flow cytometry is a quick and easy way to determine if antiretroviral drugs are restoring CD4 numbers, it is not diagnostic for HIV infection. There are many reasons why an individual may have low CD4 counts. (**C**) This answer is incorrect, because even though syncytial formation is seen in Herpes simplex virus (HSV) infections, syncytial formation is only seen when a T-tropic/CXCR4 HIV strain is responsible for infection. Therefore, it is not an initial diagnostic test that is used because it would not detect M-tropic/CCR5-HIV strains. However, this test could be used to determine if the type of HIV strain that is responsible for infection in an individual patient is a T-tropic/CXCR4 strain, which has a more negative prognosis. (**E**) This answer is incorrect, because HIV has an RNA genome that would not be amplified by PCR. RNA must first be reverse transcribed before it can be amplified through PCR. RT-PCR can be used diagnostically if the EIAs that are initially used for diagnosis are inconclusive.

HIV-1/2 antigen/antibody combination immunoassay

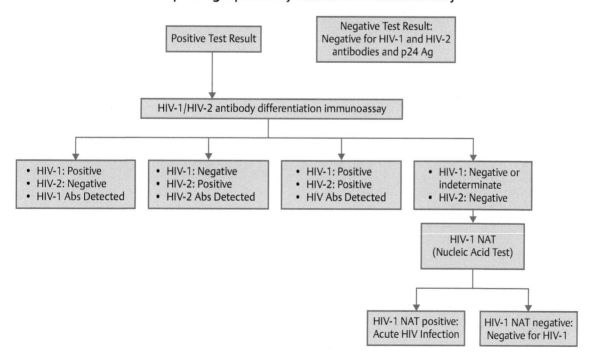

83

46. Correct: *LYST* (B)

(**B**) This child has Chédiak–Higashi syndrome, which is an autosomal recessive disease that leads to severe immunosuppression due to mutations in the *LYST* gene. Mutations in the *LYST* gene result in aberrant lysosome generation and function. These individuals have impaired neutrophil intracellular killing, and NK cell and CTL function, due to their inability to release cytotoxic granules. Partial oculocutaneous albinism and a silver sheen to the hair are common in these patients. (**A**) This answer is incorrect, because mutations in *ELANE* are associated with an autosomal dominant congenital neutrophil deficiency, which is associated with repeated respiratory and skin infections. However, since the parents are fine medically and do not appear to have a mutation in *ELANE*, one can limit this option as an unlikely candidate to be responsible for the child's immunodeficiency. (**C**) This answer is incorrect, because mutations in *WASP* lead to Wiskott–Aldrich syndrome, which is an X-linked immunodeficiency that presents with recurrent respiratory symptoms, and deficient CTL function in males. Since the patient is female, it makes this mutation unlikely. (**D**) This answer is incorrect, because mutations in *NEMO* lead to ectodermal issues (such as sparse hair, misshaped teeth, and hyperhidrosis), which are not described in this patient. *NEMO* mutations lead to a loss of NF-kB activation, which is important for both innate and adaptive immune cell activation and leads to increased opportunistic infections. (**E**) This answer is incorrect, because mutations in *NADPH oxidase* that result in immunodeficiency are X-linked, and the patient is female. Mutations in this gene result in chronic granulomatous disease (CGD), which leads to an inability of phagocytes to kill engulfed pathogens and increases in the survival of catalase-producing *Staphylococcus aureus* within the neutrophils.

47. Correct: Chédiak–Higashi syndrome (D)

(**D**) This patient has Chédiak–Higashi syndrome, in which lysosome generation and function is inhibited due to mutations in the *LYST* gene. Along with repeated infections and partial oculocutaneous albinism, the identification of giant azurophilic granules in granulocytes is pathognomonic for Chédiak–Higashi syndrome. (**A**) This answer is incorrect, because individuals with Wiskott–Aldrich syndrome have marked thrombocytopenia, which is not seen in the lab values. (**B**) This answer is incorrect, because individuals with CGD do not have a decrease in neutrophil numbers. In patients with CGD, their neutrophils are deficient in the ability to kill the pathogens that they engulf. (**C**) This answer is incorrect, because individuals with Kostmann's syndrome have significantly decreased numbers of neutrophils

(<5%), which is not seen in the lab values. (**E**) This answer is incorrect, because even though individuals with Griscelli's syndrome have similar symptoms as patients with Chédiak–Higashi syndrome, these patients do not have giant intracellular granules in the granulocytes.

48. Correct: Giant azurophilic cytoplasmic granules in granulocytes (E)

(**E**) This child has Chédiak–Higashi syndrome, which is an autosomal recessive disease that manifests when a child inherits two mutated copies of the *LYST* gene. These children have decreased neutrophil killing and NK and CTL cytotoxic ability due to aberrant fusion of vesicles and failure to transport lysosomes to the appropriate site of action. Patients with this disease have giant cytoplasmic granules in granulocytes due to the inappropriate fusion of lysosomes and endosomes. (**A**) This answer is incorrect, because Auer rods in a blast form are associated with leukemia. Patients with Chédiak–Higashi syndrome are at risk for eventually entering the "accelerated phase" of the disease in which there is uncontrolled proliferation of lymphohistiocytes and infiltration of numerous organs. Patients in the accelerated phase present with fever, lymphadenopathy, hepatosplenomegaly, more severe thrombocytopenia, and bleeding, which is not consistent with this patient's presentation. (**B**) This answer is incorrect, because this is the description of RBCs that can be seen in autoimmune anemia, which is inconsistent with the presentation of this child. (**C**) This answer is incorrect, because this is a usual description of lymphocytes in a peripheral blood smear. Lymphocyte numbers are not significantly affected by mutations in the *LYST* gene, but their cytolytic function is decreased. (**D**) This answer is incorrect, because this is a description of platelets found associated with Wiskott–Aldrich syndrome. Like patients with Chédiak–Higashi syndrome, patients with Wiskott–Aldrich syndrome manifest with recurrent respiratory infections. However, Wiskott–Aldrich syndrome is an X-linked disease that presents in boys (in contrast to our patient) and typically presents with severe eczema as well.

49. Correct: 25% (B)

(**B**) The child suffers from Chédiak–Higashi syndrome, which is an autosomal recessive disease that affects microtubule reorganization which impacts normal lysosome generation and function. Therefore, these children are immunodeficient because they have decreased neutrophil killing ability and decreased CTL and NK cell cytolytic ability. Based on mendelian genetics, since neither parent appears to have an immunodeficiency, the child has a 25% (1/4) chance of receiving the mutated form of *LYST* gene responsible for this disease from both the mother and the father. See Punnett's square below:

Father (*LYST/LYST**) × Mother (*LYST/LYST**)
Potential offspring

LYST/LYST (*wildtype*)	*LYST/LYST** (*carrier*)
LYST/LYST* (*carrier*)	*LYST*/LYST** (*disease*)

(**A**) This answer is incorrect, because the mother and father are both carriers and therefore there is a statistical chance of passing on the mutated LYST gene. (**C, D**) These answers are incorrect, because autosomal recessive diseases cannot be inherited in that pattern, unless one of the parents harbored two copies of the mutated LYST gene. Since both parents are reported to have no significant medical history, it is highly unlikely that one of them has two mutated copies of the LYST gene. (**E**) This answer is incorrect, because for the likelihood to be 100%, both parents would have to have two copies of mutated LYST genes and therefore would have symptoms of Chédiak–Higashi. Since both parents are healthy, this is highly unlikely.

50. Correct: Neutrophils (C)

(**C**) This patient suffers from leukocyte adhesion deficiency (LAD) (type I), which results in the inability of neutrophils to extravasate from the blood to the site of infection. The mutation is in CD18, which is required for the tight binding of neutrophils to endothelial cells that precedes diapedesis and chemotaxis to the site of infection. (**A, B, D, E**) These answers are incorrect, because the predominant cell types that are unable to extravasate to the site of infection are neutrophils in this disease. Other cell types have secondary mechanisms for reaching the site of infection.

51. Correct: Encapsulated organisms (C)

(**C**) Individuals with leukocyte adhesion deficiency (LAD) are highly susceptible to encapsulated organisms, including gram-positive organisms, such as *Staphylococcus aureus* and gram-negative bacilli. These infections typically manifest as skin, respiratory tract, bowel, and perirectal infections. (**A, B, D, E**) These answers are incorrect, because individuals with LAD do not have major increases in susceptibility to these organisms. The predominant issues are with encapsulated organisms and gram-negative bacilli.

52. Correct: Leukocyte adhesion deficiency (E)

(**E**) This child suffers from leukocyte adhesion deficiency (LAD). This disease is due to a mutation in CD18 that results in the loss of the ability of neutrophils to leave the blood and go to the site of infection. Because of this inability, these children are highly susceptible to skin and mucosal infections, and have impaired wound healing. A hallmark presentation of this disease is the absence of pus (neutrophil infiltration) at the site of infection, as seen above. Also, delayed separation of the umbilical cord and omphalitis are common in these patients. (**A**) This answer is incorrect, because bare lymphocyte syndrome (BLS) manifests with the loss of HLA class I and/or class II molecules. Individuals with this disease manifest with more of severe combined immunodeficiency (SCID) phenotype than is presented here. They commonly present with pneumonia, bronchitis, gastroenteritis, and/or septicemia. (**B**) This answer is incorrect, because individuals with chronic granulomatous disease (CGD) produce cells that are capable of intracellular killing by phagocytes. They commonly present with pneumonia, abscesses, supportive adenitis, osteomyelitis, bacteremia, and superficial skin infections like cellulitis. Unlike in LAD, leukocytosis is not frequently reported. (**C**) This answer is incorrect, because individuals with Kostmann's syndrome are deficient in the ability to produce neutrophils. Therefore, they are severely neutropenic, and do not display increased neutrophil numbers. (**D**) This answer is incorrect, because in individuals with myeloperoxidase deficiency that have symptoms typically present with infections due to different candidal strains. Patients with myeloperoxidase deficiency are susceptible to mucocutaneous, meningeal, bone infections, and sepsis.

53. Correct: CD18 (B)

(**B**) Individuals with leukocyte adhesion deficiency (LAD) do not express CD18, which results in the inability of neutrophils to extravasate out of blood vessels to the site of infection. (**A**) This answer is incorrect, because the absence of CD3+ cells would indicate an absence of T cells that could be associated with multiple immunodeficiencies, including DiGeorge's syndrome. (**C**) This answer is incorrect, because the absence of CD20+ cells would indicate an absence of B cells that would be associated with a B cell immunodeficiency, such as Bruton's XLA. (**D**) This answer is incorrect, because the absence of CD56 would indicate an absence of NK cells, which would result in patients who present with exacerbated infections with herpesviruses and human papillomaviruses. (**E**) This answer is incorrect, because the absence of CD95 (also called FAS) results in autoimmune lymphoproliferative disease. CD95 is important for inducing apoptosis and its absence results in uncontrolled expansion of cells of the immune system.

54. Correct: CD40L (A)

(A) This child has hyper-IgM syndrome. Individuals with this disease present with increased IgM levels and little to no other isotypes due to the absence of CD4+ T cell help, which is required for the B cell to undergo isotype switch from IgM to another isotype (e.g., IgG, IgA, IgE). CD40L on the T cell interacts with CD40 on the B cell in the presence of cytokines to induce class switch recombination. The trace amounts of IgG in this child are maternally derived from before birth. (B) This answer is incorrect, because mutations in *ATM* result in ataxia-telangiectasia. ATM is involved in the repair of double-stranded DNA breaks and its loss impairs not only the development of B and T cells, but also the ability of B cells to undergo class switch. These individuals also have low lymphocyte counts and normal neutrophil numbers, which is not compatible with the laboratory findings in this patient. (C) This answer is incorrect, because mutations in *TACI* are associated with both common variable immunodeficiency (CVID) and selective IgA deficiency (sIgAD). In CVID, the presentation is much later in life (usually past adolescence with many presenting in their 20s) and individuals with sIgAD do not have decreases in IgG and IgE as is seen in this patient. (D) This answer is incorrect, because mutations in *BTK* result in a block in B cell development at the pre-B cell stage. These individuals are deficient in all isotypes of antibody, since very few B cells are produced, which is not consistent with the laboratory findings in this patient. (E) This answer is incorrect, because mutations in *STAT3* result in HIES. Individuals with HIES are deficient in the generation of Th17 cells and manifest with extremely high levels of IgE and eczema, which is not seen in this patient.

55. Correct: Streptococcus pneumoniae (D)

(D) This individual has hyper-IgM syndrome, which puts him at a significantly increased risk of sinopulmonary infections (pneumonia, sinusitis, and otitis media) predominantly caused by encapsulated bacteria, such as *Streptococcus* and *Staphylococcus*. In addition, these individuals are immunocompromised and are susceptible to opportunistic infections, such as *Pneumocystis jirovecii* pneumonia (as described as the presenting feature in this patient above). Additional immunodeficiencies that have a significantly increased risk of infections with *Streptococcus* and *Staphylococcus* include: XLA, common variable immunodeficiency (CVID), complement deficiencies, and XL-EDA-ID. (A) This answer is incorrect, because the following immunodeficiencies have a significantly increased risk for infections with *Mycobacterium* infections: severe combined immunodeficiency (SCID), XL-EDA-ID, and chronic granulomatous disease (CGD). There is a report of a slightly elevated risk of *Mycobacterium* infection in hyper-IgM syndrome, but this is not nearly as common as *Streptococcus* and *Staphylococcus*. (B) This answer is incorrect, because the following immunodeficiencies have a significantly increased risk for infections with *Candida albicans*: APECED, HIES, SCID, MHC II deficiency, XL-EDA-ID, Wiskott–Aldrich syndrome, and myeloperoxidase deficiency. (C) This answer is incorrect, because the following immunodeficiencies have a significantly increased risk for infections with human papillomavirus: NK T cell deficiency and WHIM (*w*arts, *h*ypogammaglobulinemia, *i*mmunodeficiency, and *m*yelokathexis) syndrome. (E) This answer is incorrect, because the following immunodeficiencies have a significantly increased risk for infections with *A. fumigatus*: CGD, hyper-IgM syndrome, SCID, and leukocyte adhesion deficiency (LAD).

56. Correct: Decreased memory B cells (A)

(A) This individual has hyper-IgM syndrome, which manifests with increased susceptibility to encapsulated bacteria and presents typically as pneumonia, sinusitis, and otitis media. The lymphocyte counts are in the normal range, since there is no apparent effect on T and B development, but the ability of CD40L on the T cell binding to CD40 on the B cell to promote a T-dependent antibody response is absent. Therefore, the B cell does not receive signals through CD40 that are required for isotype switch and the generation of memory B cells. (B) This answer is incorrect, because antigen-presenting cells that lack HLA class I have bare lymphocyte syndrome (BLS), which results in a decrease in T cell numbers (CD8+ T cells), without any significant effect on B cell antibody production. (C) This answer is incorrect, because high levels of AFP are found in individuals with ataxia-telangiectasia. In addition to increased AFP, individuals with ataxia-telangiectasia have decreased lymphocyte numbers and significant problems with motor skills and coordination, which are not seen in this child. (D) This answer is incorrect, because antibodies specific for IgA are associated with sIgAD. This child has immunoglobulin deficiencies of IgG, IgE, and IgA, so this child does not have sIgAD. (E) This answer is incorrect, because the presence of p24 antigen would reveal that the child is infected with HIV. While infants with HIV are highly susceptible to opportunistic infections, as seen in this child, one would expect decreases in T cell counts, which are not seen in this child.

57. Correct: Chronic granulomatous disease (C)

(C) This patient has chronic granulomatous disease (CGD). In this disease, patients predominantly are deficient in NADPH oxidase, which is required for respiratory burst and neutrophil killing. Therefore, neutrophils can get to the site of infection and engulf these organisms, but not kill them. The neutrophils can then take these organisms to secondary sites in which the infection is eventually walled off by the immune system forming granulomas. Patients with this disease have an increased risk of developing pneumonia, abscesses, osteomyelitis, sepsis, and cellulitis. Additionally, the NBT test is the oldest and best-known laboratory confirmatory test for CGD. Since the neutrophils are unable to induce the respiratory burst, they are unable to reduce yellow NBT to blue/black formazan precipitates, as seen in this patient. (**A**) This answer is incorrect, because individuals with this disease have a deficiency in the ability of phagocytes to get to sites of infection. Like patients with CGD, they have abnormal wound healing, with infections of the skin and respiratory tract. However, because the neutrophils in these patients are capable of intracellular killing, they would be positive by the NBT reduction test. (**B**) This answer is incorrect, because individuals with Job's syndrome (HIES) have a deficiency in STAT3, which results in an inappropriate skewing of Th cells to Th2 cells. Like patients with CGD, they have increased risk of infections with *Aspergillus fumigatus*. However, patients with HIES have characteristic facial anomalies (broad nasal base and nasal bridge, protrusion of the forehead, and deep-set eyes) and high levels of IgE, which are not seen in this patient. (**D**) This answer is incorrect, because patients with Chédiak–Higashi syndrome have deficiencies in neutrophil and cytotoxic T cell killing due to an inability to inhibit inappropriate fusion of vesicles and failure for lysosomes to reach the appropriate site of action. In addition, the presence of neutrophils, eosinophils, and other granulocytes with giant azurophilic granules in peripheral blood smears are pathognomonic for Chédiak–Higashi syndrome. (**E**) This answer is incorrect, because individuals with a TLR deficiency would also be positive by the NBT assay. Like individuals with CGD, individuals with TLR deficiencies can demonstrate an increased risk of cellulitis and sepsis with normal lymphocyte numbers and immunoglobulin levels. However, patients with TLR deficiencies will be positive by the NBT assay and will not develop granulomas as seen in many older patients with CGD.

58. Correct: Job's syndrome (C)

(**C**) This child has Job's syndrome (or HIES). Patients with this disease commonly present early in life with recurrent cutaneous and pulmonary infections, eczema, and elevated IgE levels in their serum. Facial dysmorphism, including a broad nasal base and nasal bridge, protrusion of the forehead, and deep-set eyes are common in individuals with this disease. Also, many times, due to the loss of strong inflammatory responses in these individuals, the abscesses (commonly caused by *Staphylococcus aureus*) will be "cold" in that they will not have hallmarks of inflammation, such as erythema and warmth. (**A**) This answer is incorrect, because while individuals with severe atopic dermatitis may have recurrent *S. aureus* skin lesions, they tend to be more superficial. Furthermore,

individuals with atopic dermatitis do not have the associated facial dysmorphism and associated respiratory diseases, and do not have as high of a level of eosinophilia as is seen in Job's syndrome. (**B**) This answer is incorrect, because even though individuals with Wiskott–Aldrich syndrome have significant eczema and elevated IgE levels, they have a significant thrombocytopenia that is not mentioned in this patient. Furthermore, patients with Wiskott–Aldrich syndrome tend not to develop abscesses, as is seen in individuals with Job's syndrome. (**D**) This answer is incorrect, because individuals with severe combined immunodeficiency (SCID) will have a loss of lymphocytes, which is inconsistent with this patient. At times, SCID patients can have desquamative skin rashes, but these rashes are typically distinguishable from the eczematic rashes found in other immunodeficiencies. (**E**) This answer is incorrect, because Omenn's syndrome is a disease that results from deficiencies in either RAG1 or RAG2 that manifest with a loss of B cells and most T cells. Since this patient has normal numbers of lymphocytes, this answer is highly unlikely. Individuals with Omenn's syndrome produce some autoreactive T cells that proliferate extensively, resulting in overall lymphadenopathy, eosinophilia, and hepatosplenomegaly.

59. Correct: Th17 cells (D)

(**D**) This patient has Job's syndrome (or HIES). This disease manifests with recurrent eczema, abscesses, and respiratory infections caused by *S. aureus*. In the most common form, patients with this disease have an autosomal dominant mutation in STAT3, which results in the inability to generate Th17 cells. The loss of Th17 cells results in a skew to the Th2 phenotype, which promotes eosinophilia and the production of high levels of IgE, which are not beneficial in protecting from *S. aureus* skin infections. (**A**) This answer is incorrect, because individuals with the autosomal dominant from of Job's syndrome have a deficit in production Th17 cells, but do not directly impact Th1 generation. There may be an overall decrease in IFN-γ production, but this is not due to a loss of STAT3; this is likely due to an overproduction of Th2 cells, which limits Th1 generation. (**B**) This answer is incorrect, because patients with Job's syndrome have a significant increase in the differentiation of naïve CD4+ T cells to Th2 cells. This increase in Th2 cells diminishes the inflammatory immune response and increases class switch recombination to the IgE isotype. (**C**) This answer is incorrect, because Th9 cells are thought to be predominantly involved in promoting allergic inflammation. While not specifically investigated in Job's syndrome, increases in Th9 cells are associated with increases in IgE in allergic patients, indicating that these cell types would be either not affected and/or increased in patients with Job's syndrome. (**E**) This answer is incorrect, because Treg cells are critical in promoting immune tolerance and protecting individuals from the generation of autoimmunity. Individuals with Job's syndrome may have only a slight association with developing auto-immune diseases, and these associated autoimmune diseases do not present until much later in life.

60. Correct: Elevated eosinophil numbers (E)

(**E**) This patient is presenting with autosomal domi-nant Job's syndrome (or HIES). Individuals with this syndrome have mutations in STAT3 that result in the loss of the Th17/Th2 balance in which Th2 cells predominate. The elevations in Th2 cells result in significantly increased levels of IgE and eosino-phils. (**A**) This answer is incorrect, because indi-viduals with Job's syndrome have increased IgE levels, not decreased IgE levels as described above. (**B**) This answer is incorrect, because there are no significant alterations in lymphocyte numbers and/ or distribution in individuals with Job's syndrome. (**C**) This answer is incorrect, because individuals with decreased glucose-6-phosphate dehydrogenase levels have an X-linked disease that can rarely result in deficiencies in granulocyte killing functions. Those individuals who manifest with decreased killing functions can have infections with *S. aureus*. (**D**) This answer is incorrect, because complement levels are unaffected in Job's syndrome. In some respects, this makes sense, because there is a huge propensity for B cells to switch to IgE, which is not an activator of complement.

61. Correct: *RAG1/2* (B)

(**B**) This child has Omenn's syndrome, which is a form of SCID in which mutations in *RAG1* and/or *RAG2* lead to the loss of B cells, with the development of some CD8+ T cells and a restricted repertoire of CD4+ T cells that tend to be self-reactive and proliferate to a substantial degree to generate lymphadenopathy and hepatosplenomegaly. These patients tend to have sig-nificant susceptibility to respiratory infections and chronic diarrhea, and a failure to thrive. An important diagnostic clue to Omenn's disease is the presence of a diffuse, exudative erythroderma that is not seen in other forms of SCID. The dermatitis initially resembles eczema, but progresses to desquamation. (**A**) This answer is incorrect, because mutation in *ADA* results in SCID with the absence of both B and T cells. The loss of ADA results in the accumulation of toxic metabo-lites in developing T and B cells that leads to the loss of both these cell types and a resulting SCID phenotype. This patient had the hallmarks of SCID, but did not have the loss of both T and B cells that is seen in ADA-SCID. Furthermore, skin lesions are not associated with ADA-SCID. (**C**) This answer is incorrect, because mutations in *STAT3* lead to Job's syndrome (HIES). Patients with Job's syndrome have multiple skin lesions, which are typically skin abscesses caused by infection with *Staphylococcus aureus* and an increased propensity for respiratory infections. However, these

patients have normal lymphocyte numbers; it is just that their T cells are unable to differentiate into Th17 cells due to the loss of STAT3. (**D**) This answer is incorrect, because mutations in *WASP* result in the generation of Wiskott–Aldrich syndrome. This syn-drome is characterized with eczema and a mild SCID-like immunodeficiency due to a lack of normal B and T cell activation. However, they have normal lympho-cyte numbers and a thrombocytopenia, with unusu-ally small platelets. The lab results from this patient are inconsistent with this finding. (**E**) This answer is incorrect, because mutations in *ZAP-70* result in an SCID-like immunodeficiency in which there are no CD8+ T cells produced, with some nonfunctional CD4+ T cells produced. While the lab results regarding the T cells may be somewhat consistent with this finding, in patients with ZAP-70 deficiency, there are normal numbers of B cells, which is not found in this patient. Furthermore, patients with ZAP-70 deficiency do not typically show the presence of lymphadenopathy and hepatosplenomegaly. This is found in Omenn's syn-drome patients due to the inappropriate expansion of the few self-reactive T cells that are produced.

62. Correct: Eosinophilia (D)

(**D**) This patient has Omenn's syndrome, which is an SCID phenotype caused by mutations in *RAG1/2*. This patient manifests with the loss of all B cells and with very few CD8+ T cells and the generation of a few oligoclonal CD4+ T cells that are self-reactive. These self-reactive CD4+ T cells predominantly dif-ferentiate to the Th2 phenotype, which results in an eosinophilia. (**A**) This answer is incorrect, because even though the child has an SCID phenotype, he also has erythroderma and desquamation, which are seen in Omenn's syndrome. Also, patients with Omenn's syndrome have some CD4+ T cells, which tend to be self-reactive. (**B**) This answer is incor-rect, because thrombocytopenia is not a hallmark of Omenn's syndrome. Wiskott–Aldrich syndrome, which can manifest with eczema and a milder SCID phenotype, is characterized by a thrombocytopenia with unusually small platelets, which would put this disease in this child's differential diagnosis, but it is not the most likely diagnosis. (**C**) This answer is incorrect, because Omenn's syndrome is character-ized by the presence of oligoclonal self-reactive, not polyclonal self-reactive, T cells. (**E**) This answer is incorrect, because Omenn's syndrome is not charac-terized by the loss of neutrophils. There could be a decrease in neutrophil numbers if the child is cur-rently undergoing an overwhelming infection, but this is not described in the current situation.

63. Correct: A bone marrow transplant (A)

(**A**) This patient has Omenn's syndrome, which results in an SCID phenotype with the loss of B cells, CD8+ T cells, and the expansion of an oligoclonal population of CD4+ T cells due to a leaky mutation in the genes encoding for RAG1/RAG2. The only cure for these patients is an allogeneic bone marrow transplant to replace the hematopoietic stem cells with functioning RAG genes. (**B**) This answer is incorrect, since HISG is not a cure and does not positively impact the T cell deficiencies in this patient. However, HISG can be used to hopefully control infections until a bone marrow transplant can take place. (**C**) This answer is incorrect, because the lack of a functioning thymus is not the inherent problem in this individual. A thymus transplant may be beneficial in DiGeorge's syndrome, if a thymus is absent. However, in this situation, a functioning thymus is irrelevant if *RAG1/2* is mutated. (**D**) This answer is incorrect, because GM-CSF injections are used in the treatment of neutrophil deficiencies to increase neutrophil production. In this case, there is no inherent defect in neutrophils and/or their production. (**E**) This answer is incorrect, because systemic corticosteroid treatments can be used to control the autoreactive T cells, but they do not correct the inherent immunodeficiency.

64. Correct: Lymphoma (A)

(**A**) This child has ataxia-telangiectasia due to mutations in the *ATM* gene. Individuals with this disease have cells that are susceptible to inappropriately repaired double-stranded DNA breaks, which are important during the development of lymphocytes. Due to this inappropriate repair, they are much more susceptible to lymphoma and leukemia development. (**B**) This answer is incorrect, because this patient has ataxia-telangiectasia, which is associated with the development of respiratory tract infections. Despite its overall decrease in B and T cell numbers, patients with this disease do not demonstrate an increased rate of infections outside of the respiratory tract. (**C**) This answer is incorrect, because autoimmune diseases are associated with other immunodeficiencies, such as deficiencies in FoxP3, AIRE (autoimmune regulator), and C3 (complement 3). The mutation in ataxia-telangiectasia (in addition to the neurological and vascular effects) results in decreases in B and T lymphocytes, but does not affect their tolerance induction. (**D**) This answer is incorrect, because anemia is not associated with ataxia-telangiectasia. This disease results in the dilation of capillaries, but does not affect the production and/or levels of RBCs. (**E**) This answer is incorrect, because granuloma formation is associated with the chronic granulomatous disease (CGD), which is an X-linked disorder that tends to result in increases in *S. aureus* infections and granuloma formation, which is not seen in this patient.

65. Correct: Ataxia-telangiectasia (D)

(**D**) This child has ataxia-telangiectasia, which presents with loss of motor control and dilated blood vessels on exposed areas of the skin, in addition to immunosuppression. The immunosuppression is due to DNA damage repair issues that result in a decrease in both B and T cell numbers, decreased immunoglobulin level, and increased susceptibility to recurrent sinopulmonary infections and bronchiectasis. (**A**) This answer is incorrect, because even though ZAP-70 deficiency results in an immunosuppression due to decreased numbers of T cells, ZAP-70 deficiency is not associated with underlying neurological conditions and/or telangiectasia. Children with ZAP-70 deficiency present with symptoms similar to SCID, but may be milder. (**B**) This answer is incorrect, because even though patients with Omenn's syndrome have decreases in B cell and T cells, they present with eosinophilia and significant erythroderma and desquamation of the skin that is not described in this patient. Furthermore, Omenn's syndrome is apparent within the first few months of life, and this child is 10 years old. (**C**) This answer is incorrect, because while individuals with bare lymphocyte syndrome (BLS; either class I or class II) can present similarly to SCID, with patients presenting with viral, bacterial, protozoal, and/or fungal infections and failure to thrive, it is not associated with underlying neurological conditions and/or telangiectasia. (**E**) This answer is incorrect, because individuals with Wiskott–Aldrich syndrome have normal levels of B and T cells, eczema, and thrombocytopenia that are not seen in this patient. Additionally, individuals with this disease present with hemorrhagic diathesis, persistent eczema, and viral, bacterial, and fungal infections.

66. Correct: Repair of double-stranded DNA breaks (A)

(**A**) This individual has ataxia-telangiectasia, in which the ability to appropriately repair double-stranded DNA breaks is defective. Therefore, individuals with this disease have lower levels of B cells and T cells, with a greater impact on CD4+ T cells. Due to the greater impact on CD4+ T cells, the CD4:CD8 ratio in these patients is often <1. Mutations in the ATM gene in these individuals also leads to loss of coordination and motor function (ataxia) as well as dilation of capillaries to form telangiectasias of blood vessels that are primarily seen on exposed skin areas and the bulbar conjunctivae. (**B**) This answer is incorrect, because when antigen presentation is defective, T cell development is also affected since developing thymocytes are selected on HLA class I and II. Individuals with deficiencies in antigen presentation, such as bare lymphocyte syndrome (BLS), show overall decreases in T cell numbers, without neurologic effects and/or telangiectasia that is seen in this patient. (**C**) This answer is incorrect, because immunological deficiencies associated with cytoskeletal reorganization result in Wiskott–Aldrich syndrome. This X-linked immunodeficiency presents with normal numbers of B and T cells, but has eczema and opportunistic infections. Defective WASP is unlikely in this child, since the patient is female and neurological defects are not associated with Wiskott–Aldrich syndrome. (**D**) This answer is incorrect, because individuals with deficiencies in isotype switch (such as in X-linked hyper-IgM syndrome) have normal B and T cell numbers and present with recurrent bacterial infections with encapsulated bacteria. Defects in isotype switch are unlikely the overriding issue in this patient at this time, since individuals with hyper-IgM syndrome have normal B and T cell numbers and do not manifest with neurological defects. (**E**) The answer is incorrect, because ZAP-70 deficiency results in deficient signaling through the T cell receptor and therefore affects T cell development without affecting B cell development. ZAP-70 is a kinase that transmits signals after TCR engagement to induce normal T cell development and T cell activation. Individuals with this deficiency demonstrate an inability to control live attenuated vaccines and present with opportunistic infections. Furthermore, these patients do not produce CD8+ T cells and produce CD4+ T cells that are nonfunctional, which is inconsistent with the ratio of CD4:CD8 T cells listed above.

67. Correct: *FOXP3* (E)

(**E**) This child has IPEX (immune dysregulation, polyendocrinopathy, enteropathy, X-linked) syndrome, which is due to a mutation in the *FOXP3* gene. Mutations in *FOXP3* result in the loss of functional Tregs, which cause autoimmune disease and allergic inflammation. Patients with this disease typically present with a triad of symptoms: enteropathy (manifested by diarrhea), early-onset endocrinopathies, such as thyroiditis or type I diabetes, and dermatitis (which typically is an eczematous rash). Laboratory findings indicate excessively high IgE serum levels and eosinophilia. (**A**) This answer is incorrect, because deficiencies in RAG1/2 can result in Omenn's syndrome in which the patients have low levels of T and B cells, and manifest with erythroderma, desquamation, chronic diarrhea, and eosinophilia. While this patient has eosinophilia and chronic diarrhea, he has normal levels of lymphocytes, suggesting that he is unlikely to have Omenn's syndrome. (**B**) This answer is incorrect, because mutations in *FASL* result in autoimmune lymphoproliferative syndrome (ALPS). Individuals with this disease manifest with lymphadenopathy due to excessive proliferation of lymphocytes and have an increased risk of tumor development (due to loss of antitumor immune activity) and autoimmunity. While ALPS has an increased association with type I diabetes development, ALPS does not typically present with early-onset type I diabetes or the presence of eosinophilia with elevated IgE, as is seen in this patient. (**C**) This answer is incorrect, because individuals with mutations in *AIRE* result in chronic mucocutaneous candidiasis (CMC), hypoparathyroidism, and eventually adrenal insufficiency, which is inconsistent with the presentation in this child. (**D**) This answer is incorrect, because mutations in *NOD2* is associated with the development of Crohn's disease, since NOD2 is important for maintaining homeostasis and dampening inflammation in the gut. Deficiencies in NOD2 are not associated with the other symptoms presented in this child, such early-onset diabetes and dermatitis.

68. Correct: Treg cells (D)

(**D**) This child has immune dysregulation, polyendocrinopathy, enteropathy, and X-linked (IPEX) syndrome, which results in the loss of Treg cells that control autoimmune responses and GI homeostasis. Tregs produce high levels of TGF-beta and IL-10 that help to regulate the rest of the immune response. In their absence, individuals with this disease typically manifest with either thyroiditis and/or early-onset type I diabetes, eczema with high levels of IgE and eosinophilia, and enteropathy characterized by chronic diarrhea and failure to thrive. (**A**) This answer is incorrect, because while decreases in Th1 differentiation can result in elevated levels of IgE and eosinophilia (due to an inappropriate skew to Th2 cells), decreases in the IFN-γ produced by Th1 cells are associated with disseminated *Salmonella* and nontuberculous mycobacterial infections, which are not seen in this patient. (**B**) This answer is incorrect, because decreases in Th2 cells would result in eosinopenia and a decrease in IgE levels, due to the loss of isotype switch to IgE, which are not seen in this patient. (**C**) This answer is incorrect, because the loss/decreased production of Th17 cells results in Job's syndrome (HIES). While these patients do have high levels of IgE, eczema, eosinophilia, and recurrent infections, they do not have a propensity for early-onset type I diabetes or thyroiditis as is seen in this patient. (**E**) This answer is incorrect, because the loss of Tfh cells would significantly impact the ability of B cells to generate a productive antibody response, since Tfh provide help for germinal center B cells and facilitate the generation of long-lived plasma cells and memory B cells. This patient, with the exception of high IgE levels, does not appear to have any unusual T-dependent antibody response.

69. Correct: CD4+CD25+ (A)

(**A**) This child has immune dysregulation, polyendocrinopathy, enteropathy, and X-linked (IPEX) syndrome, which harbors a mutation in *FOXP3* critical for the generation of Treg cells. Treg cells are CD4+ T cells characterized by their expression of CD25 and FOXP3. They are producers of high levels of TGF-beta that actively dampen inflammatory responses in the GI tract and negatively regulate the activity of self-reactive T cells that escape central tolerance mechanisms in the thymus. Therefore, males born with this X-linked disease are prone to early-onset autoimmune-induced type I diabetes (as seen here) and thyroiditis, eczema, and enteropathy. (**B**) This answer is incorrect, because these markers are found on NK cells. NK cell deficiency manifests with recurrent, severe herpes infections (CMV, VZV, HSV, EBV) and papillomavirus infections, which are not indicated in this child. (**C**) This answer is incorrect, because these two markers can be found on human plasma cells. The inability to generate plasma cells and high levels of antibody are seen in immunodeficiencies such as common variable immunodeficiency (CVID). This disease typically manifests after adolescence and has been genetically linked to deficiencies in *TACI*. (**D**) This answer is incorrect, because these markers are found in activated cytotoxic T cells that can induce death of cells through FAS/FAS ligand interactions. The loss of this cell type can be seen in autoimmune lymphoproliferative syndrome (ALPS) in which there are deficiencies of FAS or FAS ligand expression. Individuals with this disease manifest with lymphadenopathy due to excessive proliferation of lymphocytes and have an increased risk of tumor development (due to loss of antitumor immune activity) and autoimmunity. ALPS does not typically present with early-onset type I diabetes or the presence of eosinophilia with elevated IgE levels, as is seen in this patient. (**E**) This answer is incorrect, because these markers are seen in activated CD4+ T helper cells. CD154 is also called CD40 ligand and is absent in patients with hyper-IgM syndrome. CD40L on activated CD4+ T cell engages CD40 on B cells to induce isotype switch and promote the production of memory B cells. Individuals deficient in CD154 (CD40L) are unable to promote T-dependent antibody responses and are highly susceptible to GI and respiratory infections due to their inability to undergo isotype switch to IgA.

70. Correct: Eczematic lesions on the skin (C)

(**C**) This child has immune dysregulation, polyendocrinopathy, enteropathy, and X-linked syndrome (IPEX). In addition to the symptoms above, this disease is characterized by the presence of eczematic lesions on the skin of affected boys. (**A**) This answer is incorrect, because this is a feature of Chédiak–Higashi syndrome. This is an immunodeficiency characterized by defective killing by neutrophils and CTLs. These patients manifest with recurrent pyogenic infections (especially *Staphylococcus* and *Streptococcus* species). (**B**) This answer is incorrect, because this is a feature of multiple diseases, including congenital agranulocytosis. These patients manifest with a severe neutropenia, with a buildup of neutrophil precursors in the bone marrow. These patients are susceptible to severe bacterial and fungal infections very early in life. (**D**) This answer is incorrect, because this is a feature of DiGeorge's syndrome that results in the loss of the production of T cells, which is inconsistent with this patient. Individuals with this disease have a defect in the development of the third and fourth pharyngeal pouches during development and abnormal thymus development, as well as hypoparathyroidism and cardiovascular and facial anomalies. (**E**) This answer is incorrect, because this is a phenotype of both DiGeorge's syndrome and SCID, which can have the absence of a thymic shadow. In DiGeorge's

syndrome, it is due to abnormal development of the thymus, while in SCID, atrophy of the thymus is from the lack of T cell precursors populating the organ. Individuals with either of these diseases will have a lymphopenia, which is not seen in this patient.

71. Correct: CD4-CD8- (A)

(**A**) This child has autoimmune lymphoproliferative syndrome (ALPS), which demonstrates a signature increase in double-negative (CD4– CD8–) T cells in the peripheral blood of these patients. Individuals with ALPS present with lymphadenopathy and splenomegaly, due to the inappropriate expansion of lymphocytes due to the absence of FAS protein. Individuals with this disease also develop autoimmune reactions, commonly against RBCs and platelets, which manifest as anemia and thrombocytopenia, as described above. Finally, individuals with ALPS typically produce normal levels of IgM, but have increased levels of IgG, IgA, and IgE, as seen above. (**B**) This answer is incorrect, because patients with ALPS do not characteristically show an increase in CD8+ cytotoxic T cells specifically. (**C**) This answer is incorrect, because individuals with ALPS actually have a decrease in the percentage of circulating regulatory T cells. This decrease in Tregs likely contributes to the increase in autoimmunity in addition to the loss of autoreactive lymphocyte deletion by FAS-mediated apoptosis. (**D**) This answer is incorrect, because an increase in this phenotype of cells may be seen in individuals in hyper-IgM syndrome, in which there is a mutation in the gene encoding CD154 (also known as CD40 ligand). The loss of a functional CD40L results in the production of extremely high levels of IgM, with the loss of IgG, IgA, and IgE, which is not seen in this patient. (**E**) This answer is incorrect, because this phenotype is characteristic of anergic T cells. There is a loss of normal control of autoreactive cells in individuals with ALPS, so there is no expectation that this population would be increased. In fact, the opposite would be anticipated.

72. Correct: FAS (C)

(**C**) This individual has autoimmune lymphoproliferative syndrome (ALPS). Individuals with this disease have mutations that result in nonfunctional FAS and, therefore, lose FAS-mediated apoptosis. FAS-mediated apoptosis is important for deleting self-reactive lymphocytes and controlling lymphocyte proliferation. These patients present with lymphadenopathy, splenomegaly, eczema, autoimmune reactions against RBCs and platelets, and normal levels of IgM, with increased levels of IgG, IgA, and IgE, as seen above. (**A**) This answer is incorrect, because loss of a functioning CD40L results in hyper-IgM syndrome. In hyper-IgM syndrome, B cells do not receive stimulation from CD40L on activated T cells and are unable to undergo isotype switch and develop memory B cells. While these patients can manifest with self-reactive antibodies against RBCs and platelets, they do not produce high levels of IgG, IgA, and IgE isotypes, as is seen in this individual. (**B**) This answer is incorrect, because *STAT3* mutations are associated with the generation of Job's syndrome, which has eczema and high levels of IgE. However, these individuals also have an eosinophilia, which is not described in this patient. Furthermore, this individual has increases in multiple isotypes that are not seen in Job's syndrome. (**D**) This answer is incorrect, because mutations in *WASP* are associated with Wiskott–Aldrich syndrome. These patients also have eczema and thrombocytopenia, but with unusually small platelets, which is not described for this patient. Furthermore, they have aberrant isotype distribution with low to normal levels of IgG, which is not evident in this patient. (**E**) This answer is incorrect, because mutations in *TACI* have been associated with common variable immunodeficiency (CVID), which presents with lymphadenopathy and splenomegaly. However, individuals with this disease have decreases in all antibody isotypes, as there is a loss of the ability of B cells to mature into plasma cells that secrete high levels of immunoglobulins.

73. Correct: Hodgkin's lymphoma (A)

(**A**) This child has autoimmune lymphoproliferative syndrome (ALPS). Children with this syndrome have a significant increased risk of developing either Hodgkin's or non-Hodgkin's lymphoma. (**B**) This answer is incorrect, because type I diabetes is not associated with ALPS, but is associated with mutations in FOXP3 as is seen in immune dysregulation, polyendocrinopathy, enteropathy, and X-linked (IPEX) syndrome. (**C**) This answer is incorrect, because Crohn's disease is not associated with the FAS mutation, but is associated with mutations in NOD2, which is important for maintaining homeostasis and dampening inflammation in the gut. (**D**) This answer is incorrect, because mutations in the complement pathway are associated with increased susceptibility and severity of infections with *Neisseria* species. (**E**) This answer is incorrect, because changes in gross motor functions are not associated with mutations in *FAS*, but rather with mutations in *ATM* as is seen in the immunodeficiency, ataxia-telangiectasia.

74. Correct: Adrenal insufficiency (A)

(**A**) This child suffers from polyglandular autoimmune syndrome, which is an immunodeficiency that results in the loss of T cell tolerance induction in the thymus and manifests with autoimmune diseases. The main three manifestations are mucocutaneous candidiasis (which normally presents first), hypoparathyroidism, and adrenal insufficiency (which usually develops later). This patient already manifests with mucocutaneous candidiasis (history of thrush and current infection of nailbeds) and hypoparathyroidism (physical manifestations and the presence of self-reactive antibodies against CaSR). Patients are susceptible to recurrent infections and the development of multiple types of autoimmune reactions. (**B**) This answer is incorrect, because patients with Job's syndrome (HIES) present with eosinophilia. Like individuals with polyglandular autoimmune syndrome, they are at an increased risk of developing candidiasis, but hypoparathyroidism does not present with Job's syndrome. (**C**) This answer is incorrect, because patients with Chédiak–Higashi syndrome may manifest with silver hair and/or hair with a silver sheen to it. Individuals with this disease have issues with cytotoxic killing by both neutrophils and cytotoxic T cells, and subsequently have an increased risk with *Staphylococcus* and *Streptococcus* infections. (**D**) This answer is incorrect, because cleft palate is associated with patients with DiGeorge's syndrome. Patients with DiGeorge's syndrome have a developmental defect of the third and fourth pharyngeal pouches during gestation. These patients can manifest with cardiac issues and facial anomalies, such as cleft palate. In addition, like patients with polyglandular autoimmune syndrome, individuals with DiGeorge's syndrome can present with hypoparathyroidism and recurrent infections. However, in patients with DiGeorge's syndrome, it is due to the loss of thymus tissue and decreases in T cell development, not the loss of central tolerance induction in the thymus. In patients with polyglandular autoimmune syndrome, the resulting hypocalcemia can be due to self-reactive antibodies against the CaSR, which disturb the feedback mechanisms that regulate calcium absorption. (**E**) This answer is incorrect, because patients with Job's syndrome (HIES) and/or Wiskott–Aldrich syndrome can present with eczema. Like individuals with polyglandular autoimmune syndrome, they are at an increased risk of developing recurrent infections, including *Candida* infections, but hypoparathyroidism does not present with either of these diseases.

75. Correct: *AIRE* (C)

(**C**) This patient has polyglandular autoimmune syndrome. Individuals with this disease have a mutation in the gene *AIRE* (autoimmune regulator). The AIRE protein is expressed in the thymus, lymph nodes, pancreas, adrenal cortex, and fetal liver. This protein acts to increase the expression of self-antigens in the thymus so that developing T cells that are specific for self-antigen will be deleted. Therefore, individuals with mutations in this gene have an increased risk of developing autoimmune diseases, as well as hyperparathyroidism, adrenal insufficiency, and mucocutaneous candidiasis. (**A**) This answer is incorrect, because even though mutations in *STAT1* are associated with the autosomal dominant form of chronic mucocutaneous candidiasis (CMC), individuals with mutations in *STAT1* do not develop the other symptoms described.

Furthermore, this is an autosomal dominant inherited mutation, and would be evident in at least one of her parents, which is not described here. (**B**) This answer is incorrect, because even though mutations in *ZAP-70* can lead to increases in candidiasis, the autoimmune reactions that develop tend to be autoimmune cytopenias. (**D**) This answer is incorrect, because while patients with deficiencies in myeloperoxidase have increased risk of cutaneous fungal infections, the additional symptoms described are not associated with myeloperoxidase deficiency. (**E**) This answer is incorrect, because patients with mutations in *STAT3* have Job's syndrome (HIES) and present with an increased risk of *Candida* infections. They also present with high levels of IgE, eosinophilia, and eczema, which are not described in this patient.

76. Correct: C1 inhibitor (D)

(**D**) This patient has hereditary angioedema that is caused by a deficiency in C1INH of the classic and lectin complement pathway. C1INH not only controls these complement pathways, but also controls kinin-generating and fibrinolytic pathways. C1INH inhibits numerous plasma proteases, and its control of the kinin-generating pathways is most often associated with the pathogenesis of hereditary angioedema. (**A**) This answer is incorrect, because properidin is an important regulator of the alternative pathway of complement. This deficiency does not present as described above, but is associated with increased *Neisseria* infections, especially *Neisseria meningitidis*. Patients with this deficiency also may have recurrent otitis media and pneumonia. (**B**) This answer is incorrect, because myeloperoxidase deficiencies manifest with infections due to different *Candida* species. Patients with myeloperoxidase deficiency are susceptible to mucocutaneous, meningeal, bone infections, and sepsis. (**C**) This answer is incorrect, because these individuals present with HIES (Job's syndrome). These individuals present with eczematous lesions, not edematous lesions. Individuals with this disease have a deficiency in STAT3, which causes a loss of Th17 production and an excess of Th2 cells that leads to eosinophilia and high IgE levels, which are inconsistent with this patient. (**E**) This answer is incorrect, because NADPH oxidase deficiencies affect phagocyte killing function. Mutations in this gene result in chronic granulomatous disease (CGD), which leads to an inability of phagocytes to kill engulfed pathogens and increases the survival of catalase-producing *Staphylococcus aureus* within the neutrophils. This disease does not result in the symptoms described above.

77. Correct: Recombinant C1INH (B)

(**B**) This individual is suffering from an acute attack of edema due to the lack of C1INH. This patient has hereditary angioedema, in which patients lacking C1INH are prone to acute outbreaks of angioedema of the skin, the GI tract, and the upper airway. Common triggers are dental procedures, stress, and other unknown factors. (**A,C,E**) These answers are incorrect, because all of these drugs would target a type I hypersensitivity-mediated allergic reaction, which is not the case. The lack of a pruritic rash and epidemiology suggest that her symptoms are not mediated by an anaphylactic reaction. Therefore, these drugs would have no effect on the angioedema seen in this patient. (**D**) This answer is incorrect, because during an acute attack of angioedema in patients with hereditary angioedema, an appropriate treatment is a bradykinin β2-receptor antagonist to reverse the effects of the loss of C1INH activity. Bradykinin is a key mediator of the symptoms seen in hereditary angioedema, so an agonist to the bradykinin β2-receptor would increase the severity of symptoms, not reduce them. The bradykinin β2 receptor antagonist, icatibant, has been successfully used to decrease the symptoms in these patients during an acute angioedema attack.

78. Correct: Complement 3 (C3) (A)

(**A**) This answer is correct, because this child is suffering from systemic lupus erythematosus (SLE), which is associated with the loss of C3 of the complement pathways. The loss of C3b as an opsonin for the removal of immune complexes significantly contributes to the pathology associated with this disease. The history of *Streptococcus pneumoniae* also points to a C3 deficiency, since C3 is especially important in the immune response against this encapsulated pathogen. (**B**) This answer is incorrect, because IFN-α is increased in SLE, not decreased. The increased levels of IFN-α are also thought to significantly contribute to the pathology associated with this disease. (**C**) This answer is incorrect, because CD40 ligand is not expressed in hyper-IgM syndrome. These individuals are susceptible sinopulmonary infections caused by encapsulated bacteria such as *Streptococcus* and *Staphylococcus*. While individuals with hyper-IgM syndrome can produce autoimmune reactions against cells of the blood (RBCs, platelets, neutrophils), this immunodeficiency is not associated with the development of SLE. (**D**) This answer is incorrect, because C9 is part of the terminal pathway of the complement pathway. Individuals with deficiency of C9 are not associated with the development of SLE or infections with *Streptococcus*, but are at a significantly increased risk of infections and meningitis caused by *Neisseria meningitidis*. (**E**) This answer is incorrect, because IL-17 deficiency due to the loss of Th17 cell generation is associated with an increased risk of developing recurrent infections with *Staphylococcus* species, which is not apparent above. Furthermore, individuals with Job's syndrome (HIES) do not develop IL-17-producing Th17 cells due to a deficiency in STAT3. The lack of STAT3 results in an inappropriate shift to Th2 development, with the development of eosinophilia, high IgE levels, and severe, recurrent eczema.

79. Correct: Stabilize the C3 convertase of the alternative pathway (A)

(A) This individual has a properdin deficiency. Since the individual has a normal CH50, but an abnormal/low AH50, this points to a deficiency specific to the alternate pathway. Properdin deficiency is an X-linked disease that commonly presents with an inability to control *Neisseria meningitides* infections. However, recurrent otitis media and pneumonia have been associated with properdin deficiency, as well. (B) This answer is incorrect, because it describes the action of C1INH of the classical pathway. Deficiencies in C1INH result in hereditary angioedema, which manifest in acute attacks of angioedema affecting the skin, GI, and upper airways. (C) This answer is incorrect, because this description refers to C3. A deficiency in C3 would affect both the alternate and classical pathway laboratory results, so this cannot be the correct answer. C3 is a critical molecule in all pathways of complement activation to both act as an opsonin and perpetuate the complement pathway to generate C5 to initiate the terminal pathway of the complement pathway. (D) This answer is incorrect, because it describes factor H. Factor H regulates C3 and the loss of factor H leads to uncontrolled activation of the alternative pathway, which depletes the levels of C3. The loss of C3 due to exhaustion of the alternate pathway would deplete C3 available for the classical pathway of complement, which is inconsistent with the laboratory findings described above. (E) This answer is incorrect, because this description refers to the molecule CD59 which prevents polymerization of C9 and the formation of the membrane attack complex (MAC). Deficiencies in CD59 expression due to mutations affecting the GPI anchor that attaches CD59 to the cell result in paroxysmal nocturnal hemoglobinuria.

80. Correct: Decreased HLA class I expression by flow cytometry (B)

(B) This individual has a deficiency in HLA class I, which is a form of bare lymphocyte syndrome (BLS). Individuals with this disease tend to either present with an SCID phenotype (as described above) or present toward the end of their first year with significant upper and lower respiratory infections. Many times, the loss of HLA class I is due to mutations in either TAP1/2 or tapasin. TAP1/2 are involved in peptide transport into the endoplasmic reticulum so that peptides can be loaded onto HLA class I. Tapasin is an integral part of the peptide loading complex that is responsible for appropriate loading of peptides into HLA class I. Absence of any of these proteins results in the retention of HLA class I in the endoplasmic retention and the loss of HLA class I from the cell surface. The laboratory findings highlight the importance of HLA class I for positive selection of CD8+ T cell development and its relative lack of importance for CD4+ T cell and B cell activation. Individuals with this disease

can also present with necrotizing granulomatous skin lesions. (A) This answer is incorrect, because HLA class I is not important for B cell development or the T-dependent antibody response. Since CD4+ T cells are normal in individuals with HLA class I deficiency, the levels of antibody are normal. (C) This answer is incorrect, because this lab result is associated with Chédiak–Higashi syndrome. In this disease, both cytotoxic T cells and neutrophils have a defect in cytotoxic ability due to aberrant fusion of vesicles and failure to transport lysosomes to the appropriate site of action. Individuals with this disease have decreased immune responses, but have normal numbers of lymphocytes. (D) This answer is incorrect, because HIV infection leads to decreases specifically in the CD4+ T cell subset, not the CD8+ T cell subset. Also, there is no indication in the child's history to indicate any exposure to HIV. (E) This answer is incorrect, because a decrease in CH50 would not explain deficiencies in the CD8+ T cell compartment seen in this patient. While CH50 may be decreased during overwhelming infections, this answer does not explain all of the information that was provided and, therefore, is not the best answer.

81. Correct: HLA class II deficiency (D)

(D) This patient has a deficiency in the expression of class II. Individuals with HLA class II deficiency have an SCID-like phenotype with recurrent infection, chronic diarrhea, and failure to thrive. Due to the absence of HLA class II, CD4+ T cells do not develop in the thymus. Therefore, the numbers of CD4+ T cells, but not CD8+ T cells, is decreased. Since CD4+ T cells are not required for B cell development, the number of peripheral B cells can be normal. However, due to the importance of CD4+ T cells for T-dependent antibody production, these patients present with hypogammaglobulinemia. (A) This answer is incorrect, because individuals with ZAP-70 deficiency manifest with absent CD8+ T cells and nonfunctional CD4+ T cells, which is not seen in this patient. (B) This answer is incorrect, because individuals with Bruton's XLA have a block in B cell development. Therefore, patients with Bruton's XLA have no B cells and little to no significant immunoglobulin levels, with normal T cell responses. (C) This answer is incorrect, because individuals with Wiskott–Aldrich syndrome have normal B and T cell numbers. Like patients with HLA class II deficiency, they have significantly decreased levels of immunoglobulin. However, as stated above, they have normal number of lymphocytes: it is just that the B and T cells cannot develop the immunological synapse needed to develop an effective T-dependent antibody response, which leads to the low levels of immunoglobulin. (E) This answer is incorrect, because even though individuals with common variable immunodeficiency (CVID) also present with hypogammaglobulinemia and normal numbers of B cells, this disease does not typically present until after the first decade of life. Furthermore, individuals with CVID have normal numbers of CD4+ T cells, which is inconsistent with this patient.

Chapter 5

Hypersensitivity Reactions

Michelle Swanson-Mungerson

LEARNING OBJECTIVES

- ▶ Identify the mechanism, symptoms, and treatments associated with type I hypersensitivity and transfusion reactions.
- ▶ Identify the mechanisms, symptoms, and genetics associated with type II hypersensitivities and hemolytic disease of the newborn.
- ▶ Identify the mechanism and symptoms associated with

  - – type II hypersensitivity and transfusion reactions.
  - – type III hypersensitivity reactions and the Arthus reaction.
  - – type III hypersensitivities and serum sickness.
  - – type IV hypersensitivity reactions.

5.1 Questions

Easy	Medium	Hard

1. A 25-year-old woman presents to her primary care physician in the fall with a chief complaint of rhinorrhea, watery eyes, and sneezing. She states that she had these same symptoms last fall, but they went away in the winter, so she assumed she just had a cold previously. Vital signs reveal a temperature of 37.0°C (98.6°F), a heart rate of 85 beats per minute, and a respiratory rate of 21 breaths per minute. A radioallergosorbent test (RAST) reveals a positive reaction against ragweed. Which of the following additional clinical findings would you expect to be present in this patient?

A. Enlarged nasal turbinates with a bluish-gray mucosa

B. A nonpruritic raised rash on the extremities

C. Systemic joint pain

D. Erythematous mucosa in the nasal turbinates

E. Significant cervical and axillary lymphadenopathy

2. A 12-year-old boy is brought to the emergency department by his mother due to a rapid onset of swelling of the lips and trouble breathing. The child had been eating chocolate-covered peanuts as an after-school treat when the symptoms began. Vital signs reveal a temperature of 37.0°C (98.6°F), a blood pressure of 90/60 mm Hg, a heart rate of 124 beats per minute, and a respiratory rate of 35 breaths per minute. Physical exam reveals cyanosis, and lung auscultation reveals both inspiratory and expiratory wheezing with minimal air exchange and retraction. The most appropriate immediate treatment for this patient is:

A. Corticosteroids

B. Epinephrine

C. Cromolyn sodium

D. Leukotriene inhibitor

E. Antihistamines

3. A 6-year-old child is brought to the emergency department by ambulance due to trouble breathing and a systemic rash. The child had been eating celery with peanut butter at lunch when her symptoms began. Vital signs reveal a temperature of 37.0°C (98.6°F), a blood pressure of 85/62 mm Hg, a heart rate of 124 beats per minute, and a respiratory rate of 35 breaths per minute. Physical exam reveals cyanosis, and lung auscultation reveals both inspiratory and expiratory wheezing with minimal air exchange and retraction. Which of the following cytokines would have blocked the development of Th cells that promote this type of reaction?

A. Interleukin (IL)-2

B. IL-4

C. IL-10

D. Interferon-gamma (IFN-γ)

E. Thymic stromal lymphopoietin

4. A 22-year-old woman presents to the emergency department after being found unconscious next to a bike trail. Vital signs indicate a temperature of 37.0°C (98.6°F), a blood pressure of 85/62 mm Hg, a heart rate of 124 beats per minute, and a respiratory rate of 35 breaths per minute. Physical exam reveals that her right arm is significantly swollen, and she exhibits an urticarial, pruritic rash over her entire body. Upon regaining consciousness, the patient indicates that she had been running on the bike trail when she was stung by a bee on her right arm. Which of the following isotypes is responsible for triggering this physiologic response to the bee venom?

A. IgA

B. IgG

C. IgM

D. IgD

E. IgE

5. A 34-year-old man is brought to the emergency department after being stung by a wasp while biking. He initially complained of his left calf hurting and some swelling, but within 10 minutes he was having trouble breathing and became dizzy. Vital signs indicate a temperature of 37.1°C (98.8°F), a blood pressure of 80/59 mm Hg, a heart rate of 130 beats per minute, and a respiratory rate of 39 breaths per minute. Physical examination reveals a generalized urticarial rash and significant swelling of his left calf. Respiratory examination reveals mild wheezing with mild subcostal retractions. What second messenger is critical for activating the effector cell to induce these overall physiologic symptoms?

A. Calcium

B. Cyclic adenosine monophosphate (cAMP)

C. Magnesium

D. Histamine

E. Zinc

6. An 8-year-old boy is brought in the spring to his primary care physician by his mother with a chief complaint of constant nasal drainage and watery, itchy eyes. Vital signs reveal a temperature of 37.0°C (98.6°F), a heart rate of 85 beats per minute, and a respiratory rate of 21 breaths per minute. Physical examination reveals swollen conjunctivae and dark areas of skin under his eyes. Nasal discharge is clear and the nasal mucosa is swollen and bluish in color. Patient history is significant for a less severe case of constant nasal drainage last spring, but it went away in the summer. The patient is sent for additional testing to identify the agent responsible for initiating this response. Which one of the following diagnostic tests is best associated with the mechanism responsible for the reaction?

A. Radioallergosorbent test (RAST)

B. Induration

C. RIST score

D. Mantoux skin test

E. Wheal-and-flare reaction

7. An 18-year-old woman presents to her primary care physician with a chief complaint of "tightness" in her chest when she goes outside. She had been fine all summer, but the symptoms started this fall. Vital signs reveal a temperature of 37.0°C (98.6°F), a heart rate of 85 beats per minute, and a respiratory rate of 21 breaths per minute. Physical findings are unremarkable. Patient history is significant for similar findings last fall, but it went away in the winter and she had forgotten about it until now. The patient denies having these symptoms when she is indoors, but notices the tightening in her chest when she sits outside on her deck and/or she rides in her car with the windows down. The most appropriate daily management for this patient is the use of a:

A. Muscarinic receptor agonist

B. β-2-adrenergic receptor antagonist

C. Leukotriene inhibitor

D. GABA receptor antagonist

E. Histamine receptor agonist

8. A 22-year-old man presents to the emergency department with a chief complaint of a scratchy mouth and throat, wheezing, and a rash. Vital signs indicate a temperature of 37.1°C (98.8°F), a blood pressure of 78/61 mm Hg, a heart rate of 125 beats per minute, and a respiratory rate of 37 breaths per minute. Physical exam reveals generalized urticarial rash and swelling of the lips and tongue. Lung auscultation reveals both inspiratory and expiratory wheezing. Patient history is significant in that the symptoms started within 15 minutes of eating shrimp at a local restaurant. Which of the following cell type infiltrates in the mucosa is critical for leading to the immediate physiologic symptoms seen in this patient?

A. Mast cells

B. M1 macrophages

C. Neutrophils

D. Natural killer (NK) cells

E. Th1 cells

9. A 24-year-old woman presents to her primary care physician complaining that every time she goes to her friend's apartment, she develops itchy, watery eyes and nasal drainage and starts to sneeze. She reveals that the symptoms did not start until her friend adopted a cat from the local shelter. Vital signs reveal a temperature of 37.0°C (98.6°F), a heart rate of 85 beats per minute, and a respiratory rate of 21 breaths per minute. Physical examination is unremarkable.

Which of the following cytokines is critical for the sensitization phase of this pathological condition?

A. IL-1β

B. IL-4

C. IL-23

D. Tumor necrosis factor-alpha (TNF-α)

E. IFN-γ

10. A 48-year-old man presents to his primary care physician complaining that every time he mows the lawn, he starts sneezing and develops nasal drainage and itchy, watery eyes. Vital signs reveal a temperature of 37.0°C (98.6°F), a heart rate of 85 beats per minute, and a respiratory rate of 21 breaths per minute. Physical examination is unremarkable. Which of the following therapeutics directly blocks the release of the mediators by the effector cell in this response?

A. Antihistamines

B. Corticosteroids

C. Cromolyn sodium

D. Humanized anti-IgE antibody

E. Leukotriene receptor antagonist

11. A 55-year-old man presents to the emergency department with a chief complaint of sudden lip and tongue swelling after eating cookies with walnuts in them. While traveling to the emergency department, the patient started experiencing shortness of breath and difficulty swallowing. Upon arrival, vital signs reveal a temperature of 37.1°C (98.8°F), a blood pressure of 100/72 mm Hg, a heart rate of 120 beats per minute, and a respiratory rate of 35 breaths per minute. Physical exam identifies swelling of the lips and tongue, and lung auscultation indicates both inspiratory and expiratory wheezing. Which of the following treatments directly inhibits the mediator responsible for the patient's symptoms?

A. Cromolyn sodium

B. Epinephrine

C. Hyposensitization

D. Omalizumab

E. Antihistamines

12. A 42-year-old woman presents to her primary care physician with a chief complaint of sneezing, nasal congestion, and itchy eyes when she visits her parents. Her symptoms started after they adopted a German shepherd puppy. Vital signs reveal a temperature of 37.0°C (98.6°F), blood pressure of 120/80 mm Hg, a heart rate of 80 beats per minute, and a respiratory rate of 20 breaths per minute. Physical exam is unremarkable and the patient denies having these symptoms unless she is in her parent's house. Which of the following treatments directly inhibit the immunoglobulin molecule that ultimately induces the symptoms in this patient?

A. Cromolyn sodium

B. Omalizumab

C. Corticosteroids

D. Epinephrine

E. Montelukast

13. A 7-year-old girl is brought to the pediatrician's office with a 2-month history of persistent nasal drainage, cough, and difficulty breathing that started in April. Vital signs reveal a temperature of 37.0°C (98.6°F), a heart rate of 90 beats per minute, and a respiratory rate of 30 breaths per minute. Physical examination reveals enlarged nasal turbinates and bluish-gray mucosa. Lung auscultation reveals mild inspiratory and expiratory wheezing. Which of the following mediators is responsible for activation of the nasal endothelium to enhance the extravasation of leukocytes during the activation phase of this response?

A. IL-5

B. IL-13

C. Eosinophil chemotactic factor of anaphylaxis (ECF-A)

D. Leukotriene B

E. Tumor necrosis factor-alpha (TNF-α)

14. A 24-year-old man previously presented to his primary care physician with an onset of rhinitis, sneezing, and itchy and watery eyes in the spring. After tests, he was diagnosed with an allergy to tree pollen. Hyposensitization therapy was initiated and has been continued for 2 years. He recently met with his primary care physician and stated that the symptoms have continuously decreased to the point that he has minimal symptoms in the spring. Based on the patient's current symptoms, which of the following lab results would be consistent with these findings?

A. An increase in the measured diameter of the wheal-and-flare on a skin prick test

B. A decrease in mast cell–associated IgE by immunohistochemistry

C. An increase in the circulating levels of IL-4 by enzyme immunoassay

D. A decrease in the measured diameter of the induration after allergen exposure

E. An increase in the level of allergen-specific IgG by enzyme immunoassay

15. A 22-year-old woman presents to the emergency department after being found unconscious next to a bike trail. Vital signs indicate a temperature of 37.0°C (98.6°F), a blood pressure of 85/62 mm Hg, a heart rate of 124 beats per minute, and a respiratory rate of 35 breaths per minute. Physical exam reveals that her right arm is significantly swollen, and she exhibits an urticarial, pruritic rash over her entire body. Upon regaining consciousness, the patient indicates that she had been running on the bike trail when she was stung by a bee on her right arm. Which of the following method is most likely to identify bee venom–specific IgE antibodies in the serum of this individual?

A. Western blot analysis

B. Immunoelectrophoresis

C. Radioallergosorbent test (RAST)

D. Direct immunofluorescent assay

E. Flow cytometry

16. A 32-year-old pregnant woman presents to her obstetrician for her first obstetrics appointment with her husband. Blood tests indicate that the mother has type A-negative blood (AO [CdE/cde]) and the father has type B-positive blood (BO [cDE/CdE]). Which of the following possible children are most likely to induce an anti-Rh antibody response in the mother?

A. AO (cdE/cDE)

B. AO (cdE/CdE)

C. OB (cde/cDE)

D. OO (CdE/CdE)

E. AB (CdE/cDE)

17. A male baby is born displaying the following symptoms: splenomegaly, jaundice, and a hemorrhagic, nonblanching rash. Lab values are as follows:

- Erythrocyte count: 2.2 million/mm^3
- Hematocrit: 28%
- Hemoglobin: 7 g/dL
- Platelets: 100,000/mm^3
- Leukocyte count: 9,000/mm^3
- Bilirubin: 3.7 mg/dL
- Glucose-6-phosphate dehydrogenase (G6PDH): 12.1 U/g Hb

Microscopic examination of the blood sample indicates that the red blood cells (RBCs) are normal in appearance, with no Downey cells and/or endothelial cells with an owl's eye appearance. Which of the following is the most likely diagnosis of this child?

A. Hemolytic disease of the newborn (HDN)

B. Hereditary spherocytosis

C. G6PDH deficiency

D. Cytomegalovirus infection

E. Fanconi's anemia

18. A female baby is born with jaundice and splenomegaly. The newborn is negative for syphilis, toxoplasmosis, human immunodeficiency virus (HIV), rubella, cytomegalovirus, and herpes simplex-2. No genetic abnormalities are suspected. Laboratory analysis of the blood reveals the following:

- Blood type: O-positive
- Erythrocyte count: 3.1 million/mm^3
- Hematocrit: 32%
- Hemoglobin: 8 g/dL
- Platelets: 110,000/mm^3
- Leukocyte count: 8,000/mm^3
- Bilirubin: 3.4 mg/dL
- G6PDH: 12.2 U/g Hb

This is the mother's third pregnancy and second live birth. Her blood type is A-negative. Which of the following isotypes is responsible for inducing the symptoms and laboratory results in this newly born child?

A. IgA

B. IgM

C. IgG

D. IgD

E. IgE

19. A 32-year-old woman is 12 weeks pregnant with her first child and is in a minor car accident. She is taken to the emergency department for evaluation. Vital signs reveal a temperature of 37.0°C (98.6°F), a heart rate of 60 beats per minute, and a respiratory rate of 16 breaths per minute. The woman experiences uterine bleeding, but there still is a fetal heartbeat. Laboratory results indicate that she has an A-negative blood type (AO [Cde/CdE]), while her husband has an O-positive blood type (OO [CDe/CDe]). With this information in hand, you treat the pregnant mother, put her on bed rest, and have her follow up with her obstetrician in 48 hours. The mechanism of action for the appropriate treatment is to bind:

A. Maternal RBC to prevent the fetus from developing an immune response

B. Maternal IgG to sterically hinder this IgG from binding fetal RBCs

C. Fetal RBC to block the mother from inducing an immune response

D. The Fc of maternal IgG to block it from crossing the placenta

E. Fetal RBC to block these cells from entering the mother's circulation

20. A 32-year-old woman (G4P1) undergoes an emergency cesarean section since the fetus demonstrated signs of distress during labor. Due to significant blood loss in the mother, the mother receives a transfusion of type O-negative blood, which matches her own blood type. The child is born manifesting with jaundice and hepatosplenomegaly. The newborn is negative for syphilis, toxoplasmosis, HIV, rubella, cytomegalovirus, and herpes simplex virus-2. Other pertinent laboratory results are shown below:

- Hematocrit: 28%
- Hemoglobin: 7 g/dL
- Platelets: 95,000/mm^3
- Bilirubin: 2.9 mg/dL

Which of the following is the most likely genetic makeup of the father?

A. AA (CDe/cDE)

B. AA (CDE/cde)

C. AB (Cde/cDe)

D. AO (Cde/CdE)

E. OO (CDe/CDe)

21. A 32-year-old man is brought to the emergency department after cutting his leg in an accident at a construction site. Upon the arrival, the patient is weak from loss of blood and his vital signs reveal a temperature of 37.0°C (98.6°F), a heart rate of 50 beats per minute, and a blood pressure of 105/60 mm Hg. The wound is repaired and the patient is given a blood transfusion of type A-negative blood. Within 15 minutes, the patient complains of a feeling of heat along the arm in which the blood is being transfused and pain in his chest. New vital signs indicate a temperature of 39°C (102.2°C), a heart rate of 110 beats per minute, and a blood pressure of 95/55 mm Hg. Additional review of the patient's chart indicates that his blood type is O-negative. Which of the following lab results would be consistent with the most likely diagnosis?

A. Elevated hematocrit levels

B. Decreased complement levels

C. Elevated hemoglobin levels

D. Decreased bilirubin levels

E. Elevated histamine levels

22. A 44-year-old woman is undergoing chemotherapy for metastatic breast cancer. Her oncologist notes that the patient is anemic and orders that the patient receives two units of packed RBC to counteract the anemia. Within 10 minutes of receiving the RBCs, the patient complains of chills and a feeling of tightening in the chest. Vital signs reveal a temperature of 39.5°C (103.1°C), a heart rate of 115 beats per minute, and a blood pressure of 90/55 mm Hg. Review of the patient's chart indicates that she has a type O blood and she was incorrectly given type B blood. Which of the following isotypes is responsible for initiating these symptoms in this patient?

A. IgA

B. IgG

C. IgM

D. IgD

E. IgE

23. A 26-year-old man, a renal allograft recipient of the B-positive blood group, received a kidney from an O-positive donor. The patient was transfused with type B-positive packed RBCs during and after surgery. Graft function was normal by day 5 and postoperative recovery was normal. On day 10, the patient showed declining hemoglobin levels, and after an additional transfusion with type B-positive RBCs, the hemoglobin levels fell quickly, while bilirubin levels and the patient's temperature climbed over the next 12 hours. This patient is experiencing which of the following types of hypersensitivities?

A. Type I

B. Type II

C. Type III

D. Type IV

E. Type V

24. A 42-year-old woman receives her tetanus booster at her primary care physician's office and returns 4 hours later complaining of significant pain in the deltoid muscle at the site of injection. Vital signs reveal a temperature of 37°C (98.6°C), a heart rate of 75 beats per minute, and a blood pressure of 120/80 mm Hg. Physical exam reveals edema and erythema at the site of injection without induration. The most likely direct cause of the swelling and edema is:

A. Histamine released by activated mast cells

B. C5a production that induces the release of vasoactive substances

C. Platelet accumulation and retardation of blood flow

D. Monocyte and lymphocyte infiltration

E. Formation of large antibody/antigen complexes

25. After a potential exposure to diphtheria, a 55-year-old man receives his diphtheria booster at his primary care physician's office. Three hours later, the man returns to the office complaining of significant pain in arm that received the shot. Vital signs reveal a temperature of 37°C (98.6°C), a heart rate of 75 beats per minute, and a blood pressure of 120/80 mm Hg. Physical exam reveals edema and erythema at the site of injection without induration. This patient is experiencing which of the following types of hypersensitivities?

A. Type I

B. Type II

C. Type III

D. Type IV

E. Type V

26. A 43-year-old woman receives her tetanus booster at her local pharmacy and later presents to her primary care physician complaining of significant pain in her left arm. Vital signs reveal a temperature of 37°C (98.6°C), a heart rate of 75 beats per minute, and a blood pressure of 120/80 mm Hg. Physical exam reveals edema and erythema at the site of injection on her left arm. Which of the following time frames below is consistent with this presentation?

A. 10–30 minutes

B. 1–4 hours

C. 3–5 days

D. 7–10 days

E. 10–14 days

27. A 34-year-old man presents to the urgent care with a deep laceration in his foot after stepping on a rusty nail in his barn. The wound was thoroughly cleaned and a tetanus booster was administered. Two hours later, the man comes back to the urgent care complaining of significant pain, swelling, and redness at the site of injection. Based on the reaction that this man is having, it is highly unlikely that he is deficient in which of the following complement proteins?

A. C1

B. C9

C. Properdin

D. Mannose Binding Lectin (MBL)

E. Factor B

28. A 42-year-old man presents to the emergency department complaining of fever, joint pain, and an itchy rash. Patient history is significant for being stung by a scorpion 2 weeks ago while on a morning walk with his dog. The patient receives Centruroides (horse scorpion antivenom) and his vital signs and symptoms return to normal at that time. At his current visit, vital signs reveal a temperature of 37.4°C (99.4°C), a heart rate of 72 beats per minute, and a respiration rate of 18 breaths per minute. Physical examination reveals an erythematous rash over his body, enlarged lymph nodes, and splenomegaly. Which of the following laboratory results would you expect to find decreased in this patient?

A. Albumin

B. Hematocrit

C. Complement

D. Serum creatinine

E. Immunoglobulin

29. A 45-year-old man presents to the emergency department with pain and swelling in his arm, muscle cramps, chills, fever, and vomiting. The patient indicates that he was moving a pile of wood when he was bit by a black spider with an orange hourglass marking. The patient was treated with Lactrodectus antivenom, monitored and was discharged after 2 hours of normal vital signs. Ten days later, the man presents to his primary care physician complaining of fever and joint pain. Vital signs reveal a temperature of 37.5°C (99.5°C), a heart rate of 75 beats per minute, and a respiration rate of 16 breaths per minute. Which of the following symptoms would you expect upon physical examination?

A. Jaundice

B. Nonpruritic rash

C. Induration at the injection site

D. Conjunctivitis

E. Lymphadenopathy

30. A 62-year-old man reports to the emergency department complaining of severe pain, cramping, and tingling in his left leg. He had been doing yard work when he felt a sharp pain in his left toe. After removing his boot, a black spider crawled out with orange markings under its belly. Vital signs reveal a temperature of 98.6°F (37°C), a heart rate of 71 beats per minute, and a respiration rate of 18 breaths per minute. Patient history is significant for a previous bite by a black widow spider 3 years ago in which he received antivenom for the black widow spider venom and recovered, but he developed serum sickness against the antivenom 12 days later. Your main concern with the treatment for the current bite is that the antivenom will:

A. Initiate a delayed-type hypersensitivity reaction

B. Lead to splenic rupture

C. Activate mast cells to induce anaphylaxis

D. Induce serum sickness in a shorter period of time

E. Be unable to adequately neutralize the venom

31. A 10-year-old girl presents to her pediatrician with an itchy rash on both of her legs. Vital signs are normal. Physical examination reveals a red, vesicular rash on both of her legs. Patient history is significant in that she just returned from a camping trip 2 days ago in the woods where she went hiking while wearing shorts. Which of the following cytokines is critical for initiating this response?

A. IL-1

B. IL-4

C. IL-17

D. IFN-γ

E. Tumor necrosis factor-alpha (TNF-α)

32. Prior to enrollment in medical school, medical students are required to undergo a Mantoux test. What is the defining characteristic that is measured as part of this test?

A. Vascular permeability

B. Hyperemia of superficial capillaries

C. Cellular infiltration

D. Loss of RBCs

E. Histamine release

33. A 46-year-old woman presents to her primary care physician with a chief complaint of a red, itchy, and flaky rash on her left finger where she normally wears her wedding band. She has been unable to wear her wedding band, which is made of 14 carat gold, but is able to wear a platinum ring on her other hand without any symptoms. Vital signs are unremarkable. Physical examination reveals a raised, red rash on the indicated finger. Which of the following surface markers would you expect to be expressed on the cell type that drives this response?

A. IgE

B. CD3

C. CD20

D. CD23

E. CD56

34. A 10-year-old boy is brought to his pediatrician by his mother, since she is concerned that he has numerous hard, raised, red lesions that appeared 2 days after a hiking trip in the woods. Vital signs are unremarkable and physical examination reveals hard, erythematous lesions on both of his hands and arms. Which T helper cell is critical in promoting this response?

A. Th1

B. Th2

C. Th9

D. Th17

E. TFh (T follicular helper T cell)

35. A 33-year-old man presents to the emergency department with a chief complaint of rash, fatigue, and that his "arms kept feeling as if they were asleep." Vital signs are unremarkable, but physical examination reveals three patches of a pale, flat rash on the arms of the patient. Patient history is significant for the patient owning an armadillo for the past 5 years. Due to the potential for this rash to be caused by *M. leprae*, a skin biopsy is taken. To distinguish between the tuberculoid and the lepromatous forms of leprosy, you also perform a lepromin skin test. If the individual has tuberculoid leprosy, what is the time frame within which you would expect to see a positive result in the lepromin skin test?

A. 10–30 minutes
B. 1–4 hours
C. 2–3 days
D. 5–7 days
E. 10–14 days

5.2 Answers and Explanations

| Easy | Medium | Hard |

1. Correct: Enlarged nasal turbinates with a bluish-gray mucosa (A)

(A) This patient suffers from seasonal allergies (a type I hypersensitivity), which are caused by Th2-dependent reactions that result in enlarged nasal turbinates with a bluish-gray mucosa. (B) The answer is incorrect because this type of rash is consistent with type IV hypersensitivity due to the influx of immune cells, particularly effector T cells, to the tissue site of the allergic reaction. (C) The answer is incorrect because joint pain is not associated with type I hypersensitivities, but can be associated with type III hypersensitivities which are antibody reactions against soluble antigens that lead to the formation of immune complexes that can deposit in joints to cause inflammation and joint pain. (D) The answer is incorrect because this symptom is associated with sinusitis due to infection. Since the patient's symptoms have seasonality to them and demonstrate specificity for ragweed, her symptoms are likely due to an allergic reaction, not an infection. As stated above, a bluish-gray mucosa is consistent with rhinitis due to seasonal allergies. (E) The answer is incorrect because lymphadenopathy is associated with infectious rhinitis and is not typically associated with seasonal allergies.

2. Correct: Epinephrine (B)

(B) This patient has a severe type I hypersensitivity reaction to the peanuts that he ate and is having significant trouble breathing. Therefore, in this situation, you would administer epinephrine to rapidly increase blood pressure by stimulating vasoconstriction and reversing the effects of histamine on smooth muscle constriction of the respiratory tract. (A) This answer is incorrect because the corticosteroids would not reverse the effects of the histamine that has already been released by the mast cells. Corticosteroids are overall broad spectrum immunosuppressive agent that inhibits immune cells, as well as many inflammatory mediators including activation of the arachidonic acid pathways that generate leukotrienes, thromboxanes, and prostaglandins by mast cells. The administration of corticosteroids would not immediately reverse the symptoms in this patient; however, it can be used to treat later stages of allergy. (C) This answer is incorrect because cromolyn sodium stabilizes mast cell degranulation. In this patient, the mast cells have already degranulated and therefore this drug will not treat the life-threatening symptoms. (D) This answer is also incorrect because the immediate symptoms are predominately caused by the actions of histamines. This drug can be used in later stages of allergy. (E) This answer is incorrect because even though antihistamines would be beneficial, antihistamine drugs act to compete with histamine receptors to prevent symptoms. Since the patient already has severe symptoms, the most appropriate immediate treatment acts to reverse the effects of the histamine that has already stimulated the histamine receptors on the smooth muscle cells. Once the patient is stabilized, antihistamines, leukotriene antagonists, and corticosteroids can be administered to block the later activation of mast cells that occurs while the allergen is being removed from the system.

3. Correct: Interferon-gamma (IFN-γ) (D)

(D) IFN-γ inhibits the development of Th2 cells that promote type I hypersensitivity reactions. This girl is undergoing anaphylaxis, which is caused by IgE-mediated activation of mast cells. (A) This answer is incorrect because IL-2 is a cytokine that is critical for the initial activation of CD4+ Th cells and does not directly block the differentiation of Th2 cells. (B, C, E) These answers are incorrect because these cytokines promote Th2 differentiation and would promote, not block, the development of a Th2-dependent type I hypersensitivity.

4. Correct: IgE (E)

(E) IgE produced during the sensitization phase of the allergic response is bound by mast cells via the Fcε receptor, which significantly enhances the half-life of IgE. Upon re-exposure, the allergen binds to IgE bound to the mast cell, which activates the mast cell to degranulate and release histamine along with other allergy mediators. (A) This answer is incorrect because IgA is not involved in allergic responses.

IgA is important in mucosal immunity and is secreted in bodily fluids, such as colostrum, breast milk, sweat and tears. (**B**) This answer is incorrect because IgG is not involved in type I hypersensitivity reactions, but it can be involved in type II and type III hypersensitivity reactions. (**C**) This answer is incorrect because this IgM not involved in type I hypersensitivity reactions, but it can be involved in type II and type III hypersensitivity reactions. (**D**) This answer is incorrect because IgD is only secreted in low levels and its function remains unknown. It is expressed on the surface of mature B cells where it has a role in binding antigen.

5. Correct: Calcium (A)

(**A**) Divalent cations are important sources of second messengers in immune cells. Calcium is critical to induce the degranulation of mast cells after the allergen binds IgE that is bound to FcεR on the surface of mast cells. Degranulation leads to the release of histamines and inflammatory cytokines by mast cells to induce the physiologic symptoms described above. (**B**) This answer is incorrect because cAMP is not activated by the FcεR. However, cAMP is an important second messenger in response to many cell surface receptors found on immune cells, including chemokine receptors. (**C**) This answer is incorrect because magnesium as a second messenger is associated with augmenting T cell activation. (**D**) This answer is incorrect because histamine is the end product released after FcεR signaling and is not used as a second messenger by FcεR. (**E**) This answer is incorrect, even though FcεR activation can result in the release of zinc in waves. However, the physiological significance in regards to mast cell activation is not yet identified.

6. Correct: Wheal-and-flare reaction (E)

(**E**) Individuals with suspected allergies are given a skin prick test, where an individual is exposed to a panel of allergens to identify the in vivo cause of the patient's symptoms. A small amount of allergen is injected subcutaneously and will induce a wheal (local swelling; edema)-and-flare (vasodilation; redness) reaction within 10 to 15 minutes, which is caused by histamine-induced edema. The reaction is compared to an injected negative control (allergen diluent) and a positive control (histamine). (**A**) This is not the best answer because, although the radioallergosorbent test (RAST) measures allergen-specific IgE, it is less sensitive than a skin prick test and it can give false positive/negatives. (**B**) This answer is incorrect because induration is caused by cellular infiltration during type IV hypersensitivity, such as seen in a positive tuberculin test. (**C**) This answer is incorrect because RIST measures total serum levels of IgE, not allergen-specific IgE, so it is limited in its value regarding the identification of the causative allergen. (**D**) This answer is incorrect because the Mantoux skin test is used to diagnose tuberculosis, not allergy.

7. Correct: Leukotriene inhibitor (C)

(**C**) The patient suffers from allergy-induced bronchoconstriction, likely due to an allergen that is specifically produced during the fall months. Under physiologic conditions, bronchoconstriction is induced by muscarinic receptors and relaxed by stimulation through β-adrenergic receptors. During an allergy-induced bronchoconstriction, the bronchoconstriction can instead be caused by histamine stimulation of histamine receptors and/or leukotrienes C and D activation of leukotriene receptors. Therefore, the use of a leukotriene inhibitor, such as Montelukast, can be used in the daily treatment of allergy induced asthma. (**A**) This answer is incorrect because a muscarinic receptor agonist would induce smooth muscle contraction, not relax the bronchioles. (**B**) This answer is incorrect because a β-2-adrenergic receptor antagonist could cause vasoconstriction and bronchoconstriction. In comparison, many sufferers of allergy-induced asthma use "rescue inhalers" that are comprised of β-adrenergic agonists to treat immediate airway attacks. (**D**) This answer is incorrect because GABA receptors are not expressed in the lungs and would not have a significant effect on allergy-induced asthma. (**E**) This answer is incorrect because an agonist to histamine receptors would increase bronchoconstriction (see earlier in text), not relax the smooth muscles.

8. Correct: Mast cells (A)

(**A**) During an allergic response, allergen-induced crosslinking of IgE on the surface of mast cells activates mast cells to release histamine that constricts the airways. (**B**) This answer is incorrect because M1 macrophages are pro-inflammatory and are associated with the development of nonallergic asthma and inflammation, while M2 macrophages are associated with the development of IgE-driven allergies. (**C**) This answer is incorrect because, while there is neutrophil infiltration in the mucosa of individuals with allergies, this cell type is not responsible for the immediate symptoms seen in this patient. (**D**) This answer is incorrect because NK cell infiltration is not consistently increased in allergies. (**E**) This answer is incorrect because Th2 cells, not Th1 cells, predominate in the T cell infiltrates in the mucosa to produce Th2 cytokines that exacerbate the response. Furthermore, the immediate physiologic symptoms that are seen in this patient are due to histamine, not Th1 or Th2 cell cytokines.

9. Correct: IL-4 (B)

(**B**) IL-4 is a critical cytokine in allergy for not only driving Th2 cell differentiation, but also promoting allergen-activated B cells to undergo isotype switching to IgE. The IgE produced will bind the Fcε receptors on mast cells so that with re-exposure to the same allergen, the mast cell will become activated to release histamine and other mediators of the allergic response (the activation phase). (**A, C**) These answers are incorrect because both IL-1β and IL-23 promote the differentiation of Th17 cells. Th17 cells may contribute to allergic rhinitis and asthma, but are not critical for the sensitization phase of allergies. (**D**) This answer is incorrect because TNF-α is not important in the sensitization phase of this disease. TNF-α, a pro-inflammatory cytokine, is involved in the activation phase (not the sensitization phase) in the allergic response by activating the endothelium for extravasation of circulating leukocytes to the tissue site of mast cell activation. (**E**) This answer is incorrect because IFN-γ inhibits, not promotes, the development of Th2 development, which are critical in an allergic reaction.

10. Correct: Cromolyn sodium (C)

(**C**) Cromolyn sodium stabilizes mast cell membranes and therefore prevents degranulation after mast cell activation. This drug must be administered prophylactically in order to be effective. (**A**) This answer is incorrect because, although they will block the activity of histamine once released from the activated mast cells, antihistamines do not inhibit the degranulation and release of histamines. (**B**) This answer is incorrect in that corticosteroids are important for preventing the arachidonic acid pathways and the generation of late-phase reactants, such as leukotrienes B, C, and D, prostaglandins and thromboxanes. However, corticosteroids do not block the degranulation of mast cells. (**D**) This answer is incorrect because humanized anti-IgE antibody (omalizumab) does not directly block degranulation and the subsequent release of mediators by mast cells. Omalizumab instead blocks the ability of IgE to bind to the Fcε R on mast cells and, thus, indirectly blocks mast cell activation and the release of mast cell granules. (**E**) This answer is incorrect because a leukotriene receptor antagonist blocks the actions of the leukotrienes produced after mast cell activation; it does not affect the activation and/or degranulation of mast cells.

11. Correct: Antihistamines (E)

(**E**) All of the treatments that are listed can be used in the treatment of the symptoms of an allergic response, but only antihistamines directly compete with the physiologic cause of the symptoms (histamine binding to H1 or H2 receptors) on effector cells. (**A**) This answer is incorrect because it functions to stabilize mast cell membrane and thus prevents degranulation and release of histamine. (**B**) This answer is incorrect because epinephrine is used to counteract the effects of histamine, but it does not inhibit histamine binding to its receptors. (**C**) This answer is incorrect because this treatment (also known as allergy shots) does not directly inhibit histamine action. This treatment changes

the immune response over a period of months to years from an IgE response to an IgG response against the allergen, so it cannot result in an allergy reaction. (**D**) This answer is incorrect because it does not directly inhibit histamine action. Omalizumab (humanized anti-IgE antibody) blocks the ability of IgE to bind to the Fcε receptor on mast cells to inhibit mast cell activation.

12. Correct: Omalizumab (B)

(**B**) Omalizumab is a humanized anti-IgE antibody that binds to the Fc region of human IgE. Due to the localization of the drug's binding site on IgE, it inhibits IgE from binding to the Fcε receptor expressed on the surface of mast cells. By inhibiting IgE binding, mast cells are not activated to release histamine and other physiologic mediators of the allergic response. (**A**) This answer is incorrect because cromolyn sodium stabilizes mast cell membranes and inhibits mast cell degranulation; it does not inhibit mast cell activation. (**C**) This answer is incorrect because corticosteroids do not affect mast cell activation. Corticosteroids prevent the activation of arachidonic acid pathways that result in the production of leukotrienes, prostaglandins, and thromboxanes. (**D**) This answer is incorrect because epinephrine targets and reverses the effects of histamine on cells, like epithelial cells and smooth muscle cells, that contribute to allergic symptoms. (**E**) This answer is incorrect because montelukast is a leukotriene receptor antagonist that blocks the ability of the leukotrienes produced by activated mast cells that bind CysLT1 to induce some of the symptoms associated with allergies.

13. Correct: Tumor necrosis factor-alpha (TNF-α) (E)

(**E**) Tumor necrosis factor-alpha (TNF-α) produced by mast cells during the activation phase of the type I hypersensitivity reaction activates the endothelium to increase the expression of adhesion molecules, which allows leukocytes to bind the endothelium and extravasate into the tissue site of the response. (**A**) This answer is incorrect because IL-5 is a cytokine that promotes eosinophil production and activation, but does not enhance the extravasation of leukocytes. (**B**) This answer is incorrect because IL-13 promotes and amplifies Th2-mediated responses by increasing Th2 cell differentiation and promoting B cell isotype switching to IgE. (**C**) This answer is incorrect because ECF-A is an important chemotactic factor released by activated mast cells to recruit primarily eosinophils to the tissue site of response. However, ECF-A stimulates receptors expressed on eosinophils; it does not activate the endothelium. (**D**) This answer is incorrect because leukotriene B causes neutrophil chemotaxis by stimulating receptors on neutrophils, and does not significantly affect adhesion molecule expression on endothelial cells.

14. Correct: An increase in the level of allergen-specific IgG by enzyme immunoassay (E)

(E) Hyposensitization (allergy shots) works by shifting the antibody response to an allergen from IgE to IgG, so that IgG can bind and neutralize the allergen before it can react with IgE bound to mast cells. Thus, the mast cells are not activated with allergen exposure so the patient has reduced symptoms. Therefore, an increase in the level of allergen-specific IgG detected by enzyme immunoassay (EIA) would be consistent with the patients decrease in symptoms. (A) This answer is incorrect because if the patient's symptoms are diminished, you would expect a decrease in the diameter of the wheal-and-flare (less swelling) on the skin prick test. (B) This answer is incorrect because hyposensitization does not influence the ability of IgE to bind to Fcε receptors on mast cells. Therefore, there is no expectation that the hyposensitization protocol would decrease mast-cell associated IgE. (C) This answer is incorrect because you would expect to see a decrease, not an increase, in the levels of IL-4 by EIA. IL-4 is secreted by activated Th2 cells to drive IgE responses, and also by activated mast cells. With hyposensitization, IL-4 levels drop in these patients since this therapy reprograms the Th response against the allergen to switch from a Th2 to Th1 response. (D) This answer is incorrect because induration is an indication of cellular infiltration that occurs during a type IV hypersensitivity reaction, which is not the cause of allergies.

15. Correct: Radioallergosorbent test (RAST) (C)

(C) Radioallergosorbent test (RAST) uses known allergens to identify the presence of allergen-specific IgE in the serum of patients. (A) This answer is incorrect because western blotting is not used for this type of analysis, since it is expensive, laborious, and insensitive, relative to the RAST and other EIA tests. Western blots can be used to identify the presence of antibodies that are specific for certain antigens diagnostically, but it is not logical to use this assay to identify allergen-specific IgE due to the limitations raised above. (B) This answer is incorrect because immunoelectrophoresis is used to identify the presence or absence of immunoglobulin isotypes in serum. It is not used to identify allergen (antigen)-specific immunoglobulins. (D) This answer is incorrect because direct immunofluorescent assays detect antigens in patient tissue. An invasive tissue biopsy would not be taken from a patient suspected of allergy to identify the presence of IgE on mast cells. Furthermore, it would not identify the antigen specificity of the IgE. (E) This answer is incorrect because flow cytometry is used to analyze for the presence of surface or intracellular markers on single cells, not secreted antigen-specific antibody.

16. Correct: AO (cdE/cDE) (A)

(A) This possible genetic make-up of an offspring from these two parents is the most likely to induce an anti-Rh antibody response, since the child will produce Rh-positive RBCs. The mother will not have antibodies against the A antigen on these RBCs, since they are "self." Therefore, the likelihood that there RBCs will be quickly removed from the mother's bloodstream is low and will allow ample time for the mother to induce an antibody response against the fetal RBCs, if she is exposed to fetal blood. (B, D) These answers are incorrect because this child will not induce an anti-Rh response, since the child will be negative for Rh factor. (C) The answer is incorrect because this child will be positive for Rh factor, but these RBCs will be type B and the mother will have isohemaggluttinins against these RBCs. The mother's preformed isohemagglutinins against type B sugars on the RBCs will likely lead to their expedient removal from the mother's system before she can mount an immune response against the Rh factor on the surface of the fetal RBCs. Therefore, it is not the most likely genetic makeup to an induce an anti-Rh responses when compared to A. (E) The answer is incorrect because this child will be positive for Rh factor, but these RBCs will be type AB and the mother will have isohemaggluttinins against these RBCs. The mother's preformed isohemagglutinins will lead to their removal from the mother's system before she can mount an immune response against the Rh factor on the surface of the fetal RBCs.

17. Correct: Hemolytic disease of the newborn (HDN) (A)

(A) The child was born with hemolytic disease of the newborn (HDN), due to a type II hypersensitivity that the mother mounted against the Rh antigen on the RBCs of the developing fetus. The mother's IgG crossed the placenta to bind fetal RBCs expressing the Rh antigen which lead to their destruction. This explains the anemia and petechial rash identified in this newborn. The destruction of the RBCs leads to the increased bilirubin levels in this infant. The removal of RBCs by reticuloendothelial cells helps to explain the increase in spleen size. (B) This answer is incorrect because this disease manifests with malformed RBCs that look like small spheres when viewed under a microscope. Since microscopic examination indicated that the RBCs looked normal, it makes this disease as a cause of the anemia to be highly unlikely. (C) This answer is incorrect because the baby was born with normal levels of G6PDH. While G6PDH deficiency is in the differential for babies born with anemia and signs of jaundice, the additional symptoms and enzymes level do not support this answer as the most likely diagnosis. (D) This answer is incorrect because the child does not show any indication of cytomegalovirus infection. In newborns born with

CMV infection, the newborn could be asymptomatic, but there were no Downey cells and/or cytomegalic endothelial cells (endothelial cells with an owl's eye appearance) under microscopic examination. Additionally, increase in leukocyte numbers would be expected in the presence of infection, and since the leukocyte is normal, it further decreases the likelihood that this diagnosis is correct. (**E**) This is not the best answer because individuals with Fanconi's anemia have impaired bone marrow function that leads not only to anemia, but also to low numbers of platelets and neutrophils. This child does not demonstrate a decrease in neutrophils and also doesn't demonstrate physical abnormalities, such as irregular skin coloring, and malformed thumbs or forearms, which is typically seen in Fanconi's anemia.

18. Correct: IgG (C)

(**C**) This child is anemic with jaundice and splenomegaly, because the mother produced an IgG response against the Rh antigen in a previous pregnancy. The mother does not express Rh factor (Rh-negative) and therefore sees the Rh on the infant's RBCs as foreign. Anti-Rh IgG can cross the placenta and react with the infant RBC, leading to its clearance and subsequent anemia in the newborn. (**A, B, D, E**) These answers are incorrect because these isotypes are incapable of crossing the placenta to react against the fetal RBCs.

19. Correct: Fetal RBC to block the mother from inducing an immune response (C)

(**C**) In this case, it would be appropriate to administer MICRhoGAM (a smaller amount of RhoGAM) to the mother in order to prevent the mother from inducing an antibody response against the Rh antigen on the fetal RBCs. Due to the trauma from the car accident and bleeding, there will likely be exposure of the mother to some fetal RBCs. Since the mother is A-negative and the father is O-positive with two alleles of "D," the fetal RBCs will be positive for Rh-factor. MICRhoGAM (and RhoGAM) works by binding to the fetal RBC to effectively "mask" the Rh antigen on the surface of fetal RBC and to accelerate the clearance of Rh-positive RBC from the mother's circulation. By masking the Rh antigen and accelerating the removal of these cells, the likelihood of the mother inducing an anti-Rh-immune response is minimized. (**A**) This answer is incorrect because MICRhoGAM (and RhoGAM) is an anti-Rh antibody and since the mother is Rh-negative, there is no Rh factor on the surface of the maternal RBC. (**B, D**) These answers are incorrect because MICRhoGAM (and RhoGAM) is an IgG molecule that binds to the Rh factor on fetal RBC; it is not an immunoglobulin that recognizes another IgG to block it from crossing the placenta. (**E**) This answer is incorrect because MICRhoGAM (and RhoGAM) does not influence the ability of fetal

RBC to enter the mother's circulation. MICRhoGAM (and RhoGAM) acts to accelerate the clearance of fetal RBC from the maternal circulation.

20. Correct: OO (CDe/CDe) (E)

(**E**) The mother has been pregnant 4 times and had one successful pregnancy. During these pregnancies, she likely was exposed to fetal RBCs, which may have expressed the Rh antigen. Therefore, the mother became sensitized to Rh factor and produced IgG against Rh factor that is causing the current newborn's jaundice, hematosplenomegaly, and anemia. Since the mother has type O-negative blood, she has a preformed isohemagglutinins against sugars on type A and type B blood. Therefore, fetal RBCs with type A or type B blood will be typically be bound by the mother's isohemagglutinins against the fetal RBCs and they will be removed from the mother's blood before an immune response can be mounted. If the fetus has type O blood and is Rh-positive, there are no isohemagglutinins to remove the RBCs and there is a much greater chance that the mother will mount an immune response against the fetal RBCs that are of the O type. Furthermore, the genes encoding Rh factor are inherited en bloc with "D" encoding Rh factor and is a dominant trait. Individuals that inherit two copies of "d" will be Rh-negative. Therefore, a father that has type O blood and has two copies of dominant "D" encoding the Rh factor is the most likely genetic makeup of this father. (**A, B, C**) These answers are incorrect because the mother would have isohemagglutinins against the type A or type AB blood produced from this father, so they are less likely to induce an anti-Rh response. (**D**) This answer could yield an offspring with type O blood (if the fetus receives O from the mother and O from the father), but this potential genetic makeup of the father would yield all offspring with the mother that are Rh-negative and would not induce an anti-Rh response.

21. Correct: Decreased complement levels (B)

(**B**) This patient is undergoing an acute hemolytic transfusion reaction due to an incorrect match of the blood type of the patient with the transfused blood. Since the patient has type O blood, he has isohemagglutinins of the IgM isotype that are specific for the A antigen on the donors blood type. The preformed isohemagglutinins bind to the donor RBCs and activate a systemic complement cascade reaction, which leads to the patient's symptoms. The complement is used so quickly, the overall levels of complement in the blood will be low, since the complement is being used more quickly than new complement can be produced. (**A**) This answer is incorrect because the RBCs in this patient are being destroyed and therefore will decrease hematocrit levels. (**C**) This answer is incorrect because the RBCs in this patient are being destroyed and therefore will decrease hemoglobin levels. (**D**) This answer is incorrect because you would expect increased bilirubin levels after significant RBC lysis. (**E**) This answer is incorrect because these anaphylactic symptoms are due to a type II hypersensitivity, which produces anaphylatoxins through complement activation. IgE mediates a type I hypersensitivity, which leads to increases in histamine levels. Therefore, even though this patient is displaying symptoms of anaphylaxis, the mechanism in this patient is IgE and histamine independent.

22. Correct: IgM (C)

(**C**) The patient is undergoing an acute hemolytic transfusion reaction due to an incorrect match of the blood type of the patient with the transfused blood. Since the patient has type O blood, she has isohemagglutinins of the IgM isotype that are specific for the B antigen on the donor's blood type. The preformed isohemagglutinins bind to the donor RBCs and activate a systemic classical complement cascade reaction, which leads to the patient's symptoms. (**A**) This answer is incorrect because this isotype does not induce anaphylactic responses towards antigens on RBCs. (**B**) This answer is incorrect because isohemogglutinins predominantly mediate this response, not IgG molecules on initial exposure to these antigens and therefore it is not the best answer. (**D**) This answer is incorrect because secreted IgD does not significantly contribute to the immune response. IgD mainly serves as an antigen receptor on the surface of naïve, mature B cells. (**E**) This answer is incorrect because IgE does not initiate an acute hemolytic transfusion reaction. IgE can induce anaphylaxis as part of a type I hypersensitivity, but not type II hypersensitivity such as this one.

23. Correct: Type II (B)

(**B**) This patient is undergoing a minor histoincompatability reaction. When the recipient received the kidney from an individual with type O-positive blood, there were lymphocytes that "piggybacked" in on the transplant that were specific for the "B" antigen on the recipients RBCs. It took 7 to 10 days for the B cells from the donor to mount an immune response against the type B blood, and that is why there was not an immediate reaction (as would have been seen in a Major histoincompatability reaction). When the patient received additional packed type B-positive RBCs on day 10, the antibodies from the donor lymphocytes were already made against the RBCs to quickly result in a decrease in hemoglobin and increase in bilirubin levels. (**A**) This answer is incorrect because type I hypersensitivities are associated with allergic reactions and histamine-mediated symptoms. In this case, the symptoms are due to the activation of the complement cascade. (**C**) This answer is incorrect because type III hypersensitivities are against *soluble* antigens, not the

insoluble antigens seen on the surface of RBCs. (**D**) This answer is incorrect because type IV hypersensitivities are cell-mediated reactions (not antibody-mediated reactions, such as with types I–III) and are responsible for contact dermatitis and tuberculin reactions. (**E**) This answer is incorrect because type V reactions (which are mainly categorized as this type of hypersensitivity in Europe) are essentially type II reactions in which the antibody is specific for a receptor and activates the receptor upon binding. An example of this category of hypersensitivity is exemplified by antibodies produced against the thyroid-stimulating hormone receptor in Grave's disease.

24. Correct: C5a production that induces the release of vasoactive substances (B)

(**B**) This patient is undergoing a classic Arthus reaction, which is a type III hypersensitivity. After the injection of the booster, residual tetanus-specific IgG binds to the newly injected antigen to form antibody complexes. These complexes themselves do not cause the swelling and edema, but rather activate the complement cascade to generate C3a and C5a which induce the release of vasoactive substances that cause the swelling and edema. (**A**) This answer is incorrect because the reaction induced after the booster shot is a type III hypersensitivity, not a type I hypersensitivity. In type I hypersensitivities (allergies), secondary exposure to the allergen crosslinks allergen-specific IgE on mast cells to release histamine and other mediators that can cause edema and swelling. (**C**) This answer is incorrect because, while this does occur as part of the Arthus reaction, it does not cause swelling and edema. The platelet accumulation and retardation of blood flow can result in the formation of thrombi rich in platelets and leukocytes that can induce necrosis. (**D**) This answer is incorrect because monocyte and lymphocyte infiltration causes induration in type IV hypersensitivities, but this not an example of a type IV hypersensitivity. (**E**) This answer is incorrect because, as mentioned above, the formation of large antibody/antigen complexes does not directly cause the swelling and edema, but it does initiate the complement cascade to generate C5a. Because of this fact, (**E**) is not the best answer and (**B**) is the best answer.

25. Correct: Type III (C)

(**C**) The patient is experiencing an Arthus reaction against the diphtheria antigens in the booster. This is an example of type III hypersensitivity in which antibodies against a *soluble* antigen to form antibody/antigen complexes, which lead to the activation of complement, platelet aggregation, edema, pain, and sometimes necrosis. (**A**) This answer is incorrect because type I hypersensitivities are IgE mediated and are directed towards allergens, such as pollen, grass, bee venom, etc. (**B**) This answer is incorrect because type II hypersensitivities are directed at *insoluble* antigens. Examples include hemolytic diseases of the newborn and blood incompatibility reactions. (**D**) This answer is incorrect because type IV hypersensitivities are cell-mediated reactions (not antibody-mediated reactions, such as with types I–III) and are responsible for contact dermatitis and tuberculin reactions. (**E**) This answer is incorrect because type V reactions (which are mainly categorized as this type of hypersensitivity in Europe) are essentially type II reactions in which the antibody is specific for a receptor and activates the receptor upon binding. An example of this category of hypersensitivity is exemplified by antibodies produced against the thyroid-stimulating hormone receptor in Grave's disease.

26. Correct: 1–4 hours (B)

(**B**) This patient is experiencing an Arthus reaction against the tetanus booster. In this type III hypersensitivity reaction, preformed serum antibody specific for tetanus toxoid binds to the tetanus toxoid to form immune complexes that activate the complement cascade. Signs of this type of reaction occur within 1 to 4 hours after injection of the antigen, with the maximum intensity at several hours. (**A**) This answer is consistent with IgE-mediated allergic responses (type I hypersensitivity), but the reaction against the tetanus booster in this situation is not IgE-mediated and would not be this fast. (**C**) This answer is incorrect because the time frame is too late. This time frame is more consistent with a secondary serum sickness reaction that could occur within 3 to 5 days due to a memory response against the antigen. Like an Arthus reaction, serum sickness is a type III hypersensitivity reaction, but it is typically against antivenoms or against an antigen that is administered intravenously, not into the muscle. (**D, E**) These answers are incorrect because these time points are too late to be associated with an Arthus reaction. In individuals who are undergoing a primary immune response to an antigen, it will take 7 to 10 days to produce significant levels of antigen-specific IgM in the serum and 10 to 14 days to see the production of antigen-specific IgG.

27. Correct: C1 (A)

(**A**) This patient is undergoing an Arthus reaction (local type III hypersensitivity) against the tetanus toxoid from the booster immunization. The man's preformed, tetanus-specific IgG bound to the tetanus toxoid in the vaccine forms immune complexes that result in the activation of the classical pathway of complement. If the individual was deficient in C1, he would be unable to induce the classical pathway of complement to induce the resulting symptoms described above. (**B**) This answer is incorrect because C9 is part of the membrane attack complex (MAC) of the classical, alternative, and MBL complement pathways, and is not critical in mediating the symptoms

of the Arthus reaction. (**C**) This answer is incorrect because properdin is critical for the alternative pathway of complement that is not important for mediating this type III hypersensitivity reaction. (**D**) This answer is incorrect because MBL is important for initiating the MBL, not classical, pathway of complement and therefore is not important in initiating an Arthus reaction against the tetanus toxoid. (**E**) This answer is incorrect because Factor B is critical for the alternative pathway of complement that is not important for mediating this type III hypersensitivity reaction.

28. Correct: Complement (C)

(**C**) This patient is undergoing a type III hypersensitivity against the horse antiserum, resulting in a disease called serum sickness. The patient's immune system recognizes the horse immunoglobulin that he received two weeks ago to neutralize the scorpion venom and has generated antibodies against the horse Ig to form large complexes. At the height of the type III hypersensitivity response, complement cannot be made as quickly as it is used, so therefore, the serum will indicate an overall decrease in complement levels. Therefore, (**C**) is correct because complement levels are decreased in the serum. (**A**) This answer is incorrect because during serum sickness, the large anti-horse venom/venom complexes can become deposited in the glomeruli of the kidney and decrease kidney function. The loss of kidney function during serum sickness can cause a transient albuminuria in the patient. (**B**) This answer is incorrect because while there may be a hematuria, changes in hematocrit are not associated with serum sickness. (**D**) This answer is incorrect because during serum sickness, the large anti-horse venom/venom complexes can become deposited in the glomeruli of the kidney and decrease kidney function. The loss of kidney function during serum sickness can cause elevations in serum creatinine levels in the patient. (**E**) This answer is incorrect because during serum sickness there is a hypergammaglobulinemia in the patient due to the immune response to the horse antivenom.

29. Correct: Lymphadenopathy (E)

(**E**) This individual has serum sickness, which is caused by immunoglobulins made by the patient that recognize the black widow antivenom that they received in the emergency department ten days ago. Serum sickness manifests with fever, lymphadenopathy, erythematous and urticarial rashes, painful joints, and edema. (**A**) This answer is incorrect because serum sickness does not induce jaundice, as this is a type III hypersensitivity reaction that will not result in anemia and/or increases in bilirubin, as can sometimes be seen in type II hypersensitivity reactions. (**B**) This answer is incorrect because in serum sickness, patients experience a pruritic, erythematous rash, not a nonprurititc rash. (**C**) This answer is incorrect because induration is an influx of lymphocytes and monocytes that are seen in type IV hypersensitivities which are not antibody mediated. (**D**) This answer is incorrect because this is associated with type I hypersensitivities, which are IgE mediated. This type of response is due to the patient making IgM and IgG against the horse antivenom against the black spider. This type of hypersensitivity does not impact the eye and/or conjunctivitis.

30. Correct: Induce serum sickness in a shorter period of time (D)

(**D**) Serum sickness is a type III hypersensitivity response that is mediated by the production of IgM and IgG against the antivenom. Since the antivenom is a T-dependent antigen, it results in the formation of memory B cells that will react more quickly and with a greater magnitude upon subsequent exposure. Therefore, the next time this individual is exposed to the antivenom, the memory B cells will produce a much quicker and greater response against the antivenom that will result in more immune complexes being formed in a shorter time. Therefore, the patient would manifest with much greater symptoms within a few days, compared to within a few weeks as is seen during a primary serum sickness episode. (**A**) This answer is incorrect because serum sickness is a type III hypersensitivity that is mediated by antibody, not a delayed-type hypersensitivity (type IV) that is mediated by T cells. (**B**) This answer is incorrect because even though the reticuloendothelial system and the spleen are important for removing immune complexes, there is no evidence that splenic rupture occurs in response to serum sickness and therefore is not the best answer. (**C**) This answer is incorrect because serum sickness is induced by IgM/IgG complexing with antigen—it is not an IgE mediated response that results in mast cell activation to induce anaphylaxis. (**E**) This answer is incorrect because the immune response against the antivenom will not influence the ability of the antivenom to bind and neutralize the toxin in the venom.

31. Correct: IFN-γ (D)

(**D**) The child is undergoing a type IV hypersensitivity reaction, likely due to poison ivy exposure in the woods on her camping trip. type IV hypersensitivity reactions are driven by Th1 cells that produce IFN-γ. (**A**) This answer is incorrect because IL-1 is important for the elicitation phase of the type IV hypersensitivity response, not the initiation of a type IV hypersensitivity. (**B**) This answer is incorrect because IL-4 is important for promoting antibody responses that are critical in types I to III hypersensitivity reactions in which antibody is critical to mediate these responses. Type IV hypersensitivities are dependent on Th1-mediated activation of CD8+ T cells, macrophages, and keratinocytes that mediate the swelling and itchiness associated with type IV hypersensitivity reactions to poison ivy. (**C**) This answer is incorrect because IL-17 is produced by Th17 cells, which are more associated with the development of autoimmune diseases and fighting fungal infections. (**E**) This answer is incorrect because like IL-1, TNF-α is important for the elicitation phase of the type IV hypersensitivity response, not the initiation of it.

32. Correct: Cellular infiltration (C)

(**C**) The Mantoux test is performed by injecting a small amount of tuberculin intradermally on the arm to induce a type IV hypersensitivity reaction. Forty-eight to 72 hours later, the amount of induration, which is indicative of cellular infiltration, is measured to determine if the individual has an immune response against the tuberculin antigen. (**A**) This answer is incorrect because, while swelling (or vascular permeability) can be associated with type IV hypersensitivities, it is the induration that is noted as a positive response. (**B**) This answer is incorrect because, while erythema (or hyperemia of superficial capillaries) can also be seen in response to tuberculin antigen, as stated above, it is the induration that is measured and significant in the Mantoux test. (**D**) This answer is incorrect because anemia can be associated with other types of hypersensitivities (e.g., type II hypersensitivities), but it is not measured and/or significant in the type IV hypersensitivity that is seen in a Mantoux test. (**E**) This answer is incorrect because histamine is not a cause of a type IV hypersensitivity reaction. Many of the symptoms mediated in type I hypersensitivity are induced by histamine release, but not in a type IV hypersensitivity reaction.

33. Correct: CD3 (B)

(**B**) This woman is experiencing a type IV hypersensitivity response to the nickel that is found in her wedding band. type IV hypersensitivity reactions are driven by Th1 cells that produce IFN-γ to activate CD8+ T cells and macrophages. Th1 cells (and CD8+ T cells) express CD3 as part of the T cell receptor complex to transmit the activating signal after T cell receptor engagement. (**A**) This answer is incorrect because IgE can only be expressed on B cells and B cells do not drive a type IV hypersensitivity. IgE is an important driving factor of type I hypersensitivities by binding to the Fcε receptor (CD23) on mast cells to activate the mast cells upon allergen exposure. (**C**) This answer is incorrect because CD20 is expressed on B cells, which are important for types I to III hypersensitivities, but have little to no significant impact on type IV hypersensitivities. (**D**) This answer is incorrect because CD23 is an IgE receptor found on mast cells and basophils and is used to activate mast cells in response to allergen exposure. (**E**) This answer is incorrect because CD56 is a marker that is expressed on NK cells which do not significantly promote the type IV hypersensitivity response.

34. Correct: Th1 (A)

(**A**) Th1 cells promote a type IV hypersensitivity that is causing the symptoms in this patient through the production of IFN-γ that activates macrophages and causes the induration seen in this child after exposure to poison ivy. (**B**) This answer is incorrect because Th2 cells induce antibody production that contributes to types I to III hypersensitivities. (**C**) This answer is incorrect because Th9 cells produce IL-9 and IL-10 which have recently found to be associated with Th2-mediated diseases such as atopy and in protective immune responses against helminthes. (**D**) This answer is incorrect because Th17 cells produce IL-17, which are important in promoting immune responses against fungi, certain extracellular pathogens, and in some cases promoting autoimmune responses. (**E**) This answer is incorrect because these TFh cells are important for the formation and maintenance of the germinal center during T-dependent antibody responses.

35. Correct: 2–3 days (C)

(**C**) To distinguish between the two types of leprosy, a lepromin skin test is performed to determine if the individual is mounting a Th1-mediated response that is consistent with the tuberculoid leprosy. This Th1-mediated response will manifest as a type IV hypersensitivity, which exhibits within 2 to 3 days after lepromin injection. (**A**) This answer is incorrect because this time frame is consistent with an IgE-mediated allergic response (type I hypersensitivity), but the reaction against lepromin is not IgE-mediated and therefore would not be this quick. (**B**) This answer is also too early because the lepromin skin test induces a delayed-type hypersensitivity reaction which takes 48 to 72 hours to develop in patients with tuberculoid leprosy. This time frame is consistent with an Arthus reaction (type III hypersensitivity) that could occur within 1 to 4 hours after exposure to antigen. (**D, E**) These answers are incorrect because they are too late to be associated with a type IV hypersensitivity reaction. The time frame in (**D**) is consistent with the time it would take to develop IgM during a primary immune response and (**E**) is consistent with the amount of time that it would take to detect IgG in the serum of individuals after exposure to antigen. Neither of these time points is applicable, since this response is mediated by a cell-mediated immune response, not an antibody response.

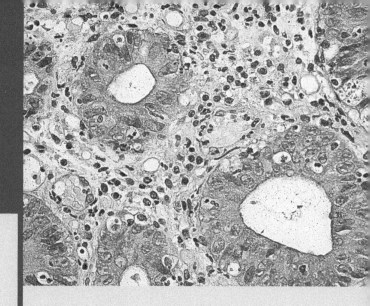

Chapter 6

Transplant Rejection and Cancer Immunology

Michelle Swanson-Mungerson

LEARNING OBJECTIVES

- ▶ Identify the symptoms, laboratory results, genetics, and treatments associated with transplant reactions.
- ▶ Identify the immune mechanisms responsible for cancer surveillance and cancer destruction by the immune system.

6.1 Questions

Easy	Medium	Hard

1. A 56-year-old woman receives a heart transplant from a donor with a compatible blood type. During the operation, the heart failed to generate a normal rhythm and biventricular failure ensued. After 3 additional hours of medical intervention, the heart became discolored and edematous with multiple petechiae. This patient is most likely experiencing which of the following types of transplant rejection?

A. Hyperacute

B. Acute

C. Chronic

D. Graft-versus-host

2. A 58-year-old man with end-stage renal disease undergoes a kidney transplant from an HLA-matched brother. Initially after perfusion, urine output is approximately 150 mL urine per hour. However, 3 hours later, urine production ceases. A duplex scan of the transplanted organ shows normal perfusion of the renal artery and vein, but signs of rejection are observed. The graft was most likely rejected as a result of:

A. Gammadelta T cell-mediated cytotoxicity

B. Complement-mediated toxicity

C. CD8+ T cell-mediated cytotoxicity

D. NK-cell-mediated cytotoxicity

E. Antibody-dependent cell-mediated cytotoxicity (ADCC)

3. A 33-year-old man presents to the emergency department with fulminant hepatic failure due to hepatitis B infection. The patient is admitted and within 24 hours receives a liver from an ABO-compatible individual. Within 90 minutes after the completion of surgery, the patient develops a fever of 39.2°C (102.5°F), and an elevated heart rate. An ultrasound of the transplanted organ reveals thrombosis of the portal vein. The liver was removed and the patient was placed on dialysis until a new ABO-compatible liver became available. Histological examination of this organ would most likely reveal:

A. Infiltration of CD4+ T cells

B. Formation of granulomas

C. Immunoglobulin deposition

D. Fibrotic scar formation

E. Infiltration of macrophages

4. A 62-year-old woman with end-stage kidney failure due to diabetic nephropathy undergoes a kidney transplant from an HLA-matched sister. Initial urine output is approximately 160 mL urine per hour after perfusion. However, 2 hours later, the patient develops oliguria and lab results demonstrate significantly elevated creatinine levels with decreased levels of complement. What is the most appropriate treatment for this patient?

A. Immunosuppress entire immune system with glucocorticoids

B. Removal of the transplanted kidney

C. Immunosuppress T cells with cyclosporin A

D. Inactivate the complement pathway with recombinant factor H

E. Plasmapheresis to remove donor-derived antibodies

5. A 25-year-old woman reports to her cardiologist 2 weeks after a heart transplant with a chief complaint of shortness of breath and a "heart flutter" of 4-day duration. Physical exam reveals normal vital signs, but her respiratory rate is 33 breaths per minute and auscultation reveals an irregular heartbeat. Hematoxylin and eosin staining of an endomyocardial biopsy reveals significant infiltration of mononuclear cells with myocyte necrosis. The most likely type of transplant rejection that is occurring is a:

A. Type I hypersensitivity

B. Type II hypersensitivity

C. Type III hypersensitivity

D. Type IV hypersensitivity

6. A 42-year-old man presents to his transplant nephrologist 3 weeks after a kidney transplant from his HLA-matched brother with a chief complaint of fever and fatigue of 3-day duration. Physical exam reveals a temperature of 38.3°C (101°F) and mild lymphadenopathy. Laboratory values indicate elevated creatinine in the blood, proteinuria, and the absence of anti-HLA I and II antibodies in the serum. The cytokine that directly promotes the most likely type of transplant rejection that is occurring is:

A. Interferon-gamma (IFN-γ)

B. Interleukin (IL)-1

C. Transforming growth factor-beta (TGF-β)

D. IL-4

E. Lymphotoxin-α

7. A 25-year-old man presents for a follow up appointment with his transplant nephrologist after an HLA-matched kidney transplant 3 months ago. The patient reports that he is feeling well, without any significant complications from the transplant. He states that he has been taking tacrolimus and mycophenolate, as prescribed. Urinalysis indicates elevated creatinine and protein. A biopsy of the transplanted kidney is ordered and histological analysis indicates the deposition of C4d on endothelial cells of the peritubular capillaries and significant infiltration of mononuclear cells including cells that have an eccentric nucleus with significant cytoplasm. Which of the following treatments will best target the source of graft destruction?

A. Immunosuppress entire immune system with glucocorticoids

B. Immediate removal of organ

C. Immunosuppress T cells with cyclosporin A

D. Inactivate the complement pathway with recombinant factor H inhibitor

E. Plasmapheresis to remove donor-specific antibodies

8. A 55-year-old man receives an HLA-matched liver transplant 45 days ago due to end-stage liver damage. He presents to his liver transplant specialist for follow-up complaining of fever, malaise, and abdominal pain of 4-day duration. Physical examination reveals a temperature of 38.9°C (102°C) and jaundice. Laboratory findings indicate:

- AST: 1,222 U/L
- ALT: 851 U/L
- Alkaline phosphatase: 367 U/L
- Bilirubin: 5.1 mg/dL
- Donor-specific antibodies: negative
- CMV-specific antibody: negative
- EBV-specific antibody: negative
- HCV-specific antibody: negative
- Anti-HBsAg antibody: negative

Histological examination of a liver biopsy derived from the patient demonstrates destructive nonsuppurative cholangitis, endotheliitis, and the absence of C4d deposition on endothelial cells. Which of the following pathological findings is most likely to be present? The predominant infiltration of cells with:

A. Eccentric nucleus and significant cytoplasm

B. A ground glass appearance

C. A multilobed nucleus

D. A large round nucleus with a large nucleus/ cytoplasm ratio

E. A dark granular center but no nucleus

9. A 49-year-old woman presents to her transplant nephrologist 4 weeks after a kidney transplant from her HLA-matched sister complaining of lower back pain on the side of the transplant, fever, and fatigue. The symptoms are of 3-day duration. Physical exam reveals a temperature of 38.9°C (102.0°F) and mild lymphadenopathy. Relevant laboratory values are below:

- Serum:
  - Creatinine: 4.7 mg/dL
  - Anti-HLA I and II antibodies: negative
- Urine:
  - Protein: 1,500 mg/dL in 24 hour

In this type of rejection, which of the following cytokines is directly toxic to the graft cells?

A. Interferon-alpha (IFN-α)

B. IL-2

C. IL-17

D. Tumor necrosis factor-alpha (TNF-α)

E. TGF-β

10. A 64-year-old man presents to his primary care physician for his annual physical. Patient history is significant for a successful kidney transplant 3 years ago. The man has elevated blood pressure, but other vital signs are normal. Physical exam is unremarkable. Laboratory results indicate elevated creatinine. Subsequently, a kidney biopsy is performed, which demonstrates thickening of the glomerular basement and interstitial fibrosis. Recipient antibodies that predominantly recognize _____ contribute to the rejection of this graft.

A. HLA class I

B. CD3

C. Integrin β4

D. HLA class II

E. Kidney injury molecule-1 (KIM-1)

11. A 58-year-old woman presents to her primary care physician for her annual physical. Patient history is significant for a kidney transplant 4 years ago. Physical exam reveals a blood pressure of 150/95 mm Hg, but other vital signs are normal. Physical exam is unremarkable. Laboratory results indicate elevated creatinine levels. A kidney biopsy reveals thickening of the glomerular basement, interstitial fibrosis, and the presence of nodular aggregates of lymphocytes and monocytes. Which of the following is produced by infiltrating immune cells to stimulate collagen production by fibroblasts in the kidney?

A. IFN-γ

B. IL-6

C. TGF-β

D. IL-8

E. Epidermal growth factor (EGF)

115

12. A 49-year-old man presents to his primary care physician with a chief complaint of dizziness and chest pain of 1-week duration. Patient history is significant for a kidney transplant 5 years ago without complication. Vital signs indicate that his blood pressure is 170/100 mm Hg. Laboratory results indicate elevated creatinine levels. Which of the following findings is most likely to be observed in a biopsy from this patient?

A. Focal cellular infiltrates of lymphocytes

B. Contracted glomeruli with a lobular pattern

C. Dilation of vascular lumen

D. Deposition of IgM on glomeruli

E. Apoptotic myofibroblasts

13. An 11-year-old girl receives a bone marrow transplant from her HLA-matched sister. However, 15 days later she develops a fine, erythematous rash on the palms of her hands and soles of her feet, which spreads to her trunk. Physical examination reveals hepatomegaly and lymphadenopathy. This girl is most likely experiencing which of the following types of transplant rejection?

A. Hyperacute

B. Acute

C. Chronic

D. Graft-versus-host

14. An 8-year-old boy receives a bone marrow transplant from his HLA-matched sister. Three weeks later, the boy develops diarrhea, and a rash that starts on the palms of his hands and soles of his feet, which later appears on his abdomen. The child is administered cyclosporin and glucocorticoids and the symptoms begin to recede. Which of the following markers is expressed on the cell type that directs the most likely response occurring in this patient?

A. CD3

B. CD11b

C. CD20

D. CD34

E. CD56

15. A 14-year-old boy with aplastic anemia is treated with an allogeneic bone marrow transplant from his HLA-matched sister. Twenty-two days after transplant, the patient develops diarrhea with abdominal pain and a maculopapular rash that started on the face and neck, before the soles of his feet and palms of his hands began to demonstrate a similar rash. An increase in which of the following cell types is most likely to be observed?

A. B cells

B. Red blood cells

C. CD4+ T cells

D. Monocytes

E. Platelets

16. A 56-year-old man with acute myeloblastic leukemia undergoes pre-transplant conditioning with total body radiation and cyclophosphamide. After these treatments, the man receives a hematopoietic cell transplant from his HLA-matched sister. Five weeks later, he develops diarrhea with abdominal pain, a maculopapular rash on his face, ears, and neck. What is the most appropriate treatment for this patient?

A. Plasmapheresis to remove antibodies specific for recipient HLA

B. Immediate removal of organ

C. Administration of rituximab (anti-CD20 monoclonal antibody)

D. Inactivate the complement pathway with a C1 inhibitor

E. Immunosuppress entire immune system with glucocorticoids

17. A 52-year-old man is scheduled to receive a kidney transplant from his brother. Which of the following laboratory tests would best identify a cellular response against his brothers' cells?

A. Enzyme-linked immunosorbent assay (ELISA)

B. Polymerase chain reaction (PCR)

C. Complement-dependent cytotoxicity (CDC)

D. Flow cytometry

E. Mixed lymphocyte reaction (MLR)

18. A 38-year-old woman requires a kidney transplant. She has been pregnant three times and there is concern that she may possess anti-HLA antibodies from these pregnancies that could increase the risk of grant rejection. Which of the following laboratory tests is most commonly used to identify anti-HLA antibodies before a transplant?

A. Ouchterlony

B. Complement-dependent cytotoxicity (CDC)

C. Polymerase chain reaction (PCR)

D. Radioallergosorbent test (RAST)

E. Western blot analysis

19. A 54-year-old man presents to his primary care physician with a 1-month history of a painful bump under his left armpit, night sweats, and fevers that "come and go." At the time of exam, the man's temperature is 38°C (100.4°F). Physical exam demonstrates the presence of a painful, enlarged lump under his left armpit. Biopsy of the lump reveals disruption of normal lymph node architecture with overwhelming numbers of large, non-cleaved cells with round nuclei. Flow cytometric analysis of cells from the tumor is shown below:

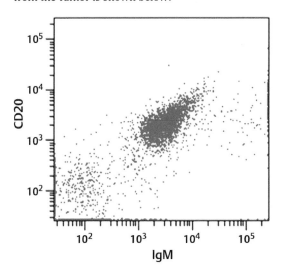

Which of the following cytokines promotes the generation of the critical effector cell that directs the most likely immune response against this tumor?

A. IL-4

B. IL-6

C. IL-10

D. IL-12

E. IL-23

20. A 48-year-old woman presents to her primary care physician complaining of a lump on her left breast that she noticed 2 weeks ago. Physical exam reveals a hard, single immobile mass with irregular borders. Analysis of a tumor biopsy reveals both carcinoma cells and tumor infiltrating cells. A deficiency in which of the following transcription factors would most likely significantly increase the risk that the patient will not mount an effective antitumor immune response?

A. STAT6

B. GATA3

C. T-bet

D. RORγT

E. C-Maf

21. A 28-year-old man presents to his primary care physician complaining of a large bump below his ear. Patient history is significant for 2 months of night sweats, intermittent fevers, and a 15-pound weight loss. Physical exam reveals a temperature of 38°C (100.4°F) and enlarged cervical and supraclavicular nodes. Tissue biopsy reveals the presence of Reed–Sternberg cells with surrounding lymphocytes, eosinophils, and histiocytes with collagen deposition. Which of the following cytokines is produced by tumor cells to limit the antitumor response?

A. IL-1

B. IL-2

C. IL-10

D. IFN-γ

E. TNF-α

22. A 30-year-old man presents to his primary care physician with a 9-month history of night sweats, weight loss, and intermittent fever. Physical exam reveals extensive lymphadenopathy. Lab results indicate that he is negative for HIV and other potential infectious causes for the lymphadenopathy. Biopsy results indicate the loss of normal lymphoid architecture and the presence of a few large cells with a bilobed nucleus, and an owl-eye appearance with a clear halo surrounding the nuclei. These large cells are surrounded by a significant number of infiltrating cells. Which of the following infiltrating cells would most likely negatively impact the prognosis for this patient?

A. Monocytes

B. T cells

C. Neutrophils

D. Natural killer (NK) cells

E. B cells

23. A woman presents to her gynecologist complaining of pelvic pain, heavy bleeding during her period, in addition to bleeding between periods for the past 3 months. Patient history is significant for fleshy, cauliflower-like raised lesions on the woman's vulva 4 years ago. A Pap test is taken and the results indicate abnormal epithelial cells. A colposcopic biopsy reveals projections of keratinized, squamous epithelium that is invading the underlying cervical stroma. A vaccine for which of the following viruses can protect against this type of tumor?

A. Hepatitis B virus

B. Epstein–Barr virus (EBV)

C. Human herpesvirus 6 (HHV-6)

D. Hepatitis C virus

E. Human papillomavirus (HPV)

24. A 65-year-old man presents to his primary care physician with a chief complaint of blood in his urine, abdominal pain, and a 25-pound weight loss over the past 3 months. Patient history is significant for smoking, hypertension, and obesity. He denies changing his eating or exercise habits to account for his weight loss. Physical exam reveals a temperature of 38°C (100.4°F) and an abdominal mass. Radiographic analysis of the kidney identifies a renal mass, which upon further investigation is identified as a malignant carcinoma. Which of the following markers are most likely to be found in the biopsy on immune cells that are responsible for killing tumor cells in a TAP1/2-independent manner?

A. CD8

B. CD20

C. CD34

D. CD56

E. CD86

25. A 43-year-old woman presents to her dermatologist with a chief concern over a dark freckle that has been getting larger in the last few months. Patient history is significant for years of sun exposure without wearing sun screen and her father had melanoma diagnosed in his 60s. Physical exam reveals a large, asymmetrical nevus with varying color and border irregularities. Treatment includes the administration of a monoclonal antibody specific for human PD-L1. Which of the following outcomes would most likely be an unintended consequence of this drug?

A. Increase in autoimmune reactions, such as hepatitis

B. Decreased metastasis due to blocking the interaction of the tumor with adhesion molecules

C. Fever and arthralgia due to a type III hypersensitivity reaction

D. Decreased angiogenesis and tumor regression

E. Increased risk of Neisseria infection due to low complement levels

26. A 72-year-old man presents to his primary care physician concerned over a few painless bumps that have appeared over the last few months. Patient history is significant for a 15-pound weight loss over the last few months without changing exercise and diet. Physical exam is remarkable for enlarged cervical and axillary lymph nodes that are firm, rounded, nontender, and mobile upon palpitation. A peripheral blood smear reveals a significant lymphocytosis with small lymphocytes. Flow cytometric analysis reveals that the majority of cells is positive for CD20, CD5, and expresses low levels of surface immunoglobulin that all contain the kappa light chain. Based on the most likely diagnosis, the patient is treated with a therapeutic monoclonal antibody to eradicate the tumor. The increased expression of which of the following molecules on the surface of the tumor cells would most likely inhibit the efficacy of the drug used in this therapy?

A. Fc gamma receptor (FcγR)

B. Surface immunoglobulin

C. CD20

D. Complement receptor 3 (CR3)

E. CD59

27. A 58-year-old man presents to his dermatologist with a large freckle on the side of his nose that has gotten larger and changed color over the past summer. Patient history is significant for years working in the sun as a farmer. When asked, the farmer states that he never wore sunscreen or a hat. Physical exam reveals an asymmetrical nevus that is 8 mm in diameter and has irregular borders with color variegation. Treatment includes the administration of a monoclonal antibody, ipilimumab. The administration of ipilimumab results in the activation of which of the following cell types?

A. Neutrophils

B. Macrophages

C. Cytotoxic T cells

D. Mast cells

E. B cells

28. As part of a normal mammogram screening, a mass with a poorly defined margin is observed in a 55-year-old woman. She follows up with her primary care physician in which a physical exam reveals a hard, single immobile mass with irregular borders. The tumor is removed and analysis of the biopsy reveals carcinoma cells that are HER2+. Based on these findings, which of the following monoclonal antibody therapies would be the best option to directly target the cancerous cells?

A. Omalizumab

B. Rituximab

C. Adalimumab

D. Abatacept

E. Trastuzumab

29. A 57-year-old man presents to his primary care physician with a 6-week history of fever, a painful bump near the back of his chin and night sweats. At the time of exam, the man's temperature is 38.3°C (101°F). Physical exam shows an enlarged cervical lymph node. Biopsy of the lump reveals disruption of normal lymph node architecture with overwhelming numbers of large, non-cleaved cells with round nuclei. Flow cytometric analysis of cells from the tumor is shown below:

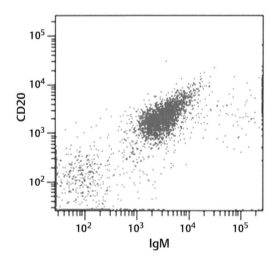

Which of the following drugs would be most beneficial for treating this patient?

A. Omalizumab

B. Rituximab

C. Adalimumab

D. Abatacept

E. Trastuzumab

30. A 61-year-old Florida native presents to her primary care physician concerned over a mole that has gotten considerably larger since her last visit 6 months ago. Physical exam reveals a multicolored, asymmetric nevus with irregular borders which is 8 mm in diameter. Which of the following cytokines is most critical for the immune response that targets the cells in this lesion?

A. TGF-β

B. IFN-γ

C. IL-4

D. IL-10

E. IL-17

6.2 Answers and Explanations

Easy	Medium	Hard

1. Correct: Hyperacute (A)

(**A**) This patient is undergoing a hyperacute rejection of the transplanted heart. Hyperacute rejections are due to the presence of preformed antibodies that recognize antigens on the surface of the transplanted tissue. These antibodies are typically due to either previous transplants, blood transfusions, and/or pregnancies. Hyperacute rejections occur within hours of transplantation and typically, the only choice is to remove the transplanted organ. (**B**) This answer is incorrect because acute transplant rejections occur within several days, not hours. Furthermore, acute transplant rejections tend to be mediated by T cells (even though humoral acute rejection is documented). (**C**) This answer is incorrect because the time frame is incorrect for chronic transplant rejection. (**D**) This answer is incorrect because the rejection is due to antibodies in the *recipient* responding to antigens on the donor tissue. In graft-versus-host rejection, a T cell mediated response from the donor is initiated against the recipient tissue (not the donated tissue). Graft-versus-host rejection predominates as a complication in hematopoietic stem cell transplants and/or bone marrow transplants.

2. Correct: Complement-mediated toxicity (B)

(**B**) This patient is undergoing hyperacute transplant rejection. Hyperacute transplant rejection is caused by preformed antibodies in the recipient that bind to antigens that are found on endothelial cells of the transplanted organ. These antibodies are of the IgM and IgG isotype and are effective in activating complement that results in destruction of the graft cells. (**A**) This answer is incorrect because gammadelta T cells can be cytotoxic, but do not contribute to hyperacute transplant rejection. (**C**) This answer is incorrect because

119

CD8+ T cells do not significantly contribute to hyper-acute transplant reactions, in part because the CD8+ T cells would not be activated to the level of causing transplant rejection within this time frame. However, CD8+ T cells significantly contribute to acute trans-plant reactions. (**D**) This answer is incorrect because while NK cells can recognize the absence of host HLA on transplanted tissue, they do not cause organ dete-rioration to this degree and in such a short amount of time. Furthermore, the case states that the kidney was received from an HLA-matched donor, which would suggest that NK cell activation would not be significant in this patient. (**E**) This answer is incorrect because antibody-dependent cell-mediated cytotoxicity (ADCC) uses IgG binding to Fc receptor cells on killer cells (such as NK cells, macrophages, etc.) and takes hours for the cells to become activated to induce cyto-toxicity. Therefore, ADCC would not cause this level of extensive damage in this short of a time frame. During hyperacute responses, the presence of preformed anti-bodies and complement in the recipient exist make it possible for this immune reaction to occur and induce significant damage in such a short amount of time.

3. Correct: Immunoglobulin deposition (C)

(**C**) This patient is undergoing hyperacute rejection of the liver. The rapid rejection is due to preformed antibodies against antigens found on the endothelial cells of the transplanted tissues. Immunoglobulin deposits on these endothelial cells to activate the complement cascade that results in the swelling and hemorrhage of tissue, decreased blood flow and necrosis of the transplanted organ. (**A**) This answer is incorrect because CD4+ T cells are involved in acute transplant rejection, which occurs within days (not hours) of transplantation. During acute rejec-tion, there is an infiltration of both CD4+ and CD8+ T cells into the rejected tissue. However, due to the rapid nature of this rejection, there is not sufficient time for the activation of these cells of the adaptive immune system. (**B**) This answer is incorrect because the formation of granulomas is associated with chronic rejection of transplants. The onset of chronic rejection is insidious with subclinical microvascular inflammation and takes months to years to occur. (**D**) This answer is incorrect because fibrotic scar for-mation is a response seen in chronic inflammation, whereas this patient is undergoing a hyperacute response. (**E**) This answer is incorrect because infil-tration of macrophages is associated with cytotoxic-ity seen in acute transplant rejection. During acute rejection, CD4+ T cells become Th1 cells that produce IFN-γ to activate macrophages. These macrophages contribute to the pathology seen in acute rejection.

4. Correct: Removal of the transplanted kidney (B)

(**B**) This patient is undergoing a hyperacute rejec-tion of the engrafted kidney, which is due to

antibody-mediated activation of complement. Unfortunately, the appropriate treatment for this patient is to remove the engrafted kidney. (**A**) This answer is incorrect because glucocorticoids will depress immune cell function (both innate and adap-tive), but will not significantly impact the comple-ment pathway that has already been initiated by preformed antibodies and preformed complement. Therefore, this treatment will not significantly impact the ongoing complement-mediated destruc-tion. (**C**) This answer is incorrect because T cells do not contribute to hyperacute graft rejection. There-fore, decreasing their activity through the adminis-tration of cyclosporin A will not impact the ongoing complement-mediated destruction of the engrafted tissue. (**D**) This answer is incorrect because factor H inactivates the alternative pathway of comple-ment, not the classical pathway of complement that is important in hyperacute graft rejection. (**E**) This answer is incorrect because the antibodies mediat-ing this reaction are *recipient* derived. If identified early enough, plasmapheresis can be used to try to remove recipient-derived antibodies to decrease the amount of immediate destruction of the organ. How-ever, plasmapheresis is used in conjunction with other treatments to decrease B cell activity and anti-body secretion. In this patient, the damage is likely too severe for this approach to work.

5. Correct: Type IV hypersensitivity (D)

(**D**) This patient is undergoing an acute cardiac allograft rejection, which is a type IV hypersensitiv-ity. Acute allograft rejection is typically mediated by infiltrating CD4+ and CD8+ T cells that promote the destruction of the graft. (**A**) This answer is incor-rect because type I hypersensitivities are allergic responses (such as seasonal allergies). This hyper-sensitivity is mediated by allergen-specific IgE mol-ecules that activate mast cells to release histamine and other chemical mediators to induce symptoms of allergies, such as runny nose, watery/itchy eyes, and even asthma. (**B**) This answer is incorrect because type II hypersensitivities are mediated by IgM and IgG antibodies that are specific for insoluble anti-gens. Examples of type II hypersensitivities are ABO transfusion reactions and anti-Rh antibodies that can cause the destruction of fetal red blood cells in hemolytic disease of the newborn. There are forms of antibody-mediated acute rejection, but they are more common in kidney transplants. (**C**) This answer is incorrect because type III hypersensitivities are mediated by IgM and IgG antibodies that are specific for soluble antigens. Examples of type III hypersen-sitivities are serum sickness and the Arthus reaction.

6. Correct: Interferon-gamma (IFN-γ) (A)

(**A**) This patient is undergoing acute rejection of the transplanted kidney. This is a type IV hypersensitiv-ity reaction that is mediated by CD4+ Th1 cells that produce IFN-γ that further activates alloreactive CD8+ T cells, NK cells, and macrophages. (**B**) This answer is incorrect because while IL-1 can promote the production of fever, IL-1 does not directly promote acute transplant rejections. (**C**) This answer is incorrect because TGF-β is produced by regulatory T cells during acute rejection that attempt to control the pro-inflammatory T cells that are promoting graft rejection. (**D**) This answer is incorrect because IL-4 promotes antibody-mediated transplant rejections. While acute transplant rejection can be mediated by HLA-specific antibodies, the absence of these antibodies in the serum of this patient makes it unlikely that this patient is undergoing acute rejection due to the humoral immune response. Furthermore, IL-4 dampens or blocks the development of Th1 cells, and therefore would have a dampening effect on acute cell-mediated transplant rejection. (**E**) This answer is incorrect because lymphotoxin-α is not thought to directly promote acute graft rejection. Lymphotoxin-α may influence CD8+ T cell function. However, this is not the best answer since it has no effect on the CD4+ T cells that drive cell-mediated acute allograft rejections.

7. Correct: Plasmapheresis to remove donor-specific antibodies (E)

(**E**) This patient has antibody-mediated acute allograft rejection. Antibody-mediated graft rejection is more common in kidney transplants, as compared to lung or liver transplants. Patients undergoing antibody-mediated acute rejection can be treated with plasmapheresis to remove the donor-specific antibodies that are causing damage to the graft via complement-mediated destruction. However, plasmapheresis is typically used in conjunction with other treatments to decrease B cell activity and antibody secretion. (**A**) This answer is incorrect because even though glucocorticoids will dampen the entire immune system, it will not target the anti-donor antibodies that have already been produced and are causing destruction of the kidney allograft. This will likely be added to the treatment, but will not specifically target the antibodies causing destruction. (**B**) This answer is incorrect because the graft is not irreversibly damaged, the patient is still asymptomatic, and there is still time to control the immune response before the transplanted organ becomes inadequate. The patient will likely have his immunosuppression medications increased in an effort to control the B cells and plasma cells that are producing the antibodies to mediate the damage. (**C**) This answer is incorrect because the use of a T cell-specific inhibitor will not be useful in inhibiting the B cells and plasma cells that are producing anti-donor antibodies to mediate the rejection of the kidney allograft. (**D**) This answer is incorrect because factor H inactivates the alternative pathway of complement, not the classical pathway of complement that is important in antibody-mediated acute graft rejection.

8. Correct: A large round nucleus with a large nucleus/cytoplasm ratio (D)

(**D**) This patient is undergoing acute cell-mediated liver rejection. Therefore, it is most likely that there would be a significant infiltration of T lymphocytes, with potentially some neutrophils and eosinophils. The T cells drive the antigraft response in this rejection and are histologically characterized by a large round nucleus with a large nucleus/cytoplasm ratio. (**A**) This answer is incorrect because this description is indicative of plasma cells, which are more likely to be present in antibody-mediated acute rejection. Since the pathology results indicate that the biopsy is negative for the presence of C4d deposition, the likelihood that the rejection is occurring is due to antibody-mediated acute rejection is significantly decreased. (**B**) This answer is incorrect because this description is indicative of CMV-infected cells. CMV infection can cause significant problems in transplants. However, this patient is seronegative for CMV-specific antibodies and therefore this is unlikely the cause of the physical and biochemical changes in this patient. (**C**) This answer is incorrect because this description defines neutrophils. In liver biopsies during acute cell-mediated rejection, there may be an infiltration of neutrophils that may contribute to the inflammation and damage seen after transplant. However, it would not be the dominant infiltrating cell type. (**E**) This answer is incorrect because this description is indicative of platelets. While platelets are very important in the hyperacute rejection process, their importance in acute rejection is not as significant. Furthermore, platelets in the response appear to be more important in antibody-mediated rejections.

9. Correct: Tumor necrosis factor-alpha (TNF-α) (D)

(**D**) This patient is undergoing acute transplant rejection of the kidney allograft. During allograft rejection that is mediated through cellular immunity (generation of Th1 cells and activation of cytotoxic T cells), TNF-α is produced that can bind to TNF-receptors to induce apoptosis of cells from the allograft. (**A**) This answer is incorrect because IFN-α is not directly cytolytic. IFN-α is produced by nucleated cells after exposure to virus or other inflammatory signals, resulting in increased expression of HLA class I. The IFN-α-dependent increase in HLA class I enhances the visibility of the allograft to cytotoxic T cells, but is not directly cytolytic. (**B**) This answer is incorrect because IL-2 is a growth factor for Th1 cells, cytotoxic T cells, and NK cells that promote allograft rejection. It is not directly cytolytic. (**C**) This answer is incorrect because while IL-17 can contribute to allograft rejection, it is thought to be important in recruiting leukocytes to the site of rejection and may be more important in antibody-mediated acute allograft rejection than in cell-mediated allograft rejection. Furthermore, IL-17 is not thought to be cytolytic. (**E**) This answer is incorrect because TGF-β is an anti-inflammatory cytokine made by T-regulatory cells that dampen allograft rejections.

10. Correct: HLA class I (A)

(**A**) This patient is undergoing chronic rejection of the transplanted kidney. The initial indications for chronic kidney rejection are hypertension, elevated creatinine and protein in the urine. This destruction is mediated by a combination of cell-mediated and humoral immune responses against the transplanted organ. HLA class I on the transplanted organ is recognized by the recipient B cells and can initiate an immune response against the HLA I found on the graft. (**B**) This answer is incorrect because CD3 is a molecule expressed on T cells that would not be expressed on the donor graft. (**C**) This answer is incorrect because while integrin β4 is expressed on cells in the kidney, it is not typically a target of the immune system during renal graft rejection. (**D**) This answer is incorrect because it would be unlikely that the transplanted kidney would express HLA class II, as the expression of HLA class II is typically restricted to antigen presenting cells. However, HLA class I is expressed on nucleated cells and thus would be expressed on the donor kidney cells and available to be recognized by the immune system. (**E**) This answer is incorrect because even though KIM-1 is a diagnostic marker for kidney injury, it is not typically a target of the immune system during renal graft rejection.

11. Correct: TGF-β (C)

(**C**) This individual is undergoing a chronic rejection of the transplanted kidney. TGF-β plays a critical role in stimulating the fibroblasts to form collagen as part of the extracellular matrix leading to fibrosis and scar formation. (**A**) This answer is incorrect because IFN-γ increases the expression of HLA class I, which can contribute to graft rejection, but not by inducing fibroblasts to produce collagen. (**B**) This answer is incorrect because IL-6 is a pro-inflammatory cytokine that inhibits the functions of regulatory T cells and enhances the activation of alloreactive T cells. (**D**) This answer is incorrect because IL-8 is an important chemokine that recruits neutrophils and granulocytes to the graft that can contribute to graft destruction, but not through the activation of fibroblasts to produce collagen. (**E**) This answer is incorrect because even though EGF is a fibrogenic cytokine, there is controversy whether EGF significantly contributes to the damage seen in chronic transplant rejection. However, EGF is thought to positively contribute to renal tube repair and/or regeneration, which ultimately enhances the recovery of kidney function after transplant.

12. Correct: Focal cellular infiltrates of lymphocytes (A)

(**A**) This individual is undergoing chronic kidney rejection in which both the innate and adaptive immune response coordinate a slow attack that results in fibrosis and loss of graft function. In biopsies from organs undergoing chronic graft rejection, it is common for the presence of focal cellular infiltrates of lymphocytes and plasma cells. These cells are perpetuating the constant attack on the organ that ultimately will result in the loss of graft function. (**B**) This answer is incorrect because during chronic renal graft rejection, the glomeruli become enlarged with a lobular pattern; in severe cases, global sclerosis may be seen. (**C**) This answer is incorrect because during chronic renal graft rejection, there is a progressive thickening and narrowing of the vascular lumen due to continuous endothelial inflammation and injury. (**D**) This answer is incorrect because since this is a chronic rejection, any deposition of antibody on the glomeruli will be of the IgG isotype. Renal graft nephropathy may be positive for IgG, fibrin and C3 deposition. (**E**) This answer is incorrect because in chronic rejection, there is constant proliferation of myofibroblasts (not apoptosis).

13. Correct: Graft-versus-host (D)

(**D**) This patient is undergoing a graft-versus-host response in which T cells that are donor-derived begin to attack the recipient. The onset of rash, splenomegaly, hepatomegaly, lymphadenopathy, diarrhea, and anemia are characteristic of this response. (**A**) This answer is incorrect because hyperacute rejections are antibody-mediated rejections that result in complement activation and destruction of the transplanted material within *hours*, not 15 days. (**B**) This answer is incorrect because an acute allograft rejection is when the host rejects the transplanted tissue. In this patient, engrafted cells from the donor are attacking recipient cells. (**C**) This answer is incorrect because this is a response in which the cells from the recipient start to attack the transplanted tissue. Furthermore, the timing of this response is off, since chronic rejection occurs after months to years, not the two weeks as is seen in this patient.

14. Correct: CD3 (A)

(**A**) This child is undergoing a graft-versus-host response in which T cells from the donor, which express CD3, are directing an immune response against the HLA antigens of the recipient. Common signs of graft-versus-host disease (GVHD) include hepatomegaly, splenomegaly, lymphadenopathy, diarrhea, anemia, weight loss, and a characteristic rash 10 to 28 days after transplant, which is characterized as a fine, diffuse, erythematous rash. The rash begins on the neck, ears, shoulders, palms of the hands and soles of the feet, and then spreads to the trunk of the individual. (**B**) This answer is incorrect as CD11b is expressed on monocytes, neutrophils, NK cells, granulocytes, and macrophages. None of these cells are responsible for directing the graft-versus-host reaction, which is a type IV hypersensitivity that is directed by T cells. (**C**) This answer is incorrect because CD20 is expressed on B cells. B cells do not significantly contribute to the graft-versus-host response. (**D**) This answer is incorrect because CD34 is expressed on hematopoietic stem cells. While these cells are critical for the establishment of a successful graft to restore the immune system in the recipient, they are not responsible for mediating the attack on the recipient cells. (**E**) This answer is incorrect because CD56 is expressed on NK cells. Even though NK cells participate in the type IV hypersensitivity response, NK cells do not direct type IV hypersensitivities.

15. Correct: CD4+ T cells (C)

(**C**) This patient is undergoing an acute episode of graft-versus-host disease (GVHD). Donor-derived T cells that were introduced with the hematopoietic stem cells are reacting against the host HLA molecules of the recipient to cause destruction. In these patients, there is significant proliferation and expansion of donor-derived CD4+ and CD8+ T cells. (**A**) This answer is incorrect because the numbers of circulating B cells in individuals undergoing acute GVHD tend to be unchanged or even decreased. Since GVHD is a type IV hypersensitivity, B cell contribution to the response is minimal. (**B**) This answer is incorrect because anemia is commonly seen in GVHD. Therefore, a decrease, not an increase in the number of red blood cells is expected. (**D**) This answer is incorrect because the numbers of monocytes are typically unchanged in individuals undergoing GVHD. (**E**) This answer is incorrect because GVHD can demonstrate cytopenia, especially thrombocytopenia. Therefore, a decrease, not an increase in the number of platelets is expected.

16. Correct: Immunosuppress entire immune system with glucocorticoids (E)

(**E**) This patient is undergoing a graft-versus-host response. In graft-versus-host disease (GVHD), T cells mediate a type IV hypersensitivity reaction that can be suppressed with glucocorticoids. Additionally, drugs that specifically inhibit T cell activation and responses can be used to dampen the response of donor-derived T cells attacking the recipient of the graft. (**A**) This answer is incorrect because a graft-versus-host reaction is mediated by T cells, not B cells and antibody. Therefore, since the response is mediated by T cells against HLA antigens, plasmapheresis to remove antibodies would not be helpful. (**B**) This answer is incorrect because this is a systemic response in which donor-derived T cells attack HLA molecules throughout the body. The skin, GI

and liver are the primary targets of a graft-versus-host reaction, and, therefore, patients with GVHD demonstrate maculopapular rashes, diarrhea, and elevated bilirubin levels. (**C**) This answer is incorrect because rituximab attacks B cells and leads to their removal from the host. As described earlier, B cells do not significantly contribute to the graft-versus-host response and therefore would not be helpful in this situation. (**D**) This answer is incorrect because complement does not significantly contribute to the graft-versus-host response. It has important implications in other transplant rejections (such as hyperacute and antibody-mediated acute responses), but is not important in GVHD.

17. Correct: Mixed lymphocyte reaction (MLR) (E)

(**E**) The mixed lymphocyte reaction (MLR) determines if either the recipient and/or donor will mount a cellular (T cell-mediated) response against each other and predicts whether the transplanted tissue will be rejected. In a two-way MLR, both donor and recipient cells are incubated with one another in the presence of 3H-thymidine. If the cells proliferate, the 3H-thymidine will be taken into the cells and the level of 3H-thymidine incorporation is proportional to the amount of proliferation. In a one-way MLR, either the donor or the recipient cell is fixed by biochemical means so that it cannot proliferate. Therefore, the proliferation of the non-"fixed" cell can be measured to determine if either the donor cells will respond to fixed recipient cells or the recipient cells can be tested to observe the response against fixed donor cells. If there is 3H-thymidine incorporation detected, these data suggest that either the recipient or the donor will generate a response, which suggests that there will be a graft reaction. Due to the fact that this response takes ~5 days, it is not useful in cadaver-derived organs. However, in transplants in which the donor is living, this is a highly useful assay, since it will identify responses to both major and minor HLA molecules. (**A**) This answer is incorrect because an ELISA does not demonstrate whether a cellular response will occur between the recipient and donor. It is useful for identifying the presence of anti-HLA antibodies in the recipients, as part of the crossmatch test. (**B**) This answer is incorrect because the polymerase chain reaction (PCR) cannot predict whether a cellular response will take place. PCR amplification and sequencing is extremely helpful in determining if there are variations of the HLA molecules between donor and recipient and also have some level of predictive value, but it cannot demonstrate a cellular response. (**C**) This answer is incorrect because complement-dependent cytotoxicity (CDC) identifies the presence of preformed antibodies specific for proteins on the recipient cells. After the incubation of patient sera with donor cells, rabbit complement is added to analyze the level of cytotoxic death induced by the classical complement pathway. As with options A and D, this assay analyzes for the presence of preformed antibodies in the recipient serum against donor cells and can be useful in crossmatch testing, but is not a readout of a cellular response. (**D**) This answer is incorrect because flow cytometry can be used as a crossmatch test. It identifies the presence of preformed antibodies in the patient that bind to the surface proteins on the donor cells. Due to the ability to rapidly test and analyze the results, this assay is helpful in deceased-donor allografts.

18.   Correct: Complement-dependent cytotoxicity (CDC) (B)

(**B**) There are three assays that are used to identify the presence of anti-HLA antibodies in a potential allograft recipient: complement-dependent cytotoxicity (CDC), Flow cytometry, and ELISA. While all three assays will detect the presence of antibodies specific for HLA, only the CDC assay is a functional assay that shows the ability of the antibodies to induce lysis in the presence of complement. (**A**) This answer is incorrect because the ouchterlony is an assay that is commonly used clinically to diagnose and aid in the prognosis of fungal infections. (**C**) This answer is incorrect because the polymerase chain reaction (PCR) does not identify the presence of circulating, preformed HLA-specific antibodies. PCR amplification and sequencing is extremely helpful in determining if there are variations of the HLA molecules between donor and recipient and also have some level of predictive value, but it cannot detect the presence of antibodies specific for HLA. (**D**) This answer is incorrect because the RAST is an ELISA-based assay that looks for the presence of allergen-specific IgE in the serum of individuals. It has no use in pre-transplant match testing. (**E**) This answer is incorrect because even though Western blot analysis can identify the presence of certain serum antibodies, it is expensive, less sensitive, and requires technical expertise. This assay would not be a good choice for the needs of this patient.

19.   Correct: IL-12 (D)

(**D**) Th1 cells direct the immune response against tumor cells through the production of IFN-γ. The cytokine that promotes the differentiation of a naïve CD4+ T cell into a Th1 cell is IL-12 and therefore is the correct answer. (**A, C**) These answers are incorrect because IL-4 and IL-10 promote the generation of Th2 cells which antagonize Th1 effector cell function. Furthermore, IL-10 is known to directly suppress the antitumor response. (**B, E**) These answers are incorrect because IL-6 and IL-23 promote the development of Th17 cells. While Th17 cells can contribute to the antitumor response, these cells are thought to be more important in the generation of autoimmune responses.

20.   Correct: T-bet (C)

(**C**) This patient has breast cancer and Th1 responses are beneficial for disease regression and/or stabilization. T-bet is a transcription factor that is not only critical for the generation for Th1 cells, but also IFN-γ production by tumor-specific CD8+ T cells. The loss of T-bet would put an individual at an increased risk of tumor development, in part due to a deficient Th1/Cytotoxic T lymphocyte (CTL) response. (**A**) This answer is incorrect because STAT6 is a signal transduction molecule that dimerizes to act as a transcription factor to promote Th2 development and dampen Th1 development. (**B, E**) These answers are incorrect because both of these transcription factors promote Th2 development, which are not protective against the development of tumors. (**D**) This answer is incorrect because RORγT is a transcription factor that is important for the development of Th17 cells. While Th17 cells can influence the antitumor response, Th1 cells are critical in mounting an optimal antitumor response.

21.   Correct: IL-10 (C)

(**C**) This patient has Hodgkin's lymphoma. IL-10 is produced by many tumor cells, especially lymphomas, to promote survival of the tumor and to limit the antitumor response induced by CD4+ Th1 cells and tumor-specific cytotoxic T lymphocytes (CTLs). Furthermore, IL-10 can inhibit NK cell killing and taken together dampen the functions of many of the most important immune cells responsible for killing malignant cells. (**A**) This answer is incorrect because IL-1 is a pro-inflammatory cytokine that would enhance the activities of innate immune cells that contribute to the tumor microenvironment, not dampen the tumor response. (**B**) This answer is incorrect because IL-2 promotes the proliferation of both CD4+ and CD8+ T cells and NK cells. Low levels of IL-2 promote the development of regulatory CD4+ T cells, while high levels of IL-2 can enhance the generation of antitumor responses. Therefore, the production of IL-2 by the tumor cell would likely enhance the tumor response, not limit the tumor response. Patients with metastatic melanoma and renal cell carcinoma have been treated with a recombinant form of IL-2 (aldesleukin) with some success. (**D**) This answer is incorrect because IFN-γ is produced by immune cells to significantly enhance the effector functions of cytotoxic CD8+ T cells and other cytotoxic cells such as NK cells to kill tumor cells. Therefore, tumor cells do not produce this cytokine to limit the antitumor response. (**E**) This answer is incorrect because TNF-α is a pro-inflammatory cytokine that has been used clinically to enhance the destruction of the tumor through its effects on immune cells, the tumor cells themselves, and the tumor vasculature.

22. Correct: Monocytes (A)

(**A**) This patient has Hodgkin's lymphoma, which is characterized by the presence of Reed–Sternberg cells, which are large cells of the B cell lineage that have an owl's eye appearance and bilobed nucleus. The presence of infiltrating monocytes likely is promoting a tumor microenvironment that dampens the antitumor immune response. Monocyte/macrophages can differentiate in to M1 (pro-inflammatory) or M2 (anti-inflammatory) phenotypes. Many times, infiltrating monocytes adopt a M2 phenotype that dampens the infiltrating antitumor immune response. Furthermore, many of these infiltrating monocytes express PD-L1, which binds to PD-1 on tumor infiltrating lymphocytes to dampen the immune response. (**B**) This answer is incorrect because the presence of tumor-infiltrating T cells in the biopsy would indicate that the immune response is trying to destroy the tumor. However, the tumor microenvironment can dampen the responses of these tumor infiltrating T cells. Nevertheless, the presence of these lymphocytes suggests a better prognosis, not a worse prognosis. (**C**) This answer is incorrect because the presence of neutrophils indicates the possibility of an antitumor response, which has a better prognosis. (**D**) This answer is incorrect because the presence of NK cells portends a better prognosis, as these cells can recognize tumor cells that down-regulate HLA class I and are unable to be attacked by CD8+ T cells. (**E**) This answer is incorrect because the presence of tumor-infiltrating B cells in the biopsy would be indicative that the immune response is trying to destroy the tumor. However, the tumor microenvironment can dampen the responses of these tumor infiltrating B cells. Nevertheless, the presence of these lymphocytes suggests a better prognosis, not a worse prognosis.

23. Correct: Human papillomavirus (HPV) (E)

(**E**) This patient suffers from cervical carcinoma, which is 95% associated with human papillomavirus (HPV) infection. This patient has a history of genital warts from HPV that puts her at an increased risk for cervical cancer. The generation of HPV vaccines has significantly decreased the incidence of HPV infection and HPV-associated disease. (**A**) This answer is incorrect because hepatitis B infection is associated with the development of liver cancer. There is a vaccine for hepatitis B; however, it does not protect against the development of cervical carcinoma. (**B**) This answer is incorrect because Epstein–Barr virus (EBV) is associated with the development of tumors of the immune system, such as Burkitt's lymphoma and Hodgkin's lymphoma. Even though there are vaccines currently in clinical trials, there currently is no approved vaccine against EBV. (**C**) This answer is incorrect because human herpesvirus-6 (HHV-6)

causes Kaposi's sarcoma, which is a tumor of epithelial cells like HPV, but the epithelial cells are not typically genital in origin. Furthermore, there is no approved vaccine against HHV6. (**D**) This answer is incorrect because hepatitis C is associated with the development of liver cancer (like hepatitis B). However, in contrast to hepatitis B, there is no vaccine to protect against infection with this virus.

24. Correct: CD56 (D)

(**D**) NK cells are critical in promoting the destruction of tumor cells, especially those tumor cells that decrease HLA class I. TAP-1/2 is responsible for promoting cytosolic peptides from proteasome degradation into the endoplasmic reticulum. The loss of TAP1/2 activity results in the loss of HLA class I loading and decreased HLA class I on the surface of tumor cells. Therefore, tumor cells that have decreased class I activate NK cells and are subsequently lysed by these cells. (**A**) This answer is incorrect because CD8+ T cells recognize tumor cells that express tumor antigen in the context of HLA class I. Therefore, if the cells have downregulated TAP1/2 activity, tumor antigens will *not* be loaded into HLA class I and CD8+ T cells will not be able to recognize these cells. (**B**) This answer is incorrect because CD20 is expressed on B cells. B cells recognize tumor antigens in their native context and do not require processing for recognition. Therefore, the absence of TAP1/2 activity is irrelevant for B cell activation. Furthermore, for B cells to activate tumor-specific CD4+ T cells within the tumor, the B cells present antigens derived from the exogenous pathway of antigen presentation, which does not require TAP1/2 function. (**C**) This answer is incorrect because CD34 is found on hematopoietic stem cells, which can be found in bone marrow and in the circulation in low numbers. These cells can differentiate into NK cells, but in the stem cell state do not have effector function. (**E**) This answer is incorrect because CD86 is found on the surface of activated antigen presenting cells. This surface molecule is important to serve as a costimulatory molecule to stimulate CD28 found on CD4+ and CD8+ T cells that contribute to the antitumor responses.

25. Correct: Increase in autoimmune reactions, such as hepatitis (A)

(**A**) The drug targets PD-L1, which is a protein that is important for maintaining peripheral immune tolerance. PD-L1 is expressed on nonlymphoid organs and nonhematopoietic cells (placenta, lung, heart, and liver). PD-L1 binds to PD-1 on activated cytotoxic T cells to decrease their activation and inhibit cytotoxic T lymphocyte (CTL)-mediated lysis. Therefore, in cancer treatments, a monoclonal antibody against PD-L1 blocks this interaction and increases the activity of tumor-specific CTL's. However, one common side effect of this drug is the loss of peripheral tolerance and reactions of the immune system against the liver, resulting in hepatitis. Additional immune-mediated adverse reactions when using antibodies to either PD-L1 or PD-1 are immune-mediated pneumonitis, colitis, endocrinopathies, rash, and encephalitis. (**B**) This answer is incorrect because PD-L1 is a marker expressed on many nonimmune cells to prevent T cell activation, but is not used as an adhesion molecule. Numerous adhesion molecules are being considered to treat cancer by inhibiting tumor metastasis. Many of these treatments have shown promise in animal studies and currently are in clinical trials. (**C**) This answer is incorrect because PD-L1 is a cell surface molecule and type III hypersensitivities are against soluble antigens. (**D**) This answer is incorrect because PD-L1 is not a receptor that promotes angiogenesis and therefore, there is no expected change in angiogenesis after this treatment. (**E**) This answer is incorrect because the mechanism of action of the anti-PD-L1 antibody is to block the PD-1/PD-L1 interaction. It does not extensively induce complement and therefore, the patient does not become immunocompromised due to a deficient amount of complement available for activation.

26. Correct: CD59 (E)

(**E**) The presentation of the patient is consistent with chronic lymphocytic leukemia (CLL), which can be treated with rituximab (anti-CD20) monoclonal antibody. Rituximab works by multiple mechanisms, including complement activation, antibody-dependent cell-mediated cytotoxicity (ADCC) and direct signaling through CD20. Some rituximab-resistant CLL cells express increased levels of CD59. CD59 is an important negative regulator of the complement cascade, and therefore, increasing the levels of CD59 decreases the level of rituximab-dependent complement activation. (**A**) This answer is incorrect because increasing the level of FcγR on the surface of the lymphoma cells does not have any significant effect on rituximab therapy. However, increased levels of FcγR on NK cells, macrophages, and other potential killer cells that can mediate ADCC could enhance the therapeutic benefit of rituximab. (**B**) This answer is incorrect because surface immunoglobulin expression is neither targeted by rituximab nor has a significant impact on the clinical efficacy of this drug. (**C**) This answer is incorrect because increasing the levels of CD20 would make the tumor cells more easily recognized by rituximab. Therefore, increasing the levels of CD20 would increase the efficacy of rituximab, not decrease the efficacy of the monoclonal antibody. (**D**) This answer is incorrect because enhancing the levels of CR3 is not expected to affect any of the mechanisms by which rituximab leads to the destruction of B cell tumors. CR3's normal function is to stimulate phagocytosis, and does not directly regulate the complement cascade so the increased

expression of CR3 would not impede the complement pathway induced by rituximab.

27. Correct: Cytotoxic T cells (C)

(**C**) The administration of ipilimumab targets the CTLA-4 molecule on CD8+ cytotoxic T cells, as well as CD4+ T cells. CTLA-4 signaling negatively regulates T cell responses and anti-CTLA-4 monoclonal antibodies which block CTLA-4 binding to B7 results in a loss of negative regulation by CTLA-4. The administration of ipilimumab, which is a monoclonal antibody that binds CTLA-4 without inducing CTLA-4 signaling, leads to an increase in the activation of both CD4+ and CD8+ T cells in melanoma patients. The enhanced T cell activation in ipilimumab-treated patients results in a regression and/or containment of the tumor. (**A**) This answer is incorrect because CTLA-4/B7 engagement is not a controlling factor for neutrophils. After crosslinking of Mac-1 on neutrophils, human neutrophils have been demonstrated to increase B7 family members, but the administration of a blocking CTLA-4 monoclonal antibody would not affect the neutrophil. Instead ipilimumab would affect the target cell that the neutrophil interacts with through B7. (**B**) This answer is incorrect because macrophages are antigen presenting cells that express B7 family members after activation. Therefore, the administration of ipilimumab targets the cell that the macrophage would interact with and not directly affect the activation of macrophages. (**D**) This answer is incorrect because mast cells do not express CTLA-4. However, mast cells do express PD-L1 and are potential targets of melanoma monoclonal antibody treatments that target PD-1 and/or PD-L1. (**E**) This answer is incorrect because activated B cells also are antigen presenting cells that express B7 family members that interact with CTLA-4 and CD28 on T cells. Therefore, the drug is targeting the T cells, not the antigen presenting cell or the cell that provides B7 to stimulate CTLA-4.

28. Correct: Trastuzumab (E)

(**E**) This answer is correct, because trastuzumab targets HER2 that is expressed on the surface of the breast cancer tumor cells. trastuzumab leads to the death of breast cancer cells by increasing antibody-dependent cell-mediated cytotoxicity (ADCC) of breast cancer tumor cells and by blocking HER2 signaling that promotes tumor growth. (**A**) This answer is incorrect because Omalizumab is a monoclonal antibody that recognizes IgE and is used to treat type I hypersensitivity reactions. Omalizumab inhibits the binding of IgE to the FcεR1 on the surface of mast cells and basophils, thereby inhibiting the activation of these cells and histamine release. (**B**) This answer is incorrect because rituximab is used to treat B cell lymphomas. Rituximab recognizes CD20 on the surface of B cells (including B cell lymphomas) and kills these cells through complement activation, ADCC, or through direct stimulation of CD20. (**C**) This answer is incorrect because adalimumab is used to treat multiple inflammatory diseases, including rheumatoid arthritis, plaque psoriasis, ulcerative colitis, and Crohn's disease. Adalimumab targets TNF-α and decreases immune-mediated inflammatory reactions. (**D**) This answer is incorrect because abatacept is used to treat rheumatoid arthritis by targeting B7 family members. Abatacept is a CTLA-4 fusion protein that binds B7 family members on antigen presenting cells and inhibits the stimulation of CD28 on T cells. Thus, T cell activation is diminished and patients with rheumatoid arthritis demonstrate an improvement of symptoms.

29. Correct: Rituximab (B)

(**B**) This answer is correct, because rituximab is used to treat B cell lymphomas. The pathology results combined with the data demonstrating that almost all of the cells are B cell-derived indicate the presence of a B cell lymphoma. Rituximab recognizes CD20 on the surface of B cells and kills these cells through complement activation, antibody-dependent cell-mediated cytotoxicity (ADCC), or through direct stimulation of CD20. Rituximab is currently used to treat multiple types of B cell lymphomas, including non-Hodgkin's lymphoma, chronic lymphocytic leukemia (CLL), and also nontumor conditions, such as rheumatoid arthritis. (**A**) This answer is incorrect because Omalizumab is a monoclonal antibody that recognizes IgE and is used to treat type I hypersensitivity reactions. Omalizumab inhibits the binding of IgE to the FcεR1 on the surface of mast cells and basophils, thereby inhibiting the activation of these cells and histamine release. (**C**) This answer is incorrect because adalimumab is

used to treat multiple inflammatory diseases, including rheumatoid arthritis, plaque psoriasis, ulcerative colitis, and Crohn's disease. Adalimumab targets TNF-α and decreases immune-mediated inflammatory reactions. (**D**) This answer is incorrect because abatacept is used to treat rheumatoid arthritis by targeting B7 family members. Abatacept is a CTLA-4 fusion protein that binds B7 family members on antigen presenting cells and inhibits the stimulation of CD28 on T cells. Thus, T cell activation is diminished and patients with rheumatoid arthritis demonstrate an improvement of symptoms. (**E**) This answer is incorrect because trastuzumab targets HER2 that is expressed on the surface of breast cancer tumor cells. Trastuzumab leads to the death of breast cancer cells by increasing ADCC of breast cancer tumor cells and by blocking HER2 signaling that promotes tumor growth.

30. Correct: IFN-γ (B)

(**B**) Th1 cells direct the immune response against tumor cells through the production of IFN-γ. IFN-γ is critical for activating macrophages, NK cells, and tumor-specific CD8+ cytotoxic T cells that are responsible for destroying the altered cancer cells. (**A**) This answer is incorrect because TGF-β is known for promoting melanoma cell growth, while inhibiting the function of infiltrating immune cells. Therefore, TGF-β decreases the antitumor response that is required to contain and eradicate this lesion. (**C, D**) These answers are incorrect because IL-4 and IL-10 promote the generation of Th2 cells which antagonize Th1 effector cell function. Furthermore, IL-10 is known to directly suppress the antitumor response. (**E**) This answer is incorrect because IL-17 is produced by Th17 cells that can contribute to the antitumor response. However, these cells are thought to be more important in the generation of autoimmune responses.

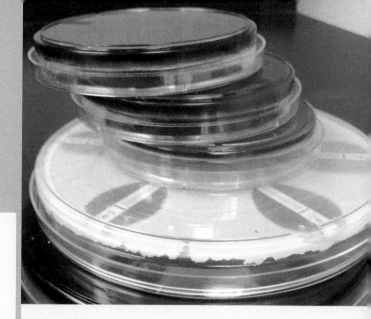

Chapter 7

General Microbiology

Melphine M. Harriott, Thomas C. Bolig, and Matthew P. Jackson

LEARNING OBJECTIVES

▶ Describe the laboratory diagnosis and antimicrobial testing methods for bacteria, viruses, fungi, yeast, and parasites.

▶ Discuss the etiology, epidemiology, pathogenesis, clinical manifestations, complications, diagnosis, and treatment and prevention of:

- infections of the genital tract.

- upper and lower respiratory tract infections.

- bloodstream and lymphatic system infections.

- infections of the head and neck.

- infectious diarrhea and dysentery.

- foodborne illness.

- eye infections.

- skin, soft tissue, joint, muscle, and bone infections.

- meningitis, meningoencephalitis, encephalitis, myelitis, and brain lesions.

▶ Describe the common HIV/AIDS-related opportunistic infections.

▶ Compare and contrast the structure and function of bacterial, viral, fungal, yeast, and parasitic cells.

▶ Discuss virulence mechanisms and correlate virulence mechanisms with specific pathogens.

▶ Discuss antimicrobial mechanism of action, spectrum of activity, common adverse effects, and resistance mechanisms.

▶ Discuss the steps of viral replication.

▶ List the normal microbiota for each organ system and explain the roles played in health and disease by the normal microbiota.

▶ Explain the role of immunopathogenesis in the development of post-infectious diseases.

▶ Describe bacterial metabolism, growth, and genetics.

▶ Compare and contrast the different methods of sterilization and disinfection.

7.1 Questions

Easy	Medium	Hard

1. A 25-year-old woman visits her doctor with a 5-day history of abdominal pain, dysuria, and vaginal discharge. She is sexually active and has several male partners. Her vital signs are normal. Bimanual pelvic exam shows cervical motion tenderness and mucopurulent vaginal discharge is noted. Which of the following bacteriology media plates would best isolate the most likely agent of this infection?

A. Blood agar

B. Eosin methylene blue (EMB)

C. MacConkey agar

D. Regan–Lowe agar

E. Thayer–Martin agar

Consider the following case for questions 2 to 3:

A 50-year-old woman, who has been incarcerated for the past 5 years, is brought to the prison hospital with a cough productive of bloody sputum. She reports experiencing a persistent cough for approximately 2 months, but in the last few days she has noticed an increase in sputum production with the presence of blood. She claims she has lost approximately 20 pounds in the past few months and has had night sweats for about 1 month. She smokes 20 cigarettes per day but the rest of her medical history is unremarkable. On examination, she appears thin and frail. Her vital signs are normal. Her lung exam is notable for decreased breath sounds, diffusely. A chest radiograph demonstrates a cavity infiltrate of the right upper lobe.

2. Which of the following bacteriology media plates would best isolate the most likely agent of this infection?

A. Buffered charcoal yeast extract (BCYE) agar

B. Hektoen agar

C. Lowenstein–Jensen (LJ) agar

D. Sabouraud Dextrose agar

E. Thiosulfate citrate bile salts sucrose (TCBS) agar

3. Which of the following microscopic methods would best confirm the identity of the most likely pathogen of this infection?

A. Gram stain

B. Kinyoun stain

C. Potassium hydroxide (KOH) preparation

D. Trichrome stain

E. Tzanck smear

4. A 34-year-old woman presents with fever, fatigue, and weight loss. She has previously been diagnosed as HIV positive. She has lost 10 pounds over the past month. Her temperature is 38.8°C (101.8°F). She is ill appearing and pale. On examination, the liver edge is below the costal margin. Her CD4 count is 36 cells/μL. Blood cultures are positive after 2 weeks and the Gram stain is negative for organisms but the acid-fast stain demonstrates the organism as shown below:

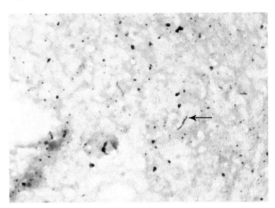

Which of the following characteristics of this pathogen prevented it from appearing in the Gram stain?

A. A thick peptidoglycan layer

B. Lack of a cell wall

C. Lipopolysaccharide (LPS)

D. Mycolic acid in the cell wall

E. Teichoic acid

5. A 24-year-old woman presents to her primary care physician with a cough of 2-week duration and sinus pressure. She states that she had a sore throat a week ago and the cough at that time was nonproductive but now she is producing a small amount of sputum. At the time of examination her temperature is 37.8°C (100°F). Scattered rales in the left lower lung field are present. A chest X-ray reveals patchy infiltrates in the left lower lobe. The cold agglutinin IgM titer is elevated. Which of the following must be added to the media to support the growth of the most likely agent of this infection?

A. Charcoal

B. Hemin

C. Serum

D. Yeast extract

E. 7.5% salt

6. A 68-year-old woman with end stage renal disease comes to the emergency department with fever, chills, and fatigue. She is currently on peritoneal dialysis. On examination, her temperature is 39.4°C (102.9°F) and tachypnea and tachycardia are noted. She is admitted to the hospital for possible sepsis. After 24 hours, Gram stain from blood cultures demonstrates the presence of pink, rod-shaped organisms. Based on the Gram stain results, which of the following is most likely to be the causative agent of this infection?

A. *Candida albicans*

B. *Klebsiella pneumoniae*

C. *Listeria monocytogenes*

D. *Neisseria meningitidis*

E. *Staphylococcus aureus*

7. A 7-year-old girl wakes up in the morning complaining of a sore throat. Her temperature at the time is 38°C (100.4°F). She stays home from school and refuses to eat all day. Later that evening when her mother went to check on her, she felt warmer than before and was complaining that her throat hurt so badly she couldn't sleep. Her mother takes her to the urgent care clinic and her temperature is noted to be 38.9°C (102.2°C). On examination, the girl's throat is notably erythematous with white exudate on both tonsils. Cervical lymphadenopathy is present. A swab of the throat is obtained and sent for culture. The throat culture grows β-hemolytic, gram-positive cocci. The most likely agent of this infection is:

A. Bacitracin resistant

B. Catalase negative

C. Coagulase positive

D. Novobiocin resistant

E. Optochin sensitive

Consider the following case for questions 8 to 9:

A previously healthy 77-year-old man is brought to the emergency department with tachypnea and severe chest discomfort. He states that a few days ago he started experiencing chills, a productive cough, and pain in his side. On examination, his temperature is 38.9°C (102°F) and his pulse is 125 per minute. Chest auscultation demonstrates significant bilateral crackles with expiratory wheezes and a chest radiograph shows bilateral, diffuse pulmonary infiltrates with effusion. A sputum Gram stain is shown below:

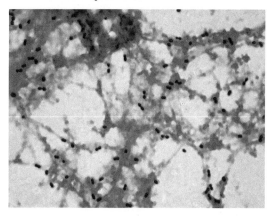

8. Which of the following is the most likely agent of this infection?

A. *Bacillus anthracis*

B. *Corynebacterium diphtheriae*

C. *Haemophilus influenzae*

D. *Pseudomonas aeruginosa*

E. *Streptococcus pneumoniae*

9. A microbroth dilution was set up for the *S. pneumoniae* isolate, as seen in the image below. For Row E, levofloxacin, what is the minimal inhibitory concentration (MIC)?

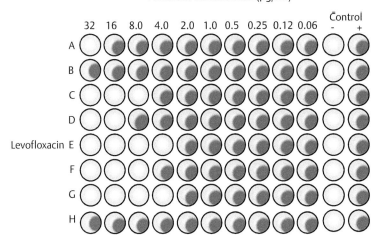

Antibiotic concentration (µg/mL)

A. 32 µg/mL

B. 4.0 µg/mL

C. 2.0 µg/mL

D. 0.12 µg/mL

E. 0.06 µg/mL

10. A medical student is participating in a summer research project and is given the task of developing a compound that targets only gram-positive bacteria. Which of the following components should she focus her research on?

A. Chitin

B. Lipopolysaccharide (LPS)

C. Lipoteichoic acid

D. Mycolic acid

E. Peptidoglycan

11. A 6-year-old boy presents with a 1-day history of bloody diarrhea and vomiting. He had recently visited an apple orchard and consumed unpasteurized apple cider. His stool culture grows a sorbitol negative (non-fermenting) organism on MacConkey with sorbitol agar. The organism is subsequently found to produce a toxin. The activity of this toxin is most similar in activity to:

A. Ciprofloxacin

B. Erythromycin

C. Penicillin G

D. Trimethoprim–sulfamethoxazole (TMP–SMX)

E. Vancomycin

12. A 31-year-old woman has sudden onset of a runny nose, "stuffed sinuses," sore throat, and feels more tired than normal. A few days ago her husband came home from work with similar symptoms. She does not have a fever and the drainage from her nose is clear. She treats her symptoms with over-the-counter cold medications. After a week, the woman is back to her normal state of health. Which of the following is a characteristic of the causative agent of this infection?

A. Cell membrane contains ergosterol

B. Cell wall contains NAG–NAM

C. Contains a protein shell that protects the genome

D. Genome is composed of DNA and RNA

13. A 41-year-old man is referred to an ophthalmologist for left eye pain and decreased vision. He has no history of trauma to the eye. He does have a history of frequent cold sores. Fluorescein staining of eye showed the findings seen below:

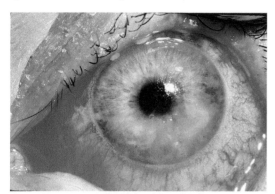

Source: Management of Eyelid and Periorbital Trauma. In: Codner M, McCord C, Hrsg. Eyelid & Periorbital Surgery. 2nd Edition. Thieme; 2016. doi:10.1055/b-005-148980

The man was prescribed acyclovir and instructed to follow up with the ophthalmologist in a month. Which enzyme is required for activity of acyclovir?

A. Integrase

B. Neuraminidase

C. Reverse transcriptase

D. RNA polymerase

E. Thymidine kinase (TK)

14. An investigator is developing a compound that targets HIV gp120. Which of the following steps of the cell cycle will be inhibited by this compound?

A. Attachment to the host cell

B. Capsid uncoating

C. Exit from the host cell

D. Penetration of the host cell

E. Replication of genome

Consider the following case for questions 15 to 17:

A 14-year-old boy goes camping with his Boy Scout troop. They camp close to a stream and the boys frequently visit the shore to observe a family of beavers who were building a dam. A week after he returns, the boy complains of abdominal cramps, watery diarrhea, and foul-smelling flatulence. After 3 days of symptoms, his mother takes him to his pediatrician. The boy admits to his doctor that he drank water from the stream while camping. The physician orders a stool culture, ova and parasite (O&P) examination, and fecal fat test.

15. Ideally, how many stool specimens should be submitted for O&P examination for this patient?

A. One specimen

B. Two specimens, collected the same day

C. Three specimens, collected the same day

D. Three specimens, collected on 3 separate days

16. Which of the following is the best stain to visualize the causative from a stool specimen?

A. Acid-fast

B. Calcofluor-white

C. Giemsa

D. Gram stain

E. Trichrome

17. Identification of which of the following structures in the stool would be diagnostic?

A. Adult worm

B. Gametocyte

C. Larva

D. Sporozoite

E. Trophozoite

18. A 56-year-old woman presents with multiple wounds on her forearm. She has a history of injury to her hand while trimming the bushes in her yard. She states that initially she had one small pimple on her hand and eventually several nodule-like lesions appeared on her arm. She is concerned because it is summer and she is embarrassed to have her arms uncovered. She is otherwise feeling well. Her vital signs are normal. On examination, four shallow ulcers are noted along the lymphatic channel, and a small amount of clear drainage is present. Her physical exam is otherwise unremarkable. A biopsy from the ulcer shows yeast cells with elongated daughter yeast budding from the mother cell. Which one of the following would best confirm that this pathogen is a dimorphic fungus?

A. Demonstration of sexual and asexual reproduction

B. Conversion of yeast cells to fungal form

C. Detection of (1-3)-β-D-glucan

D. Fluorescence of lesion with Wood's lamp

E. Lactophenol cotton blue preparation from the ulcer

19. A 4-year-old boy from Somali is adopted by a family in the United States. As part of the adoption process, the boy is given a routine physical exam along with laboratory testing. The boy is healthy and has no complaints. His physical exam is unremarkable. However, the family is concerned about the laboratory tests below:

- Sputum AFB stain × 3: No AFB seen
- Sputum AFB culture × 3: No growth after 6 weeks
- Interferon-gamma (IFN-γ) release assay: Positive
- Tuberculosis (TB) skin test: Positive
- Chest X-ray: Normal

What is the most appropriate management for this boy's condition?

A. This boy has active TB disease and must be treated

B. This boy has latent TB infection and should be treated

C. This boy is likely infectious and should be in respiratory isolation

D. This boy likely has active TB and the cultures should be repeated

E. This boy has disseminated TB and CT scans should be ordered

20. A 68-year-old patient with stage IV non-Hodgkin's lymphoma (NHL) has been treated for pneumonia for the past 8 days with minimal improvement. Despite therapy, a histopathological specimen of the lung reveals the following:

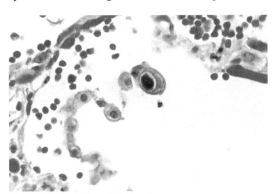

Source: CDC/Dr. Edwin P. Ewing, Jr.

In addition to the pneumonia, over the past few days the patient has noticed a decrease in visual acuity in her left eye. On examination of the eye, the sclera and conjunctivae are non-erythematous with no lesions or exudates. The pupils are round and reactive to light with a small left afferent pupillary defect. Visual acuity testing shows 20/20 on the right and 20/100 on the left. Fundoscopic exam reveals cotton wool exudates, hemorrhage, and findings indicative of a small field of necrotizing retinitis in the mid-periphery of the left retina. Given these findings, what medication should the patient be started on?

A. Acyclovir

B. Antiretroviral therapy

C. Foscarnet

D. Isoniazid

E. Trimethoprim–sulfamethoxazole (TMP–SMX)

21. A 53-year-old man presents to his primary care physician for discoloration of his right first and second toenails. The patient states that for the last few months he has noticed that his toenails have thickened and become discolored. He also reports a slight odor in his right foot and admits to having a similar problem in the past. He denies any pain, numbness, or paresthesia. The patient has an allergy to fluconazole but otherwise has no significant history. Physical exam reveals opaque and faintly yellow discolored first and second toenails with hyperkeratosis and onycholysis of the first toenail. The rest of his exam is within normal limits. A lactophenol cotton blue preparation of colonies grown from subungual scrapings reveals the following:

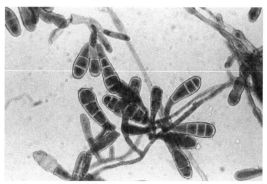

Source: CDC/Dr. Lucille K. Georg

Which enzyme is inhibited by the most appropriate therapy for this patient?

A. 1,3 β-glucosidase
B. 14-α-demethylase
C. Dihydrofolate reductase
D. DNA polymerase
E. Squalene epoxidase

22. A 29-year-old woman returns 1 week after vacationing in Costa Rica. She felt feverish and broke into a sweat a few days prior to presentation but recovered quickly. She presents to an outpatient clinic feeling feverish again and reports chills, headache, myalgias, and arthralgias. She denies vision changes, shortness of breath, chest pain, nausea, vomiting, or diarrhea. The patient's vital signs are as follows:

• Temperature: 39.3°C (102.7°F)
• Heart rate: 98 beats per minute
• Blood pressure: 119/61 mm Hg
• Respiratory rate: 13 breaths per minute

Thick and thin Giemsa-stains and polymerase chain reaction (PCR) confirm *Plasmodium vivax* infection. G6PD testing was negative. In addition to chloroquine, which of the following drugs should be included in the management of this infection?

A. Artemether
B. Atovaqone
C. Metronidazole
D. Primaquine
E. Quinidine

23. A 46-year-old woman is on mechanical ventilation in the intensive care unit after a motor vehicle accident. On the fourth day of hospitalization, the patient develops a fever (38.7°C [101.7°F]), tachycardia (heart rate, 122 beats per minute), hypotension (blood pressure, 88/59 mm Hg), and acute kidney injury (serum creatinine 7.0 mg/dL). Blood cultures are drawn and empiric broad-spectrum antibiotic therapy is initiated. Chest X-ray reveals new pulmonary infiltrates. Gram stain from bronchial suction reveals numerous gram-negative rods. About 48 hours later, blood cultures grow *Pseudomonas aeruginosa*. Which of the following components of the bacterial cell wall is most likely responsible for this infection?

A. Lipid A
B. Lipoteichoic acid
C. O antigen
D. Peptidoglycan
E. Pyoverdin

Consider the following case for questions 24 to 25:

A 20-year-old college student presents to the university student health service. The patient reports to the health care provider that he has developed a fever, malaise, and cough productive of scant, whitish sputum over the last few days. Rales are heard in the right posterior lung field. Chest X-ray reveals a patchy consolidation in the right lower lobe. Cold agglutinins are elevated. The patient is started on a 3-day course of antibiotics and quickly recovers.

24. Which of the following organisms is the most likely infectious etiology?

A. Influenza A virus
B. *Legionella pneumophila*
C. *Mycobacterium tuberculosis*
D. *Mycoplasma pneumoniae*
E. *Streptococcus pneumoniae*

25. Which of the following antibiotics is ineffective against this pathogen?

A. Azithromycin
B. Ceftriaxone
C. Doxycycline
D. Erythromycin
E. Levofloxacin

135

26. A homeless veteran, admitted 4 days ago, dies after his clinical status rapidly deteriorates. Chest radiograph reveals collections of tiny, uniform, and discrete pulmonary opacities throughout both lungs (see chest X-ray image below). An IFN-γ release assay is positive. Autopsy revealed lymphematogenous spread of small, caseating granulomas throughout the patient's body. Gram stains from lung tissue demonstrate that no organisms are present. Blood cultures are no growth to date.

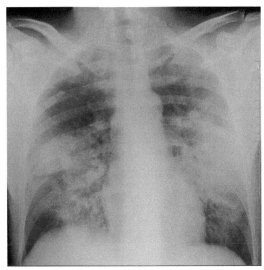

Source: Case 214. In: Yu E, Jaffer N, Chung T et al., Hrsg. RadCases. Emergency Radiology. 1st Edition. Thieme; 2015

Why is the most likely causative agent of this infection not visualized on Gram stain?

A. Lipoteichoic acid present in the cell wall

B. Lacks a cell wall

C. Muramic acid absent in the cell wall

D. Mycolic acid present in the cell wall

Consider the follow case for questions 27 to 28:

A 34-year-old woman with type 1 diabetes mellitus presents to the emergency department with a 2-day history of headache, nasal congestion, and progressively worsening facial pain. The pain is localized to the area surrounding her nares and left nasolabial fold with tenderness to palpation over the left maxillary sinus. The patient has a documented history of noncompliance with her insulin. Her hemoglobin A1C is 12.8% and her blood glucose is 457 mg/dL. Inspection of the nares reveals a black eschar on the medial wall of the left nostril with sloughing of the nasal septum. The area surrounding the eschar was biopsied, and a histopathological specimen of the tissue is given below:

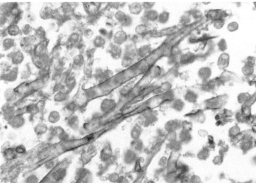

Source: CDC/Dr. Libero Ajello

27. The patient is immediately started on intravenous (IV) antimicrobial therapy by the otolaryngologist. Which of the following is the most likely agent of this infection?

A. *Aspergillus fumigatus*

B. *Blastomyces dermatitidis*

C. *Candida albicans*

D. *Entamoeba histolytica*

E. *Histoplasma capsulatum*

F. *Malassezia furfur*

G. *Mucor circinelloides*

28. What is the mechanism of action of the best treatment of choice for the most likely causative agent?

A. Decreases synthesis of mycolic acids

B. Forms pores in the cell membrane

C. Inhibits DNA-dependent RNA polymerase

D. Inhibits the synthesis of β-glucan

Consider the following case for questions 29 to 30:

A 63-year-old man with a history of type 2 diabetes mellitus and peripheral artery disease is on the general medicine unit for treatment of a right foot ulcer. The area around the ulcer is erythematous and tender to touch. Bone is palpated when a draining sinus tract is probed. Roentgenogram and magnetic resonance imaging are suggestive of osteomyelitis of the right first and second metatarsals. Biopsy and microbiological tests of bone and surrounding soft tissue reveal gram-positive cocci in clusters that are catalase and coagulase positive.

29. What organism is most likely responsible for this patient's osteomyelitis?

A. *Clostridium perfringens*

B. *Pseudomonas aeruginosa*

C. *Staphylococcus aureus*

D. *Staphylococcus epidermidis*

E. *Streptococcus agalactiae*

30. Antimicrobial susceptibility testing of the causative agent demonstrates resistance for oxacillin. Which of the following agents has activity against this pathogen?

A. Cefoxitin

B. Ceftaroline

C. Ceftazidime

D. Ceftriaxone

E. Cefuroxime

31. The incidence of vancomycin-resistant *Staphylococcus aureus* and vancomycin-resistant *Enterococcus* infections is increasing. Van-A is one of the resistance genes acquired by these organisms. What is the mechanism of action of Van-A resistance?

A. Alteration of peptidoglycan precursors

B. Augmented transport of drug out of the cell

C. Cleavage of a β-lactam ring

D. Methylation of ribosomal subunit

E. Mutation of a penicillin binding protein (PBP)

Consider the following case for questions 32 to 33:

A 31-year-old woman presents to a family medicine clinic for a new patient visit. The patient feels that she is in good health, but recently has been experiencing a decrease in exercise tolerance. She also now sleeps on two pillows because it seems to help with her sleep. On further questioning by the physician, the patient mentions that she moved to the United States from rural India 15 years ago and that she may have had an episode of untreated "strep throat" as a child. On examination, vital signs are stable (temperature, 37.6°C [99.7°F]; heart rate, 72 beats per minute; blood pressure, 109/74 mm Hg; body mass index, 22). HEENT (Head, ears, eyes, nose, throat) findings are unremarkable. There is a 3/6 mid-diastolic, low-pitched, rumbling murmur heard best at the cardiac apex. Lungs sounds are vesicular. Wheezes, rales, and rhonchi are absent. The rest of the exam is negative.

32. What is the most likely diagnosis?

A. Aortic regurgitation

B. Aortic stenosis

C. Mitral stenosis

D. Pulmonary stenosis

E. Tricuspid stenosis

33. What virulence factor is most likely responsible for the development of mitral stenosis in this patient?

A. Erythrogenic toxin

B. IgA protease

C. M protein

D. Protein A

E. Streptolysin O

34. A 16-year-old girl presents to the emergency department with fever, headache, photophobia, vomiting, and a rash involving her abdomen, chest, and arms. The lesions of this rash are small, red, flat, nonblanching, and nontender. She has hypotension and tachycardia. Brudzinski's sign is positive.

Lumbar puncture results:

* Opening pressure: 24 cm H_2O
* Glucose: 20 mg/dL
* Protein: 53 mg/dL
* WBCs: 190/mm³ (97% neutrophils)
* Xanthochromia: negative

Gram stain of the CSF is shown below:

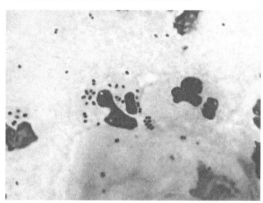

The patient's immunizations are up to date. She has a history of meningitis and sepsis caused by the same pathogen when she was 10 years old. Otherwise, her past medical history is unremarkable. After treatment with antibiotics, she is referred to a specialist for immunodeficiency testing. Which of the following immunodeficiency is most likely present in this patient?

A. C5 to C9 deficiency

B. Chronic granulomatous disease

C. Common variable immunodeficiency

D. Leukocyte adhesion deficiency type I

E. Selective IgA deficiency

137

35. Bacterial growth in a chemostat is used to maintain which of the following growth phases?

A. Autolysis

B. Death

C. Exponential

D. Lag

E. Stationary

36. An urban hospital has an outbreak of infections characterized by watery diarrhea that was traced back to health care staff. Isolates of the infectious agent required culture in an environment devoid of oxygen. Which of the following is the most likely nosocomial disease?

A. Cystitis

B. Pneumonia

C. Pseudomembranous colitis

D. Scalded skin syndrome

E. Thrush

37. Which of the following antibiotics is effective due to the differences between eukaryotic cells and prokaryotic cells at translation?

A. Amphotericin B

B. Ciprofloxacin

C. Gentamicin

D. Methicillin

E. Trimethoprim–sulfamethoxazole (TMP–SMX)

38. Which of the following antibiotics is effective due to the differences between eukaryotic cells and prokaryotic cells at replication?

A. Amphotericin B

B. Ciprofloxacin

C. Gentamicin

D. Methicillin

E. Trimethoprim–sulfamethoxazole (TMP–SMX)

39. DNA sequence comprising a cluster of structural genes preceded by a promoter and controlled by a common regulatory protein defines which of the following?

A. Intron

B. Operator

C. Operon

D. Regulon

E. Transposon

40. The addition of DNAase to growth medium would inhibit bacterial gene transfer by which of the following processes?

A. Competence

B. Conjugation

C. Lysogeny

D. Transduction

E. Transformation

41. Which of the following would convert a non-toxigenic strain of *Corynebacterium diphtheriae* to diphtheria toxin production?

A. Conjugation

B. Fur-mediated repression

C. Mutation

D. Transduction

E. Transformation

42. A conjugal mating experiment that was performed using two different strains of *Escherichia coli* resulted in the production of an F′ (prime) strain. The series of events that most likely preceded formation of this strain would be:

A. Conjugation of two F′ (prime) strains

B. Formation of an Hfr followed by an Hfr × F⁻ mating

C. Resolution of an Hfr

D. Resolution of an Hfr followed by an F′ (prime) × F⁻ mating

E. Resolution of F+ from the chromosome

43. Transposons contribute to bacterial virulence by transferring genes for which of the following?

A. Antibiotic resistance

B. Conjugation

C. Invasion

D. Missense mutation

E. Toxin production

44. Sterilization of surgical instruments by the use of super-heated steam (autoclaving) is necessary due to the risk of contamination with bacteria producing which of the following structures?

A. Capsule

B. Endospores

C. Lipopolysaccharide (LPS)

D. Mycolic acid

E. Peptidoglycan

45. An asymptomatic woman reported to her physician after her partner revealed that he had been diagnosed with a bacterial sexually transmitted infection. Her physician collected an endocervical swab that was transported to the lab where it was transferred to a confluent layer of monkey kidney cells. Intracytoplasmic inclusions were isolated and subjected to a nucleic acid amplification test (NAAT) to detect a specific 23S ribosomal RNA target. Which of the following is the correct molecular diagnostic test?

A. DNA sequencing

B. Hybridization

C. Multilocus sequence typing

D. Pulsed field gel electrophoresis

E. Transcription-mediated amplification

7.2 Answers and Explanations

Easy	Medium	Hard

1. Correct: Thayer–Martin agar (E)

(**E**) This woman most likely has gonorrhea, a common sexually transmitted infection caused by *Neisseria gonorrhoeae*, a gram-negative diplococcus. Typical findings in females include mucopurulent or purulent vagina, urethral or cervical discharge, vaginal bleeding, fullness or tenderness of the adnexa, abdominal pain, and cervical motion tenderness. *N. gonorrhoeae* grows best on Thayer–Martin agar (answer choice E) or Martin–Lewis agar, which are selective media for pathogenic *Neisseria*, such as *N. gonorrhoeae* and *N. meningitidis*. Both media are similar to chocolate agar but, unlike chocolate agar, contain antibiotics to inhibit the growth of normal microbiota of the urogenital tract. *N. gonorrhoeae* will grow on chocolate agar, which is supplemented with X (hemin) and V (nicotinamide adenine dinucleotide) and Thayer–Martin agar. Additionally, *Neisseria* species require increased carbon dioxide to grow. Note: Clinically, *Chlamydia* may present in a similar manner, but *Chlamydia* does not grow on artificial media. (**A**) Blood agar is a nonselective and differential agar that supports the growth of a wide variety of organisms. *N. gonorrhoeae*, however, does not grow on blood agar. Pathogenic *Neisseria* species are fastidious (i.e., require complex nutritional needs); media including chocolate and Thayer–Martin agar provide enhanced nutrients that blood agar does not. See Appendix F for a summary of common media used in the clinical microbiology laboratory. (**B, C**) Eosin methylene blue (EMB) and MacConkey agars are selective media for enteric gram-negative bacteria. *Neisseria* is gram-negative but is not an enteric pathogen; hence it does not grow on EMB media. or MacConkey. Both lactose and sucrose fermentation can be detected on EMB agar. Organisms that ferment both lactose and sucrose are blue or black. Organisms that do not ferment lactose or sucrose are clear or colorless. On this media, *E. coli* (a lactose and sucrose fermenter) produces a characteristic green metallic sheen (see image [i] at the end of this answer). MacConkey agar is differential for lactose reactions only. Lactose positive organism (fermenters) are pink and lactose negative organism (non-fermenters) are clear or colorless (see image [ii] at the end of this answer). (**D**) Regan–Lowe agar is a media used for the isolation of *Bordetella* species, including *B. pertussis*, the agent of whooping cough. The media contains antimicrobials to inhibit the growth of normal microbiota and beef extract to provide the growth components needed for the organism to grow. This media is selective for *Bordetella* species, which are usually respiratory pathogens. The urogenital pathogen, *N. gonorrhoeae*, would not grow on this media.

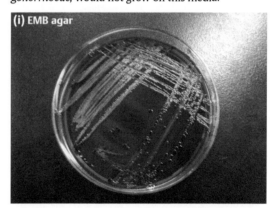

(i) EMB agar

(ii) MacConkey

Lactose positive (fermenter)	Lactose negative (non-fermenter)

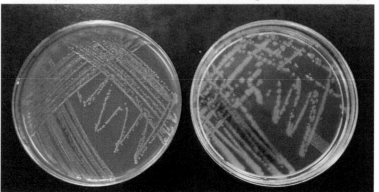

2. Correct: Lowenstein–Jensen (LJ) agar (C)

(**C**) This woman most likely has tuberculosis (TB) as indicated by the fever, night sweats, chest pain, and hemoptysis. The chest X-ray assists in this diagnosis as cavitary lesions may be seen in TB. One of the selective media that may be used for the isolation of *Mycobacteria tuberculosis*, the agent of TB, is Lowenstein–Jensen (LJ) agar. This media is egg based and contains malachite green to inhibit the growth of other microbes. (**A**) Buffered charcoal yeast extract (BCYE) is a selective medium for the isolation *Legionella pneumophila*, a gram-negative rod. This media contains L-cysteine and yeast extract to support the growth of *Legionella* species. Charcoal is added to the media to remove toxic products produced by the bacteria during metabolism. *Legionella* infections may manifest as atypical or consolidation pneumonia. In this case the patient's history of incarceration, hemoptysis, weight loss, and night sweats point toward *M. tuberculosis* as the causative agent. BCYE does not support the growth of *M. tuberculosis*. (**B**) Hektoen agar is a selective and differential media for enteric gram-negative bacilli, including *E. coli*, *Shigella*, and *Salmonella*. Lactose, sucrose, and hydrogen sulfide (H$_2$S) reactions can be seen on this medium. Lactose and sucrose fermenters are orange or salmon colored and lactose and sucrose non-fermenters are bluish-green. Organisms that produce H$_2$S will have a black center (see image at the end of this answer). In this case, the woman has a respiratory infection and not gastrointestinal infection. *M. tuberculosis*, the agent of this infection, will not grow on Hektoen agar. (**D**) Sabouraud Dextrose agar is used for the isolation of yeast and mold. Bacteria are inhibited on this medium due to the addition of antibiotics. While it is possible that the symptoms described in the stem may be due to a fungal agent, such as *Histoplasma capsulatum*, it is more likely with the patient history that *M. tuberculosis* is the causative agent. *M. tuberculosis* will not grow on Sabouraud Dextrose agar. (**E**) Thiosulfate citrate bile salts sucrose (TCBS) agar is selective and differential for the growth of pathogenic *Vibrio* species. *V. cholerae* and other non-cholerae species are agents of gastrointestinal infections. Additionally, some *Vibrio* species, especially *V. vulnificus* is the agent of skin and soft-tissue infections. These organisms do not typically cause respiratory infections. TCBS will not support the growth of the respiratory pathogen *M. tuberculosis*.

Hektoen agar

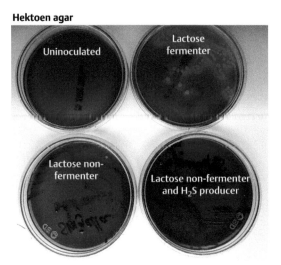

3. Correct: Kinyoun stain (B)

(**B**) This woman most likely has tuberculosis (TB) as indicated by the fever, night sweats, chest pain and hemoptysis. The chest X-ray assists in this diagnosis as cavitary lesions may be seen in TB. The best stains to visualize *M. tuberculosis*, the agent of TB, are the Kinyoun (answer choice B) and Ziehl–Neelsen stains, which are commonly referred to as acid-fast stains (also called acid-fast bacilli [AFB] stains). For both stains the primary stain is carbol-fuschin (red color), the decolorizer is acid-alcohol, and the counterstain in malachite green. The difference between the two stains is that for the Ziehl–Neelsen stain the slides containing the patient specimen or the culture isolate are heated prior to staining in order for the stain to penetrate the waxy cell wall. The Kinyoun stain is often referred to as the "cold" stain because heating is not required; instead the concentration of the primary stain is increased to allow stain penetration. With both these stains, *Mycobacterium* species, including *M. tuberculosis* appear as pink/red rods (bacilli) (see image at the end of this answer) because they retain (hold fast) the color of the primary stain even in the presence of the acid-alcohol decolorizer, hence they are referred to as AFB. (**A**) *Mycobacteria* do not Gram stain because the Gram stain reagents are unable to penetrate the waxy cell wall. (**C**) KOH preparations are used to visualize yeast and fungi, especially from clinical specimens. The KOH dissolves keratin and cellular debris, allowing for better visualizing of these pathogens. (**D**) The trichrome stain is used for the identification of parasites, not *Mycobacteria*. (**E**) The Tzanck smear is the classic method of evaluating vesicular material from herpes simplex, herpes zoster, and varicella infections. For this test, the fluid from the vesicle is removed and smeared on slide. The slide is fixed with methanol and then stained with Giemsa or another method. While this method has been largely replaced by other methods (such as direct fluorescent antibody tests), it is a classic test used for the identification of members of the herpes family of viruses.

AFB positive slide

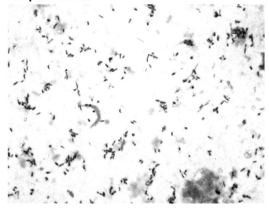

4. Correct: Mycolic acid in the cell wall (D)

(**D**) This woman has AIDS and her low CD4 count puts her at risk for mycobacterial infections. The acid-fast stain shows a pink, rod-shaped bacterium that is characteristic of *Mycobacterium* species. One of the characteristic features of *Mycobacterium* species is the presence of mycolic acid (answer choice D), a fatty acid, in their cell wall (see image at the end of this answer). The Gram stain reagents are unable to penetrate the lipophilic cell wall; therefore, acid-fast stains must be used. Mycolic acid also facilitates resistant to chemicals and some antibiotics and assists the organism in evasion from the host immune system. This woman likely has a disseminated *Mycobacterium avium-intracellulare* complex (MAC) infection. Infections are typically associated with immunocompromised individuals, especially in AIDS when the CD4 count is less than 50 cells/μL. Infections are often nonspecific and include the symptoms described in this case, as well as abdominal pain, diarrhea, and shortness of breath. This pathogen can be recovered from blood and occasionally from bone marrow and is an acid-fast bacillus. (**A**) A thick peptidoglycan layer is a characteristic of gram-positive cell walls. *Mycobacteria* are more similar to gram-negative bacteria because the peptidoglycan layer is not as dense. (**B**) This woman is unlikely to have a *Mycoplasma* or *Ureaplasma* infection, which are typically agents of urogenital infections (both) and respiratory infections (*Mycoplasma*). *Mycoplasma* and *Ureaplasma* are unique bacteria because they do not have a cell wall; hence they do not pick up the Gram stain, which relies on characteristics of the cell wall, especially peptidoglycan. Mycobacteria, on the other hand, do have a cell wall. (**C**) Lipopolysaccharide (LPS) is part of the outer cell membrane of gram-negative bacteria. LPS is composed of lipid A, a core polysaccharide. Some mycobacteria species may have LPS. However, LPS is not the reason mycobacteria do not Gram stain. This mycolic acid is the major reason for the inability of these organisms to uptake Gram stain. (**E**) Teichoic acid is composed of polymers of phosphates, carbohydrates, and amino acids that are covalently linked to peptidoglycan. Teichoic acid is found in the cell wall of gram-positive bacteria, not mycobacteria.

Mycobacterial cell wall

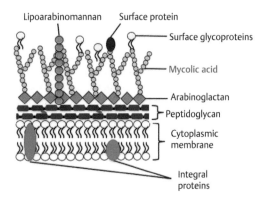

5. Correct: Serum (C)

(**C**) This is a case of atypical pneumonia. Symptoms include nonproductive cough and imaging may reveal patchy infiltrates. A positive cold agglutinin test is not specific for *Mycoplasma*, but is often positive during infections with this organism. *Mycoplasma* does not have a cell wall and culture of these organisms in the clinical laboratory can be difficult. *Mycoplasma* has complex nutritional requirements (fastidious) and must have sterols and lipids to grow. Serum supplies the required lipids and must be added to the media. (**A**) Charcoal is added to some media including Buffered Charcoal Yeast Extract (BCYE) agar, which supports the growth of *Legionella*. *Legionella* produces toxic metabolites as it grows and the charcoal is added to the media to remove these compounds. *Legionella* may present as atypical pneumonia that may progress to consolidation. The cold IgM in this case indicates that *Mycoplasma* and not *Legionella* is the most likely agent. (**B**) Hemin (also called X factor) is a part of blood agar and chocolate agar. This is not a requirement for the growth of *Mycoplasma*. Hemin is necessary for the growth of *Haemophilus* species, including *H. influenzae*, which is a respiratory pathogen. *H. influenzae* typically does not present as atypical pneumonia, as observed in this case. (**D**) Yeast extract is added to many different types of microbiological media used to grow clinically significant bacteria. Yeast extract provides essential nutrients for bacterial growth but is not required for the growth of *Mycoplasma*. (**E**) Salt is added to several types of media, including mannitol salt agar, a selective and differential media for pathogenic staphylococci. The high concentration of salt prevents the growth of other organisms. *Staphylococcus aureus* may cause respiratory tract infections, including pneumonia, but not usually atypical pneumonia as seen in this case. *Mycoplasma*, the agent of the infection in this case, will not grow on media with high salt. Note that enterococci and *Vibrio* also grow in elevated salt concentrations.

141

6. Correct: *Klebsiella pneumoniae* (B)

(**B**) The Gram stain shows pink, rod-shaped organisms that is characteristic of gram-negative rods (bacilli). Of the answer choices, only *K. pneumoniae* is a gram-negative rod. See Appendix G for a summary of select clinically significant pathogens and their corresponding Gram stain reactions. The Gram stain is the most important differential stain for bacteriology. The procedure is as follows: (1) fix the specimen to a microscope slide with heat or ethanol; (2) add the primary stain, crystal violet, which will bind to peptidoglycan; wash with water; (3) add iodine, a mordant that forms a complex with crystal violet; wash with water; (4) add alcohol decolorizer (a thick gram-positive cell wall will trap the crystal violet-iodine complex within the cell whereas a thin gram-negative cell wall will lose the crystal violet-iodine complex); wash with water; (5) add safranin, the counterstain that stains the cell wall of gram-negative organisms; gram-positive organisms will retain the primary stain. To summarize, gram-positive organisms stain purple (retains primary stain) whereas gram-negative organisms stain pink (retains counterstain). In addition to the color, morphology can be visualized. The basic shapes of bacteria are cocci (round), bacilli (rod-shaped), coccobacilli (short round rods), and spirochetes. See Appendix H for a summary of Gram stain reactions and common morphologies. (**A**) *Candida albicans* is a yeast. Yeast is oval, and budding forms may be seen microscopically. Yeast retains the crystal violet of the Gram stain procedure and is larger than cocci. See Appendix H for Gram stain examples. (**C**) *Listeria monocytogenes* is a gram-positive rod. The organism in this case is a gram-negative rod. (**D**) *Neisseria meningitidis* is a gram-negative diplococcus, not a rod. (**E**) *Staphylococcus aureus* is a gram-positive coccus. The organism in this case is a gram-negative rod.

7. Correct: Catalase negative (B)

(**B**) This girl most likely has "strep throat" caused by *Streptococcus pyogenes*, a β-hemolytic (see image [i] at the end of this answer) gram-positive coccus. This organism is also referred to as group A streptococci. Catalase is an enzyme produced by many clinically significant bacteria. Very few pathogenic bacteria are catalase negative. This is a key test to differentiate streptococci, which are catalase negative, from staphylococci, which are catalase positive. The enzyme catalase in the presence of hydrogen peroxide forms water and oxygen. After a colony grows on an agar plate, the organism to be tested is smeared on a glass slide and hydrogen peroxide is added to the slide. The presence of bubbles indicates a positive result (see image [ii] at the end of this answer). See image [iii] for a chart summarizing the biochemical identification of gram-positive cocci. (**A**) Bacitracin is an antimicrobial agent and in small concentrations (0.04 U) it can be used to identify *S. pyogenes*; however, *S. pyogenes* is bacitracin susceptible (sensitive). For this test, an inoculum of the bacteria to be tested is streaked on a blood agar plate. A small paper disc impregnated with bacitracin is sterilely placed on top of the bacteria. The plate is incubated overnight and then evaluated. If there is growth of bacteria onto the disk, the organism is resistant to bacitracin. If the growth of the organism is inhibited in the area surrounding the disk, a small zone of no growth will be seen (zone of inhibition). This means the organism is susceptible (sensitive) to the bacitracin (see image [iv] at the end of this answer). Several different tests to identify pathogens are performed in a similar manner. (**C**) Coagulase is a test utilized for the identification of *Staphylococcus aureus*, which is coagulase positive. Coagulase is produced by the organism and can convert fibrinogen to fibrin. This is not a useful test for the identification of streptococci since all streptococci, including *S. pyogenes*, are negative for coagulase. There are several methods of testing coagulase. For the tube coagulase test, serum (usually rabbit serum) is added to a test tube. The organism to be tested is grown on agar plates and then added to the serum. The tube is incubated for 4 to 24 hours and then evaluated for the formation of a clot, which would indicate a positive test (see image [v] at the end of this answer). (**D**) Novobiocin is set up in a similar manner, as described in the explanation for answer choice **A**. Novobiocin is mainly used for the identification of *Staphylococcus saprophyticus*, which is novobiocin resistant. (**E**) Optochin (ethylhydrocupreine hydrochloride) is used for the identification of *Streptococcus pneumoniae*, which is optochin sensitive. Other streptococci, including *S. pyogenes*, are optochin resistant. The optochin test is set up in a similar manner as the bacitracin test (see answer choice A).

(i) Types of homolysis

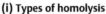

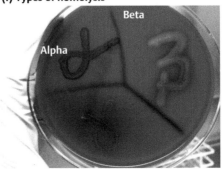

Alpha – partial hemolysis of red blood cells; greenish zone surrounds colonies

Beta – complete hemolysis of red blood cells; can see through agar plate

Gamma – no hemolysis; no change in the in the area of growth

(ii) Slide catalase test

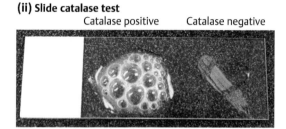

Catalase positive   Catalase negative

(iii)

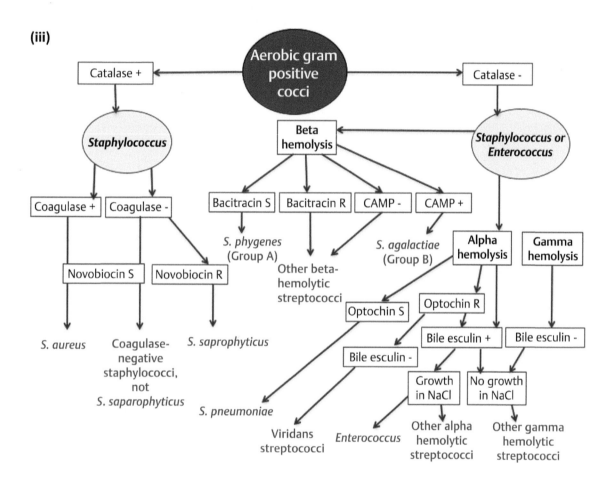

(iv) Bacitracin

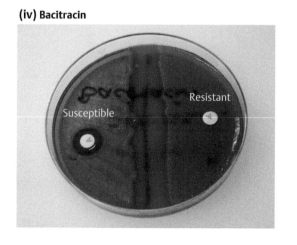

(v) Tube coagulase

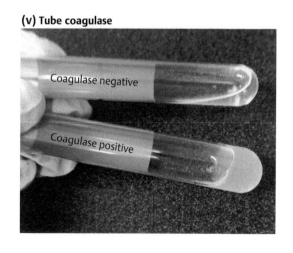

8. Correct: *Streptococcus pneumoniae* (E)

(**E**) This man is most likely to have pneumonia caused by *S. pneumoniae*, the most common bacterial agent of pneumonia. This organism has a very characteristic Gram stain morphology and typically appears as gram-positive cocci in pairs (diplococci) and can also be in chains. They are often lancet shaped or shaped like eyes, as seen in the image in the question stem. See Appendix G for a summary of select clinically significant pathogens and their corresponding Gram stain reactions. (**A**) *Bacillus anthracis* is a gram-positive rod with spores. This organism is a rare agent of pneumonia and is associated with inhalation of the spores, which are associated with herbivores, such as sheep and goat. As a result, infections are also referred to as Woolsorter's disease. Inhalation anthrax is very serious, and individuals are typically much more critical than described in this question stem. Often mediastinal widening and pleural effusions are seen on imaging. (**B**) *Corynebacterium diphtheriae*, a gram-positive rod (without spores), is the agent of diphtheria that affects the pharynx. The pseudomembrane on the throat may block the airways, leading to respiratory distress. Pneumonia, as presented in this case, is not a usual finding. (**C**) *Haemophilus influenzae* is an agent of respiratory infections but is often associated with individuals with underlying conditions, such as chronic obstructive pulmonary disease. *H. influenzae* is a gram-negative coccobacilli or short rod. (**D**) *Pseudomonas aeruginosa* is often associated with respiratory infections in cystic fibrosis patients and patients with ventilators (ventilator-associated pneumonia or VAP). *P. aeruginosa* is a gram-negative rod.

9. Correct: 4.0 µg/mL (B)

(**B**) The MIC is the lowest antimicrobial concentration that completely inhibits visible bacterial growth. Bacterial growth can be visualized by the turbidity in the well. A turbid or cloudy well indicates growth. In the image presented in the question, the lowest concentration of levofloxacin that inhibits the growth of the *S. pneumoniae*, resulting in a clear well and lack of turbidity is 4.0 µg/mL. The minimal inhibitory concentration (MIC) value can be compared with standards to determine if the organism is susceptible, intermediate, or resistant to a certain antimicrobial. The Clinical and Laboratory Standards Institute defines these terms as follows: Susceptible means bacterial resistance is absent or at clinically insignificant levels. The antimicrobial agent in question may be an appropriate choice for that particular bacterium. Resistant means the organism is not inhibited by serum-achievable levels of the drug. Test results correlate with a resistance mechanism that renders treatment success doubtful. Intermediate means that the antimicrobial agent in question may not be an appropriate choice for treating the infection. The antimicrobial agent may still be effective against the testing isolate, but possibly less so than against a susceptible isolate. The purpose of susceptibility testing is to predict whether the bacterium is capable of expressing resistance to the antimicrobial agents that are potential choices as therapeutic agents for managing the infection. The tests are performed under standardized conditions to ensure reproducibility. Most susceptibility assays are performed on automated systems in the clinical laboratory. However, three manual assays that are still performed include the microbroth dilution assay as seen in the question, the Epsilometer test (E-test), and the Kirby–Bauer test. For the microbroth dilution test, different concentrations of antibiotics are placed in microdilution tray. A suspension of the bacterial organism is also added to each well and incubated overnight. The plate is then evaluated for growth or lack of growth in well (turbidity indicates growth). The MIC can then be determined. The E-test uses the principle of a predefined antibiotic gradient on a plastic strip to generate MIC value and it is processed like the disc diffusion. After incubation, the MIC is read where the growth and inhibition edge intersects the strip (see image [i] at the end of this answer). For the Kirby–Bauer test, antimicrobial agents are impregnated on filter paper discs. The culture plate with bacteria and discs are incubated overnight. The zone of inhibition is measured and then compared to standards to determine if the drug is susceptible or intermediate (see image [ii] at the end of this answer). (**A, C, D, E**) These answers are incorrect. The MIC is 4.0 µg/mL.

(i) E-test

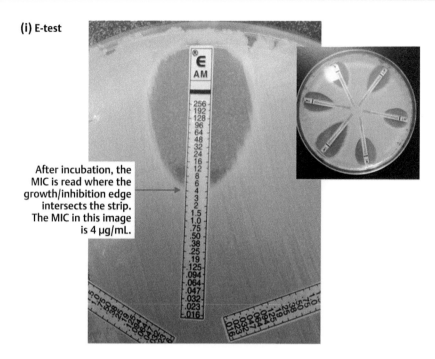

After incubation, the MIC is read where the growth/inhibition edge intersects the strip. The MIC in this image is 4 µg/mL.

(ii) Kirby-Bauer

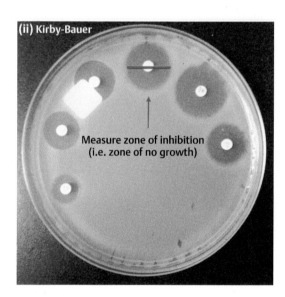

Measure zone of inhibition (i.e. zone of no growth)

10. Correct: Lipoteichoic acid (C)

(**C**) Key differences between gram-positive and gram-negative bacteria are their cell wall features. Gram-positive bacteria have a thick peptidoglycan layer. Protruding from the peptidoglycan of gram-positive bacteria, but not gram-negative bacteria, are lipoteichoic acid and teichoic acid (see image [i] at the end of this answer). These structures are polymers of phosphates, carbohydrates, and amino acids that are covalently linked to peptidoglycan (teichoic acid) or lipids (lipoteichoic acid). They promote adhesion and anchor the cell wall to the cell membrane. (**A**) Chitin is an essential component of the cell wall of fungi and yeast. It is composed of N-acetylglucosamine (NAG). Chitin chains are cross-linked covalently to β (1,3)-glucan. Chitin provides structural support for fungal and yeast cells. (**B**) Lipopolysaccharide (LPS) is found in the outer membrane of gram-negative bacteria (see image [ii] at the end of this answer). Only gram-negative bacteria have an outer membrane. LPS is composed of lipid A, a core polysaccharide, and O-antigen, a polysaccharide. LPS (also known as endotoxin) can induce endotoxic shock. (**D**) Mycolic acid is a fatty acid found in the cell wall of mycobacteria, not gram-positive bacteria. (**E**) Peptidoglycan is found in almost all clinically significant bacterial cell walls (except *Mycoplasma* and *Ureaplasma*). Peptidoglycan is a network of polymers composed of alternating and repeating units of the carbohydrates NAG and N-acetylmuramic acid (NAM). These carbohydrates form a linear chain and the NAG–NAM units are linked by a β-1,4 glycosidic bond. The cell wall functions to provide shape and protection to the bacterial cell.

(i)

Gram positive cell wall

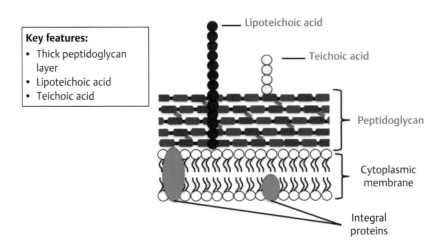

Key features:
- Thick peptidoglycan layer
- Lipoteichoic acid
- Teichoic acid

Lipoteichoic acid

Teichoic acid

Peptidoglycan

Cytoplasmic membrane

Integral proteins

(ii)

Gram negative cell wall

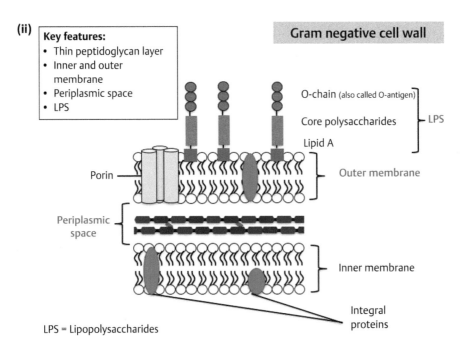

Key features:
- Thin peptidoglycan layer
- Inner and outer membrane
- Periplasmic space
- LPS

O-chain (also called O-antigen)

Core polysaccharides — LPS

Lipid A

Porin

Outer membrane

Periplasmic space

Inner membrane

Integral proteins

LPS = Lipopolysaccharides

---

11. Correct: Erythromycin (B)

(**B**) This boy most likely has an infection with *Escherichia coli* O157:H7 and the lack of sorbitol fermentation is the key in identifying this organism. Infections are transmitted by undercooked meat (typically ground beef) and unpasteurized products, such as apple cider. This organism produces a toxin, the Shiga-like toxin that targets the 28S RNA of the 60S subunit of the host cell ribosome. This in turn inhibits protein synthesis (translation). Antibiotics can also target ribosomes (of bacterial cells), resulting in inhibition of protein synthesis. Classes of antibiotics that are translation inhibitors include the macrolides, such as erythromycin (answer choice B). Macrolides, oxazolidiones (linezolid), chloramphenicol, lincosamides (clindamycin), and streptogramins (dalfopristin/quinupristin) target the bacterial 50S ribosome. Aminoglycosides, gycylcyclines (tigecycline), and tetracyclines also inhibit translation, but target the 30S ribosome. The spectrum of activity of erythromycin is mainly limited to gram-positive organisms, *Chlamydia*, *Mycoplasma*, and spirochetes. See Appendix I for a summary of antibacterial agents' mechanism of action and spectrum of activity. (**A**) Ciprofloxacin is a fluoroquinolone that targets DNA gyrase and topoisomerase, resulting in inhibition of bacterial DNA replication, not translation (protein synthesis). Ciprofloxacin has activity against anaerobes, streptococci, and many gram-negative organisms. (**C**) Penicillin G is a β-lactam antibiotic that targets bacterial cell wall synthesis by blocking transpeptidases (PBPs). Transpeptidases catalyzes cross-links between rows and layers of peptidoglycan. Penicillin has activity against several organisms including enterococci, *Listeria*, streptococci, *Neisseria meningitidis*, and spirochetes. (**D**) Trimethoprim–sulfamethoxazole (TMP–SMX) is a folate synthesis inhibitor that has a broad spectrum. This agent has good urinary penetration and is often used for uncomplicated urinary tract infections. (**E**) Vancomycin is a glycopeptide that targets bacterial cell wall synthesis by binding to the terminal D-alanine. Vancomycin mainly targets gram-positive organisms, including staphylococci, streptococci, and enterococci. Oral vancomycin can be used in the treatment of *Clostridioides (Clostridium) difficile* infections.

12. Correct: Contains a protein shell that protects the genome (C)

(**C**) The causative agent of this infection is most likely to be a virus. Rhinovirus, coronavirus, and enterovirus are the most frequent pathogens of the "common cold," which is most likely what this woman has. Viruses are obligate intracellular organisms that need host cell enzymes (such as DNA polymerase) and machinery (such as ribosomes) to complete their life cycle. A virus core is composed of DNA or RNA (not both) and encased in a protein shell (answer choice C) or the capsid that protects the genome. Some viruses have an outer lipid bilayer or envelope, but not all of them (see image at the end of this answer). See Appendix N for a list of the clinically significant viruses and their properties. (**A**) The cell wall of mold and yeast, not viruses, contains ergosterol. This infection is unlikely to be due to a mold or yeast. Most fungal respiratory infections affect immunocompromised individuals and are more serious than described in this case. (**B**) Bacterial cell walls are composed of NAG and NAM. This infection is unlikely to be due to a bacterial pathogen because of the description of the symptoms (clear nasal drainage, lack of fever) and rapid improvement in her health without antimicrobial agents. (**D**) Viral genomes are composed only of RNA or DNA (not both).

Viral structure: envelope

- Composed of
  - Lipids
  - Glycoproteins
  - Proteins
- Function:
  - Attachment and entry to host cell (initiate infection)
- Composition
  - Combination of host and viral proteins

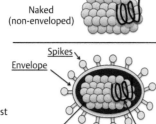

13. Correct: Thymidine kinase (TK) (E)

(**E**) This man has keratitis with herpes simplex virus (HSV), most likely HSV-1. Classic findings of ocular infections with HSV are dendrites seen on the epithelium or cornea, as seen in the image in the question stem. The most common antiviral agent used in the treatment of herpes infections is acyclovir, a nucleoside analogue. This drug is a prodrug that must be converted to be active and needs thymidine kinase (TK) (answer choice E). Viral TK catalyzes the reaction that allows synthesis of DNA from a salvage pathway. Viral TK allows herpes viruses to replicate in nerve cells in spite of the low amount of DNA precursors. Additionally, viral TK is required to activate acyclovir by phosphorylating acyclovir monophosphate. (**A**) Integrase is produced by retroviruses including HIV and facilitates the integration of viral DNA into the host cell chromosome. Integrase is not produced by HSV. (**B**) Neuraminidase is an enzyme produced by influenza virus. At the end of replication cycle, influenza virus buds from host cell. As the virus buds, it binds to the surface sialic acid. Sialic acid is the receptor for influenza virus and therefore neuraminidase cleaves sialic acids and allows release of newly synthesized viral particle. (**C**) Reverse transcriptase is produced by retroviruses (and hepatitis B virus). Reverse transcriptase can covert RNA to DNA (RNA-dependent DNA polymerase) and can also be used to replicate the DNA (DNA-dependent DNA polymerase). (**D**) RNA polymerase is used to copy RNA from an RNA template. This is an enzyme that only RNA viruses make. It is also called replicase (i.e., enzyme used to replicate their genome). Host cells do not contain RNA-dependent RNA polymerases, so RNA viruses encode their own replicases. Herpes virus is a DNA virus and does not have RNA polymerase.

14. Correct: Attachment to the host cell (A)

(**A**) The general steps of viral replication include (1) recognition of the target cell, (2) attachment, (3) penetration, (4) uncoating, (5) gene expression (replication/transcription/translation), (5) virion assembly and maturation, and (6) viral release by lysis or budding. gp120 is on a HIV envelope protein that plays a vital role in the attachment to the host cell (answer choice A). gp120 recognizes and binds to CD4 on T cells. gp120 then undergoes conformational change that allows binding to co-receptor (CCR5 or CCR4). (**B, C, E**) gp120 does not play a role in uncoating of the capsid, replication of the genome, or exit from the host cell. (**D**) Fusion and penetration into the host cell is mediated by gp41 (also called fusion peptide).

15. Correct: Three specimens, collected on 3 separate days (D)

(**D**) This boy has the classic clinical findings of giardiasis, caused by the flagellated, protozoan parasite, *Giardia lamblia*. Ideally, three stool specimens

147

collected over 2 or 3 days are needed for O&P examination because parasites, especially protozoa, may be intermittently shed in the stool, and collection of multiple specimens over several days will increase the chances of recovery. For helminth infections, one stool specimen may be enough to recover the parasite. Beavers are classically associated with *Giardia* infections and in this case, the beavers may have contaminated the water consumed by the boy, leading to his infection. (**A, B, C**) For protozoa infections, multiple samples over multiple days will increase the chance of recovering the parasite.

16. Correct: Trichrome (E)

(**E**) This boy is infected with *Giardia lamblia*, a parasite. The trichrome stain is the classic stain used for the diagnosis of parasites in the stool. The trichrome stain incorporates three colors. Different regions of the parasite will differentially stain. (**A**) Acid-fast stains are used for *Mycobacterium*. Some bacteria, such as *Nocardia*, will stain with a modified version (varying concentrations of decolorizer) of the acid-fast stain. Some parasites, notably *Cryptosporidium*, *Cyclospora*, and *Cystoisospora* also stain with a modified acid-fast stain. All three of these parasites do cause diarrhea and may be associated with contaminated water; however, the symptoms are more consistent with *Giardia* in this case, hence trichrome stain is a better answer choice. (**B**) Calcofluor-white is a fluorescent stain that binds to chitin, which is only found in the cell wall of fungi and is therefore used for the identification of fungi, not parasites. (**C**) The Giemsa stain is used for blood parasites, such as *Plasmodium*, the causative agent of malaria. This stain would not be useful for the diagnosis of gastrointestinal parasites recovered from the stool. (**D**) The Gram stain is the classic stain used to visualize bacteria, not parasites. Typically, Gram stains are not performed on stool specimens because the amount of normal bacterial microbiota is so immense that it would not be beneficial in detecting pathogenic bacteria.

17. Correct: Trophozoite (E)

(**E**) This boy is infected with *Giardia lamblia*, a protozoan parasite. Amoebas and flagellates have two main morphological forms (see image [i] at the end of this answer), cysts and trophozoites (answer choice E). Cysts are the immotile stage that is protected by a resistant wall and lives in the environment. This is most often the infective form of the parasite. The trophozoite is the motile stage that feeds and multiplies within the host. This is usually the diagnostic form of the parasite. However, both cysts and trophozoites may be recovered from clinical specimens. See Appendix P for an overview of the classification of clinically significant protozoa and worms. (**A**) Adult worms are seen in nematode, cestode, and trematode infections, not protozoan infections. Worms have three major forms: eggs (also called ova),

larvae, and adult worms (see image [ii] at the end of this answer). (**B**) A gametocyte is the form of *Plasmodium* that is part of the sexual cycle of the parasite. The gametocytes may be male or female. The gametocyte may be ingested by the *Anopheles* mosquito when the mosquito bites a human (see image [iii] at the end of this answer). (**C**) Larva is the intermediate phase of nematodes, cestodes, and trematodes, but not protozoa. Some organisms have multiple larval phases. The host that harbors the larval phase is called the intermediate host. The host that harbors the adult worms is called the definitive host. (**D**) Sporozoites are morphologic forms of Apicomplexia, including *Plasmodium*. In *Plasmodium*, the sporozoite matures in the mosquito and is transmitted to humans (see image [iv] at the end of this answer). Upon the bite, the sporozoite form of the parasite enters the human liver and develops into schizonts that have merozoites.

(i) Parasite-life cycle overview: amoebas and flagellates

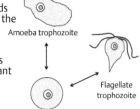

- Trophozoite
  - Motile stage that feeds and multiplies within the host
- Cysts
  - Immotile stage that is protected by a resistant wall
  - Iifective

Amoeba trophozoite

Flagellate trophozoite

Cyst

(ii) Parasite-life cycle overview: nematodes, cestodes, and trematodes

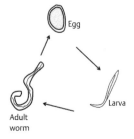

- Eggs (ova)
- Larva
  - An immature stage in the development of a worm before becoming a mature adult
- Adult worm

Egg

Larva

Adult worm

(iii) Parasite-life cycle overview: apicomplexica

- Morphological forms that are important for diagnosis include
  - Trophozoites (ring from)
  - Schizonts
  - Merozoites
  - Gametocytes

Trophozoite (ring form)

Schizont

Ruptured RBC with merozoites

Gametocyte

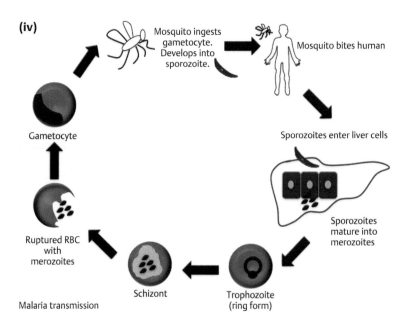

(iv)

Mosquito ingests gametocyte. Develops into sporozoite.

Mosquito bites human

Gametocyte

Sporozoites enter liver cells

Ruptured RBC with merozoites

Sporozoites mature into merozoites

Schizont

Trophozoite (ring form)

Malaria transmission

---

18. Correct: Conversion of yeast cells to fungal form (B)

(**B**) This patient has lymphocutaneous sporotrichosis, which is caused by the dimorphic fungus *Sporothrix schenckii*. The pathogen enters the skin following trauma. The hallmark of infection is a primary lesion at the point of entry and secondary lesion along the lymphatic channel. Usually the individual is otherwise well, and very few systemic manifestations are seen. *S. schenckii* yeast have a characteristic appearance and are budding yeast cells that are elongated, giving a "cigar body" appearance (see image at the end of this answer). This organism is dimorphic, that is, it grows as a mold at 25°C (room temperature). This is the form that exists in the environment. The spores of the mold can be traumatically inoculated into a wound as in this case, leading to an infection. At body temperature (37°C), the organism is a budding yeast. To confirm that this yeast seen in tissue is dimorphic, the conversion of the yeast cells to fungal form is necessary (answer choice C). This is accomplished by incubating the plates at 25°C. Other clinically significant dimorphic fungi include *Blastomyces dermatitidis*, *Coccidioides immitis*, *Histoplasma capsulatum*, and *Paracoccidioides brasiliensis*. Since conversion can take time, more rapid diagnostic tools are currently used for identification, including molecular methods. (**A**) Fungi are capable of both sexual and asexual reproduction. Sexual reproduction involves meiosis followed by fusion of protoplasm and nuclei of the mates. In contrast, asexual reproduction involves only mitosis. Demonstration of sexual and asexual reproduction would not aid in determining if this pathogen is dimorphic. (**C**) β-D-glucan is a component of fungal cell walls and this test, if positive, is a nonspecific indicator of a fungal infection. The β-D-glucan tests will not indicate if the pathogen is dimorphic. Keep in mind that this test may not detect some fungi, including zygomycetes and *Cryptococcus*. (**D**) A Wood's lamp is an UV light that is useful for the diagnosis of some fungal infections because infected skin will fluoresce under this light. For example, skin infections with *Malassezia furfur* will emit a yellow or orange fluorescence and dermatophytic infections with *Microsporum* will emit apple green fluorescence. A Wood's lamp is not used in the diagnosis of *Sporothrix* infections. Furthermore, it would not indicate whether the yeast was dimorphic. (**E**) Lactophenol cotton blue is a stain used to visualize hyphae or other morphologic forms from culture. Staining the yeast from the ulcer would not aid in determining if the pathogen is dimorphic.

S. schenckii yeast cells

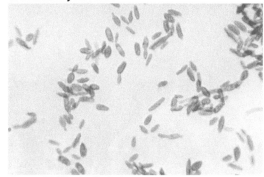

Source: CDC/Dr. Lucille K. Georg

---

19. Correct: This boy has latent TB infection and should be treated (B)

(**B**) It is important to differentiate tuberculosis (TB) latent infection from TB disease. Following inhalation of *Mycobacteria tuberculosis*, bacteria enter the alveoli and subsequently reproduce and survive in macrophages. A lesion or granuloma begins to form. At this point, a person may have an infection or

149

disease. In an infection (latency), the bacteria cease to grow and the lesion calcifies. However, in a small percentage of cases this can be reactivated resulting in disease. In disease, the lesion liquefies and the bacterium is coughed up; additionally, the organism may disseminate via the blood to other organs. This boy likely has latent TB infection as indicated by the positive IFN-γ release assay and the positive skin test. The Centers for Disease Control and Prevention (CDC) does not recommend routine testing of low-risk individuals. However, this boy is from a geographic region with a high incidence of TB. The CDC does recommend treatment of latent TB to prevent the spread of the organism to other individuals. Hence, answer choice B is correct. The tuberculin skin test (Mantoux or purified protein derivative) is used to determine if an individual is infected with *M. tuberculosis* and is positive approximately 3 to 9 weeks after infection and thereafter. The reaction is due to cellular immunity and hypersensitivity response. IFN-γ release assays include the QuantiFERON-TB Gold and the T-SPOT assay. The QuantiFERON-TB Gold quantifies release of IFN-γ from lymphocytes in whole blood from patients incubated with three *M. tuberculosis* antigens. The T-SPOT measures T cell response to *M. tuberculosis* antigens. A positive reaction for the skin test or the IFN-γ release assay will indicate if an individual has been infected, but will not differentiate between latent infection and disease. (**A, D**) This boy does not have TB disease and does not need to be treated and the cultures do no need to be repeated. In patients with TB disease, the granuloma is not contained and the necrotic tissue undergoes liquification. The material drains into the bronchus or blood vessels. In disease, the chest X-ray is most often abnormal and cultures and AFB stains for *M. tuberculosis* are often positive. (**C**) Patients with latent TB infection are not infectious and cannot transmit the disease to others because the granuloma containing the bacterium undergoes fibrosis and calcification, and the bacterium is contained. (**E**) This boy does not have disseminated TB. He is otherwise well and his chest X-ray is normal. Moreover, the positive IFN-γ release assay and TB skin test indicate latent infection.

20. Correct: Foscarnet (C)

(**C**) The clinical scenario describes a patient who has cytomegalovirus (CMV) pneumonia. The histopathological specimen in the image presented in the question demonstrates the classic owl's eye appearance of inclusion bodies in CMV infected cells. Ganciclovir is a first-line therapy for CMV. This patient has most likely failed the treatment with ganciclovir and has now developed CMV retinitis. Foscarnet is the drug of choice after failing to respond to ganciclovir. (**A**) Acyclovir is often used to treat varicella zoster virus and herpes simplex virus (HSV) infections. It has no activity against CMV. (**B**) This patient is immunocompromised because of NHL and has histopathological evidence of CMV infection. There is no indication for antiretroviral therapy. (**D**) Isoniazid is an antitubercular medication. There is no evidence to suggest disseminated TB. (**E**) Trimethoprim–sulfamethoxazole (TMP–SMX) is a folate synthesis inhibitor. It has no antiviral activity.

21. Correct: Squalene epoxidase (E)

(**E**) This patient has onychomycosis or a fungal infection of the toenails. Nail thickening (hyperkeratosis), discoloration, and splitting of the nails (onycholysis) are common findings of a chronic toenail infection. The lactophenol cotton blue preparation shows hyphae consistent with a dermatophyte infection (*Epidermophyton*, which is a dermatophyte, affects the nail and skin). Oral medications, terbinafine and itraconazole, are first-line drugs to treat onychomycosis. These two drugs are equal in efficacy, but it would be best to avoid itraconazole due to the allergy to fluconazole. Terbinafine prevents the synthesis of lanosterol, a precursor to ergosterol, by inhibiting the enzyme squalene epoxidase (answer choice E). (**A**) Many fungi possess the ability to degrade β-glucan. 1,3 β-glucosidase hydrolyzes chains of β-glucan. There are currently no antifungals targeting this enzyme, however, there is interest in developing an agent that utilizes this enzymatic activity. (**B**) 14-α-demethylase is inhibited by azole medications, such as fluconazole. 14-α-demethylase converts lanosterol to ergosterol. This patient has an allergy to fluconazole. (**C**) No known antifungal class targets dihydrofolate reductase. Dihydrofolate reductase converts dihydrofolic acid to tetrahydrofolic acid, which is a precursor metabolite used in nucleic acid synthesis. Trimethoprim–sulfamethoxazole (TMP–SMX), an antibacterial medication, inhibits dihydrofolate reductase. (**D**) The primary function of DNA polymerase is to synthesize DNA. The antiviral medications foscarnet and cidofovir are viral DNA polymerase inhibitors. There are no known antifungal agents that target DNA polymerase.

22. Correct: Primaquine (D)

(**D**) Malaria treatment can be complicated, but, in general, chloroquine is the first-line treatment for patients with chloroquine-sensitive organisms. Chloroquine reduces parasitemia by killing merozoites. It does not have activity against hypnozoites in the liver of patients with *Plasmodium vivax* or *Plasmodium ovale* infections. The addition of primaquine prevents recurrence of malaria in these patients. Primaquine prevents recurrence of *P. vivax* and *P. ovale* by killing hypnozoites in the liver. (**A**) Artemether is an artemisinin often reserved for chloroquine-resistant *P. falciparum*. (**B**) Atovaquone is often used in combination with proguanil to treat uncomplicated, chloroquine-resistant *P. falciparum* infections. This antimalarial combination is also commonly used as chemoprophylaxis for *P. falciparum*. It does not have activity against hypnozoites. (**C**) Metronidazole has antiprotozoal activity and is frequently used to treat anaerobic bacterial infections. However, it does not have antimalarial activity. (**E**) IV quinidine is typically reserved for severe *P. falciparum* infections resistant to chloroquine. Cardiac monitoring should be administered because quinidine prolongs the QT interval, which may lead to arrhythmias, particularly torsades de pointes.

23. Correct: Lipid A (A)

(**A**) The development of fever, hypotension, acute kidney injury (sharp elevation in creatinine), new lung infiltrates, and positive Gram stain and blood culture are consistent with sepsis from bacteremia secondary to ventilator-associated pneumonia (VAP). *Pseudomonas aeruginosa*, a gram-negative rod, is a frequent pathogen in VAP. Gram-negative bacteria have endotoxin, also called lipopolysaccharide (LPS), located in the outer membrane of the cell wall. LPS is composed of lipid A and O antigen. Lipid A induces fever and sepsis by stimulating activated macrophages to secrete TNF-α and IL-1. (**B**) Lipoteichoic acid induces sepsis by the same mechanism as endotoxin (LPS). However, lipoteichoic acids are present in gram-positive bacteria only. The patient in this question has a *P. aeruginosa* infection, which is a gram-negative rod. (**C**) Endotoxin is composed of lipid A and O antigen. O antigen is important in the identification of some gram negatives (especially *Neisseria* species). O antigen, since it is a polysaccharide, is weakly immunogenic and does not induce septic shock. (**D**) Peptidoglycan is an integral component of the cell wall of both gram-positive and gram-negative bacteria. The complex network of N-acetylglucosamine (NAG) and N-acetylmuramic acid (NAM) provides the rigid structure of the cell wall. Endotoxin and lipoteichoic acids, which are the major inducers of sepsis, can be found attached to the cell walls of gram-negative and gram-positive bacteria, respectively. (**E**) *P. aeruginosa* produces pyoverdin, a blue–green pigment (see image at the end of this answer). Pyoverdin does not play a role in the pathogenesis of sepsis.

***P. aeruginosa*: pyoverdin**

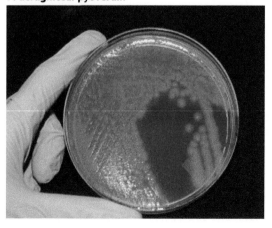

24. Correct: *Mycoplasma pneumoniae* (D)

(**D**) *Mycoplasma pneumoniae* is a respiratory pathogen that causes "atypical pneumonia." The course is mild and self-limited; chest X-ray often reveals findings that look worse than the patient does clinically. Cold agglutinins, IgM autoantibodies to red blood cells, are nonspecific serologic markers used in the diagnosis of *M. pneumoniae*. An elevated cold agglutinin titer supports the diagnosis of *M. pneumoniae*. (**A**) Influenza A virus is a highly contagious respiratory pathogen. Infections often occur in outbreaks in the late fall and winter. Patients often present with fever, malaise, upper and lower respiratory symptoms, and myalgia. Primary influenza pneumonia is rare in otherwise healthy adults. The patient in the question stem does not have myalgia and has laboratory and radiological findings more consistent with *M. pneumoniae*. (**B**) *Legionella pneumophila* is also a cause of "atypical pneumonia." However, the fact that the patient is in college does not have any GI manifestations, and has elevated cold agglutinins makes *Legionella* less likely. Also, a water source (e.g., air conditioners producing sprinklers in the grocery store) is usually associated with *Legionella*. (**C**) The clinical manifestation of tuberculosis (TB), caused by *Mycobacterium tuberculosis*, is more indolent than seen in this case. Some of the common symptoms of TB include fever, night sweats, weight loss, and hemoptysis. Epidemiologic risk factors, such as incarceration, HIV infection, homelessness, immigration from area with high prevalence or incarceration, are not mentioned in this question stem, making this an unlikely answer choice. (**E**) *Streptococcus pneumoniae* is the number one cause of "typical" community-acquired pneumonia (CAP). It would be very unlikely that a 20-year-old college student would develop CAP without mentioning some of predisposing factors (i.e., immunodeficiency, lung disease) in the question stem. Additionally, the clinical presentation would most likely be more severe.

25. Correct: Ceftriaxone (B)

(**B**) *Mycoplasma pneumoniae* is notable for not having a cell wall. Ceftriaxone, a third-generation cephalosporin, is a β-lactam antibiotic. It's mechanism of action involves binding to PBPs, which prevent transpeptidation of cell wall precursors thus preventing cell wall synthesis. Ceftriaxone and all other β-lactams do not have any antimicrobial activity against *M. pneumoniae*, since it does not have a cell wall. See Appendix I for a summary of antibacterial agents' mechanism of action and spectrum of activity. (**A, D**) Azithromycin and erythromycin are macrolide antibiotics. They bind to the 50s ribosomal subunit that inhibits the action of peptidyltransferase. Macrolides binding of this subunit prevents formation of new peptide bonds and translocation of the translational apparatus Azithromycin is effective against *Mycoplasma*. (**C**) Doxycycline is a tetracycline derivative. This drug binds to the 30S ribosomal subunit which prevents tRNA from binding at the A-site of the mRNA-ribosome translational complex. This ultimately prevents protein synthesis. Doxycycline can be used to treat infections with *M. pneumoniae*. (**E**) Levofloxacin is a fluoroquinolone that is effective against *M. pneumoniae*. Fluoroquinolones inhibit topoisomerase II, a DNA gyrase. Topoisomerase II relieves strain as DNA is being unwound by helicase. The inability of topoisomerase II to relieve DNA supercoils inhibits DNA synthesis.

26. Correct: Mycolic acid present in the cell wall (D)

(**D**) This man most likely has pulmonary tuberculosis (TB) caused by *Mycobacterium* tuberculosis as indicated by the positive IFN-γ release assay and chest X-ray. *M. tuberculosis* is an acid-fast bacillus that does not Gram stain well (i.e., not gram positive or gram negative) because its cell wall has a high lipid content. The fatty acid that gives *M. tuberculosis* its acid-fast property is mycolic acid. (**A**) Lipoteichoic acids are found in gram-positive bacteria. This is not a component of mycobacteria cell walls. (**B**) Mycobacteria do have cell walls. It is the mycolic acid component of the cell wall that makes them acid-fast. *Mycoplasma pneumoniae* is unique for not having a cell wall. (**C**) *Chlamydia trachomatis* and not *M. tuberculosis* fails to Gram stain because its cell wall lacks muramic acid.

27. Correct: *Mucor circinelloides* (G)

(**G**) The above scenario describes mucormycosis in a patient with diabetes. Mucormycosis is most often caused by *Mucor* and *Rhizopus* species. These fungi will often first come into contact with skin, nasopharyngeal, or oropharyngeal mucosa. They then invade and proliferate blood vessel walls where an excess of glucose and ketones exist. Symptoms such as headache, facial pain, orbital pain, and cranial nerve paralysis (e.g., CNN III, IV, VI, or VII) are seen. Physical exam findings classically include a black eschar. Mucormycosis is a medical emergency with high morbidity and mortality that must be treated surgically (removal of the necrotic, infected tissue by an experienced otolaryngologist) and medically (IV amphotericin B). This patient's chronically elevated blood glucose (evident by her history, Hemoglobin A1C, and current blood glucose), symptoms, physical exam findings, and laboratory findings all point to mucormycosis. The histopathology shows broad, ribbon-like, non-septated branching hyphae, indicative of a *Mucor* or *Rhizopus* infection. (**A**) The microscopic appearance of *Aspergillus fumigatus* is septate hyphae that branch at 45-degree angles. The patient's medical history and clinical findings indicate zygomycetes are more likely to be causing this infection. (**B**) *Blastomyces dermatitidis* is an endemic mycosis. This dimorphic fungus can be found primarily in Central America and areas east of and surrounding Ohio and Mississippi rivers. *B. dermatitidis* exists as a large, round

yeast with broad-based budding in human tissue. The patient history, clinical scenario, and histopathology point toward *Mucor* as an agent of this infection. (**C**) Candidal infections do not typically present with a black eschar. *Candida* is most commonly associated with mucocutaneous thrush. On pathologic examination, *Candida* is described as small budding yeast with pseudohyphae. (**D**) *Entamoeba histolytica* is a protozoan that causes amebiasis, a disease which causes dysentery and right upper quadrant pain due to liver abscesses. Histology would show multinucleated amoeba with phagocytosed red blood cells in its cytoplasm. *E. histolytica* is not known to cause sinus infections as seen in this case. (**E**) *Histoplasma capsulatum*, an endemic mycosis of the Mississippi and Ohio River valleys, most frequently causes pneumonia, but systemic histoplasmosis can also be seen. *Histoplasma* are much smaller than *Mucor* spp. and would be seen located inside macrophages. This infection described in this case is unlikely to be caused by *Histoplasma*. (**F**) *Malassezia furfur*, a noninvasive fungus limited to cutaneous areas, causes tinea versicolor. Tinea versicolor is a condition where hyper and/or hypopigmented patches appear on a person's skin (most prominently on the trunk). A characteristic "spaghetti and meatball" pattern is often used to describe its appearance on a KOH preparation.

28. Correct: Forms pores in the cell membrane (B)

(**B**) Mucormycosis requires prompt administration of IV amphotericin B. This medication's antifungal property is due to alteration of the fungal cell membrane. Amphotericin B is a polyene that inserts into the cell membrane, creating pores through which electrolytes can freely pass. The ability of electrolytes to move across the cell membrane causes cell lysis. Amphotericin B will also, however, create holes in renal tubules, making this drug nephrotoxic. Amphotericin B is used clinically for serious systemic mycoses. (**A**) Isoniazid (also known as isonicotinylhydrazide, INH) inhibits a reductase that leads to decreased synthesis of mycolic acids. Mycolic acids are only present in mycobacteria, making this drug highly specific for *M. tuberculosis*. In this case a fungal agent is the most likely causative agent. (**C**) Rifampin's mechanism of action is to inhibit DNA-dependent RNA polymerase. Inhibition of bacterial DNA-dependent RNA polymerase halts the synthesis of mRNA. Rifampin does not have antifungal activity. (**D**) Echinocandins (caspofungin, micafungin, and anidulafungin) act by inhibiting the production of β-glucan, an essential component of the fungal cell wall. These agents are not effective against zygomycetes.

29. Correct: *Staphylococcus aureus* (C)

(**C**) Colonizers of the skin are often responsible for osteomyelitis. In this case, a skin and soft-tissue infection was contiguous with bone. The finding of gram-positive cocci in clusters that are catalase and coagulase positive is consistent with the lab findings

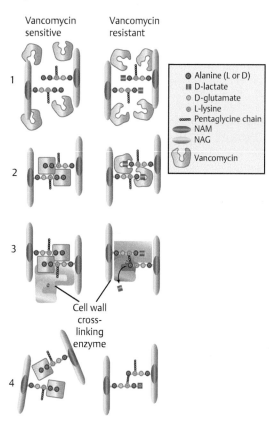

for *S. aureus.* (**A**) Clostridia are gram-positive rods. *Clostridium perfringens* causes gas gangrene. (**B**) *Pseudomonas aeruginosa* is a gram-negative rod. It is not a typical agent of osteomyelitis, but has been associated with osteomyelitis, following a puncture wound. (**D**) *Staphylococcus epidermidis* is coagulase negative, not coagulase positive. (**E**) Streptococci are catalase negative. The agent in this case was catalase positive, indicating staphylococci and not streptococci as the likely agent.

30. Correct: Ceftaroline (B)

(**B**) The first generation cephalosporins (cefazolin, cephalothin, cephalexin) cover mainly gram-positive organisms (but not methicillin-resistant staphylococci). The second generation cephalosporins (cefuroxime, cephamycins including cefoxitin and cefotetan) cover both gram-positive (but not methicillin-resistant staphylococci) and gram-negative organisms, but not *Pseudomonas aeruginosa.* The third generation cephalosporins (cefotaxime, ceftriaxone, ceftazidime, cefixime) cover mainly gram-negative organisms including *P. aeruginosa.* The fourth generation cephalosporins (cefepime) have similar activity to the third generation. The fifth generation cephalosporins (ceftaroline; answer choice B) is mainly reserved for the treatment of methicillin-resistant *Staphylococcus aureus* (MRSA). (**A, C, D, E**) None of these agents are effective against methicillin-resistant *S. aureus.* See Appendix I for a summary of antibacterial agents' mechanism of action and spectrum of activity.

31. Correct: Alteration of peptidoglycan precursors (A)

(**A**) The mechanism of action of vancomycin, a glycopeptide, is binding to D-alanyl-D-alanine (D-ala:D-ala), a component of peptidoglycan. When vancomycin is bound to D-ala-D-ala, the cell wall cannot properly form. Van-A confers vancomycin resistance by altering the peptide D-ala:D-ala to D-ala:D-lac. Vancomycin is unable to effectively bind to D-ala:D-lac (see image at the end of this answer). (**B**) Efflux pumps are a general mechanism of resistance that is frequently utilized by gram-negative bacteria. For example, gram-negative bacteria can become resistant to tetracyclines due to augmented transport (efflux pump). Some gram-positive bacteria also utilize efflux pumps. For example, macrolide resistance in gram-positive bacteria may be mediated by efflux pumps. This is not usually a method of vancomycin resistance. (**C**) This choice describes

a resistance mechanism to β-lactam antibiotics. Although vancomycin inhibits cell wall synthesis, it's mechanism of action is different. (**D**) Methylation of 23S rRNA confers erythromycin (macrolide) resistance. (**E**) Penicillin binding protein (PBP) mutations prevent the binding of β-lactam antibiotics to PBP. The PBP2a mutation in methicillin-resistant Staphylococcus aureus (MRSA) confers resistance to almost all β-lactam antibiotics.

32. Correct: Mitral stenosis (C)

(**C**) This patient's presentation history and physical exam findings are suggestive of mitral valve stenosis, which may present with a diastolic murmur. Exercise intolerance, due to impaired left ventricular filling, is often the initial presenting symptom. Also, mentioned in the history is two-pillow orthopnea. Her past medical history is suggestive of rheumatic fever secondary to streptococcal pharyngitis. Almost all cases of mitral valve stenosis are caused by commissure (fibrosis) of the mitral valve leaflets that occur after the initial insult of acute rheumatic fever. The chronic sequelae of streptococcal pharyngitis, caused by *Streptococcus pyogenes* (group A streptococci [GAS]), are prevented by prompt administration of antibiotics when a diagnosis of strep pharyngitis is made. Molecular mimicry plays an important role in the pathogenesis of rheumatic fever. Antibodies for GAS cross-react with host antigens in cardiac tissue. Mitral stenosis is classically associated with rheumatic heart disease. (**A**) In aortic regurgitation an early diastolic decrescendo murmur is heard best at the left sternal border. (**B, D**) In aortic stenosis and pulmonary stenosis, a systolic murmur is most often present. (**E**) In tricuspid stenosis the diastolic murmur is best heard along the left sternal border in the fifth or sixth intercostal space.

33. Correct: M protein (C)

(**C**) *Streptococcus pyogenes* (also called group A streptococci) is a gram-positive coccus in chains that is responsible for rheumatic fever. The M protein is a virulence factor found on the cell surface that helps *S. pyogenes* evade phagocytosis. Antibodies produced against M protein may cross-react with human tissues, especially cardiac tissue, leading to rheumatic fever. Hence, rheumatic fever is an autoimmune disease. (**A**) Erythrogenic toxin is expressed by *S. pyogenes* and causes the rash of Scarlet fever. It has a mechanism of action similar to toxic shock syndrome toxin produced by *Staphylococcus aureus* and nonspecifically activates T cells, resulting in a pro-inflammatory cytokine response. (**B**) IgA protease cleaves the IgA expressed by mucosal surfaces. Respiratory pathogens such as *Streptococcus pneumoniae*, *Haemophilus influenzae*, *Neisseria gonorrhoeae*, and *Neisseria meningitidis* are known to produce IgA protease in order to colonize mucosal surfaces. *S. pyogenes* typically does not produce IgA protease. (**D**) Protein A binds IgG and is a virulence factor expressed by *S. aureus* to avoid opsonization. (**E**) Streptolysin O mediates β-hemolysis on blood agar plates and is produced by *S. pyogenes*. The antibodies to streptolysin O (ASO titers) are a serologic marker used for the diagnosis of rheumatic fever and poststreptococcal glomerulonephritis. Streptolysin O has no known role in the pathogenesis of rheumatic fever or poststreptococcal glomerulonephritis.

34. Correct: C5 to C9 deficiency (A)

(**A**) This patient's clinical presentation is consistent with meningococcal meningitis. The CSF fluid analysis (low glucose, high protein, neutrophilic predominance) and Gram stain are indicative of bacterial meningitis. Extracellular and intracellular gram-negative diplococci in CSF fluid are suggestive of *Neisseria meningitidis*. A patient with recurrent *Neisseria* infections raises suspicion for C5 to C9 deficiency. (**B**) Chronic granulomatous disease increases susceptibility to catalase positive organisms, especially *Staphylococcus aureus* and gram-negative enteric organisms, such as *Serratia* and *Klebsiella*. Although, *N. meningitidis* may be

infrequently associated with chronic granulomatous disease, this organism is more likely to be associated with complement deficiencies. (**C**) Common variable immunodeficiency patients are predisposed to infections of the respiratory tract and develop bronchiectasis. Common variable immunodeficiency is not specifically associated with an increased risk for *Neisseria* infections. (**D**) Patients with leukocyte adhesion deficiency type I typically have a history of recurrent skin and mucosal infections. These patients have increased neutrophils in their blood, but no neutrophils at sites of infection (impaired neutrophil migration and chemotaxis). In this case, neutrophils are present in this patient's CSF. (**E**) Most patients with selective IgA deficiency are asymptomatic. A minority of patients may be predisposed to respiratory and gastrointestinal infections.

35. Correct: Exponential (C)

(**C**) The exponential or log phase is when active bacterial growth is occurring. Bacterial cells double by fission with growth rates dependent on temperature and nutrient availability. A chemostat is a bioreactor that maintains constant nutrient levels through the input of fresh media and the removal of bacterial waste products. This maintains a steady-state cell growth to optimize yields. See image at the end of this answer for an overview of the bacterial growth cycle. (**A**) Bacterial autolysis is the enzyme-induced destruction of the cell often in response to an environmental signal. In *Bacillus subtilis*, signal transduction induces production of an autolysin that facilitates the release of spores from the mother cell. In *Streptococcus pneumoniae*, the lytA gene is transcribed along with recA. Cell lysis releases *S. pneumoniae* DNA for genetic exchange. (**B**) Death phase results from the depletion of nutrients and the accumulation of organic acids that cause cell damage. Autolysis may play a role in the death phase with certain bacteria. (**D**) Lag phase is the first stage of bacterial growth in liquid culture. Bacterial cells are adapting to the growth media, temperature, and oxygenation prior to entering the exponential phase. (**E**) Stationary phase results from the depletion of nutrients and/or the accumulation of toxic products through fermentation.

Bacterial growth curve

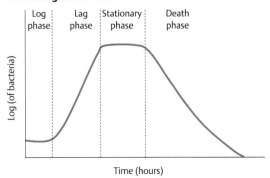

36. Correct: Pseudomembranous colitis (C)

(C) *Clostridioides (Clostridium) difficile* is an anaerobic gram-positive bacillus that causes pseudomembranous colitis. *C. difficile* produces spores which may be transmitted in the hospital setting. (A) Nosocomial cystitis is typically seen in catheterized patients with facultative gram-negative rods, such as *Escherichia coli, Proteus mirabilis, Klebsiella pneumoniae,* and *Pseudomonas aeruginosa.* The gram-positive coccus *Enterococcus faecalis* is another etiologic agent of nosocomial cystitis. (B) Pneumonia acquired in an institutional setting may be caused by the gram-negative, aerobic, pleomorphic rod *Legionella pneumophila. L. pneumophila* can grow inside amebae that reside in stagnant fresh water. Common sources are the cooling towers of air conditioning units, respiratory therapy equipment, and shower heads. (D) Scalded skin syndrome is a nosocomial infection of neonates caused by specific exfoliative-producing strains of *Staphylococcus aureus. S. aureus* is a facultative gram-positive coccus. (E) Thrush is an overgrowth of endogenous strains of the fungus *Candida albicans* in the oral cavity of immunocompromised patients. It is not a typical nosocomial pathogen.

37. Correct: Gentamicin (C)

(C) Gentamicin is an aminoglycoside that inhibits the 30S subunit of the prokaryotic ribosome. (A) Amphotericin B is an antifungal agent that binds to ergosterol in fungal cell membrane forming pores. (B) Ciprofloxacin is a fluoroquinolone that inhibits prokaryotic DNA gyrase and topoisomerase. (D) Methicillin is a β-lactam antibiotic that interferes with cell wall synthesis. (E) Trimethoprim–sulfamethoxazole (TMP–SMX) is an inhibitor of dihydrofolate reductase that interferes with folic acid synthesis. See Appendix I for a summary of antibacterial agents' mechanism of action and spectrum of activity.

38. Correct: Ciprofloxacin (B)

(B) Ciprofloxacin is a fluoroquinolone that inhibits prokaryotic DNA gyrase and topoisomerase, which are enzymes utilized during prokaryotic replication. (A) Amphotericin B is an antifungal agent that binds to ergosterol in fungal cell membrane forming pores. (C) Gentamicin is an aminoglycoside that inhibits the 30S subunit of the prokaryotic ribosome. (D) Methicillin is a β-lactam antibiotic that interferes with cell wall synthesis. (E) Trimethoprim–sulfamethoxazole (TMP–SMX) is an inhibitor of dihydrofolate reductase interfering with folic acid synthesis. See Appendix I for a summary of antibacterial agents' mechanism action and spectrum of activity.

39. Correct: Operon (C)

(C) By definition, an operon has a promoter which controls transcription of a cluster of structural genes with expression controlled by an activator or repressor that binds at the operator. A classic example in bacteria is the lac operon, which encodes proteins for the modification, transport, and catabolism of lactose. (A) An intron is a nucleotide sequence within a gene that is removed by RNA splicing, following transcription and preceding translation. Introns occur in prokaryotic, eukaryotic, and viral genomes. (B) The operator is the DNA sequence that binds to a repressor or activator effecting RNA polymerase binding and transcription initiation. (D) A regulon is more than one operon at disparate locations on the chromosome regulated by a common repressor or activator. (E) Transposons are mobile genetic element comprising an antibiotic resistance gene flanked by insertion sequences. Transposons are responsible for spreading antibiotic resistance through a population of bacteria through gene transfer.

40. Correct: Transformation (E)

(E) Transformation is the transfer of naked DNA into a bacterial cell. The recipient must be made competent for transformation in the lab while some bacteria are naturally competent for DNA uptake. Because transfer involves naked DNA, it is susceptible to the action of a degradative enzyme DNAase. (A) Competence refers to the potential for a bacterial cell to undergo transformation. There are laboratory methods that can make a bacterium competent for transformation while some are naturally competent. (B) Conjugation is bacterial cell-to-cell transfer of DNA by direct contact. The process is mediated by an episome (specialized plasmid) that encodes a sex pilus and the genes for replicative transfer of the bacterial chromosome. (C) Lysogeny is the state of integrated bacteriophage DNA in the bacterial chromosome following transduction. (D) Transduction is the transfer of DNA by bacteriophage. It can be through a lytic cycle with the nonspecific uptake and transfer of DNA from donor to recipient; this is referred to as generalized transduction. Lysogeny or integration of bacteriophage DNA into the bacterial chromosome results in specialized transduction with specific segments of DNA transferred.

41. Correct: Transduction (D)

(D) Several virulence factors, including diphtheria toxin, are encoded by genes which are carried by bacteriophage. Nontoxigenic strains of *Corynebacterium diphtheriae* may be converted to toxin producers by lysogeny (integration of bacteriophage DNA into bacterial chromosome). (A) Conjugation is the process of gene transfer between bacteria by direct contact. Conjugation is mediated by an episome (specialized plasmid) that encodes a sex pilus and gene products for replicative transfer of the bacterial chromosome from donor to recipient. (B) Fur is the ferric uptake regulator protein that is responsible for repression of gene expression in some bacteria. Fur binds with Fe++ as a corepressor to the diphtheria toxin gene operator to inhibit toxin synthesis. (C) Mutation is a process of genetic change that

155

occurs at a spontaneous rate in bacterial cells due to sequence change and recombination. An accumulation of nucleotide changes in combination with selective pressure may lead to the development of antibiotic resistance but would not be a likely cause of conversion of a nontoxigenic strain to toxin production. (**E**) Transformation is the transfer of naked DNA into a bacterial cell. The recipient must be made competent for transformation in the lab while some bacteria are naturally competent for DNA uptake.

42. Correct: Resolution of an Hfr followed by an F′ (prime) × F⁻ mating (D)

(**D**) An F (fertility) episome has the capacity to integrate into the *Escherichia coli* chromosome forming an Hfr (high frequency of recombination) strain. Hfr strains have the capacity to transfer a significant portion of the host chromosome to an F⁻ recipient during conjugation. Resolution of the Hfr within the original host strain may result in the F episome carrying chromosomal gene(s) on the episome. This situation is referred to as an F′ (prime) because the episome possesses the capacity to transfer those gene(s) to and F⁻ recipient. (**A**) Conjugation of two F′ strains cannot occur due to the exclusion properties of an *E. coli* carrying the F episome. An F+, Hfr, or F′ cannot be a recipient in a conjugation experiment. (**B**) Formation of an Hfr followed by an Hfr × F⁻ mating would transfer a portion of the donor chromosome during a conjugation. Transferred genes would integrate into the recipient chromosome and the F episome sequences would be lost. An F′ is the intact episome with chromosomal gene(s). (**C**) Resolution of an Hfr creates the F′ and would precede the conjugation experiment described in the question. (**E**) Resolution of F+ from the chromosome would not result in the formation of an F′ strain because the episome is not carrying any chromosomal sequences.

43. Correct: Antibiotic resistance (A)

(**A**) Transposons comprise an antibiotic resistance gene flanked by insertion sequences that encode integrase enzymes. Transposons delivered into bacteria as part of a conjugative R (resistance) plasmid overcome host restriction barriers and hop into the chromosome. Intergeneric transfer of antibiotic resistance has been documented. (**B**) Conjugation is mating between bacteria; the transfer of genetic material by cell–cell contact. R factors may be transferred by conjugation. (**C**) Invasion is a virulence attribute of bacterial pathogens in the respiratory and gastrointestinal tract. Shigella carries the genes for invasion on a plasmid. (**D**). Transposons may induce a missense mutation by inserting into the chromosome and antibiotic resistance may arise through the accumulation of mutations. However, the two events are not linked. (**E**) Bacteria such as the enterotoxigenic *Escherichia coli* carry toxin genes on a plasmid. Transposons are not involved in conferring toxin production in prokaryotes.

44. Correct: Endospores (B)

(**B**) Endospores are produced by the soil bacteria *Bacillus* and *Clostridium* during periods of prolonged nutrient or water depravation. They are composed of the bacterial DNA, peptidoglycan, and an impermeable dipicolinic acid coat. Superheated (pressurized) steam is required to inactivate endospores due to their resistance to chemical agents and UV radiation. (**A**) Capsule is the polysaccharide coat that surrounds a number of pathogenic bacteria such as *Streptococcus pneumoniae* and *Haemophilus influenzae*. It contributes to pathogenesis but does not necessarily contribute to extraordinary resistance to killing. (**C**) Lipopolysaccharide (LPS) or endotoxin is an extracellular component of all gram-negative bacteria. The inflammatory response to the lipid A portion of LPS may induce endotoxic shock in cases of gram-negative sepsis. (**D**) Mycolic acid is one extracellular constituent of the acid-fast bacillus mycobacteria. The extracellular components of the mycobacteria render them resistant to traditional staining methods and contribute to the chronicity of infection. (**E**) Peptidoglycan comprises the cell wall of all bacteria. It is composed of repeating subunits of N-acetylmuramic acid (NAM) and N-acetylglucosamine (NAG). While it maintains bacterial shape, it is permeable and does not contribute to extraordinary resistance to killing.

45. Correct: Transcription-mediated amplification (E)

(**E**) Transcription-mediated amplification is a reverse transcriptase and RNA polymerase nucleic acid amplification test (NAAT) used to identify the specific 23S rRNA of *Chlamydia trachomatis*. *C. trachomatis* can cause asymptomatic infections and commonly occurs concomitantly with *Neisseria gonorrhoeae*. *C. trachomatis* is an obligate intracellular pathogen that forms cytoplasmic inclusions. (**A**) DNA sequencing can be used for identification of specific genes of interest, including 23S rRNA. However, it is not an amplification test used to detect a specific rRNA target. (**B**) Hybridization is used to detect specific DNA sequences with a suitable probe. DNA is digested with a restriction endonuclease and electrophoretically separated and transferred to a substrate prior to hybridization. A Southern blot is a DNA-based hybridization method. (**C**) Multilocus sequence typing is a DNA sequencing technique that is used to type multiple housekeeping gene loci. Approximately 500 base pair internal fragments of each gene are sequenced and are assigned as distinct alleles to create a profile define an isolate. (**D**) Pulsed field gel electrophoresis can be used to identify bacterial isolates based on restriction enzyme digestion and electrophoretic separation. It differs from traditional electrophoresis because the electric field applied across the gel matrix changes orientation at timed intervals. This permits the separation of large (up to 2 megabytes) DNA fragments.

Chapter 8

Nervous System Infections

Melphine M. Harriott

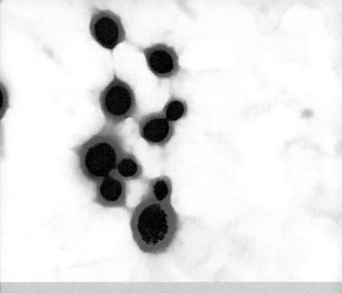

LEARNING OBJECTIVES

▶ Discuss the etiology, epidemiology, pathogenesis, clinical manifestations, complications, diagnosis, and treatment and prevention of:

- meningitis, meningoencephalitis, encephalitis, myelitis, and brain lesions.

- neurotoxin infections.

- head and neck infections.

- prion diseases.

- genital tract infections.

- congenital and neonatal infections.

- bloodstream and lymphatic system infections.

- skin, soft tissue, joint, muscle, and bone infections.

- infectious diarrhea and dysentery.

- foodborne illness.

▶ Describe prions.

▶ Describe the laboratory diagnosis and antimicrobial testing methods for bacteria, viruses, fungi, yeast, and parasites.

▶ Discuss virulence mechanisms and correlate virulence mechanisms with specific pathogens.

▶ Discuss antimicrobial mechanism of action, spectrum of activity, common adverse effects, and resistance mechanisms.

▶ Describe the common HIV/AIDS-related opportunistic infections.

▶ Explain the role of immunopathogenesis in the development of post-infectious diseases.

8.1 Questions

Easy	Medium	Hard

Consider the following case for questions 1 to 2:

A 19-year-old woman presents at 37-week gestation to the obstetrics unit following the rupture of fetal membranes, which occurred several hours earlier at home. The woman did not feel like she was in labor at the time so she did not seek medical attention. Five hours later she gives birth to a baby boy by vaginal delivery. Eight hours after birth, her newborn refuses to feed after repeated attempts. The mother reports to the nurse that the baby cries when she is holding him but settles down when he is placed in his bassinet. Blood and cerebrospinal fluid (CSF) from the infant are obtained for culture and both show gram-positive cocci in chains.

1. Which of the following is the most likely causative agent of this infection?

A. *Enterococcus faecalis*
B. *Staphylococcus aureus*
C. *Streptococcus agalactiae*
D. *Streptococcus pneumoniae*
E. *Streptococcus pyogenes*

2. The most likely etiological agent of this infection is also associated with:

A. Erythroblastosis fetalis
B. Granulomatosis infantiseptica
C. Neonatal pneumonia
D. Ophthalmia neonatorum
E. Roseola infantum

Consider the following case for questions 3 to 4:

A 5-day-old infant is brought to the emergency department because he "won't stop crying" and he "won't wake up and eat." The mother was concerned and sought medical care when she realized the baby had a fever. The baby was born full term and the mother reports that the pregnancy was uneventful, but she did have a bout of the "flu" for a few days when she was 8 months pregnant. The infant's temperature is 38.3°C (100.9°F). On examination, the infant is irritable, crying, and inconsolable. Tachypnea is noted and the clinician observes that the baby's anterior fontanel is full. A lumbar puncture is performed and after 2 days a β-hemolytic organism is recovered on blood agar. A Gram stain of the pathogen is shown below.

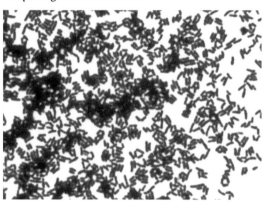

3. Which of the following is most crucial in the defense against the most likely pathogen of this infant's infection?

A. Antibody production
B. Enterocytes
C. Eosinophils
D. Macrophages
E. T lymphocytes

4. Which test would best aid in confirming the identity of the most likely pathogen?

A. Agglutination with antibodies to Lancefield group B
B. CAMP test with enhanced hemolysis in an arrowhead pattern
C. Formation of a clot with rabbit plasma
D. Production of metachromatic granules
E. Zone of inhibition around optochin disk

5. A 31-year-old woman gives birth to a healthy baby girl at 39-week gestation. The pregnancy was uneventful. On day 2, mom and baby are to be discharged from hospital; however, the baby develops a fever to 38.8°C (101.8°F). A CBC is performed and all values are within normal limits, but the baby is observed in the neonatal intensive care unit (NICU) overnight. On day 3, the baby is not feeding well, is lethargic, and has a full fontanel. A lumbar puncture is performed and the Gram stain shows few pink rod-shaped bacteria. Based on the etiological agent, which of the following is most likely mediating the pathogenesis and contributing to this infection?

A. K antigen

B. Production of an actin tail and intracellular spread

C. P-fimbria

D. Polyribosylribitol phosphate (PRP)

E. Toxin that inhibits protein synthesis

6. A previously healthy 10-month-old girl presents to the emergency department with a 1-day history of fever, vomiting, and lethargy. The child has had a few upper respiratory infections and ear infections, but her history is otherwise unremarkable. The family has not vaccinated any of their children due to religious objections. The child's temperature is 38.9°C (102°F). Physical exam reveals a positive Brudzinski's sign. An organism from the CSF does not grow on blood or MacConkey agars but does grow on media supplemented with hemin and nicotinamide adenine dinucleotide (NAD). Which of the following would most likely be observed on Gram stain from the girl's CSF?

A. Gram-positive rod

B. Gram-negative coccobacilli

C. Gram-negative diplococci

D. Gram-positive diplococci

E. Gram-positive cocci in clusters

7. A 17-year-old boy suddenly develops a severe headache. His mother gives him an over-the-counter analgesic and sends him to bed. The next morning the boy complains his headache is worse and he now has a fever. When the window blinds open, he cringes at the light. The boy's mother takes him to the emergency department. In the emergency department, the boy reports that he recently returned from summer camp and had shared a cabin with four other boys for a week. His temperature at the time of exam is 39.9°C (103.8°F). His physical exam is unremarkable. A spinal tap is performed, and cerebrospinal fluid (CSF) results are shown below:

- CSF analysis:
  - WBCs: 1,500/mm³; 95% neutrophils
  - Glucose: 22 mg/dL
  - Protein: 150 mg/dL

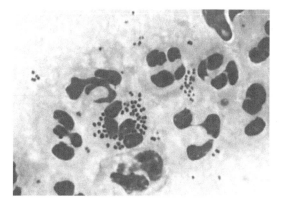

Which of the following is the most likely diagnosis?

A. *Haemophilus influenzae* type b

B. *Listeria monocytogenes*

C. *Neisseria meningitidis*

D. *Streptococcus pneumoniae*

E. *Streptococcus agalactiae*

Consider the following case for questions 8 to 9:

A 19-year-old man presents to the emergency department with fever and lethargy. His girlfriend states he appeared normal the prior evening but had complained of a severe headache. That morning she found him in bed moaning and complaining of lethargy and neck pain. His history is significant for splenectomy following a motor vehicle accident 2 years ago. At the time of examination his temperature is 40.3°C (104.5°F). In addition, nuchal rigidity and a purpuric rash on his legs and trunk are noted. CSF is obtained and the Gram stain demonstrates the presence of gram-negative cocci in pairs.

8. In addition to the most likely agent causing this infection, this man is at increased risk for developing an infection with:

A. *Actinomyces israelii*

B. *Clostridium tetani*

C. *Klebsiella pneumoniae*

D. *Neisseria gonorrhoeae*

E. *Shigella sonnei*

9. Infections with this pathogen may result in severe disease and hemorrhaging into the:

A. Adrenal glands

B. Kidneys

C. Liver

D. Pancreas

E. Spleen

10. A previously healthy 76-year-old man presents to the emergency department with fever, headache, and back and neck pain. His daughter is concerned because her father seemed lethargic and "not himself" during her daily visit. The man states the symptoms started suddenly the prior day. His temperature is 39.3°C (102.8°F) and physical exam reveals a positive Kernig's sign. A lumbar puncture is performed and the CSF Gram stain shows many PMNs and gram-positive cocci in pairs and chains. Which of the following is a characteristic of the most likely etiological agent of this infection?

A. α-Hemolytic on blood agar

B. β-Hemolytic on blood agar

C. Growth on chocolate agar but not blood agar

D. Lactose negative (non-fermenter) on MacConkey agar

E. Lactose positive (fermenter) on MacConkey agar

11. A 9-month-old infant presents to the urgent care clinic with fever and vomiting of 4-day duration. The mother states that the child refuses to eat and that he is more irritable than normal. About 2 weeks ago, the child had a runny nose. At the time of examination, the infant's temperature is 39.4°C (102.9°F) and bulging fontanels are noted. The physician sends the child to the hospital where the child is admitted. Cerebrospinal fluid (CSF) is collected and reveals normal glucose and protein levels and an elevated lymphocyte count. No organisms are seen on the Gram stain. The most likely agent of this infection is:

A. Coxsackie B virus

B. *Cryptococcus neoformans*

C. *Escherichia coli* K1

D. *Naegleria fowleri*

E. Parvovirus B19

12. During a family summer vacation, an 18-month-old girl refuses to eat and acts fussier than normal. Her mother becomes concerned when the girl develops a fever to 38.9°C (102°F) and develops a rash on her extremities. At the emergency room the girl is still febrile. Small red lesions are noted on the buccal mucosa and a maculopapular rash is present on her hands, including her palms, and her feet, including the soles. CSF is obtained and shows normal glucose and elevated protein and WBCs, with a predominance of mononuclear cells. The most likely etiological agent is:

A. Enterovirus

B. *Haemophilus influenzae* type b

C. *Neisseria meningitidis*

D. Mumps virus

E. *Streptococcus pneumoniae*

Consider the following case for questions 13 to 14:

A 40-year-old HIV-positive woman presents to the emergency department with a 1-week history of fever, malaise, and headache. Earlier that morning, her friend had stopped by to check on her and had found her confused and disoriented and brought her to the emergency department. On physical examination she is lethargic, her heart rate is 70 beats per minute, her blood pressure is 100/60 mm Hg, and her temperature is 38.3°C (100.9°F). Head CT is unremarkable. Other pertinent findings are shown below:
- CSF analysis:
  - WBCs: 207/mm^3; 76% lymphocytes
  - Glucose: 43 mg/dL
  - Protein: 150 mg/dL
- CD4 T cells: 87 cells/μL

13. After 3 days, yeast is identified from the CSF. Which of the following is most likely be seen microscopically in the CSF?

A. Budding yeast with a broad base

B. Budding yeast with hyphae and pseudohyphae

C. Clusters of yeast with short hyphae

D. Encapsulated, ovoid budding yeast

E. Large spherule containing endospores

14. The primary focus of this man's infection was most likely the:

A. Bloodstream

B. GI tract

C. Lungs

D. Mouth

E. Skin

15. An otherwise healthy 24-year-old man presents with a 5-day history of a painful lesion on his penis. Additionally, he complains of severe headache, fever, and neck stiffness. The man is sexually active and currently has several partners. He has not recently travelled outside of the United States. A scraping from the base of the lesion and CSF are obtained. CSF shows a lymphocytic pleocytosis. Which of the following is the most appropriate management for this patient?

A. Abacavir–lamivudine

B. Azithromycin

C. Acyclovir

D. Ceftriaxone

E. Penicillin

16. A woman brings her 67-year-old father to the physician because of increasing forgetfulness and paranoia. She states her father also seems to be more clumsy than usual, especially at night. The man has no prior psychiatric history. Physical examination reveals sensory ataxia. He is oriented to time and place, but has deficits in short-term memory. Laboratory results are shown below:

- CSF serology:
  - VDRL: negative
  - FTA-ABS: positive
  - *Toxoplasma gondii* antibody, IgM: negative
  - *Toxoplasma gondii* antibody, IgG: positive
  - West Nile antibody, IgM: negative
  - West Nile antibody, IgG: negative

Which of the following is the most likely diagnosis?

A. Guillain–Barré syndrome

B. Neurosyphilis

C. Rabies

D. Toxoplasmosis

E. West Nile encephalitis

17. A 38-year-old homeless man presents with a 4-day history of painful swelling of his testicle. For the past 24 hours he has also been experiencing an excruciating headache, fever, and difficulty moving his neck. The man is not up to date with vaccinations. His temperature is 38.3°C (100.9°F). On examination, his left testicle is inflamed. No lesions are observed on his penis. His CSF shows pleocytosis with a lymphocytic predominance. This infection was most likely transmitted by:

A. Contaminated food

B. Direct inoculation into the skin

C. Displacement of an endogenous strain

D. Respiratory droplets

E. Sexual transmission

Consider the following case for questions 18 to 19:

A 40-year-old woman presents with a 1-day history of fever, headache, vomiting, and abdominal cramps. Three months ago she was diagnosed with stage III breast cancer and is currently undergoing chemotherapy. A lumbar puncture is performed and the CSF shows pleocytosis with a neutrophil predominance, gram-positive rods, elevated protein, and decreased glucose.

18. The most likely virulence mechanism mediating this infection is:

A. A polysaccharide capsule

B. Intracellular survival and spread

C. Lipopolysaccharide (LPS)

D. Pili

E. Superantigen production

19. This pathogen can be best identified by growth:

A. At 42°C

B. At 4°C

C. In the absence of O_2

D. In increased CO_2

E. In the presence of high salt

20. In July, a previously healthy 73-year-old man presents with confusion, weakness in his legs, and diplopia. Within a week several other individuals who reside in the same retirement facility present with similar symptoms, myoclonus and gait disturbances. Epidemiological investigation reveals that several dead birds were found in the area surrounding the retirement home prior to and around the time this illness began in the residents. Which of the following is the most likely mechanism of transmission of this infection?

A. Direct contact with the dead birds

B. Droplet transmission from an infected human

C. Inhalation of secretions from the birds

D. Mosquito bite

E. Tick bite

21. During Christmas break, a 17-year-old boy in Michigan develops fever, headache, and vomiting. The next morning the boy's symptoms have not subsided and his father notices that he is tired, confused, and hallucinating, so he takes him to the emergency department. In the emergency department the boy's temperature is 37.8°C (100.1°F), he is not oriented to time or place, and he has a seizure while in the observation room. CSF shows elevated lymphocytes and protein levels and normal glucose levels. A CT scan shows abnormalities in the temporal lobe. The boy's medical history is unremarkable and he is up to date with childhood immunizations. Which of the following is the most likely diagnosis?

A. Enterovirus meningitis

B. *Haemophilus* meningitis

C. Herpes encephalitis

D. Subacute sclerosing panencephalitis (SSPE)

E. West Nile encephalitis

22. A 38-year-old HIV-positive man presents with headache, fever, rash, memory loss, and left-sided weakness. On examination, his temperature is 38.0°C (100.5°F). Physical exam reveals a vesicular rash on his trunk. His CD4 count is 104 cells/μL. CSF analysis shows a WBC count of 1,800 cells/mm³ with 87% lymphocytes.

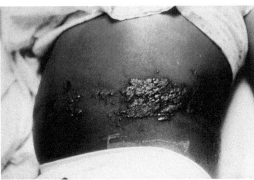

Source: CDC

Which one of the following is most likely to be seen from a skin scraping from this rash?

A. Cowdry type A bodies

B. Guarnieri bodies

C. Negri bodies

D. Torres bodies

E. Henderson–Patterson bodies

23. A 54-year-old man presents to a neurologist with weakness, pain, and tingling in his left arm and is subsequently diagnosed with neuropathy. A few weeks later he presents to the emergency department with increased pain and weakness in his arm and muscle twitching, difficulty swallowing and breathing, and increased salivation. The man is admitted and placed on ventilation. Two days after admission, the man becomes disoriented and combative. Four days following admission the man is in a coma. One week following admission, the patient dies. Autopsy shows the findings as seen in the image below taken from brain sections from the Ammon's horn, which confirm the diagnosis.

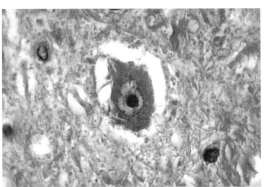

Source: CDC/Dr. Daniel P. Perl

Contact with which of the following is most likely to be in this man's history?

A. Bats

B. Birds

C. Mosquitos

D. Pigs

E. Ticks

Consider the following case for questions 24 to 25:

A 32-year-old HIV-positive man presents to the emergency department with headache, fever, nausea, and vomiting. Earlier that day, his mother had stopped by to check on him because he had been sick all week. She decided to bring him to the emergency department because he failed to recognize her and seemed to be "talking nonsense." At the time of examination, the man is disoriented, his temperature is 37.2°C (99°F), and his heart rate is 80 beats per minute. Physical examination shows posterior cervical lymphadenopathy. His CD4 count is 60 cells/μL. CT scan of his brain reveals multiple ring-enhancing lesions.

24. Which of the following is most likely to be seen from a brain biopsy?

A. Acid-fast bacilli

B. Bradyzoites within a tissue cyst

C. Encysted larvae

D. Enlarged cells with basophilic inclusions

E. Negri bodies

25. Which of the following is the most appropriate management for this patient?

A. Administration of albendazole plus praziquantel

B. Administration of clarithromycin

C. Administration of ganciclovir

D. Administration of pyrimethamine plus sulfadiazine

E. No antimicrobial agent; supportive therapy only

26. A 35-year-old man presents with seizures, headache, nausea, and vomiting. The man had worked with the Peace Corps in El Salvador and returned to the United States about 8 months ago. Brain imaging demonstrates multiple cystic lesions in the cerebral cortex with the presence of several scolices within the cavities. Which of the following is the most likely mechanism of transmission?

A. Bite from an infected raccoon

B. Direct inoculation of pathogen into skin

C. Ingestion of food contaminated with human feces

D. Ingestion of undercooked beef

E. Ingestion of undercooked pork

27. A 45-year-old man presents with a 3-day history of fever, headache, neck pain and stiffness, and photophobia. About 1 month ago he reports that he went camping in a wooded area in upstate New York. He recalls having a rash and feeling like he had the flu for a few days but then felt well again. At the time of exam, his temperature is 38.5°C (101.3°F). Physical exam reveals nuchal rigidity. IgM antibody to a spirochete was detected from his CSF. In addition to this infection, which other infection is this man most likely to have?

A. Babesiosis

B. Bartonellosis

C. Chagas disease

D. Cutaneous leishmaniasis

E. Malaria

28. A 54-year-old woman presents with intermittent fever, facial pain, headache, double vision, and dizziness. She became concerned when a black lesion appeared on her nose. On examination, a nasal eschar is noted along with significant facial edema and periorbital edema. Her serum glucose is 780 mg/dL and urine is positive for glucose and ketones. CT scan shows thickening and bony destruction of the nasal sinus cavity and thickening of the medal rectus. A biopsy of the lesion is obtained. Which of the following is most likely to be seen from the biopsy from this lesion?

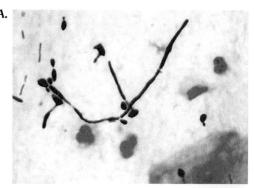
A.

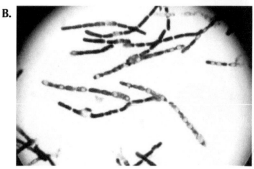
B.

Source: CDC

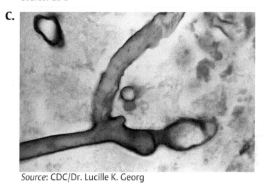
C.

Source: CDC/Dr. Lucille K. Georg

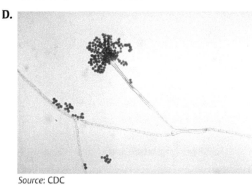
D.

Source: CDC

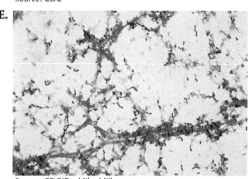
E.

Source: CDC/Dr. Mike Miller

163

29. A 13-year-old girl is brought to the emergency department with a 2-day history of fever, headache, nausea, and vomiting. On the second day of illness her mother becomes concerned because the girl seems anxious and irritable, complains that her food tastes and smells "weird," and is having difficulty recalling recent events. On examination, the child's temperature is 39.5°C (103.5°F) and blood pressure is 95/60 mm Hg. The girl is oriented to time but not place and nuchal rigidity and a positive Kernig's sign are noted. The cerebrospinal fluid (CSF) Gram stain shows many neutrophils but no organisms are seen. A Wright–Giemsa stain from the CSF shows the findings below.

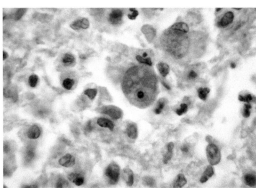

Source: CDC/Dr. Martin D. Hicklin

This girl is most likely to have a recent history of:

A. A mission trip to Haiti
B. Camping in the woods
C. Eating ice cream
D. Jet skiing in the ocean
E. Waterskiing in the lake

Consider the following case for questions 30 to 31:

A 43-year-old man presents with headache, nausea and vomiting and weakness of his right side. He has a history of a renal transplant approximately 6 months prior to the current presentation. CT and MRI reveal a lesion in the frontal lobe, suggestive of an abscess. A Gram stain from the abscess is shown below.

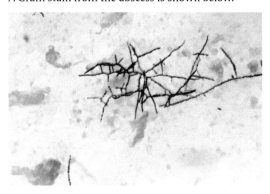

30. Which additional test would best confirm the identity of the most likely agent of this infection?

A. Endospore stain
B. Giemsa stain
C. Kinyoun stain
D. KOH preparation
E. Trichrome stain

31. The first-line therapy for this pathogen is:

A. Amphotericin B
B. Albendazole
C. Clindamycin
D. Rifampin
E. Trimethoprim–sulfamethoxazole

32. A previously healthy 38-year-old woman is brought to the emergency department by the ambulance, following a seizure. She has been experiencing a severe headache for the past few days and her husband states that she has been experiencing some memory loss. Her history is significant for poor dental hygiene and a dental extraction which occurred 3 days prior to the onset of symptoms. On examination, she does not know the day or time and is having difficulty speaking. A CT scan shows a lesion in the temporal lobe, suggestive of an abscess. Gram stain from the lesion shows gram-positive cocci in chains. Which of the following is the most likely etiological agent of this infection?

A. *Streptococcus agalactiae*
B. *Streptococcus anginosus* group
C. *Streptococcus bovis* group
D. *Streptococcus pneumoniae*
E. *Streptococcus pyogenes*

33. A 42-year-old woman presents with nausea, vomiting, and abdominal pain of 24-hour duration. In the last 12 hours she started experiencing dry mouth, difficulty with her vision, and weakness in her arms. She has no significant medical history or travel history. She has not consumed any undercooked meat or eaten outside of her home. She is the owner of a small business that preserves jams, jellies, fruits, and vegetables. Which of the following tests would best confirm the agent of this infection?

A. Double zone of hemolysis following growth in anaerobic conditions
B. Detection of pathogen specific antibodies in serum
C. Detection of toxin from serum from infected woman
D. Elek test for toxin detection from colonies growing on agar plate
E. Gram stain from vomitus or stool showing gram-positive rods with spores

Consider the following case for questions 34 to 35:

A 4-month-old girl presents with weakness and cannot lift her head on her own. She has a 5-day history of a cold and has been irritable. She has not been breastfeeding as often as usual and cannot suck well so her mother has been giving her breast milk with a syringe. She is also drooling more than normal. No one else that lives in her home is sick. The baby's temperature is 37.1°C (98.8°F). On examination, she has a decreased gag reflex, hypotonia, and poor suck.

34. Which of the following is the most likely mechanism of transmission of this infection?

A. Contaminated breast milk

B. Inhalation of dust

C. Transplacental transmission

D. Transmission during parturition

E. Transmission from another infected individual

35. The most appropriate next step in the management of this infection includes administration of:

A. Equine serum botulism antitoxin

B. Human-derived botulism immune globulin

C. Gentamicin

D. Metronidazole

E. Penicillin G

36. A 58-year-old homeless man is brought to the emergency department by the police, who found him under the influence of drugs and alcohol, missing socks and shoes, and barely responsive. On examination, his temperature is 40.1°C (104°F), his heart rate is 90 beats per minute, and his blood pressure is 60/40 mm Hg. Physical examination shows that he is having difficulty breathing, his neck is stiff and hyperextended, and he is having muscle spasms. In addition, his feet are gangrenous and ulcerated. The most likely causative agent of this infection produces a toxin that targets:

A. All neurons

B. Enterocyte neurons

C. Inhibitory interneurons

D. Motor neurons

E. Vagus nerve

Consider the following case for questions 37 to 38:

A 57-year-old man presents with a 5-day history of weakness in his legs, which has made it difficult for him to stand or walk. During the last 24 hours, he has also been experiencing shortness of breath and numbness in his fingers. About 2 weeks ago, he recalls having the "stomach flu." Several other family members also had similar diarrheal symptoms. The health department was notified and eventually epidemiological analysis showed all the infected individuals had eaten chicken potpie at the same diner.

37. Which of the following mechanisms is most likely mediating his current condition?

A. Cross-reactive antibodies that bind to peripheral nerves

B. Immune complex deposition in peripheral nerve vasculature

C. Inflammation of the peripheral nerves due to superantigen production

D. Invasion of a pathogen into peripheral nerves

E. Production of an exotoxin that inhibits acetylcholine

38. This man is most likely to have had a recent infection with

A. *Campylobacter jejuni*

B. *Escherichia coli* O157:H7

C. *Salmonella*

D. *Shigella*

E. *Vibrio cholerae*

39. Which of the following is a characteristic of abnormal prions (PrPSc)?

A. Effectively disinfected by heating to at least 80°C

B. Genome has RNA but not DNA

C. Levels remain constant throughout disease

D. Normally found in the tissues of animals and humans

E. Occur due to the misfolding of normal prions proteins

40. A 64-year-old woman has a 3-month history of progressively worsening symptoms including visual disturbances, difficulty sleeping, forgetfulness, and tremors with pronounced involuntary movements involving her entire body. Her mental status continues to deteriorate and she eventually slips into a coma and within 9 months dies of her initial symptoms. On autopsy vacuolated neurons are seen and there is an absence of an immune response. Which of the following would best confirm the diagnosis?

A. Gram stain

B. Serology

C. Toxin analysis

D. Viral culture

E. Western blot

41. A 16-year-old boy with Chiari malformation develops pseudomeningocele, following a suboccipital craniotomy. Subsequently, he undergoes a procedure for ventriculoperitoneal (VP) shunt placement. The boy is discharged home; a week following the VP shunt placement his mother notices redness along the line of the shunt. The boy also complains of a headache and has a fever. In the emergency room, the boy's temperature is 38.7°C (101.6°F) and physical exam reveals that the area along the shunt is erythematous and tender. A Gram stain from CSF from the shunt shows gram-positive cocci. Which of the following mechanisms is most likely mediating this infection?

A. Biofilm formation

B. Capsule

C. Endotoxin production

D. Exotoxin production

E. Intracellular invasion and spread

42. A previously healthy 7-month-old girl presents with a 3-day history of a runny nose and a 1-day history of fever. She was brought to the hospital by the ambulance because she experienced a seizure at home. The mother states that the baby has been fussier than normal and has been feeding less than usual. The baby attends daycare. The baby's temperature is 40.4°C (104.7°F); physical exam, CSF findings, and neurological imaging studies are unremarkable. The baby is admitted to the pediatric intensive care unit. Within 2 days she is afebrile and looks well and is ready to be discharged. Prior to discharge, the nurse notices a blanching maculopapular rash on her abdomen. The physician is not concerned about the rash and the baby is discharged home. Which of the following is the most likely agent of this infection?

A. Double-stranded DNA virus

B. Single-stranded RNA virus

C. Gram-positive cocci in pairs

D. Gram-positive rods

E. Protozoan parasite

43. A 26-year-old woman presents with weakness in her arms, malaise, dizziness, and dry mouth. She has a history of illicit drug abuse and admits to recently "skin popping" black-tar heroin. On examination, she is afebrile. She has multiple abscesses on both forearms. Material from the abscess shows large, gram-positive rods with spores. Which of the following is the most likely agent of this infection?

A. *Bacillus anthracis*

B. *Bacillus cereus*

C. *Clostridium perfringens*

D. *Clostridium botulinum*

E. *Clostridium tetani*

44. A 53-year-old man in Tanzania presents with a fever and malaise. He works as a safari tour guide and spends much of his time outdoors. Based on his symptoms he is diagnosed with malaria and treated with chloroquine. He stays home from work with a persistent fever for the next 2 weeks. During this time, he also develops a severe headache and is having difficulty sleeping. Within a few days he is hallucinating and experiencing memory loss. At the hospital his temperature is 38.9°C (102°F). Cerebrospinal fluid (CSF) is obtained and the Giemsa stain is shown below.

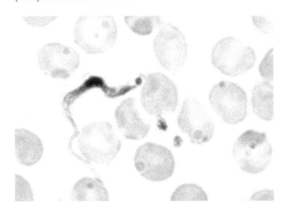

Which of the following is the most likely diagnosis?

A. African trypanosomiasis

B. Chagas disease

C. Drug-resistant malaria

D. Schistosomiasis

E. Yellow fever

8.2 Answers and Explanations

Easy	Medium	Hard

1.   Correct: *Streptococcus agalactiae* **(C)**

(C) *Streptococcus agalactiae*, also called group B streptococcus (GBS), is a gram-positive coccus in chains as described in the stem. Some women carry GBS in their gastrointestinal tract or vagina. Transmission to the newborn then occurs during passage through the birth canal resulting in infections, including meningitis, typically manifesting within the first week following birth. For this reason, routine anorectal and vaginal samples are obtained between 35 and 37 weeks gestation to screen for maternal colonization with GBS. Risk factors for neonatal GBS infections include premature delivery and prolonged rupture of membranes. Neonatal meningitis may be difficult to diagnose based on clinical manifestations alone. In this case, spinal fluid Gram stain results aid in the diagnosis. Other common bacterial agents of neonatal meningitis include *Escherichia coli* (K1, capsular serotype, and gram-negative rod) and *Listeria monocytogenes* (gram-positive rod). **(A, B, E)** *Enterococcus faecalis*, *Staphylococcus aureus*, and *Streptococcus pyogenes* are all gram-positive cocci but infrequent agents of neonatal meningitis. **(D)** *Streptococcus pneumoniae* is a gram-positive coccus in chains and pairs and is a common agent of meningitis in adults. Although there is the possibility that this pathogen may cause neonatal meningitis, in this case, since the mother had prolonged rupture of membranes, it is more likely that GBS or *E. coli* K1 is the causative agent of this baby's infection.

---

2. Correct: Neonatal pneumonia (C)

(C) The etiological agent of this infection is the gram-positive coccus *Streptococcus agalactiae* (also called group B streptococci [GBS]). This organism is an agent of neonatal meningitis, pneumonia, bacteremia, and sepsis. Infections may be transmitted to neonates during parturition, resulting in early-onset infections or by household contacts or other individuals leading to late-onset and late, late-onset infections. See the following table for the type of infections included in each category.

Category	Occurrence of infections	Type of infections
Early-onset	At birth or within 1 week after birth	Meningitis, pneumonia, sepsis
Late-onset	4 to 5 weeks after birth	Meningitis, bacteremia
Late, late-onset	**> 3 months after birth**	**Bacteremia**

(A) Erythroblastosis fetalis or hemolytic disease of the newborn occurs as a result of ABO and Rh incompatibilities between an Rh-negative mother and her Rh-positive fetus. In these cases, the mother's IgG antibodies leave the maternal circulation, cross through the placenta into the fetal circulation, and destroy the red blood cells (RBCs) of the fetus. For this reason, Rh-negative mothers are routinely given prophylactic Rho immunoglobulin at ~28 weeks gestation and shortly after delivery. **(B)** Granulomatosis infantiseptica is associated with *Listeria monocytogenes*. In adults, *L. monocytogenes* is foodborne and can then be transmitted to the fetus either in utero or perinatally. In granulomatosis infantiseptica, newborns will have abscesses or granulomas in the lungs, liver, spleen, kidney and brain. **(D)** Ophthalmia neonatorum or neonatal conjunctivitis is most often caused by *Neisseria gonorrhoeae*, a gram-negative diplococcus and *Chlamydia trachomatis*, an obligate intracellular bacteria or the viral pathogen herpes simplex virus (HSV). **(E)** Roseola infantum is caused by human herpes virus-6 (HHV-6), a double-stranded DNA virus. This virus most often affects children between the ages of 6 months and 2 years old. Infections are characterized by prolonged high fevers, which may result in febrile seizures, which are then followed by a rash.

---

3. Correct: T lymphocytes (E)

(E) This Gram stain shows gram-positive rod and the pathogen is β-hemolytic. This infection is most likely due to *Listeria monocytogenes*, an agent of meningitis in neonates, immunocompromised individuals and the elderly. This organism is a facultative intracellular pathogen and can survive and multiply in macrophages and enterocytes. Therefore, T cells are the main defense mechanism against *Listeria* and individuals with cell-mediated immune deficiencies are at a higher risk for infection with *L. monocytogenes*. Infections are transmitted to adults following ingestion of contaminated food. Commonly associated foods include unpasteurized milk and milk products, like ice cream, undercooked meat, or pre-cooked meat, such as hot dogs and deli meats. Transmission to neonates may then occur in utero resulting in early-onset infections. This usually occurs during the 3rd trimester. Infections may also occur perinatally, resulting in late-onset infections. Meningitis is a manifestation of late-onset infections. **(A)** *L. monocytogenes* is a facultative intracellular pathogen. Therefore, antibodies do not play a fundamental role in the defense against this organism. **(B, D)** *L. monocytogenes* can survive and multiply in macrophages and enterocytes. Hence, these cells are not the best defense mechanism against this pathogen. **(C)** There is no evidence to support that eosinophils are involved in the defense against *Listeria*. Eosinophils are key players in helminth infections.

---

4. Correct: CAMP test with enhanced hemolysis in an arrowhead pattern (B)

(B) The Gram stain shows gram-positive rods and the pathogen is β-hemolytic. This infection is most likely due to *Listeria monocytogenes*, an agent of meningitis in neonates, immunocompromised individuals, and the elderly. On blood agar this pathogen is β-hemolytic and looks very similar to group B streptococcus (*Streptococcus agalactiae*). The CAMP (Christie, Atkins, Munch-Peterson) test (answer choice B) can be used to assist in the identification of *L. monocytogenes*. For this test, a β-hemolytic strain of *Staphylococcus aureus* is streaked on a plate. An unknown is then streaked perpendicular to the *S. aureus* (close to but not touching). An enhanced area of hemolysis in the shape of a block or rectangle will be present where the *S. aureus* and *Listeria* meet (see image [i] at the end of this answer). **(A)** Agglutination with antibodies to Lancefield group B is a characteristic of group B streptococcus (GBS) or *Streptococcus agalactiae*. Both *L. monocytogenes*

167

and GBS are CAMP test positive.. However, GBS gives an increased hemolysis that looks like an arrow head while *Listeria* gives a block-shaped area of increased hemolysis. Additionally, *L. monocytogenes* is catalase positive and has distinct motility (tumbling motility in wet preparation and umbrella motility in semi-solid media; see image [ii] at the end of this answer) whereas GBS is catalase negative and nonmotile. **(C)** Formation of a clot within a tube containing rabbit plasma describes coagulase or clumping-factor formation, which is a characteristic of *Staphylococcus aureus*. This pathogen is a gram-positive coccus in clusters. There is a possibility that *S. aureus* may be an agent of neonatal meningitis; however, the most common

bacterial agents of neonatal meningitis are GBS, *L. monocytogenes*, and *Escherichia coli* K1. **(D)** Metachromatic granules are a characteristic of *Corynebacterium diphtheriae*, a gram-positive rod that is the agent of the oropharyngeal pseudomembranous infection diphtheria. This pathogen is not a typical agent of neonatal meningitis. **(E)** A zone of inhibition around an optochin disk (i.e., optochin susceptibility) is a characteristic of *Streptococcus pneumoniae*, a gram-positive coccus in chains and pairs. This pathogen may be an occasional agent of neonatal meningitis; however, the image in the question stem shows gram-positive rod. Furthermore, *S. pneumoniae* is α-hemolytic, not β-hemolytic as described in the stem.

Listeria monocytogenes
CAMP positive
Block head hemolysis

Negative control

(i)

CAMP Test
In the presence of *S. aureus* sphingomyelinase, CAMP factor causes an area of enhanced hemolysis

Streptococcus agalactiae
CAMP positive
Arrow head hemolysis

CAMP = Christie-Atkins-Munch-Peterson

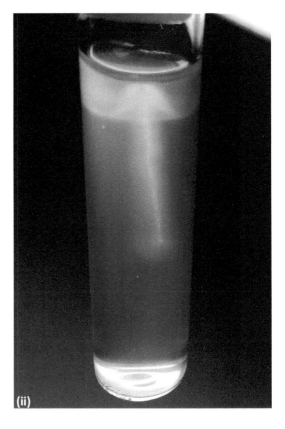

(ii)

5. Correct: K antigen (A)

(A) The pathogen causing this infection is *Escherichia coli*. *E. coli* is a gram-negative rod and will be pink or red on Gram stain. The most important virulence factor for *E. coli* strains involved in meningitis is the presence of a capsule (K antigen). Capsular strain K1 is the main serotype involved in neonatal meningitis. **(B)** Production of an actin tail and intracellular spread is a characteristic of *Listeria monocytogenes*, another agent of neonatal meningitis. *L. monocytogenes* is a gram-positive rod and is therefore purple or bluish with Gram stain. Another agent that also produces an actin tail and spreads cell-to-cell is *Shigella*. *Shigella* is a gram-negative rod and is mainly an agent of gastrointestinal infections (bacillary dysentery). **(C)** P-fimbriae are commonly found in *E. coli* strains; however, this virulence factor is thought to play a vital role in urinary tract infections rather than meningitis. **(D)** Polyribosylribitol phosphate (PRP) is a component of the capsule of *Haemophilus influenzae* type b, a gram-negative rod or coccobacillus. While it is possible that *H. influenzae* may cause neonatal infections, the most common organisms involved in neonatal meningitis include group B streptococcus (*Streptococcus agalactiae*), *L. monocytogenes*, and *E. coli* K1. **(E)** Enterohemorrhagic *E. coli* and *Shigella dysenteriae* produce the Shiga-like toxin and Shiga toxin, respectively, that inhibits protein synthesis. Strains of *E. coli* that cause meningitis do not produce this toxin. (Note: *Pseudomonas aeruginosa* and *Corynebacterium diphtheriae* also produce toxins that inhibit protein synthesis.)

6. Correct: Gram-negative coccobacilli (B)

(B) This girl has meningitis caused by *Haemophilus influenzae* type b (also called Hib). *H. influenzae*, both typable (encapsulated) and non-typable strains (nonencapsulated), may colonize the nasopharynx of healthy individuals. Infections are transmitted via respiratory droplets. *H. influenzae* capsular type b is associated with the majority of invasive infections including meningitis and infections may be prevented by vaccination. *Haemophilus* species need hemin (also called X factor) and/or nicotinamide adenine dinucleotide (NAD; also called V factor) to grow. *Haemophilus influenzae* does not grow on blood agar and MacConkey agar but will grow on chocolate agar, which is supplemented with X and V factors. *Haemophilus* are gram-negative coccobacilli or short rods. **(A)** *Listeria monocytogenes* is a gram-positive rod that is an agent of meningitis. High-risk individuals for meningitis with this pathogen include neonates, the elderly, and individuals with T cell immune deficiencies. *L. monocytogenes* grows well on blood agar and is β-hemolytic. Because it is gram-positive it will not grow on MacConkey agar, which is selective for gram-negative organisms. **(C)** A gram-negative diplococcus that is an agent of meningitis is *Neisseria meningitidis*. High-risk individuals for meningitis with this pathogen include

those living in close quarters populations such as college dorms, military barracks, and prisons. *N. meningitidis* does grow on blood agar but not on MacConkey agar (Note: *N. gonorrhoeae* does not grow on blood or MacConkey agars.) Based on the age of the patient in this case, the more likely agent is *H. influenzae* type b rather than *N. meningitidis*. **(D)** A gram-positive diplococcus that is an agent of meningitis is *Streptococcus pneumoniae*. Based on clinical presentation alone, there is a possibility that this infection could be due to *S. pneumoniae*; however, *S. pneumoniae* grows well on blood agar and is α-hemolytic. Like *H. influenzae* type b infections, invasive *S. pneumoniae* infections can be prevented by vaccination. **(E)** *Staphylococcus* species such as *S. aureus* or coagulase-negative staphylococci are gram-positive cocci in clusters that may cause meningitis in adults but are not common agents of neonatal meningitis. Coagulase-negative staphylococci are more often associated with nervous system shunts and device-related infections.

7. Correct: *Neisseria meningitidis* (C)

(C) The boy has septic meningitis, which is also referred to as purulent meningitis. Most often the etiological agents of septic meningitis are bacteria. In septic meningitis, the CSF WBC count is elevated (>1,000 WBCs/mm^3) and mostly PMNs are present as described in this case. Additionally, the glucose is usually markedly decreased while the protein is elevated. In this case the Gram stain shows gram-negative diplococci, which aids in narrowing down the causative agent, *Neisseria meningitidis*. *N. meningitidis* (also called meningiococcus) is a causative agent of meningitis in older children, young adults, and adults. Populations in close quarters, such as this boy who shared a cabin with other children, are at increased risk for meningitis with this pathogen. Transmission occurs via direct contact or respiratory droplets. Acute bacterial meningitis with this organism may be quite serious and meningococcemia may be seen concurrent with the meningitis. In these cases, purpuric or petechial lesions may be seen on the skin as a result of disseminated intravascular coagulation (DIC). **(A)** *Haemophilus influenzae* type b is an agent of meningitis in older children and adults. This pathogen is a gram-negative rod or coccobacillus (tiny rod). It is possible that this agent may be implicated in this patient's infection; however, the Gram stain showing gram-negative diplococci and the boy's recent history of being in close quarters with other children make *N. meningitidis* a more likely agent in this case. **(B)** *Listeria monocytogenes* is a gram-positive rod. This agent mainly causes meningitis in neonates, the elderly, and the immunocompromised. In healthy individuals the pathogen most often manifests as mild gastrointestinal illness. This boy does not have clinical manifestations of listeriosis and the Gram stain is not indicative of this pathogen. **(D)** *Streptococcus pneumoniae* is a gram-positive coccus in pairs and chains. This pathogen may cause meningitis in any age group, but is the most common agent of acute bacterial meningitis in adults. The Gram stain in this case confirms that *N. meningitidis* is the causative agent of this child's infection. **(E)** *Streptococcus agalactiae* (also called group B streptococcus [GBS]) is a gram-positive coccus in chains. This agent is mainly an agent of meningitis in neonates. In older children and adults, this pathogen may cause bacteremia and skin and soft-tissue infections. This is unlikely to be the agent in this case.

8. Correct: *Klebsiella pneumoniae* (C)

(C) This man has meningitis caused by *Neisseria meningitidis*, a gram-negative diplococcus (or cocci in pairs as described in the stem). Classic findings of meningitis with this pathogen include a petechial/purpuric rash. The main mechanism of virulence for this pathogen is a capsule. Certain populations are at increased risk for infections with encapsulated organisms including asplenic individuals. The only other encapsulated pathogen in the answer choices is *Klebsiella pneumoniae* (answer choice C). Cells found in the spleen, including macrophages, play an important role in mediating opsonization of encapsulated bacteria. Other individuals also at risk for infections with encapsulated bacteria include those with terminal complement deficiencies (C5–C9) and children from 6 months to 1 year of age (by this time maternal antibodies have most likely waned and the child's cell-mediated immunity is still developing). Note that *N. meningitidis* has a capsule. However, *N. gonorrhoeae* does not have a capsule. **(A, B, D, E)** *Actinomyces israelii, Clostridium tetani, Neisseria gonorrhoeae,* and *Shigella sonnei* are not encapsulated.

9. Correct: Adrenal glands (A)

(A) A serious complication of infection with *Neisseria meningitidis* is Waterhouse–Friderichsen syndrome. A classic finding of this disease is hemorrhaging into the adrenal glands. *N. meningitidis* meningitis may be present in conjunction with meningococcemia as in this case. Alternatively, meningitis or meningococcemia may be present independent of one another. The petechial rash is a classic sign of infection with this organism, but the rash is not always present. The *Neisseria* endotoxin (lipooligosaccharide [LOS]) induces disseminated intravascular coagulation (DIC). In DIC, clots form in blood vessels and bleeding from the skin occurs. This results in purpuric or petechial lesions seen in *N. meningitidis* infections. (Note: LOS is very similar in function but varies slightly in structure to the typical gram-negative lipopolysaccharide [LPS].) **(B, C, D, E)** Waterhouse–Friderichsen syndrome is characterized by hemorrhaging into the adrenal glands, *not* the kidneys, liver, pancreas, or spleen.

10. Correct: α-Hemolytic on blood agar (A)

(A) A 76-year-old man is at risk for meningitis with *Streptococcus pneumoniae* and *Listeria monocytogenes*.

S. pneumoniae is gram-positive cocci in pairs (diplococci) and chains, while *L. monocytogenes* is gram-positive rods. Hence, the most likely etiological agent of this infection is *S. pneumoniae*, which is α-hemolytic on blood agar. **(B)** Two frequent agents of bacterial meningitis that are β-hemolytic on blood agar include *L. monocytogenes* and *S. agalactiae*. *Listeria* is a gram-positive rod and *S. agalactiae* is a gram-positive coccus in chains. **(C)** Chocolate agar is enriched with X (hemin) and V (NAD) factors that are necessary for the growth of *Haemophilus influenzae*. *H. influenzae* grows well on chocolate agar but not on blood agar. Blood agar provides the X but not the V factor. (Note: V factor is found in intact RBCs, so it is present in blood agar but not readily available unless the RBCs are lysed.) *S. pneumoniae*, however, grows well on both blood agar and chocolate agar. **(D, E)** MacConkey agar is selective for gram-negative rods. Crystal violet and bile salts inhibit the growth of gram-positive organisms. Therefore, a gram-positive organism as described in the stem will not grow on MacConkey agar.

11. Correct: Coxsackie B virus (A)

(A) Non-polio enteroviruses, especially coxsackievirus (type B1) and echovirus virus, are common viral agents involved in aseptic meningitis. These are single-stranded RNA viruses. Viruses cannot be seen with light microscopy due to their small size, hence the absence of organisms on the Gram stain. The main differences in laboratory values between bacterial and viral meningitis is that in bacterial meningitis the CSF glucose is usually low and protein elevated with neutrophils being the main cell type observed. This is in contrast to viral meningitis in which the glucose is most often normal and the protein is normal or slightly elevated and the main cell types seen are mononuclear cells. Viral meningitis is often referred to as aseptic meningitis because no organisms are isolated on routine artificial (bacterial) microbiological media. **(B)** *Cryptococcus neoformans* is a yeast that may be seen as purple, oval budding structures on Gram stain. This pathogen is mainly an agent of meningitis in immunocompromised individuals, especially those with HIV. This is unlikely pathogen in this case. **(C)** *Escherichia coli* K1 is an agent of neonatal meningitis and is gram-negative rod. Most often in bacterial meningitis, the CSF glucose is decreased and protein is elevated and the major cell type seen is neutrophils (also called polymorphonuclear cells). The age of the child makes *E. coli* K1 unlikely. **(D)** *Naegleria fowleri* is a protozoan parasite that is the agent of primary amebic meningoencephalitis (PAM). This infection is transmitted following contact with contaminated water, usually following recreational activities. The organism often affects healthy young children. The age and presentation in this case are not consistent with *Naegleria* infection. **(E)** Parvovirus B19 is a rare agent of meningitis. This pathogen most often affects school-age children and results in a febrile illness with a lacy, reticular erythematous rash on the trunk and extremities and a prominent erythema on the face (resembling slapped checks). This virus may also be transferred transplacentally, resulting in congenital infections.

12. Correct: Enterovirus (A)

(A) This child most likely has hand, foot, and mouth disease (HFMD), which classically presents with an enanthem on the tongue or buccal mucosa and an exanthem on the hands and feet. HFMD is most often caused by coxsackievirus A16 and enterovirus A71. Viral meningitis may complicate the course of HFMD as described in this case. Enteroviruses, especially coxsackievirus and echovirus are commonly implicated in viral meningitis in children. Enteroviral infections are more common during the summer and fall months. There is currently no vaccination for non-polio enteroviruses. **(B, C, E)** All three of these bacterial pathogens are plausible agents of this infection, especially since this child is not up to date with vaccinations. However, the CSF analysis indicates that this infection is viral (normal glucose and protein, mononuclear cells) rather than bacterial. **(D)** Mumps virus is may cause meningitis in unvaccinated individuals. The clinical presentation in this case is not consistent with mumps meningitis.

13. Correct: Encapsulated, ovoid budding yeast (D)

(D) This infection is most likely due to the yeast *Cryptococcus neoformans* var. *neoformans* (most often referred to as *C. neoformans*). This pathogen is a common agent of meningitis in the immunocompromised, especially in HIV-positive individuals with CD4 counts greater than 100 cells/μL. *C. neoformans* is equipped with a capsule and is a budding yeast as described in answer choice D (see image [i] at the end of this answer). India ink stain is the classic test for detection of this organism and the budding yeast may be seen with the capsule (see image [i] at the end of this answer). However, the India ink test is not very sensitive; hence, this test has been largely replaced by antigen-based assays. Central nervous system (CNS) infections with this pathogen may be indolent and symptoms may occur over 1 to 2 weeks as in this case. Note that *Cryptococcus gattii* may cause similar manifestations as *C. neoformans*, but *C. gattii* infections are usually seen in the Pacific Northwest (United States) and in British Columbia, Canada. Biochemical or molecular identification can differentiate these pathogens from one another. See Appendix M for other infections that are frequently associated with HIV/AIDS. **(A)** This is a description of the yeast form of *Blastomyces dermatiditis* (broad base budding yeast, see image [ii] at the end of this answer), an endemic fungus. While this pathogen may disseminate to the CNS, it is not a common agent of CNS infections. Primary infections with *B. dermatitidis* usually manifest as pulmonary infections and then disseminate to the skin and soft tissue as well as the bone, and sometimes the CNS, especially in immunocompromised individuals. *C. neoformans* is a more common agent of meningitis

and is more likely to be causing this infection. **(B)** Budding yeast with hyphae and pseudohyphae are characteristics of *Candida albicans* (see image [iii] at the end of this answer). This pathogen is not a typical agent of meningitis. **(C)** Clusters of yeast with short hyphae is a classic description of *Malassezia furfur* (often described as spaghetti and meatballs, see image [iv] at the end of this answer). This pathogen is the agent of tinea versicolor, also referred to as pityriasis versicolor, a superficial skin infection and is not a usual agent of meningitis. **(E)** Large yeast-like spherules with endospores are a description of the yeast form of *Coccidioides immitis* (see image [v] at the end of this answer). This pathogen primarily causes respiratory infections; however, it may disseminate to the CNS as well as other organs, especially in the immunocompromised. *C. immitis* is endemic to the San Joaquin Valley in California. *C. neoformans* is a more common agent of meningitis and clinical findings and presentation in this case are more consistent with *Cryptococcus* meningitis.

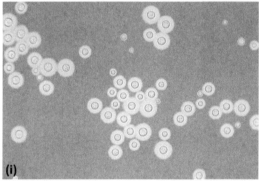

(i)
Source: CDC/Leanor Haley

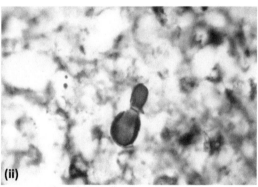

(ii)
Source: CDC/Dr. Libero Ajello

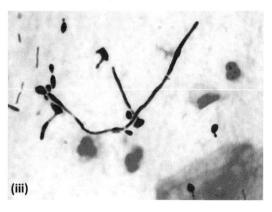

(iii)

171

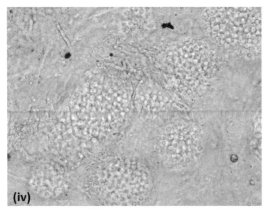

(iv)

Source: Tinea Versicolor. In: Sterry W, Paus R, Burgdorf W, Hrsg. Thieme Clinical Companions–Dermatology. 1st Edition. Thieme; 2006

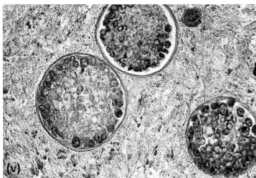

(v)

Source: CDC/Dr. Lucille K. Georg

14.   Correct: Lungs (C)

(C) This infection is due to *Cryptococcus neoformans*. Infections are transmitted via inhalation of the yeast and the primary focus of infection is the lungs. Pigeon droppings enhance growth of this pathogen in soil. The pathogen may disseminate from the lungs; the two most common dissemination sites are the central nervous system and the skin/soft tissue. **(A, B, D, E)** *Cryptococcus* is found in the soil and is then inhaled. As a result, the primary focus of infection is the respiratory tract. Hence, the bloodstream, GI tract, mouth and skin are incorrect. From the respiratory tract, the organism may disseminate to the bloodstream, GI tract, skin, or other organs.

15.   Correct: Acyclovir (C)

(C) This man most likely has concurrent genital herpes (painful genital lesions) and meningitis with herpes simplex virus-2 (HSV-2), a sexually transmitted pathogen. Herpes virus remains latent indefinitely; therefore, it is not "treatable." However, management of genital and CNS infections with HSV includes acyclovir. Meningitis usually occurs in primary infections and HSV-2 should be included in the differential diagnosis of aseptic meningitis in an otherwise healthy adult. Meningitis may be preceded by genital lesions or occur concurrently with

the lesions as in this case. **(A)** Abacavir/lamivudine is a combination agent used in the management of human immunodeficiency virus (HIV) infections. In acute HIV, meningitis with a lymphocytic predominance may be seen; however, painful genital lesions are not typical features of acute HIV. **(B)** Azithromycin is an antibacterial agent used in a number of infections, including genital infections with *Chlamydia trachomatis*. Painful genital lesions and meningitis are not typical features seen in *C. trachomatis* infections; therefore, this answer choice is unlikely. **(D)** Ceftriaxone is used in the treatment of genital infections caused by *Neisseria gonorrhoeae*. Gonorrhea often presents very similarly to *Chlamydia*. Painful genital lesions and meningitis are not characteristic of gonorrhea. Hence, this answer choice is incorrect. **(E)** Penicillin is used in the treatment of syphilis, a sexually transmitted infection caused by *Treponema pallidum*. In primary syphilis a genital lesion may be present; however, this lesion is most likely to be painless rather than painful as in this case. Meningitis may be present in primary or secondary syphilis.

16.   Correct: Neurosyphilis (B)

(B) The patient has symptoms of neurosyphilis. Neurosyphilis occurs 5 to 30 years after initial exposure and may affect any organ system including the nervous system, cardiovascular system, and skin. Manifestations of neurosyphilis may include meningitis, dementia, psychosis, general paresis, and tabes dorsalis. Because primary syphilis presents as a painless genital ulcer, patients may or may not remember the initial genital infection. The fluorescent treponemal antibody-absorbed assay (FTA-ABS) is positive in this case, which confirms this diagnosis. This test is a treponema-specific test. Nontreponema tests, such as the VDRL and RPR may be negative in late syphilis. If clinical findings are suggestive of neurosyphilis, as in this case, then it is imperative to follow up negative nontreponema tests with treponema-specific tests. **(A)** Guillain–Barré syndrome is an important cause of ascending flaccid paralysis. This disease is not directly caused by the presence of an infectious agent, but is due to an aberrant immune response to a pathogen, most notably *Campylobacter jejuni*. An antecedent infection with *C. jejuni* induces an immune response and antibodies may cross-react with gangliosides in neuronal myelin. The clinical findings in this case are not consistent with Guillain–Barré syndrome. **(C)** Rabies is a viral infection, which has a long incubation phase (3–12 months after exposure). During the neurologic phase of rabies, hydrophobia, pharyngeal spasms, hyperactivity, anxiety, and depression are common. Most often diagnosis is made postmortem by histological analysis of brain tissue. The clinical manifestations suggest that rabies is unlikely. **(D)** Toxoplasmosis is caused by the protozoan parasite *Toxoplasma gondii*. Clinical manifestations include fever, confusion, headache, and poor coordination. A large percentage of individuals have been infected at some point with this parasite but are asymptomatic. Symptomatic disease usually occurs in immunocompromised individuals and in neonates. The serology in this case indicates that the IgM is negative but the IgG is positive. IgM antibodies usually indicate an acute infection whereas IgG indicates a past infection. The positive IgG in this case most likely indicates that the patient has been exposed to *Toxoplasma* in the past. **(E)** The causative agent of West Nile encephalitis is the West Nile virus, an arbovirus that is transmitted via a mosquito bite. Clinical manifestations of encephalitis include fever, headache, and unsteady gait. More severe cases may involve muscle weakness and paralysis. The West Nile IgM and IgG antibodies are negative in this case; hence, West Nile encephalitis is most likely not the diagnosis.

17. Correct: Respiratory droplets (D)

(D) This man is most likely to have an infection with the mumps virus, which is transmitted via respiratory droplets. The hallmark feature of infection is parotitis (see image at the end of this answer). However, inflammation of the salivary glands may not always be present. Bilateral or unilateral orchitis may be present with or without the parotitis. The most common extrasalivary complication is aseptic meningitis. Mumps may be prevented with a live-attenuated virus vaccination (measles, mumps, and rubella [MMR]). This man is homeless and not up to date with vaccinations, hence he is at increased risk for mumps. **(A, B, C, E)** Contaminated food, direct inoculation into the skin, and displacement of an endogenous strain are not mechanisms of transmission of the mumps virus. Note that while none of these answer choices has been implicated as a transmission mechanisms of mumps virus, fomites (inanimate objects) have been shown to be involved in the transmission of this pathogen.

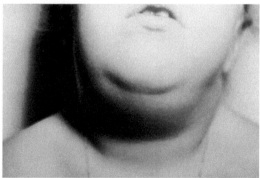

Source: CDC

18. Correct: Intracellular survival and spread (B)

(B) This infection is most likely due to *Listeria monocytogenes*, a gram-positive rod. It is an important agent of meningitis in immunocompromised individuals, such as the breast cancer patient in this case. *L. monocytogenes* can survive intracellularly within a

phagocytic cell and can then escape the phagosome and travel cell-to-cell, causing cellular destruction along its path (answer choice B). The pathogen does this by rearranging host cell actin and then creating a "tail" that allows the pathogen to propagate from one cell to another. *L. monocytogenes* is transmitted by ingestion of contaminated food and in immunocompetent individuals infections are usually limited to a mild gastrointestinal illness. However, infections may be more serious in immunocompromised individuals. **(A)** Frequent pathogens implicated in meningitis that have capsules include *Streptococcus pneumoniae, Escherichia coli* K1, *Neisseria meningitidis, Haemophilus influenzae* type b, and *Cryptococcus neoformans. Listeria monocytogenes,* however, does not have a capsule. **(C)** *L. monocytogenes* is a gram-positive bacterium; therefore, it does not have lipopolysaccharide (LPS) that is found only in gram-negative cell walls. **(D)** *N. meningitidis* and not *Listeria* have pili that facilitate in adhesion. The pili of *Neisseria* can vary the antigens on the surface which allows the organism to evade the immune system. **(E)** *Listeria* does produces a toxin called listeriolysin O (LLO), which aids the pathogen in escaping the phagosome, however, this pathogen does not produce a superantigen toxin.

19. Correct: At 4°C (B)

(B) The pathogen causing this infection is *Listeria monocytogenes*, which grows well in cold temperatures including refrigerator temperature (4°C). As a result, foods such as cold-cut deli meats and ice cream are frequently implicated in the transmission of *Listeria*. Other growth characteristics of *L. monocytogenes* include β-hemolysis on blood agar, catalase production, CAMP test positive with a rectangular hemolysis pattern (see image [i] at the end of this answer), and motility at room temperature (tumbling motility on wet preparation and cloudiness in the shape of an umbrella in semisolid media; see image [ii] at the end of this answer). **(A)** A clinically significant bacterial pathogen that grows best at 42°C is *Campylobacter jejuni*. Infections with *Campylobacter* usually result in diarrhea and CNS manifestations (Guillain–Barré syndrome) may occur as postinfectious sequelae. **(C)** The absence of O_2 indicates anaerobic growth conditions. *Listeria* is a facultative anaerobe, which means it can grow with or without oxygen but is not a strict anaerobe. There are several other bacterial pathogens that are also facultative anaerobes. However, there are very few pathogens that grow in the cold; hence B is the best answer. **(D)** Increased CO_2 represents capnophilic conditions. An example of a capnophilic pathogen is *Haemophilus* species. **(E)** There are several organisms, most notably *Enterococcus* and *Vibrio*, that may be able to survive and grow in the presence of high salt. This is not a characteristic of *L. monocytogenes*.

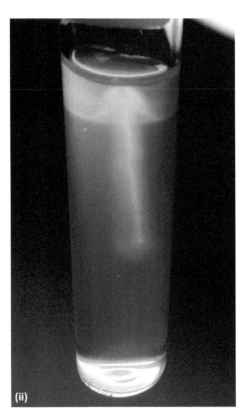

Listeria monocytogenes
CAMP positive
Block head hemolysis

CAMP Test
In the presence of *S. aureus* sphingomyelinase, CAMP factor causes an area of enhanced hemolysis

Streptococcus agalactiae
CAMP positive
Arrow head hemolysis

Negative control

(i)

CAMP = Christie-Atkins-Munch-Peterson

(ii)

20. Correct: Mosquito bite (D)

(D) This infection is most likely due to West Nile virus, a flavivirus. Infections are transmitted by the bite of an infected mosquito. Other mechanisms of transmission include vertical transmission, usually in utero. Infections occur worldwide and most often occur in the summer months, when mosquitos are abundant. Infections are most often asymptomatic but may also manifest as aseptic meningitis or more serious encephalitis, as in this case. West Nile encephalitis most often affects individuals older than 55 years of age and common manifestations include myoclonus, ascending flaccid paralysis and gait disturbances. Flaviviruses, including West Nile virus, are all single-stranded, positive-sense RNA viruses. Most of the pathogens in the flavivirus family are arthropod-borne viruses (arboviruses). **(A, C)** Birds are a reservoir for West Nile virus. To date, there is not sufficient evidence demonstrating that birds are definitely involved in the transmission of West Nile virus to humans. **(B)** Human-to-human transmission of West Nile virus has not occurred as of date. **(E)** Ticks are not involved in the transmission of West Nile virus.

21. Correct: Herpes encephalitis (C)

(C) This boy has encephalitis. Herpes simplex virus-1 (HSV-1) is the most frequent agent involved in fatal sporadic encephalitis. Most often the pathogen affects the temporal lobe, resulting in the symptoms seen in this case. **(A)** The mental status changes and CT findings indicate that this is more likely encephalitis rather than meningitis. It is worth noting that enteroviruses are also agents of encephalitis and clinical findings may be similar to those of herpes encephalitis. However, the temporal lobe abnormalities are classic findings of HSV encephalitis. Hence, this is more likely to be the diagnosis in this case. **(B)** CSF findings in this case show elevated lymphocytes, which indicate a likely viral etiology rather than a bacterial etiology. Furthermore, the boy has been vaccinated therefore *Haemophilus influenzae* is not as likely to be the etiological agent. **(D)** Subacute sclerosing panencephalitis (SSPE) is a neurological complication of measles. Infections most often occur in children who have had measles infection prior to the age of 2. SSPE occurs years following the primary infection. Infections occur in stages and progressively get worse and in many cases are fatal. The course of this patient's infection and the fact that this boy is immunized and is unlikely to have had natural disease makes this disease an unlikely diagnosis. **(E)** It is unlikely that this infection is due to West Nile virus. December in Michigan is cold and mosquitos, which are necessary for the transmission of this virus, would not be present. However, if it were summer or the boy had been in a climate with mosquitoes, arboviruses, such as West Nile virus, should be considered as possible etiologic agents of this infection.

22. Correct: Cowdry type A bodies (A)

(A) This man has encephalitis caused by varicella zoster virus. Cowdry type A inclusion bodies are characteristic of cells infected varicella zoster and herpes simplex virus. These inclusions are intranuclear and eosinophilic (see image at the end of this answer). The vesicular rash shown in the figure is along the dermatome and is characteristic of herpes zoster (shingles). The rash commonly affects the thoracic and lumbar dermatomes. Both meningitis and encephalitis are complications of shingles and are more commonly seen in immunocompromised individuals. **(B)** Guarnieri bodies are eosinophilic cytoplasmic inclusions seen in epithelial cells infected with smallpox. The rash of smallpox is vesicular and can be seen all over the body in similar stages of development. However, smallpox is eradicated due to effective worldwide vaccination efforts. Hence, smallpox virus is an unlikely agent in this case. **(C)** Negri bodies are round or oval eosinophilic inclusions found in the cytoplasm of rabies infected nerve cells. Exanthems, such as the rash seen in this patient, are not typical findings of rabies. **(D)** Torres bodies are seen in the liver during yellow fever virus infections and are intranuclear and eosinophilic inclusion bodies. Yellow fever rarely causes nervous system sequelae. **(E)** Henderson–Patterson bodies are seen in molluscum contagiosum and are eosinophilic and cytoplasmic inclusions. The lesion of molluscum contagiosum is a dome shaped papule with central umbilication that is usually skin colored. This infection is usually limited to the skin. HIV-positive individuals may have more serious infections than immunocompetent individuals. The rash in this case is characteristic of herpes zoster and not molluscum contagiosum.

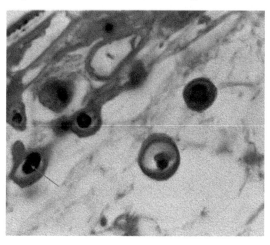

23. Correct: Bats (A)

(A) This is a case of rabies, caused by the rabies virus, an RNA virus that is transmitted via the bite of an infected animal. Common reservoirs include bats, small rodents, raccoons, skunks, dogs, and cats. The image in the question stem shows a classic finding of rabies infections, Negri bodies. Negri bodies are eosinophilic inclusion bodies that are round or oval and can be found in the cytoplasm of rabies infected nerve cells. Most often inclusion bodies are seen in the Ammon's horn of the hippocampus and the Purkinje cells of the cerebellum. The incubation phase of this but is typically 1 to 2 months but may be for several years too. Rabies begins with a prodrome phase that consists of nonspecific symptoms and then progresses to the neurological symptoms. Rabies most often manifests as encephalitic rabies with hydrophobia, increased salivation, hyperactivity, and seizures. In a smaller percentage of cases, paralytic rabies with flaccid paralysis may be seen. An important feature of rabies infection is that although the incubation phase is long, once symptoms appear the disease progresses rapidly. **(B, D)** Birds and pigs are important in the transmission of several pathogens but are not typical reservoirs of rabies. **(C, E)** Mosquitos and ticks are commonly involved in transmitting pathogens involved in nervous system infections including meningitis and encephalitis. Neither insect is involved in the transmission of rabies.

24. Correct: Bradyzoites within a tissue cyst (B)

(B) This man most likely has toxoplasmosis. In human tissue the bradyzoite form of the organism can be seen within a tissue cyst. Several clinical clues indicate this infection is most likely toxoplasmosis. Ring-enhancing lesions are characteristic findings of several conditions including toxoplasmosis. Additionally, toxoplasmosis involves posterior cervical lymphadenopathy as noted in this case. Lastly, the patient is immunocompromised with a low CD4 count and toxoplasmosis is most likely to infect immunocompromised individuals. Toxoplasmosis is caused by *Toxoplasma gondii*, a protozoan parasite. The organism is transmitted by ingestion of oocysts, which may be found in undercooked meat (most often pork or venison), ingestion of material contaminated with cat feces, blood transfusion, or transplacentally. Oocysts develop into tachyzoites (see image [i] at the end of this answer), which are most often seen in blood specimens. Tachyzoites may be passed from a pregnant woman to her fetus. The tachyzoites eventually localize to the muscle and CNS. Here they become tissue cysts with bradyzoites (see image [ii] at the end of this answer). See Appendix M for other infections that are frequently associated with HIV/AIDS. **(A)** Acid-fast bacilli, especially *Mycobacterium avium-intracellulare* complex (MAC) are important agents of infection in the immunocompromised. Infections with MAC usually manifest as lymphadenitis, pulmonary disease, or disseminated infections. Disseminated infections usually occur in AIDS when the CD4 count < 50 cells/μL and typical manifestations include fever, weight loss, night sweats, and diarrhea. There is the possibility that AFB, including MAC, *M. tuberculosis*, or other species may be involved in nervous system infections; however, the clinical findings in this case indicate that *Toxoplasma* is the more likely agent of this infection. **(C)** *Taenia solium* is the agent of neurocysticercosis. In this infection the larval form of the pathogen encysts in tissue, resulting in lesions. Infections are endemic in South and Central America, Asia, and sub-Saharan Africa. Any individual may have disseminated *T. solium* infections. It is possible that this infection could be due to *T. solium*, however, because this man is HIV-positive, there is no travel history provided, and because posterior cervical lymphadenopathy is present, *Toxoplasma* is a more likely agent. **(D)** Enlarged cells with basophilic inclusions are characteristic of cytomegalovirus (CMV) infected cells. In late-stage CMV infections, especially in AIDS with a CD4 less than 50 cells/μL, neurological manifestations, including encephalitis may occur. CNS lesions, such as described here are not typically seen in CMV encephalitis. *Toxoplasma* is a more likely agent of AIDS related encephalopathy and mass lesions. **(E)** Negri bodies are pathognomonic for infections with rabies virus and are usually seen after postmortem. None of this man's symptoms is a feature seen in rabies. Furthermore, there is no indication that HIV-positive individuals are at higher risk for rabies.

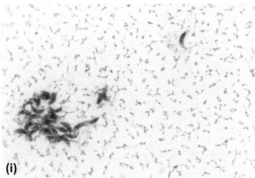

(i)

Source: CDC/Dr. L.L. Moore, Jr.

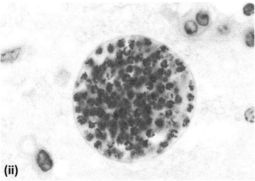

(ii)

Source: Jitender P. Dubey, USDA Agricultural Research Service

25. Correct: Administration of pyrimethamine plus sulfadiazine (D)

(D) Cerebral toxoplasmosis in HIV-positive or AIDS patients should be treated. The recommended regimen is pyrimethamine plus sulfadiazine. **(A)** Albendazole plus praziquantel is the recommend treatment for neurocysticercosis caused by the trematode *Taenia solium*. This man is more likely to have toxoplasmosis. **(B)** Clarithromycin is often used to treat *Mycobacterium avium-intracellulare* complex (MAC) infections. However, this man has toxoplasmosis and clarithromycin is not an effective agent in this case. **(C)** If this infection were due to CMV, then ganciclovir would be the agent of choice; however, this infection is due to *Toxoplasma*. **(E)** Cerebral toxoplasmosis in HIV-positive or AIDS patients should be treated; hence, this answer choice is incorrect.

26. Correct: Ingestion of food contaminated with human feces (C)

(C) This is a case of neurocysticercosis caused by *Taenia solium*, a tapeworm. Neurocysticercosis is transmitted following ingestion of food, water, or other material contaminated with the stool of an infected individual. Infections with *T. solium* can occur in two ways. This pathogen can be found in the larval form in pigs. Ingestion of undercooked pork results in gastrointestinal infections with *T. solium* (see image at the end of this answer). Infected humans release *T. solium* ova (eggs) into their stool. Ingestion of human feces containing these eggs results in the formation of larvae that embed in human tissue or cystercercosis. One of the most common locations of dissemination is the nervous system (neurocysticercosis). This organism is endemic in sub-Saharan Africa, India, and Central and South America. This pathogen should be included in the differential diagnosis of brain abscess, especially in immigrants from geographic areas in which infections are endemic. This man's travel history and CNS lesion indicate that neurocysticercosis is the most likely diagnosis. **(A)** This is a mechanism of transmission for rabies, another central nervous system infection. The symptoms of this case do not resemble rabies. **(B)** Direct inoculation via the skin is the mechanism of transmission for other worms, especially *Ancyclostoma duodenale*, *Necator americanus* (hookworms) and *Strongyloides stercoralis*. This is not a mechanism of transmission for *T. solium*. **(D)** Ingestion of undercooked beef is associated with several pathogens including another tapeworm, *Taenia saginata*. This is not a mechanism of transmission for tissue infections with *T. solium*. **(E)** Ingestion of undercooked pork is the mechanism of transmission for gastrointestinal infections with *T. solium*. This results in an individual becoming a carrier and releasing ova of *T. solium* into their stool, which if ingested can lead to cystercercosis.

Taenia Transmission

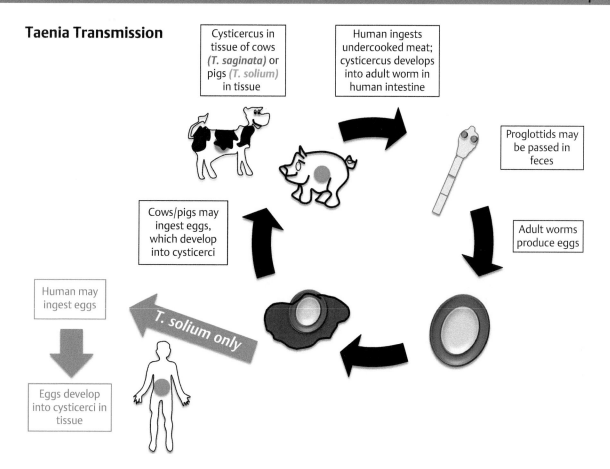

---

27. Correct: Babesiosis (A)

(A) This man's current diagnosis is most likely Lyme disease, which is caused by the spirochete *Borrelia burgdorferi*. Lyme disease is transmitted by the bite of the *Ixodes scapularis* tick, also called deer tick. This may also carry other pathogens including the protozoan parasite, *Babesia* (which causes babesiosis), *Anaplasma*, and Powassan virus. Lyme disease may be seen in many parts of the United States, but there is a higher incidence in areas of the Midwest, especially Wisconsin and the Northeast states, such as Connecticut and upstate New York. Lyme disease occurs in stages. During the first stage the classic symptoms include a target-shaped red rash, called erythema migrans and "flu-like" symptoms. During the secondary stage, the pathogen disseminates to several systems including nervous, cardiac, and musculoskeletal systems. Meningitis may be seen during this stage. The third stage of Lyme disease is characterized by chronic arthritis. Serological testing is the best mechanism of diagnosing Lyme disease. Babesiosis is a febrile illness, similar in manifestation to malaria, without the periodicity seen in malaria. Infections are best diagnosed with thick and thin blood smears to evaluate RBCs for the presence of the pathogen. **(B)** Bartonellosis is caused by the bacterial pathogen *Bartonella henselae*. This pathogen may be transmitted by a scratch from a cat or from the bite of an infected flea. Ticks are not involved in bartonellosis (also called cat scratch fever). **(C)** Chagas disease is caused by the parasite *Trypanosoma cruzi*, which is transmitted by the reduviid (also called triatomine or kissing bug), not a tick. **(D)** Leishmaniasis is caused by the parasite *Leishmania* and is transmitted by a sandfly, not a tick. **(E)** The causative agent of malaria is the parasite *Plasmodium*, which is transmitted by a mosquito bite, not a tick bite.

28. Correct: (C)

(C) Zygomycetes or *Mucorales* may result in rhino-orbital-cerebral infections (mucormycosis), as seen in this case. The image shows the broad, branching ribbon-like sparsely septate or nonseptate hyphae with wide angles that are characteristic of Zygomycetes. These infections most often affect diabetic patients in ketoacidosis, such as this patient. Zygomycetes are fungi and include several genera notably *Mucor* and *Rhizopus*. These pathogens have the unique ability to survive in the high glucose and acidic conditions seen during ketoacidosis. Fluconazole is not effective against the pathogens that cause mucormycosis, hence, liposomal amphotericin B or isavuconazole are often used in the treatment of these invasive infections. **(A)** This is an image of a budding yeast with pseudohyphae, which is characteristic of *Candida* species. *C. albicans*, the

177

most common clinical species, and usually causes mucosal infections or bloodstream infections. The invasive nature of this infection and the clinical findings seen in this case are not consistent with *Candida*. **(B)** This image shows gram-positive rods with spores which are characteristic of *Bacillus*. *B. anthracis* may cause eschar that may resemble infections of Zygomycetes. However cutaneous anthrax is usually transmitted by direct contact and may affect any individual, not just the immunocompromised. The progression of this infection and the fact this woman is in ketoacidosis make mucormycosis a more likely diagnosis. **(D)** *Aspergillus*, as seen in this image, may cause a similar infection as mucormycosis. In the case presented in the stem, the most likely diagnosis is mucormycosis, especially because the woman is a diabetic in ketoacidosis. *Aspergillus* infections are classically seen in neutropenic patients. (Note: the sporulating form of *Aspergillus* seen in this image is typically seen in culture. The tissue form of *Aspergillus* has septate hyphae with acute angle branching and is very similar microscopically to Zygomycetes.) **(E)** In the early stages of infection, rhino-orbital-cerebral infections with Zygomycetes may mimic sinusitis. One of the most common bacterial pathogens of sinusitis is *Streptococcus pneumoniae*, a gram-positive coccus in chains and pairs (i.e., diplococci), as seen in this image. It is unlikely that *S. pneumoniae* would cause such an invasive and rapidly progressive infection, as described in this case.

29. Correct: Waterskiing in the lake (E)

(E) The image in the question stem shows the trophozoite form of *Naegleria fowleri*, an amebic parasite that is found in fresh, warm water. Transmission occurs via contact with contaminated warm water sources, usually through water activities such as waterskiing (answer choice E), jumping, swimming, or diving in the water, which results in inhalation of water containing the pathogen. This pathogen is associated with primary amebic meningoencephalitis (PAM). Although any age group is at risk for infections, children contract infections at a higher rate than other age groups most likely because of their increased exposure to water activities. Following inhalation, the pathogen migrates from the olfactory mucosa to the brain via the cribriform plate of the ethmoid bone. Because of the olfactory involvement, infected individuals often complain of unusual smells or tastes, such as in this case. Infections are rapidly progressive and are most often fatal. **(A)** A mission trip to Haiti would put this girl at risk for a number of infections including cholera and other diarrheal infections and other arthropod-borne infections, such as Zika and dengue fevers. However, the image and the presentation are more consistent with *Naegleria fowleri*, which is found worldwide in fresh water sources. **(B)** Camping would most likely increase the likelihood

of arbovirus associated meningitis/encephalitis or other bacterial tick-borne infections. The image and the clinical manifestations are more consistent with *N. fowleri*. **(C)** Recently, ice cream has been associated with several incidences of *Listeria monocytogenes* outbreaks. *Listeria* is an agent of meningitis, usually in neonates, the elderly, or individuals with cell-mediated immune deficiencies. Symptoms of this case are more consistent with meningoencephalitis rather than meningitis alone. Furthermore, *Listeria* is a gram-positive rod that most likely would have been seen on Gram stain. **(D)** *Naegleria* is associated with fresh, warm water. Saltwater recreational activities may put this girl at risk for other infections, such as non-cholera *Vibrio* infections, which are agents of skin and soft-tissue infections and diarrhea.

30. Correct: Kinyoun stain (C)

(C) This infection is most likely due to *Nocardia*. *Nocardia* species will stain with the modified acid-fast stain. The stain is called modified acid-fast because the decolorizer used is a weaker acid in comparison to the traditional acid-fast stain used for *Mycobacteria*. Two acid-fast stains are the Kinyoun (answer choice C) and Ziehl–Neelsen stains. *Nocardia* typically causes pulmonary infections, which are transmitted via inhalation. But *Nocardia* may also be involved in brain abscess and skin and soft-tissue infections. Skin and soft-tissue infections are transmitted by direct contact, usually with contaminated soil. Hematogenous spread may result in disseminated infections, such as brain abscesses. Immunocompromised individuals are at increased risk for disseminated infections. Predisposing conditions for brain abscess with *Nocardia* include transplantation, HIV, and prior dental infection. Based on Gram stain it is impossible to differentiate between *Nocardia* and *Actinomyces*, which are both branching filamentous gram-positive rods. *Nocardia* is partially acid fast, but *Actinomyces* is not. Furthermore, *Nocardia* is aerobic whereas *Actinomyces* is anaerobic. *Actinomyces* also forms draining sinus tracts with "sulfur granules," which is not a characteristic of *Nocardia*. **(A)** *Nocardia* does not have spores so an endospore stain would not be valuable in the diagnosis of this infection. Clinically significant gram-positive rods with spores include *Clostridium* and *Bacillus*. **(B)** Giemsa stain would show the branching thin rods but it would not differentiate *Nocardia* from *Actinomyces*. **(D)** *Nocardia* and *Actinomyces* may be mistaken for fungi due to the branching thin rods, which resemble hyphae. A KOH preparation is a classic preparation used to visualize fungi from clinical specimens. It aids in dissolving cellular debris and keratin, allowing for better visualization of fungi. This preparation would not be beneficial in confirming the identity of *Nocardia*. **(E)** The trichrome stain is utilized for visualizing parasites. This stain would not be useful for identifying *Nocardia*.

31. Correct: Trimethoprim–sulfamethoxazole (E)

(E) The first-line agent for *Nocardia* is trimethoprim-sulfamethoxazole. Other agents that may also be used (depending on the location of infection) include carbapenems, linezolid, and minocycline. (A) Amphotericin B is an antifungal agent. Although *Nocardia* has a fungal-like morphology, amphotericin B is not effective against *Nocardia*. (B) Albendazole is used for parasites, especially helminths. This agent is not effective against *Nocardia*. (C) Clindamycin is not an agent used for infections with *Nocardia*. This agent may be effective for infections with other gram-positive rods including *Clostridium*. (D) Rifampin is used in the management of several infections including *Mycobacteria* (acid-fast bacilli). Although *Nocardia* is modified acid-fast, rifampin is not a typical agent used in treatment of *Nocardia* infections.

32. Correct: *Streptococcus anginosus* group (B)

(B) The woman has a brain abscess caused by streptococci, as indicated by the Gram stain results. Of the answer choices, the most likely agent is *Streptococcus anginosus* group, which is part of the viridans streptococci group. These organisms are commensal flora of the human oral cavity and throat, gastrointestinal tract, and vagina. They have a propensity for forming abscesses in various anatomic sites. Viridans streptococci are composed of several groups of organisms: the mitis group, the anginosus group, the mutans group, the salivarus group, and the bovis group. Within each group are several species. These organisms are mainly α-hemolytic and are involved in a variety of infections. Predisposing conditions for brain abscesses include otitis media as in this case, mastoiditis, sinusitis, dental infection, penetrating trauma or neurosurgical procedure, endocarditis, lung abscess, and immunosuppression. (A) *Streptococcus agalactiae* is also referred to as group B streptococci. This pathogen is mainly an agent of neonatal meningitis, pneumonia, and bacteremia. *S. agalactiae* is not a common agent of brain abscesses. (C) *Streptococcus bovis* group is also part of the viridans streptococci group. This group is most often involved in sepsis, endocarditis, and bacteremia. There is an association between *S. bovis* group infection and subsequent development of colon cancer. The *S. bovis* group is not commonly involved in brain abscesses. (D) *Streptococcus pneumoniae* is a common agent of bacteremia, pneumonia, otitis media, sinusitis, and meningitis. This pathogen is not a frequent agent of brain abscesses. (E) *Streptococcus pyogenes* (group A streptococci) mainly causes pharyngitis and skin and soft-tissue infections. Meningitis may occur following an ear infection; however, brain abscesses are rarely associated with *S. pyogenes*.

33. Correct: Detection of toxin from serum from infected woman (C)

(C) The infectious agent of this infection is *Clostridium botulinum*, an anaerobic gram-positive rod with spores. This is case of adult foodborne botulism and infections must be confirmed by the detection of the botulinum toxin (answer choice C). The toxin can be identified from food, serum (adults), stool (infants), gastric contents, and vomitus. The organism can be grown in culture; however, toxin detection is necessary for confirmation of *C. botulinum*. The classic presentation of adult foodborne botulism includes dry mouth, fixed and dilated pupils, and descending flaccid weakness, as seen in this case. Manifestations are due to the botulinum toxin, which inhibits acetylcholine neurotransmitter release. Adult foodborne botulism is associated with canned foods, including vegetables, fruit, and fish. This woman's occupation involves canning and there is the possibility that she consumed contaminated food, which then led to her infection. (A) *Clostridium* species, including *C. botulinum* are anaerobic gram-positive rods and can be cultured in vitro. Note that *C. botulinum* is a potential bioterrorism agent (also referred to as select agent) that must only be handled in laboratories that are equipped to work with such agents, such as the State Laboratory. A double zone of hemolysis is seen with *C. perfringens*, not *C. botulinum*, on media containing blood. (B) Serological testing for *C. botulinum* is not available. The diagnosis of botulism must include toxin detection. (D) Elek test is an immunodiffusion test for the detection of *Corynebacterium diphtheriae* toxin. This test is not used for the detection of the botulinum toxin. (E) A Gram stain from a clinical specimen is not a useful mechanism of detecting *C. botulinum* because only toxigenic strains are pathogenic. The Gram stain would not differentiate toxigenic strains from nontoxigenic strains. Infections with *C. botulinum* must be confirmed with toxin analysis.

34. Correct: Inhalation of dust (B)

(B) This baby has infant botulism or floppy baby syndrome, caused by *Clostridium botulinum*. In the past, infant infections were most often attributed to ingestion of honey. Inhalation of dust, containing *C. botulinum* spores, is now thought to be the main mechanism of transmission (answer choice B). Infections have also been linked to contaminated powdered infant formula. Classic symptoms of infection include hypotonia, poor suck, and decreased gag reflex, as described in this case. *C. botulinum* is a sporulated, anaerobic gram-positive rod that produces a neurotoxin that inhibits acetylcholine release, resulting in a flaccid descending paralysis.

(A, C, D, E) Infant infections with *C. botulinum* arise as a result of direct inhalation or ingestion of the spores. Contaminated breast milk, vertical transmission, and transmission from an adult with foodborne botulism are not means of transmission. Infections with *C. botulinum* are not communicable.

35. Correct: Human-derived botulism immune globulin (B)

(B) Administration of *the Clostridium botulinum* antitoxin is a crucial step in the management of infant or adult botulism. For infants, administration of human-derived botulism immune globulin (also referred to as BabyBIG or BIG-IV) should occur as soon as possible. **(A)** Equine serum botulism antitoxin is utilized for children older than 1 year old and adults with botulism. This antitoxin contains antibodies to several botulinum toxin types. Because this contains equine serum, there is a risk of anaphylaxis and serum sickness; therefore, this product should be avoided in cases of infant botulism, such as in this case. **(C, D, E)** There is no consensus or standard protocol for the use of antibiotics in botulism. Antibiotics may or may not be used. If antimicrobials are used, penicillin G is the preferred antimicrobial and metronidazole may be used as an alternative. However, aminoglycosides such as gentamicin should not be used in the treatment of *C. botulinum* because these agents enhance the neuromuscular blockade caused by the botulinum toxin. While there is debate on the use of antibiotics, the medical community agrees that the administration of antitoxin is necessary; hence, antibiotics (answer choices C to E) are not the best next step.

36. Correct: Inhibitory interneurons (C)

(C) This man has tetanus caused by *Clostridium tetani*. It produces a toxin that targets inhibitory interneurons and prevents these neurons from releasing GABA (γ-aminobutyric acid) and glycine inhibitory neurotransmitters. This pathogen is an anaerobic gram-positive rod with spores. Infections occur following direct contact with the spore, most often after trauma to the skin. Common symptoms include muscle rigidity/spastic paralysis with trismus (lockjaw) and risus sardonicus (see image at the end of this answer). The tetanus toxin (i.e., tetanospasmin) binds to receptors at the end of motor neurons and is transported to the CNS in a retrograde manner. The toxin is a protease that cleaves SNAREs proteins and prevents the release of GABA and glycine resulting in muscle spasms/rigidity. **(A)** *Clostridium sordellii* produces a toxin (lethal toxin) that targets may target all neurons. This pathogen causes myonecrosis, endocarditis, and other infections. It is frequently implicated in gynecological infections following childbirth, abortions, surgical procedures, infections associated with injection drug users, and infections following trauma. Based on the clinical scenario in

the question stem, this pathogen cannot be ruled out. However, the clinical manifestations of spastic paralysis, trismus, and risus sardonicus are classic findings of tetanus; hence, answer choice A is incorrect. **(B)** *Clostridium perfringens* produces an enterotoxin that targets enteric neurons. Infections result in diarrhea and not the manifestations described in this case. **(D)** The botulinum toxin, produced by *Clostridium botulinum*, predominately affects the peripheral nervous system and acts on stimulatory motor neurons at the neuromuscular junction. The botulinum toxin cleaves SNAREs and prevents the release of acetylcholine resulting in "limp" or flaccid muscles, not stiff muscles as described in this case. **(E)** *Bacillus cereus* and *Staphylococcus aureus* produce enterotoxins that target the vagus nerve, resulting in emesis following ingestion of contaminated food. The symptoms in this case are not consistent with either of these pathogens.

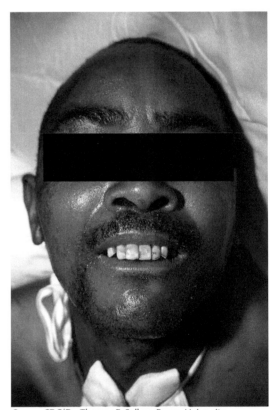

Source: CDC/Dr. Thomas F. Sellers, Emory University

37. Correct: Cross-reactive antibodies that bind to peripheral nerves (A)

(A) This man most likely has Guillain–Barré syndrome, which is a progressive ascending, symmetrical flaccid paralysis. This disease is immune-mediated and results in demyelination of neurons in the peripheral nervous system. Guillain–Barré syndrome is thought to be caused due to molecular mimicry in which the body produces antibodies to an antecedent infection with a particular pathogen. These antibodies cross-react with peripheral nerve components due to the sharing of cross-reactive epitopes. In other words, these antibodies should recognize a specific antigen, but instead these antibodies bind to a closely resembling antigens on nerve cells, which ultimately results in demyelination. **(B)** There is some evidence to support the role of immune complex (antigen-antibody) deposition in the pathogenesis and development of Guillain–Barré syndrome. However, the most widely accepted mechanism of Guillain–Barré syndrome pathogenesis is molecular mimicry; hence, answer choice B is incorrect. **(C)** Inflammation is present during Guillain–Barré syndrome, but the inflammation is not due to the production of a superantigen. **(D, E)** Guillain–Barré syndrome is due to an immune response rather than the presence of a viable pathogen that invades or produces virulence factors such as exotoxin.

38. Correct: *Campylobacter jejuni* (A)

(A) There is strong evidence demonstrating the correlation between an antecedent infection with *Campylobacter jejuni* and the development of Guillain–Barré syndrome. Other pathogens have also been linked to Guillain–Barré syndrome including cytomegalovirus (CMV), varicella zoster virus (VZV), *Mycoplasma pneumoniae*, HIV, and possibly Zika virus. *C. jejuni* is a curved gram-negative rod that is transmitted by the ingestion of contaminated food, most often unpasteurized milk or undercooked poultry. Primary infections manifest as diarrhea. **(B, C, D)** Preceding infections with *E. coli*, *Salmonella*, and *Shigella* are not associated with Guillain–Barré syndrome but are associated with reactive arthritis. **(E)** To date there is not a correlation between *Vibrio cholerae* and development of Guillain–Barré syndrome.

39. Correct: Occur due to the misfolding of normal prions proteins (E)

(E) Abnormal prions or PrPSc, arise due to the abnormal folding of the PrPc protein, which is a normal cellular protein component. The PrPc secondary structure is dominated by α-helices while the abnormal protein PrPSc secondary structure is dominated by β-pleated sheets. **(A)** Prions are not disinfected as easily as viruses or other infectious agents. They are resistant to disinfection by heat (to 80°C), formaldehyde, proteases, and ionization and UV radiation. Chemical agents used to disinfect prions include 1N sodium hydroxide (NaOH) and autoclaving in a gravity displacement autoclave at 121°C for 1 hour. **(B)** Prions do not have RNA or DNA nucleic acids. They are composed solely of proteins. **(C)** Cellular (normal) prions, PrPc levels remain the same throughout disease, but levels of abnormal PrPSc rise as prion disease progresses; therefore, this answer choice is incorrect. **(D)** Normal prions (PrPc, cellular prions) are found in the tissues of animals and humans; however, abnormal prions are not normally present in healthy individuals.

40. Correct: Western blot (E)

(E) This woman most likely has Creutzfeldt–Jakob disease (CJD), a prion disease. Diagnosis of CJD and other prion diseases includes the detection of the abnormal prion protein, which can be accomplished with Western blot or quaking-induced conversion assay. Histopathology of brain tissue of patients with prion disease typically shows amyloid plaques that arise due to the aggregation of proteins rich in β-pleated sheets, which form insoluble fibrils. These plaques cause neurons to look vacuolated. Amyloid plaques do not induce interferon and there is very little or no immune response in prion diseases. CJD usually affects individuals 50 to 70 years old and most often occurs due to the spontaneous conversion of cellular prions to the abnormal form. Other mechanisms of abnormal prion acquisition include mutations in the prion protein gene (PRNP), or transmission via injection, transplantation of contaminated tissue or contact with contaminated medical devices. **(A)** Prions are composed of only protein; therefore, the Gram stain would not be beneficial in diagnosing disease or visualizing the protein particles. **(B)** Serology is the analysis of antigens (pathogens in the patient's specimen) or antibodies (the immune response to the pathogen). Because prions are not very immunogenic, serology is not a good mechanism of detecting prion disease. **(C)** Prions do not produce toxins so this would not be a mechanism of diagnosing prion disease. **(D)** Prions are composed of only proteins and unlike viruses, these proteins are unable to grow in cell culture.

41. Correct: Biofilm formation (A)

(A) The most common pathogens associated with shunt, catheter, and line-related infections and contamination are coagulase-negative staphylococci, especially *Staphylococcus epidermidis* and the gram-positive rod, *Propionibacterium acnes* (now called *Cutibacterium acnes*). Both organisms can form a biofilm on the catheter lumen. Organisms from the biofilm can then translocate and enter the bloodstream or CNS as in this case, leading to more serious disease. Biofilms are communities of organisms that produce a three-dimensional structure on a solid surface and are encased within an extracellular matrix composed mainly of polysaccharides. Biofilms are more recalcitrant to both the host immune system and antimicrobials than planktonic organisms (non-biofilm associated). **(B)** The capsule does play a role in biofilm development; however, it is the biofilm itself that is mediating this infection. **(C)** Gram-positive bacteria, such as *Staphylococcus*, which is most likely involved in this infection, do not have endotoxin. Endotoxin is associated with the outer membrane of gram-negative organisms and is also called lipopolysaccharide (LPS). Recall that it is the lipid A portion of LPS that is toxigenic. **(D)** *S. epidermidis* and

181

other coagulase-negative staphylococci produce few exotoxins, but these toxins are not known to play a major role in the pathogenesis of these infections. Therefore, secreted toxins most likely did not play a role in this infection. **(E)** Some strains of coagulase-negative staphylococci may be invasive, but most strains are generally of low virulence and are non-invasive. In this case, the organism gained entry into the CNS via the VP shunt. The organism itself was not particularly invasive; however, the pathogen was in the "right place at the right time" and gained access to a normally sterile anatomic location.

42. Correct: Double-stranded DNA virus (A)

(A) This child is most likely to have roseola infantum (also called exanthem subitum and sixth disease). The etiological agent of this infection is most often human herpes virus-6 (HHV-6), a double-stranded DNA virus (answer choice A). Infections most often begin with an abrupt onset of high fever followed by the exanthem. Due to the high fever, seizures may occur, as seen in this case. The peak age of incidence of infection is between 6 and 12 months of age. The girl's age, the fact that she attends daycare, and her preceding upper respiratory infection make this roseola infantum the most likely diagnosis. **(B)** RNA viruses, such as arboviruses, should be included in the differential diagnosis of fever and a rash. There is nothing in this child's history to indicate exposure to an arthropod vector and the symptoms of the sudden onset of high fever and seizure indicate that the most likely diagnosis is roseola infantum. **(C)** *Streptococcus pneumoniae* is the most common gram-positive coccus in pairs and is a frequent agent of meningitis in all age groups but especially older children and adults. This child most likely does not have meningitis, as the CSF findings are normal. Classic CSF findings of bacterial meningitis include elevated cell count with a neutrophilic predominance, elevated protein, and decreased glucose. **(D)** A gram-positive rod that is frequently involved in CNS infections and should be on the differential is *Listeria monocytogenes*. However, infections in children most often occur in neonates. This child's age and clinical presentation are more consistent with roseola infantum. **(E)** A protozoan parasite that is involved in CNS infections is *Naegleria fowleri*. This organism causes primary amebic meningoencephalitis (PAM). The epidemiology and clinical findings of this case indicate that *Naegleria* is unlikely to be the agent of this infection.

43. Correct: *Clostridium botulinum* (D)

(D) This woman is most likely to have wound botulism cause by *Clostridium botulinum*, an anaerobic gram-positive rod with spores. Infections are frequently associated with intravenous drug abuse. Symptoms are similar to foodborne botulism and include fixed, dilated pupils, dry mouth, and descending flaccid paralysis. The clinical findings in this case are consistent with wound botulism. In wound botulism, the bacteria infect the skin, most often following trauma to the skin; the organism then produces the toxin in vivo. This is in contrast to adult foodborne botulism where infections arise following ingestion of the preformed toxin in the food. In both cases, the toxin blocks acetylcholine release at the neuromuscular junction, resulting in weakness, dry mouth, and flaccid paralysis. **(A)** *Bacillus anthracis* is an aerobic gram-positive rod with spores that may cause wound infections and eschar formation. Weakness of the arms and dry mouth are more likely to indicate *C. botulinum* rather than *B. anthracis*. Furthermore, in anthrax, an eschar is most often present, which is not seen in this case. A key difference between *Bacillus* and *Clostridium* is that *Bacillus* is aerobic while *Clostridium* is anaerobic. **(B)** *Bacillus cereus* is a gram-positive rod with spores and most often is an agent of foodborne gastroenteritis. It is also a rare agent of eye infections and wound infections following traumatic inoculation. The manifestations of this case indicate that *C. botulinum* rather than *B. cereus* is the more likely agent. **(C)** *Clostridium perfringens* is a large gram-positive rod with spores that causes wound infections which can lead to myonecrosis. The dizziness, dry mouth, and weakness in this woman's arms suggest that *C. botulinum* is a more likely causative agent of infection. **(E)** *Clostridium tetani* is a large gram-positive rod with spores and is associated with rigid or spastic paralysis. There is no indication that this woman is experiencing trismus or risus sardonicus which are classic findings of tetanus. Instead, the weakness with dry mouth is indicative of infection with *C. botulinum*.

44. Correct: African trypanosomiasis (A)

(A) The image shows a trypomastigote of *Trypanosoma*. Since this man is from Tanzania, this is most likely to be *Trypanosoma brucei gambiense* and *T. b. rhodesiense*, the agents of African sleeping sickness. *T. b. rhodesiense* is mainly seen in East Africa and *T. b. gambiense* is mainly seen in West Africa. Both of these pathogens are transmitted by the painful bite of a tsetse fly. The early stage of African sleeping sickness is marked by nonspecific constitutional symptoms, development of a chancre at the bite site, and lymphadenopathy. During the late stage, the pathogen affects the nervous system resulting in drowsiness, behavioral changes, difficulty walking, slurred speech, and eventually coma. **(B)** The agent that causes Chagas disease, *Trypanosoma cruzi*, looks virtually identical microscopically to *T. b. gambiense* and *T. b. rhodesiense*. However, Chagas disease is mainly seen South and Central America. Furthermore, infections are characterized by constitutional symptoms, unilateral swelling of the eyelid (Romaña's sign), and secondary sequelae such as cardiomyopathy, dysphagia, megaesophagus, and megacolon. The clinical findings and geography indicate that African sleeping sickness and not Chagas disease is most likely the diagnosis. **(C)** This infection is not due to drug-resistant malaria. Malaria usually manifests as paroxysms of fever and chills and this man has a consistent fever over several weeks. Furthermore, the image in the question stem shows a trypomastigote and not a malarial form, such as a ring form (see image [i] at the end of this answer) or gametocyte (see image [ii] at the end of this answer). Note that one species of *Plasmodium*, *P. falciparium* may cause cerebral malaria. Findings seen in cerebral malaria may be similar to those seen in this case and include delirium, seizures, and coma. **(D)** Schistosomiasis is incorrect since the image shows a trypomastigote of *Trypanosoma*. Some *Schistosoma* species are commonly seen in African countries including *S. haematobium* and *S. mansoni*. *S. haematobium* usually infects the genitourinary tract and both *S. haematobium* and *S. mansoni* may cause swimmers itch and Katayama fever. **(E)** Yellow fever is incorrect because the image points to *Trypanosoma* as the causative agent. Viruses cannot be visualized with light microscopy. Yellow fever may be seen in Africa and manifestations include a febrile illness with conjunctival injection that may progress to hepatitis or hemorrhagic fever. The symptoms in this case are not consistent with yellow fever.

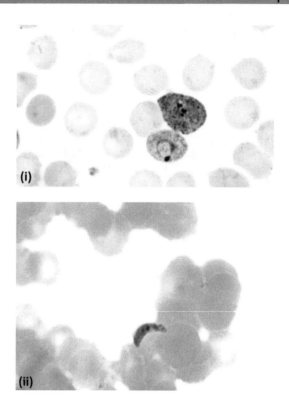

(i)

(ii)

Chapter 9

Head, Neck, and Respiratory Infections

Matthew P. Jackson, Alexander S. Maris, Melphine M. Harriott, and Thomas C. Bolig

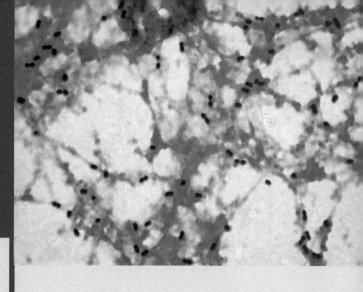

LEARNING OBJECTIVES

▶ Discuss the etiology, epidemiology, pathogenesis, clinical manifestations, complications, diagnosis, and treatment and prevention of:
  - eye infections.
  - ear infections.
  - head and neck infections.
  - upper and lower respiratory tract infections.
  - genital tract infections.
  - congenital and neonatal infections.
  - bloodstream and lymphatic system infections.

▶ Describe the laboratory diagnosis and antimicrobial testing methods for bacteria, viruses, fungi, yeast, and parasites.

▶ Discuss virulence mechanisms and correlate virulence mechanisms with specific pathogens.

▶ Discuss antimicrobial mechanism of action, spectrum of activity, common adverse effects, and resistance mechanisms.

▶ Describe the common HIV/AIDS-related opportunistic infections.

▶ Compare and contrast the structure and function of bacterial, viral, fungal, yeast, and parasitic cells.

9.1 Questions

Easy	Medium	Hard

1. A 17-month-old child who recently recovered from an upper respiratory tract infection becomes irritable, has a slight fever (37.8°C, 100.4°F), and frequently pulls at his left ear. Suspecting an infectious etiology, the pediatrician prescribes a 7-day course of amoxicillin. Four days later, the child's mother reports no improvement in symptoms and is very troubled because the boy seems to be less responsive to sound coming from his left side. The pediatrician made which of the following medical errors. Failure to:

A. Differentiate acute otitis media from otitis media with effusion

B. Perform a myringotomy on the initial visit

C. Perform a proper review of the child's immunization history

D. Prescribe the appropriate antibiotic

E. Refer the child to a hearing specialist

2. A 12-year-old boy wakes up at 2:00 a.m. with shooting pains in his right ear. The boy had returned from a 2-week summer camp near a local lake the previous weekend with daily swimming as one of the activities. He wakes his mother who notices that his ear canal is red and slightly swollen. A small amount of pus is visible on a cotton swab that she inserts into the boy's ear. His mother drives the boy to an urgent care clinic that morning where the attending physician observes gram-negative rods in the pus and prescribes antibiotic drops along with an ear canal wick. What is the most likely etiology for the boy's infection?

A. *Candida albicans*

B. Influenza H3N2

C. *Pseudomonas aeruginosa*

D. *Staphylococcus aureus*

E. *Streptococcus pneumoniae*

3. Eight days postpartum a newborn infant presents with bilateral redness of the eyes, swelling of the eyelids, and pus from his conjunctiva. Giemsa staining of the conjunctival scrapings reveal intracytoplasmic inclusion bodies in epithelial cells and direct immunofluorescent staining confirms the diagnosis. What is the most likely source of the infant's eye infection?

A. Contaminated eye drops

B. Hands of a health care worker

C. Mother's vagina

D. Predisposing respiratory tract infection

E. Transplacental passage

4. A previously healthy 14-year-old boy undergoing overnight orthokeratology wakes his father at 4:30 a.m. complaining of eye pain and adhesive secretions that prevent him from opening his right eyelid. His father rinses the boy's eyes and helps him remove the contact lenses; he notices that the lens storage case contains cloudy fluid on both sides. The boy's right cornea is severely vascularized and his conjunctiva is reddened and contains pus. His left eye appears normal and he is otherwise healthy. The ophthalmologist schedules an appointment to see his patient that morning and administers antibiotic drops to both eyes. Which of the following virulence factors could have contributed to corneal perforation if this infection was left untreated?

A. *Haemophilus influenzae* polyribitol phosphate capsule

B. *Pseudomonas aeruginosa* protease

C. *Staphylococcus aureus* exfoliative toxin

D. *Streptococcus pneumoniae* pneumolysin

E. *Streptococcus pyogenes* pyrogenic exotoxin

5. A 23-year-old woman reports to the urgent care clinic with pain and redness in her left eye. The attending physician asks the patient to remove her contact lenses for an ophthalmic examination. She notices reddening of the cornea and excessive tear formation. History reveals that the woman had been swimming in a pond the day before and felt as though there was a dirt particle under her contact lens all night. Assuming corneal trauma and a bacterial infection, the attending physician prescribes ciprofloxacin eye drops. Twenty-four hours later the woman is transported by her boyfriend to the emergency department with severe pain in her left eye. The emergency room physician notes corneal perforation and an ophthalmologist is consulted. Ultimately, the patient undergoes a corneal transplant. What is a possible postoperative complication for this patient?

A. Antibiotic resistant *Pseudomonas aeruginosa*

B. Chorioretinitis

C. Meningitis

D. Recurrence of *Acanthamoeba* infection

E. Transplant rejection

6. A 7-year-old boy is sent home with a note from the school nurse. The nurse is concerned because the boy's vision test revealed a sharp reduction in acuity compared to the test that she performed when he was in first grade. The boy's parents take him to the family physician who observes a granuloma in the peripheral fundus during an ophthalmic exam. Suspecting an infectious etiology, the physician takes a history which includes a summer vacation trip to Disney World and the adoption of a new puppy. What is the most likely etiology of this boy's condition?

A. Air contaminated with the spores of *Histoplasma capsulatum*

B. Soil contaminated with the cysts of *Acanthamoeba spp.*

C. Soil contaminated with the eggs of *Toxocara canis*

D. Water contaminated with the cysts of *Toxoplasma gondii*

E. Water contaminated with the eggs of *Schistosoma mansoni*

7. A 31-year-old HIV patient presents to his physician with white patches on his tongue that extend into his throat. He first noticed difficulty swallowing food the previous week. What is the most likely etiology for this manifestation?

A. *Aspergillus fumigatus*

B. *Candida albicans*

C. *Mucor* species

D. *Staphylococcus aureus*

E. *Streptococcus mutans*

8. A 10-year-old boy comes home from school feeling tired and complaining of a sore throat. His mother notices that his face is flushed and takes his temperature. The family pediatrician sees the boy that evening and finds that he has a fever (38.8°C, 101.9°F) and an exudate on his tonsils. She bases her diagnosis on the results of a rapid antigen test performed in the office. A throat swab is sent to the lab for a confirmatory diagnosis and antimicrobial susceptibility testing. The pediatrician will prescribe antibiotics to prevent sequelae caused by which of the following virulence factors?

A. M protein

B. Protein A

C. Pyrogenic exotoxin A

D. Streptolysin O

E. Teichoic acid

9. Fourteen students attending college in Virginia report to the campus' health clinic with similar symptoms over a 2-week period. Campus health care providers observe that all the students are experiencing a chronic cough (≥ 3-day duration), a persistent headache, and an elevated temperature (average 38°C, 100.4°F). A history reveals that the campus outbreak is limited to residents of a single dormitory. A resident director of that same dormitory had been hospitalized the previous month with Stevens–Johnson syndrome. Nasopharyngeal and oropharyngeal swabs are sent to the Centers for Disease Control and Prevention (CDC) for quantitative polymerase chain reaction. A key feature of the pathogen causing this outbreak is that it:

A. Contains mycolic acid

B. Exists as a budding yeast cell in tissue

C. Is covered with hemagglutinin

D. Is encapsulated

E. Lacks a cell wall

10. An 86-year-old man who is recovering from influenza develops a fever, shortness of breath, and chest pain. He is hospitalized with a productive cough. Sputum and blood samples show gram-positive diplococci and chest X-ray shows consolidation of the right lower lung. Which of the following is a potential complication of his infection?

A. Cystitis

B. Meningitis

C. Mucormycosis

D. Osteomyelitis

E. Rheumatic fever

11. In July 2015, New York City experienced an increased incidence of pneumonia cases reported by clinics and hospitals in the Bronx area. Patient intake histories were reviewed to ascertain common patterns of work, residence, travel, or recent hospitalization. A total of 128 people were infected with 12 deaths attributed to the outbreak. Epidemiologists traced the source to a hotel cooling tower that was dispersing pathogen-containing aerosols into the environment. Which of the following would be used to confirm the diagnosis in the exposed patients?

A. A tuberculin skin test

B. Bacterial culture from a lung biopsy

C. Giemsa stain of a thick blood smear

D. Gram stain of sputum

E. Isolation of yeast cells from lymph node biopsy

12. A 6-month-old infant is diagnosed with cystic fibrosis through genetic testing. He experiences postnatal difficulty passing meconium (meconium ileus) as well as breathing impairment within the first weeks of life. Which of the following is the most likely sequence of lung infections that this infant will suffer from throughout adolescence?

A. *Haemophilus influenzae* followed by influenza virus

B. *Coccidioides immitis* followed by *Streptococcus pneumoniae*

C. *Streptococcus pyogenes* followed by *Paragonimus westermani*

D. *Staphylococcus aureus* followed by *Pseudomonas aeruginosa*

E. *Aspergillus fumigatus* followed by *Mycobacterium tuberculosis*

13. An otherwise healthy 42-year-old woman who recently recovered from a cold sees her primary care physician because she had been experiencing a fever (39.5°C, 103.1°F), a purulent nasal discharge, and facial pain for the past 3 days. She is diagnosed with bacterial sinusitis and is prescribed a 7-day course of amoxicillin which resolves the symptoms. What is the most likely etiology of this woman's sinus infection?

A. *Actinomyces israelii*

B. *Moraxella catarrhalis*

C. *Mucor* species

D. Rhinovirus

E. *Streptococcus pneumoniae*

14. A recent immigrant from Cambodia reported to the emergency department of a New York hospital complaining of weight loss and night sweats. Her cough is productive and slightly tinged with blood. The attending physician orders a tuberculin skin test and an interferon-gamma release blood test which both show positive results. Which of the following antimicrobial agents will be one component of the treatment regimen for this patient?

A. Acyclovir

B. Fluconazole

C. Gentamicin

D. Isoniazid

E. Piperacillin

15. A 45-year-old man is hospitalized, following a motor vehicle accident. His condition requires extended mechanical ventilation. Fifteen days post-admission, he develops a fever up to 39.5°C (103.1°F) and his blood oxygen level is 86% indicating hypoxia. A chest radiograph shows atelectasis (collapsed lung). A Gram stain from a bronchoalveolar lavage (BAL) is shown below.

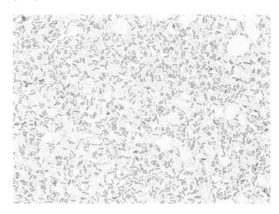

Empiric antimicrobial therapy should be initiated against which of the following?

A. *Candida albicans*

B. Methicillin-resistant *Staphylococcus aureus* (MRSA)

C. *Streptococcus pneumoniae*

D. *Pneumocystis jirovecii*

E. *Pseudomonas aeruginosa*

16. In September 2001, 22 people were infected with *Bacillus anthracis*, 11 developing the life-threatening inhalational form of the infection. Five infected individuals died of inhalational anthrax due to massive pulmonary infection and edema. The virulence factor responsible for pulmonary edema in this case can be described as edema factor plus:

A. Hyaluronic acid capsule

B. Lecithinase

C. Lipopolysaccharide

D. Metalloprotease

E. Plasminogen activator

17. A 22-year-old solider is in the hospital following a war injury. He is a veteran of the war in Iraq and his convoy was attacked with an improvised explosive device (IED). He sustained numerous injuries, including a penetrating trauma to his leg and was hospitalized for over a month. While in the hospital he develops a productive cough, chills, fever, and shortness of breath. Chest X-ray shows consolidation of left upper lobe. The sputum is sent to the lab for a Gram stain and culture. The Gram stain shows a short gram-negative rod. It was subsequently identified and antimicrobial susceptibility demonstrates resistance to several antibiotics. Which of the following is the most likely causative agent?

A. *Acinetobacter baumannii*

B. *Coccidioides immitis*

C. *Enterococcus faecium*

D. *Klebsiella pneumoniae*

E. Methicillin-resistant *Staphylococcus aureus* (MRSA)

18. Which of the following diseases has recently emerged in adult carriers who can serve as a source of infection of nonimmunized children?

A. Diphtheria

B. Influenza

C. Measles

D. Polio

E. Whooping cough

19. A 62-year-old man with periodontal disease and history of a recent tooth extraction presented to the emergency department of a local hospital with a facial abscess. Stain of pus from the abscess revealed gram-positive rods resembling fungal mycelia. Some clusters of rods appeared to have embedded yellow-colored granules. What is the most likely causative agent of this infection?

A. *Actinomyces israelii*

B. *Aspergillus fumigatus*

C. *Bacillus cereus*

D. *Clostridium perfringens*

E. *Histoplasma capsulatum*

20. A 4-year-old girl presents to the emergency department with difficulty swallowing and difficulty breathing, and fever. Her mother states that the symptoms had just begun earlier that day. At the time of examination, the girl's temperature is 40.1°C (104.2°F). On examination, the girl appears visibly ill and respiratory distress and stridor is observed. Additionally, while seated, she is leaning forward with her mouth open and drooling. Imaging findings are shown below.

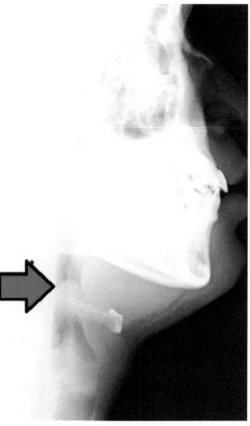

Source: Wikimedia/Med Chaos

Which of the following virulence factors is produced by the likely causative agent of this infection?

A. Hemagglutinin-neuraminidase

B. Pili that can vary antigens

C. Polyribitol phosphate capsule

D. Toxin that inhibits protein synthesis

E. Toxin that interacts with G_i protein

21. A 3-year-old boy presents to clinic with his mother with a 2-day history of increasing fussiness and "tugging on his ears." On examination, his eyes and oral cavity are unremarkable. On otoscopic exam, a bulging left tympanic membrane that is erythematous and has an air-fluid level behind it is observed; air insufflation fails to produce any movement. A minute perforation is noted from which a small amount of pus is oozing, which is collected for culture. The right tympanic membrane is unremarkable and moves appropriately on air insufflation. The remainder of the physical exam is unremarkable. The child's vaccination history is uncertain. The drainage from the boy's ear shows gram-positive cocci and a blood agar plate grows colonies that have a concave morphology and a green discoloration pattern of hemolysis. Which of the following is the most likely etiological agent of this infection?

A. *Haemophilus influenzae*

B. *Moraxella catarrhalis*

C. *Staphylococcus aureus*

D. *Streptococcus pneumoniae*

E. *Streptococcus pyogenes*

22. A 5-year-old girl who recently emigrated from Eastern Europe is brought to the clinic complaining of throat pain. Symptoms started approximately 5 days ago and include low-grade fever, malaise, and sore throat without cough. The child denies any rhinorrhea, headache, or skin rash. Her mother states that the girl developed a "strange grating sound whenever she breathes in." On examination, vitals include a temperature of 38.1°C (100.5°F), heart rate of 114 beats per minute, respiratory rate of 22 beats per minute, O$_2$ saturation of 89% on room air and a normal blood pressure for her age. Prominent cervical lymphadenopathy is noted. On opening her mouth, a grayish-white, fibrinous, friable, coalescing membrane is visualized in an erythematous posterior oropharynx. Scraping this membrane with a tongue depressor causes minor bleeding and a diminished gag response. On auscultation, breath sounds are symmetrically reduced bilaterally and normal S1 and S2 heart sounds are heard. Electrocardiogram shows sinus tachycardia without other abnormalities.

What complication of this patient's infection is most likely to contribute to her demise in the next 24 hours?

A. Cardiac dysfunction

B. Endophthalmitis

C. Neurological dysfunction

D. Skin ulcers

E. Suffocation

23. A 68-year-old nursing home resident presents to the on-site nurse with a 3-day history of low-grade fever and muscle aches. She reports that her symptoms started suddenly 2 days after her son came to visit her for Christmas, remarking that "he had to leave early because his body was hurting and he felt really tired and sweaty." She reports feeling warm though she has not taken her temperature. She has had a headache, fatigue, loss of appetite, episodic sweats, and myalgias since her symptoms started. She has not had any recent travels. On examination, her temperature is 38.8°C (101.7°F); vital signs are otherwise normal. Her sinuses are tender to palpation, clear nasal discharge is noted from the anterior nares, and the pharynx is hyperemic without exudates. Mild tender cervical lymphadenopathy is noted. The remainder of her physical exam is unremarkable, though she does report some mild chest discomfort and shortness of breath at the end of the pulmonary exam. The organism most likely causing this patient's symptoms has which of the following characteristics?

A. Circular DNA genome

B. Circular partially double-stranded DNA genome

C. Double-stranded RNA genome

D. Segmented DNA genome

E. Single-stranded segmented RNA genome

24. A 12-month-old girl is brought to the emergency department by her parents with 1 day of worsening cough and difficulty breathing. The parents report that she had been otherwise healthy until 3 days ago when she developed a low-grade fever, nasal discharge, and "stuffy" nasal breathing. They have been treating her symptomatically with acetaminophen and nasal bulb irrigation. Over the last 24 hours, the child has developed a raspy cough, labored breathing, and wheezing. On examination, a well-developed infant in moderate respiratory distress is observed. There is a mild amount of clear nasal discharge with flaring of the nares. Intercostal and subcostal retractions are prominent. The eyes are slightly sunken and the anterior fontanelle is open but slightly depressed. On auscultation, diffuse end-expiratory wheezes and a mild tachycardia is noted. The physical exam is otherwise unremarkable. Which of the following viruses is the most likely etiologic agent affecting this patient?

A. Human parainfluenza virus (HPIV)

B. Measles virus

C. Mumps virus

D. Respiratory syncytial virus (RSV)

E. Severe acute respiratory syndrome (SARS) virus

25. A 25-year-old man, a fourth year medical student, is recovering from an upper respiratory tract infection. He has had about ten days of nasal congestion, clear rhinorrhea, mild headache, sinus pressure, fatigue, malaise, mild myalgias, low-grade fever, sore throat, and a raspy cough. He has been managing with increased warm fluids, increased sleep, rigorous hand-washing, acetaminophen, and an occasional ibuprofen. He did not seek medical care because he was starting to feel better. Within a week, he is nearly back to his baseline state of health. Which of the following viruses belongs to the same viral family as the most likely etiologic agent responsible for this patient's symptoms?

A. Hepatitis C virus (HCV)

B. Hepatitis E virus (HEV)

C. Human papillomavirus (HPV)

D. Poliovirus

E. Respiratory syncytial virus (RSV)

26. A 9-year-old immigrant Caucasian boy presents to clinic with his adoptive parents to establish care. His parents report an unfortunate life-long history of poor growth and recurrent lung and sinus infections. Genetic studies are ordered and pending. He is started empirically on a vigorous nutritional regimen that includes vitamin supplementation and pancreatic enzyme replacement therapy. His parents are counseled on the fact that he may require a lung transplant soon. Which of the following organisms is most likely to cause severe lung infections in this patient population?

A. *Burkholderia cepacia*

B. *Candida albicans*

C. *Klebsiella pneumoniae*

D. *Legionella pneumophilia*

E. *Streptococcus pneumoniae*

27. A 4-year-old boy is brought by his parents to the walk-in clinic on the 4th of July with a 1-week history of low-grade fever and painful blisters. The boy attends daycare and about 1 week ago, the patient's mother noticed that he was feeling warm and was eating less than usual. The previous evening, the boy developed mildly painful blistering lesions on the palms of his hands and the soles of his feet. When questioned, the boy confirms that he's been scratching a little bit at a few of these lesions and that his throat hurts. On examination, vitals are unremarkable, including a temperature of 37.8°C (100.0°F). Vesicular lesions on erythematous bases are observed on the buccal and tongue mucosa, the palms of the hands and the soles, and dorsa of the feet. The most likely causative agent of this infection is also frequently implicated in:

A. Aortitis

B. Aseptic meningitis

C. Cirrhosis

D. Pelvic inflammatory disease (PID)

E. Shingles

28. A 22-year-old woman college student is preparing for final exams. During this time, she develops a blistering vesicular lesion on the border of her right upper lip. The genomic composition of the most likely causative agent of this infection is most similar to that of:

A. Hepatitis A virus (HAV)

B. Influenza virus

C. Measles virus

D. Parvovirus

E. West Nile virus

29. An 8-year-old boy returns from summer camp complaining of a sore throat and a red, itchy eye. His mother takes him to the pediatrician's office. The boy's mother states that the boy had been swimming frequently during camp and that several of the other boys that also attended camp were experiencing similar symptoms. The boy does not wear glasses or contact lenses and he has not travelled outside the camp he attended. His temperature at the time of exam is 38.4°C (101.1°F). Physical exam demonstrates that the boy's right eye is red with serious discharge. He denies any eye pain or photophobia. Preauricular adenopathy is also noted. Additionally, his pharynx and tonsils are red. Which of the following is the most likely causative agent of this infection?

A. Adenovirus

B. *Chlamydia trachomatis*

C. Fusarium

D. *Loa loa*

E. *Staphylococcus aureus*

30. A 2-day-old baby girl in the newborn nursery is evaluated for severe bilateral eye exudates. She has a thick, bilateral, yellow–green purulent discharge from the eyes with surrounding erythema so much so that the examiner has difficulty separating her eyelids. Visualization of the bilateral conjunctivae shows marked inflammation and hyperemia of the conjunctival blood vessels. Her vaginal birth history was unremarkable but the 19-year-old mother reports that this was an unplanned pregnancy and thus she had no prenatal care except for a third trimester ultrasound at a local emergency department. Which of the following is the most likely causative agent of this infection?

A. *Candida albicans*

B. *Chlamydia trachomatis*

C. *Neisseria gonorrhoeae*

D. *Streptococcus agalactiae*

E. *Trichomonas vaginalis*

31. A 30-year-old woman presents to the eye clinic with unilateral eye pain, decreased vision, and a serious, watery discharge from the infected eye. Her medical history is unremarkable. On examination, conjunctival injection is noted in the left eye, most prominent around the corneal limbus. Slit-lamp examination reveals punctate and diffusely branching ulcers on the corneal epithelium without penetration into the corneal stroma. Fluorescein staining of the infected eye shows a 4 mm branched, dendritic corneal lesion. The pathogen most likely responsible for this patient's acute, unilateral, ocular symptoms most likely underwent reactivation by emerging from what cell type?

A. α-Lower motor neurons

B. Peripheral blood mononuclear cells (lymphocytes)

C. Pseudounipolar primary somatosensory neurons

D. Segmented neutrophils

E. Vascular endothelial cells

32. A 36-year-old HIV-positive man presents to the walk-in clinic complaining of issues with his vision. He comments that his right eye has been "acting funny" and continues to explain that over the last couple of days he has started seeing little flashes of light and blind spots in his eye's visual field. He reports that his vision has progressively been getting blurry. He denies ocular pain, decreased extraocular movements, or symptoms in his left eye. The man is not currently taking his HIV medications and does not recall his last CD4 count. Which of the following is the most likely agent of this infection?

A. *Candida albicans*

B. Cytomegalovirus (CMV)

C. Epstein–Barr virus (EBV)

D. Human herpes virus-8 (HHV-8)

E. *Pseudomonas aeruginosa*

33. A 37-year-old woman recently returned home to Seattle after hiking in the Mojave Desert (near the Nevada/California border). Over the past several days, she has developed a fever (38.5°C, 101.3°F), cough, joint pains, and small bumps on her shins. Her physician conducts a physical exam. Her HEENT (Head, Ears, Eyes, Nose, and Throat) and cardiovascular exams are normal. Faint, end-expiratory rales are appreciated in the right lower lung field. The patient has no lymphadenopathy or hepatosplenomegaly. Abdomen is nontender. There are small, erythematous nodules near the anterior crest of the tibia bilaterally that are painful to palpation. Chest X-ray is negative. Low dose chest computed tomography (CT) scan shows right interlobular septal thickening and a small right pleural effusion. Cultures on Sabouraud dextrose agar grow hyphae with arthrospores at 25°C. How will the most likely causative agent appear on examination of the pleural fluid?

A. Encapsulated yeast

B. Septate, branching hyphae

C. Small yeast cells inside macrophages

D. Spherule containing numerous endospores

E. Yeast with broad-based budding

34. A 51-year-old Yemeni American develops fevers, rigors, nonproductive cough, and dyspnea 3 days after returning from Yemen to visit his relatives. His vital signs are: temperature, 38.2°C (101.8°F); blood pressure, 131/92 mm Hg; heart rate, 98 beats per minute; and O$_2$ saturation, 94%. The patient is suspected of having Middle East respiratory syndrome (MERS) and is admitted to the hospital. PCR is pending. Which of the following describes the causative agent of MERS?

A. Enveloped, double-stranded DNA virus

B. Enveloped, double-stranded RNA virus

C. Enveloped, single-stranded DNA virus

D. Enveloped, single-stranded RNA virus

E. Nonenveloped, double-stranded DNA virus

F. Nonenveloped, single-stranded DNA virus

G. Nonenveloped, double-stranded RNA virus

H. Nonenveloped, single-stranded RNA virus

35. A 39-year-old HIV-positive man is admitted to the hospital for declining respiratory status. According to his partner, the patient began to feel short of breath with exertion about a week ago. He subsequently developed fever, fatigue, and a nonproductive cough. This morning, he was severely dyspneic and was brought to the hospital. The patient appears in distress and is using his accessory muscles of respiration. His vital signs are: temperature, 38.9°C (102°F); blood pressure, 117/82 mm Hg; heart rate, 121 beats per minute; respiratory rate, 20 breaths per minute; and O_2 saturation, 88%. He has rales and rhonchi throughout all lung fields, bilaterally. Cardiovascular exam is unremarkable besides the tachycardia. Abdomen is nontender, nondistended, and bowel sounds present. There is no hepatosplenomegaly. No skin lesions are present, and musculoskeletal exam is within normal limits. Pertinent laboratory results are shown below:

- CBC:
  - Hemoglobin: 15 g/dL
  - WBC: 6,000 cells/mm³
  - Platelets: 217,000/mm³
- CD4 cell count: 110 cells/μL
- Microbiology:
  - (1-3)-β-D-glucan: 93 pg/mL (normal = < 31 pg/mL)
  - Interferon-gamma release assay: negative
  - Blood culture: pending
- Sputum culture: pending
  - Gram stain from sputum: mixed gram-positive and gram-negative flora
  - Acid-fast stain from sputum: no acid-fast organisms seen
- Chest X-ray:

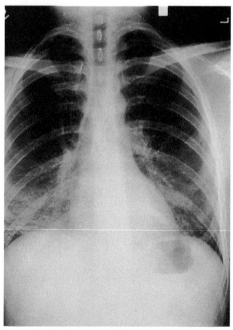

Source: CDC/Jonathan W.M. Gold, MD

High-resolution computed tomography (HRCT) scan confirms the findings visualized on chest X-ray and there is no evidence of cavitary lesions or bronchiectasis. Pulmonology is consulted for a diagnostic bronchoalveolar lavage (BAL). What is the mechanism of action of the preferred antimicrobial regimen(s) for this patient?

A. 50S ribosomal subunit inhibitor plus arabinosyltransferase inhibitor

B. Ergosterol binder

C. Ergosterol synthesis inhibitor

D. Inhibition of folic acid synthesis

E. RNA polymerase inhibitor plus mycolic acid synthesis inhibitor plus intracellular pH lowering agent plus arabinosyltransferase inhibitor

36. A 12-year-old pediatric inpatient develops a headache, sore throat, nonproductive cough, runny nasal discharge, and sneezing over a period of 5 days. Her lungs are clear to auscultation bilaterally with no wheezes, rales, or rhonchi. The rest of her medical exam remains unchanged. The medical team in charge of her care orders a molecular respiratory panel, which returns positive for rhinovirus. Why does rhinovirus rarely cause lower respiratory tract infections?

A. Does not replicate well at 37°C

B. It is acid labile

C. It is an enveloped virus

D. Lacks tropism for the lung

37. A 2-year-old boy is brought to a children's hospital to be evaluated for a cough. He has been hoarse for the last three days. The patient's mother describes the cough as "barking." An inspiratory stridor is noted at rest. The patient's lungs fields are negative for wheezes, rales, and rhonchi. The patient is up to date with his vaccinations. An X-ray shows the following:

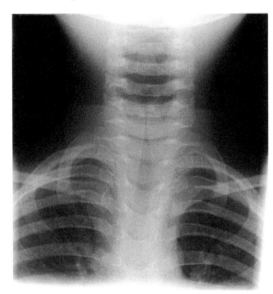

Source: Airway Disorders. In: Dyleski R, Linstrom C, Pitman M et al., Hrsg. Total Otolaryngology. Head and Neck Surgery. 1st Edition. Thieme; 2014.

Which of the following pathogens is most likely responsible?

A. Gram-negative coccobacillus

B. Gram-positive diplococci

C. Gram-positive rod

D. DNA virus

E. RNA virus

38. A 30-year-old woman presents to her physician with a sore throat of 4-day duration. One week ago she visited Las Vegas and while there she engaged in a one-time sexual encounter with a man she met at the casino. She denies vaginal intercourse but admits to participating in oral sex. Her temperature is 37.1°C (98.8°F). Examination reveals an erythematous pharynx, yellowish exudate covering the tonsillar pillars, and cervical lymphadenopathy. A throat swab was sent to the laboratory for culture and the resulting pathogen grows well on Thayer–Martin agar. Which of the following is a characteristic of the most likely agent causing this infection?

A. Antigenically variable pili

B. Exotoxin that inactivates elongation factor-2 (EF-2)

C. Latency in trigeminal ganglia

D. M protein

E. Polysaccharide capsule

39. An 11-year-old girl presents with swelling of the salivary glands. The mother states that her daughter is lethargic, complains of a headache, and has not been eating well for the past 3 days. The mother brought her daughter to the physician when she noticed swelling in her daughter's face. At the time of examination, the patient's temperature is 37.2°C (99.0°F) and severe parotitis is noted. She has not received routine childhood vaccinations. The most likely diagnosis of this infection is:

A. Diphtheria

B. Lemierre's syndrome

C. Ludwig's angina

D. Mumps

E. Sjörgen's syndrome

40. A 42-year-old woman with acute myeloid leukemia presents to the emergency department with a fever of 3-day duration. She is currently undergoing chemotherapy for the leukemia. A CBC at the time of admission demonstrates a severe reduction in neutrophils. The woman states she has had a mild cough for several weeks, but other than the fever, she has been feeling well. A chest radiograph demonstrates two cavities in the right upper lobe. A bronchoscopy with biopsy is performed and the bronchoalveolar lavage (BAL) fluid demonstrates branching, Y-shaped hyphae. Which of the following cells is primarily involved in the innate immune response to the most likely pathogen?

A. Basophils

B. Eosinophils

C. Lymphocytes

D. Macrophages

E. Neutrophils

41. A 58-year-old homeless man presents to the emergency department with fever, chest pain, and cough productive of blood-tinged sputum. On examination, the man is clearly intoxicated. He states he drinks whenever he can, but denies smoking cigarettes or using illicit drugs. His temperature is 38.9°C (102.0°F), and his respiratory rate is 29 breaths per minute. Decreased breath sounds and crackles in the right lower field are noted on lung examination. His CBC demonstrates elevated WBCs. A chest radiograph reveals an infiltrate in the right lower lobe. A sputum culture grows the organism on MacConkey agar as shown below.

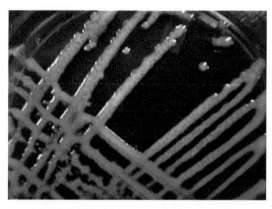

Which of the following virulence factors is produced by the likely causative agent of this infection?

A. Capsule

B. M protein

C. Pneumolysin

D. Pyoverdin

E. Toxin that binds elongation factor-2 (EF-2)

42. A previously healthy 32-year-old woman who lives in San Diego presents to her primary care physician in June with a cough of 2-week duration, sinus pressure, and pain. She states that she had a sore throat 1 week ago. The cough at that time was nonproductive, but now she is producing a small amount of yellowish phlegm. She has no sick contacts and has no recent travel history. She works in the aviary at the zoo and takes care of macaws, parrots, and parakeets. At the time of the examination, her temperature is 37.8°C (100.0°F). Scattered rales in the left lower lung field are present. A chest X-ray reveals patchy areas of consolidation in the left lower lobe. Gram stain and routine bacterial culture of sputum on blood, chocolate, and MacConkey are negative for organisms. Which of the following agents would best target the most likely causative agent of this infection?

A. Amoxicillin–clavulanate

B. Doxycycline

C. Itraconazole

D. Oseltamivir

E. Penicillin G

43. A previously healthy 61-year-old man presents with a 4-week history of a chest pain and a cough, productive of sputum. About 6 months prior, he had visited his family in Japan, and he recalls eating crabs at an oceanfront seafood restaurant. He denies night sweats or any weight loss and vitals and physical exam are unremarkable. A chest X-ray shows focal consolidation. CBC demonstrates eosinophilia and the acid-fast bacilli smear is negative. The sputum ova and parasite exam demonstrates the presence of the ovum seen below.

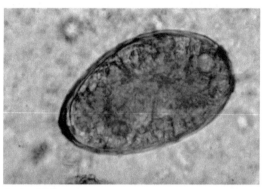

Source: CDC

Which of the following pathogens is the most likely agent of this infection?

A. *Ascaris lumbricoides*

B. *Echinococcus granulosus*

C. *Paragonimus westermani*

D. *Strongyloides stercoralis*

E. *Schistosoma japonicum*

44. A 16-year-old boy visits his primary care physician with a 4-day history of a sore throat, fever, and general malaise. He states that he is very tired and just wants to sleep. His mother notes that he has not been eating as much as he normally does. His medical history is unremarkable, he is up to date with vaccinations and is not on medication. On examination, notable pharyngeal inflammation and white tonsillar exudate is observed. In addition, he has marked posterior cervical lymphadenopathy. His temperature at the time of the examination is 38.8°C (101.8°F). A CBC demonstrates the presence of the cells shown below.

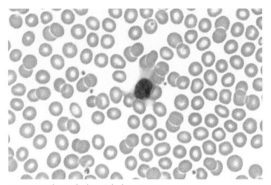

Source: Wikimedia/Dr. Erhabor Osaro

Which of the following would best confirm the diagnosis and identify the most likely agent of this infection?

A. β-Hemolytic growth on blood agar

B. Elek test positive

C. Growth on chocolate agar and not blood agar

D. Positive heterophile antibody

E. Positive DNase B antibody

45. A 5-year-old boy visits the dentist for a toothache. The child is subsequently found to have a cavity. The pathogen most likely responsible for this condition produces an enzyme that converts:

A. Fibrinogen to fibrin

B. Glucose to propionate and acetate

C. Hydrogen peroxide to water and oxygen

D. Sucrose to lactic acid

E. Urea to ammonium

9.2 Answers and Explanations

Easy	Medium	Hard

1. Correct: Differentiate acute otitis media from otitis media with effusion (A)

(A) This is most likely a case of otitis media with effusion (OME). Acute otitis media (AOM) is a common bacterial infection in the pediatric population that clinical findings include ear pain and systemic symptoms such as fever and malaise. Purulent draining may occur in AOM following perforation of the tympanic membrane. AOM is usually bacterial in etiology and may be treated with antibiotics, such as amoxicillin or amoxicillin–clavulanate. OME occurs due to the blockage of the eustachian tube due to fluids in the middle ear. OME may occur after an episode of AOM or a cold viral infection. Most often the only sign or symptom of OME is impaired hearing, which may be mild to moderate. Fever, pain, and other symptoms are usually absent. OME is mainly self-limiting; hence, a "wait and watch" approach is recommended. Antibiotics are not warranted. **(B)** Myringotomy is surgical incision and tube placement in the eardrum; although newer methods use laser incision that obviates the need for tube placement. While this is a treatment for chronic OME, it would not have been appropriate for the pediatrician to perform this procedure on the initial visit. **(C)** *Streptococcus pneumoniae* and nontypeable *Haemophilus influenzae* are the most common bacterial causes of acute otitis media in children. Current vaccine practice in the United States includes immunization against *S. pneumoniae* and *H. influenzae* type b (Hib) at 2, 4, and 6 months of age in an effort to prevent bacterial meningitis. A consequence of these vaccines is that colonization rates with *S. pneumoniae* and Hib have declined which may impact the rates of secondary infections in the respiratory tract. The Hib vaccine would not impact the colonization rate with nontypeable *Haemophilus*. Presumably the child's pediatrician would be aware of his vaccination history. **(D)** If this were a case of acute otitis media, amoxicillin would have been the most appropriate antibiotic. *S. pneumoniae* is a common bacterial etiology and although up to 40% of strains may have resistance to β-lactam antibiotics, they are still the best drug class due to the high levels that may be achieved in the middle ear fluid. **(E)** A sign of OME is hearing loss. However, because most cases resolve it would be a premature decision to refer to a hearing specialist.

2. Correct: *Pseudomonas aeruginosa* (C)

(C) This is a case of swimmer's ear (otitis externa) caused by *Pseudomonas aeruginosa*. The boy most likely contracted the infection by swimming in contaminated water while at summer camp. *P. aeruginosa* is a common inhabitant of water and can be an opportunistic pathogen. It can cause infections of the: (i) lung in cystic fibrosis patients; (ii) eye in hard contact lens wearers; and (iii) skin, also known as hot tub folliculitis. Hot tub folliculitis is analogous to swimmer's ear because it is due to environmental source, that is, contaminated water. *P. aeruginosa* produces a number of virulence factors including an ADP-ribosylating toxin, alginate that contributes to biofilm formation, and an elastase that can damage tissue. **(A)** *Candida albicans* is a common inhabitant of the skin and may be a source of skin and mucosal infections. Examples are diaper rash in an infant or vaginitis. Considering the child's history at summer camp and the relative severity of this infection, *C. albicans* is an unlikely etiology. (**B**) Influenza H3N2, one hemagglutinin and neuraminidase type that can cause influenza, is not indicated in this case. A predisposing viral infection may lead to otitis media. However, this child presented with otitis externa. (**D**) *Staphylococcus aureus* may inhabit the skin or nares of some individuals and is an agent of otitis externa. It is a potential source of endogenous infection of the eye, skin, respiratory tract, or bloodstream typically through some trauma. *S. aureus* is a highly virulent organism producing a number of cytolytic toxins, a superantigen, and protein A. This organism is a gram-positive cocci and not gram-negative rod; hence, this answer choice is incorrect. (**E**) *Streptococcus pneumoniae* is the etiologic agent of otitis media or middle ear infection. Because *S. pneumoniae* is a common resident in the upper respiratory tract it can be a source of secondary bacterial infection following a viral respiratory tract infection. There, the most common presentation would be a predisposing cold leading to fluid accumulation in the middle ear that promotes the growth of *S. pneumoniae*. This case is more likely to be otitis externa which is mainly associated with *P. aeruginosa* or *S. aureus*, not *S. pneumoniae*.

3. Correct: Mother's vagina (C)

(**C**) This is a case of inclusion conjunctivitis caused by *Chlamydia trachomatis*, a common bacterial cause of sexually transmitted infections also known as ophthalmia neonatorum. Different serovars of *C. trachomatis* have tissue tropisms for the urogenital tract or conjunctival epithelial cells. However, serovars that are typically sexually transmitted infections may cause conjunctivitis in the neonate, especially during a vaginal birth. In addition to the case presentation, the use of Giemsa stain to identify intracellular inclusion bodies and a direct fluorescent antibody test designate *C. trachomatis*. *Chlamydia* is intracellular pathogens that form glycogen-containing inclusion bodies. Because they lack a cell wall, traditional staining methods cannot be used for diagnosis. Other common agents of ophthalmia neonatorum include *Neisseria gonorrhoeae* and Herpes simplex virus-2 (HSV-2). (**A**) Contact lens wearers can be susceptible to conjunctivitis through contaminated cleaning solutions or eye drops. *Pseudomonas aeruginosa* is implicated in cases of contact lens-associated eye infections. However, there is no indication in the case that eye drops were used for this newborn boy. (**B**) Staphylococcal scalded skin syndrome (SSSS) may be transmitted to neonates by the hands of health care workers. SSSS is caused by strains of *Staphylococcus aureus* that produce exfoliative toxin. This toxin induces cleavage at the stratum granulosum causing desquamation in the infant. *S. aureus* may colonize the nares of certain individuals so outbreaks of SSSS in neonatal wards it typically traced to one individual.

In the case described in the question stem, the ocular infection was most likely vertically transmitted during parturition. (**D**) Predisposing upper respiratory tract infections (URTIs) with a virus, *Streptococcus pneumoniae* or *Haemophilus influenzae* may spread to the conjunctiva. Due to the age of the infant and no indication of a predisposing URTI, these pathogens can be ruled out. In addition, the laboratory identification required a Giemsa stain and direct fluorescent antibody test that are used for *Chlamydia*. (**E**) Transplacental passage is a means for the vertical transmission of pathogens that fall under the TORCH acronym (**T**oxoplasmosis, **O**ther [Syphilis, HIV], **R**ubella, **C**ytomegalovirus, and **H**erpes simplex-2). Transplacental passage may result in intrauterine growth restrictions, neurologic complications, and other systemic manifestations. Although inclusion conjunctivitis is vertically-transmitted, it is not passed from mother to child transplacentally.

4. Correct: *Pseudomonas aeruginosa* protease (B)

(**B**) *Pseudomonas aeruginosa* is a gram-negative rod that can inhabit a variety of environmental niches and cause opportunistic infections typically when immunocompromised. This bacterium can be a cause of bacterial conjunctivitis and keratitis in extended contact lens wearers. *P. aeruginosa* produces a number of virulence factors including exotoxin A, alginate, and proteases (answer choice A), which can contribute to tissue damage. Overnight orthokeratology is the practice of wearing contact lenses for extended periods of time to temporarily reshape the cornea and reduce refractive errors of the eye. In this case, a contaminated contact lens case permitted the growth of *P. aeruginosa*. (**A**) *Haemophilus influenzae* can be a cause of infectious keratitis and would most likely follow a secondary bacterial infection of the sinuses. However, it is not an environmental isolate and would not be expected to contaminate a poorly maintained contact lens case. The polyribitol phosphate capsule is the virulence attribute of *H. influenzae* type b that contributes to bacterial meningitis. (**C**) While *Staphylococcus aureus* is another potential cause of keratitis in contact lens wearers, the exfoliative toxin would not contribute to corneal perforation. ET is responsible for producing cleavage at the stratum granulosum causing the staphylococcal scalded skin syndrome (SSSS) in neonates. (**D**) While *Streptococcus pneumoniae* can be a cause of conjunctivitis, the predisposing condition would typically be an upper respiratory tract bacterial infection. Pneumolysin is a pore-forming cytolysin that can contribute to tissue damage during bacterial pneumonia. There is no indication this boy has any respiratory symptoms. (**E**) *Streptococcus pyogenes* causes pharyngitis, acute rheumatic fever, and the sequelae of rheumatic heart disease. It can be rare cause of bacterial conjunctivitis but would most likely follow an upper respiratory tract infection. Pyrogenic exotoxin is a superantigen that induces the nonspecific activation of T cells by non-discriminately cross-linking T cell receptor and major histocompatibility complex (MHC) class II molecule. This results in massive cytokine release causing life-threatening symptoms.

5. Correct: Recurrence of *Acanthamoeba* Infection (D)

(D) *Acanthamoeba* keratitis can be caused by contaminated contact lenses. In this case, the patient most likely encountered the parasite while swimming in a pond. The physician mistakenly assumed a bacterial infection (such as *Pseudomonas aeruginosa*, the most common cause of contact lens-associated keratitis). Unfortunately, antibiotics would not be effective against an ameba parasite permitting the infection to progress to corneal perforation. The most common cause of penetrating keratoplasty (corneal transplant) failure following *Acanthamoeba* keratitis is due to reinfection by contaminating cysts. (A) *Pseudomonas aeruginosa* would be a reasonable choice for bacterial keratitis associated with extended contact lens use. However, the history of swimming in a pond and the failure to resolve the infection with antibiotic eye drops points to a different etiology of infection. (B) Chorioretinitis is inflammation of the choroid and retina of the eye. Common infectious etiologies of chorioretinitis include cytomegalovirus (CMV) and *Toxoplasma gondii*. Infections are mostly associated with immunocompromised states, especially AIDS. Chorioretinitis symptoms are redness and light sensitivity as with keratitis but will also include impaired night vision and altered color perception. This is an unlikely complication. (C) *Acanthamoeba* may cause severe meningitis and as with this case, there is typically a history of contact with contaminated water. *Naegleria* is another parasite that can cause amebic meningitis. However, there were no signs of meningitis (headache, stiff neck, altered consciousness, etc.) in this case presentation. (E) Corneal transplant (also called penetrating keratoplasty) with localized immunosuppression has a very high success rate. Following amebic keratitis, there is the possibility of transplant reinfection due to contaminating cysts at the site of infection. However, this is unlikely.

6. Correct: Soil contaminated with the eggs of *Toxocara canis* (C)

(C) This is most likely a case of ocular toxocariasis caused by *Toxocara canis*. The boy accidentally ingested the eggs of the dog roundworm, *Toxocara canis*, and became an accidental injured host. Eggs shed by an infected dog may enter the human host through the practice of pica or geophagia. Children are most susceptible to infection; approximately 14% of the U.S. population has antibodies to *Toxocara* indicating a very high exposure rate. As the human is an unintentional host the worm larvae do not follow the normal life cycle stages. *T. canis* larvae travel through the portal circulation of the dog to the liver and lungs. From the lungs the larvae are coughed up and swallowed to complete their life cycle in the canine intestine, whereas in humans they migrate to different areas of the body. This form of parasitemia is referred to as visceral larva migrans, with the eye a possible locus of infection. Ocular toxocariasis is almost always unilateral and can be treated with corticosteroids and surgery. Note that visceral larval migrans can also be attributed to *Toxacara cati*, which is associated with cats. This organism is transmitted to humans in a similar manner as *T. canis*. (A) *Histoplasma capsulatum* is a dimorphic fungus that may cause systemic mycosis with the eye being a potential site of infection (chorioretinitis). *H. capsulatum* spores are ubiquitous in the environment with a higher risk of exposure amongst individuals who are chronically exposed to bird and bat droppings. Infection is typically unapparent in healthy individuals but dissemination may occur with immunocompromised individuals. Infection of the eye is visible as small areas of inflammation and scarring surrounding the retina. Vision may not be impacted unless the macula is affected. The boy's history and clinical findings are more consistent with *Toxocara*. (B) *Acanthamoeba* is a free-living freshwater ameba (protozoan parasite) that may cause serious infections of the eye and meningitis. A typical case presentation would be keratitis in a patient who wears contact lenses. The infection is refractory to antibiotics and may lead to rapid destruction of the cornea requiring transplant surgery (penetrating keratoplasty). This is unlikely to the cause of this boy's infection. (D) *Toxoplasma gondii* is a protozoan parasite with the sexual stage of its life cycle occurring in cats. Humans are accidental injured hosts. The tachyzoites form of the organism is found in blood and can also cross the placenta resulting in congenital infections. Other mechanisms of transmission include ingestion of the oocyte from cat feces and ingestion of bradyozoites in undercooked meat, especially lamb. Serologic studies have shown that infection rates may be as high as 50% in some countries. Eye disorders in persons infected with *T. gondii* may occur but pathology is typically unapparent in healthy individuals. Immunocompromised individuals (e.g., HIV patients) who were congenitally infected with *T. gondii* may show the severe neurologic symptoms associated with encephalitis. Primary or reactivated infections in a healthy host, such as in this case, are highly unlikely. Hence, this is not the best answer choice. (E) *Schistosoma mansoni* is a helminth parasite that causes schistosomiasis and is mainly limited to Africa. Eggs released into freshwater become miracidia which infect snails. Sporocysts of *S. mansoni* grow in the snail and are released as swimming cercariae which penetrate human skin and the larvae or schistosomule travel through the circulation to the lungs and heart. The final niche is the mesenteric circulation where paired male and female worms can produce

300 eggs per day that are released in the feces of the host. The symptoms of acute schistosomiasis include fever, myalgia, diarrhea, and respiratory symptoms. The travel history and symptoms in this case indicate that this is most likely not the infecting agent.

7. Correct: *Candida albicans* (B)

(B) This is a case of oropharyngeal candidiasis commonly referred to as thrush, caused by *Candida albicans*. *C. albicans* is a common inhabitant of the skin and oral and pharyngeal infection is usually from an endogenous source. This is an uncommon infection in healthy adults but may occur with immunocompromised individuals especially in HIV/AIDS, cancer treatments, organ transplantation, diabetes, corticosteroid use, dentures, and broad-spectrum antibiotic use. See Appendix M for the common infections associated with HIV/AIDS. **(A)** *Aspergillus fumigatus* is an environmental fungus that may cause opportunistic infections, especially in neutropenic patients. It is a source of allergic sinusitis for some individuals. *Aspergillus* may colonize a preexisting cavity leading to an aspergilloma (fungus ball) in the lungs. Invasive aspergillosis is a serious infection that may occur in profoundly immunocompromised individuals. It most commonly affects the lungs and may spread to other areas of the body. *A. fumigatus* infection does not resemble the characteristic appearance of oropharyngeal candidiasis described in this case. **(C)** *Mucor* species (and *Rhizopus* species) cause mucormycosis (also referred to as zygomycosis), a rare infection caused by fungi of the subdivision Mucoromycotina. As with candidiasis, mucormycosis is seen in patients with immunodeficiency. However, *Mucor* typically infect the sinuses or lungs causing headache, sinus pain, fever, and a cough. Left untreated in an immunocompromised patient, the fungal infection will spread to other areas of the body and can become rapidly fatal. **(D)** While *Staphylococcus aureus*, which colonizes the nares and skin of some individuals, may be a source of endogenous infections, it does not cause thrush. *S. aureus* may cause a variety of skin infections, bloodstream infections, infections of the bone and joint, and conjunctivitis. **(E)** *Streptococcus mutans* colonizes the oral cavity and can be a source of dental caries (cavities). Its niche in the oral cavity is limited to the teeth. It does not cause the characteristic white patches seen with oral candidiasis.

8. Correct: M protein (A)

(A) The boy has pharyngitis caused by *Streptococcus pyogenes* (strep throat). *S. pyogenes* is also referred to as group A *Streptococcus* and β-hemolytic *Streptococcus*. M protein (answer choice A) protrudes from the surface of the bacterial cell and undergoes a crude form of antigenic variation. The antigenic structure of M protein resembles human cardiac myosin protein which is an example of host immune response evasion by molecular mimicry. A potential complication of pharyngitis is poststreptococcal sequelae. Circulating M protein may induce the production of antibodies that cross react with human heart muscle causing cardiac damage. This is referred to as rheumatic heart disease. **(B)** Protein A is produced by *Staphylococcus aureus*. It is a surface protein that provides immune evasion capacity to the bacterial cell by binding to the Fc portion of mammalian IgG antibodies. Protein A does not have a direct role in tissue damage. **(C)** Pyrogenic exotoxin A is a virulence factor produced by *Streptococcus pyogenes*. It is a superantigen that causes the indiscriminate cross-linking of the major histocompatibility complex (MHC) of antigen-presenting cells and the T cell receptor. This nonspecific cross-linking activates a significant population of T cells causing massive cytokine release and a cascade of physiologic effects that include fever, rash, disseminated intravascular coagulation, and hypotension. The rash and fever are characteristic of scarlet fever that can follow streptococcal pharyngitis. Scarlet fever is an acute phase of a *S. pyogenes* infection and is not considered sequela, a chronic condition that follows a disease. **(D)** Streptolysin O is a pore-forming cytolysin produced by *S. pyogenes*. It has a complement-like mechanism of action with multiple receptor-binding subunits that coalesce to form a large pore in the membrane of erythrocytes. Circulating antibodies to Streptolysin O can be diagnostic for rheumatic heart disease or scarlet fever. **(E)** Teichoic acid is a cell wall component of gram-positive bacteria. They are bacterial polysaccharides composed of glycerol phosphate or ribitol phosphate and may be directly linked to peptidoglycan or to lipids (lipoteichoic acid), depending on the genus of gram-positive bacterium. Teichoic acid provides rigidity to the cell wall and may induce an inflammatory response in the host. This characteristic makes teichoic acid a virulence factor analogous to lipopolysaccharide of gram-negative bacteria.

9. Correct: Lacks a cell wall (E)

(E) These college students have atypical pneumonia caused *by Mycoplasma pneumoniae*, a unique bacterial pathogen that lacks a cell wall. Key features of the case that point to this diagnosis are:

1. Outbreak setting in close living quarters

2. Symptoms of chronic cough, headache, and fever

3. Stevens–Johnson syndrome (SJS) in an index patient. SJS is a hypersensitivity reaction affecting the skin and mucous membranes and may be caused by medications or by an infection with *M. pneumoniae*.

4. Because *M. pneumoniae* lacks a cell wall, does not cause sputum production, and is difficult to culture, naso- and oro-pharyngeal swabs are collected from patients. The polymerase chain reaction is one method used to make the diagnosis.

Pneumonia caused by *M. pneumoniae* is referred to as atypical pneumonia because it cannot be treated with cell wall-acting β-lactam antibiotics and does not produce sputum. It is also referred to as walking pneumonia because it may affect young people who can maintain normal life activities. **(A)** Mycolic acid is a significant component of the *Mycobacterium tuberculosis* cell wall, giving the pathogen resistance to phagocytosis and opsonization. A granuloma is formed in the lung, followed by a delayed-type hypersensitivity reaction as seen in the tuberculin skin test. *M. tuberculosis* is the causative agent of tuberculosis (TB). TB is unlikely in this setting and the symptoms and outbreak cluster are not consistent with the disease. Most exposures result in inapparent infections in the early stages of disease. Active TB is characterized by a productive cough, night sweats, fever, and chronic weight loss. The "wasting disease" aspect of TB is caused by the release of cytokines in response to the chronic infection. **(B)** *Blastomyces dermatitidis*, a dimorphic fungus that can cause pneumonia, grows as a broad-based budding yeast cell in tissue (see image at the end of this answer). It is not transmitted person to person but is contracted by environmental exposure to the fungal spores. The infection initiates in the lung but *B. dermatitidis* can disseminate to the skin and bone, especially in immunocompromised individuals. The outbreak pattern, patient population, and symptoms in this case presentation are not consistent with a fungal pneumonia. **(C)** Hemagglutinin is a surface glycoprotein of influenza virus that binds to sialic acid on membrane of susceptible cells. Although influenza would be readily transmitted among college dormmates, the symptoms, specimen collection, and index case of SJS do indicate this viral etiology. **(D)** Encapsulated causes of pneumonia are *Streptococcus pneumoniae* and *Haemophilus influenzae* types a–f. *S. pneumoniae* is the most common cause of bacterial pneumonia and is typically diagnosed in the elderly. The symptoms would be more pronounced and the patients would produce rusty-colored sputum. A Gram stain and culture of sputum can be diagnostic. A chest X-ray would show consolidation. *H. influenzae* can cause pneumonia, sinusitis, and conjunctivitis. Type b is the most virulent and can cause meningitis. The incidence of *H. influenzae* type b infections have declined with introduction of the vaccine in 1993. Neither of these pathogens is associated with SJS.

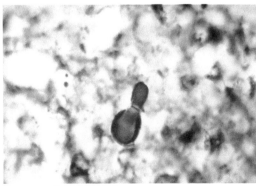

Source: CDC/Dr. Libero Ajello

10.   Correct: Meningitis (B)

(B) This man has "typical" pneumonia caused by the gram-positive diplococcus *Streptococcus pneumoniae*. *S. pneumoniae* is one of the most common causes of bacterial pneumonia, following influenza. *S. pneumoniae* is an encapsulated bacterium that can cause invasive infections including meningitis (answer choice B). It is also a cause of sinus and, particularly in children, otitis media. Introduction of a polyvalent pneumococcal conjugate vaccine (PCV) in 2000 dramatically reduced cases of invasive disease. Current vaccine compositions protect against 13 or 23 serotypes (PCV13 and PCV23, respectively). These capsular vaccines are conjugated to a protein toxoid to enhance antigen presentation and immunologic memory. Note: *Staphylococcus aureus* is also an important cause of secondary bacterial pneumonia following influenza. **(A)** Cystitis or bladder infection is a potential complication of hospitalization. The most common cause is *Escherichia coli* with other potential bacteria etiologies of hospital-acquired urinary tract infections. *E. coli* is not typical agent of pneumonia in adults and *S. pneumoniae* is not a typical agent of cystitis. **(C)** Mucormycosis is a fungal infection typically of the sinuses caused by the Mucoromycotina (zygomycetes). Mucormycosis is a rare infection most commonly seen in patients with weakened immune systems. The infection in this case is unlikely to be due to mucormycosis. **(D)** Osteomyelitis or infection of the bone most commonly follows the introduction of bacteria through trauma. The most common cause is *S. aureus*. *Mycobacterium tuberculosis*, a respiratory pathogen, may disseminate to the bone also. However, *S. pneumoniae* is not a typical agent of osteomyelitis. **(E)** Rheumatic fever is a potential sequelae of pharyngitis caused by *Streptococcus pyogenes*. Cross-reactive antibodies to *S. pyogenes* M protein may react with cardiac myosin causing tissue damage. *S. pyogenes* is not a frequent agent of pneumonia; hence, the infection in this case is unlikely to be due to *S. pyogenes*.

11.   Correct: Bacterial culture from a lung biopsy (B)

(B) This is an outbreak of atypical pneumonia caused by the gram-negative bacillus *Legionella pneumophila*. *L. pneumophila* has the unique ability to survive in the environment by inducing uptake into freshwater amebae that inhabit cooling towers. This adaptation to living inside a protozoan makes the bacterium highly virulent. *L. pneumophila* used coiling phagocytosis to media uptake into macrophages. Diagnostic testing includes culture from bronchial aspirate or biopsy (*L. pneumophila* does not typically cause a productive cough), a urine antigen test, paired serology, direct fluorescence staining, and PCR. The urine antigen test is fast method of diagnosis but does not detect all serotypes of *L. pneumophila*. Note that the urine antigen test only tests for one serotype of

L. pneumophila. Therefore, negative results do not necessarily rule out a *Legionella* infection. **(A)** A tuberculin skin test is a delayed-type hypersensitivity reaction to the purified protein derivative (PPD) of *Mycobacterium tuberculosis*. *M. tuberculosis* spreads from person to person and causes a chronic infection of the lung. Formation of the granuloma coincides with the production of cytokines that cause the systemic symptoms associated with tuberculosis. Seroconversion occurs within 2 to 12 weeks' postexposure and is seen as a positive skin test reaction (wheal) to PPD. The case described in the question stem is unlikely to be caused by *M. tuberculosis*. **(C)** Giemsa stain is used for the histopathologic diagnosis of protozoan parasites such as the *Plasmodium* species (malaria) or *Babesia microti* (babesiosis). *Legionella* diagnosis would not include a Giemsa stain from blood. **(D)** *Legionella pneumophila* does always cause a productive cough necessitating more aggressive diagnostic methods such as aspiration of pleural fluid or tissue biopsy for culture followed by fluorescent staining and PCR. Note that while most often *Legionella* presents as atypical pneumonia it may develop into a consolidation pneumonia. Furthermore, *Legionella* does not Gram stain's poorly and may be difficult to visualize; hence, Gram stain is not the best mechanism of diagnosis. **(E)** Isolation of yeast cells from lymph node biopsy suggests infection with a fungal pathogen such as *Histoplasma capsulatum*. In tissue, *H. capsulatum* is encountered as yeast cells, found within macrophages, and is most commonly associated with exposure to bird or bat droppings. While a zoonotic infection in an urban setting is possible, it is unlikely that there would have been a widespread outbreak. A typical case presentation would be an individual who is chronically exposed to pigeon or other bird (including chicken) droppings. Note that *H. capsulatum* is a dimorphic fungus that is a yeast in vivo (37°C) and a mold when grown at 30°C.

---

12. Correct: *Staphylococcus aureus* followed by *Pseudomonas aeruginosa* (D)

(D) By adolescence, a majority of cystic fibrosis patients experience lung infections with *Staphylococcus aureus* followed by *Pseudomonas aeruginosa*. Bacteria such as *S. aureus* and *Haemophilus influenzae* that are common inhabitants of the human host cause infections of the cystic fibrosis lung in childhood followed by infections with the environmental opportunistic pathogen *P. aeruginosa*. *P. aeruginosa* can cause chronic lung infections because it is can form a biofilm in the lung making it refractory to the immune response and antibiotic therapy. Another important agent of respiratory infections in cystic fibrosis patients is *Burkholderia cepacia*. **(A)** *Haemophilus influenzae* has been a common cause of upper respiratory tract infections in children causing otitis media and sinusitis. Introduction of the

H. influenzae serotype b vaccine into the pediatric immunization schedule in 1987 has dramatically reduced infections in the United States. It may be an agent of respiratory infections, especially in young patients with cystic fibrosis; however, *S. aureus* and *P. aeruginosa* are more frequent agents. Influenza virus is a cause of seasonal respiratory tract infections that may lead to a secondary bacterial infection. The most common pathogens involved in respiratory infections in cystic fibrosi patients are *S. aureus* followed by *P. aeruginosa*. **(B)** *Coccidioides immitis* is a fungal pathogen of the lower respiratory tract with geographic specificity to the southwestern region of the United States. Also known as Valley Fever, infections with coccidioidomycosis presents with a triad of symptoms including fever, joint pain, and erythema nodosum (rounded nodules on the skin). *Streptococcus pneumoniae* is the most common cause of bacterial pneumonia and may follow a viral infection. Diagnosis is made by isolation from the sputum and blood and a chest radiograph. It is possible that a cystic fibrosis patient may be infected with *S. pneumoniae*. However, the most common pathogens are *S. aureus* followed by *P. aeruginosa*. **(C)** *Streptococcus pyogenes* causes pharyngitis with the potential for poststreptococcal sequelae involving heart muscle. It is not a cause of bacterial pneumonia. *Paragonimus westermani* is a lung fluke that causes human infections in eastern Asia and South America. Humans become infected by ingestion of the *P. westermani* metacercariae (cyst stage) that have infected fresh water crabs. **(E)** The lungs of cystic fibrosis patients may be chronically colonized with *Aspergillus fumigatus*, a fungus ubiquitously found in the environment. Defective mucociliary clearance coupled with prolonged antimicrobial therapy may contribute to chronic fungal colonization. *Mycobacterium tuberculosis* spreads from person to person by droplet and causes the chronic disease tuberculosis. Because the surface coat of *M. tuberculosis* renders it resistant to a cell-mediated response, the host forms a granuloma to contain the pathogen in the lung. Granuloma formation is accompanied by a T cell-mediated cytokine response leading to the systemic symptoms associated with active tuberculosis. Fungal pneumonia followed by infection with *M. tuberculosis* is not the most common course of lung infections seen in a young person with cystic fibrosis.

---

13. Correct: *Streptococcus pneumoniae* (E)

(E) *Streptococcus pneumoniae* is one of the most common agents of bacterial sinusitis. The case presentation is typical with a predisposing viral infection that impacts the host's innate immunity permitting overgrowth of a resident bacterium. Bacterial sinusitis is a common misdiagnosis but this patient has classic symptoms of a purulent nasal discharge, face pain, and fever. **(A)** *Actinomyces israelii* is a gram-positive rod that is often described as branching or filamentous. This organism is a commensal bacterium that may cause opportunistic infections following oral or abdominal surgery. *A. israelii* is an anaerobe that can form a localized abscess containing granulomatous tissue and "sulfur granules." This pathogen is not a typical agent of bacterial sinusitis. **(B)** *Moraxella catarrhalis* is a gram-negative diplococcus that may inhabit the upper respiratory tract. It is a cause of otitis media and sinusitis but the incidence is more common in children. *S. pneumoniae* remains the most common cause in the pediatric and adult population. **(C)** *Mucor* species are members of zygomycetes class of fungi. Mucormycosis (also called zygomycoses) is a fungal infection typically of the sinuses of immunocompromised patients. The clinical findings in this case indicate that zygomycetes is not the most likely agent of this infection. The patient is otherwise healthy and antibiotics resolve the course of the infection, indicating a bacterial source. **(D)** Rhinovirus causes the common cold. It was responsible for the predisposing condition in this case.

14. Correct: Isoniazid (D)

(D) This woman's symptoms and the diagnostic assays indicate that she has an active infection with *Mycobacterium tuberculosis*. The treatment regimen is **R**ifampin, **I**soniazid (answer choice D), **P**yrazinamide, and **E**thambutol (RIPE therapy) and for 6 to 9 months. Isoniazid has selective activity against *Mycobacteria* and inhibits mycolic acid, a vital component of the cell wall. Rifampin inhibits RNA polymerase and therefore nucleic acid synthesis and also has activity against *Staphylococcus aureus* and *Neisseria meningitis*. Pyrazinamide and ethambutol inhibit *Mycobacteria* cell wall components and therefore cell wall synthesis. **(A)** Acyclovir is an antiviral DNA polymerase inhibitor used to treat herpes virus infections. **(B)** Fluconazole is used to treat fungal infections such as infections with *Candida albicans*. Fluconazole inhibits the fungal enzyme lanosterol 14-α demethylase which converts lanosterol to ergosterol. This in turns disrupts cell membrane synthesis, cytochrome P450. **(C)** Gentamicin is an aminoglycoside antibiotic that is used mainly for infections with gram-negative bacteria and some gram-positive bacteria. It may be used for endocarditis, abdominal infections, septicemia, and complicated urinary tract infections. Some aminoglycosides including amikacin and streptomycin have activity against *M. tuberculosis*, but not gentamicin. Aminoglycosides are translation inhibitors that target the 30S ribosome. **(E)** Piperacillin is a β-lactam antibiotic. It is often used in combination with the β-lactamase inhibitor tazobactam. Piperacillin–tazobactam is used to treat infections with many organisms including *Pseudomonas aeruginosa*. β-Lactam antibiotics inhibits the bacterial cell wall. This agent does not have activity against *M. tuberculosis*.

15. Correct: *Pseudomonas aeruginosa* (E)

(E) *Pseudomonas aeruginosa* is a gram-negative rod and is the most common cause of late-onset ventilator-associated pneumonia (VAP). Late-onset is defined as an infection that occurs for 5 or more days, following admission in the hospital. This would be considered a case of late onset VAP occurring over 2 weeks following mechanical ventilation. Other than *P. aeruginosa*, the other frequent pathogens of late-onset VAP include *Staphylococcus aureus*, *Escherichia coli*, *Klebsiella pneumoniae*, *Enterobacter* species, *Serratia marcescens*, and *Acinetobacter baumannii*. Empiric antimicrobial therapy should target these agents and may include cefepime, piperacillin–tazobactam, meropenem, levofloxacin, or vancomycin. **(A)** *Candida albicans* is a fungal pathogen and may be a colonizer of the respiratory tract. Yeast may be potential pathogens of VAP but are not typical agents. *C. albicans* stains gram-positive and both budding yeast and hyphal forms would be seen in the Gram stain. Fluconazole and other azoles as well as amphotericin B are effective against *C. albicans*. **(B)** Although *P. aeruginosa* is the predominating pathogen associated with late-onset VAP, methicillin-resistant *S. aureus* (MRSA) must also be considered. This pathogen has been implicated with increasing frequency in hospital-acquired infections. *S. aureus* is a gram-positive coccus and vancomycin would be considered as part of the antimicrobial regimen for MRSA. **(C)** *Streptococcus pneumoniae* is a gram-positive coccus in pairs and chains and a potential pathogen responsible for rapid (early)-onset VAP. *S. pneumoniae* is also the most common cause of community-acquired pneumonia. *S. pneumoniae* are typically susceptible to β-lactam antibiotics. **(D)** *Pneumocystis jirovecii* is a fungal agent that causes interstitial pneumonia in immunocompromised individuals. *P. jirovecii* pneumonia (formerly *Pneumocystis carinii* pneumonia or PCP) is a presenting manifestation of AIDS. Trimethoprim–sulfamethoxazole can be used as a prophylactic agent and for treatment of *Pneumocystis* pneumonia. *P. jirovecii* is not a typical agent of VAP.

16. Correct: Metalloprotease (D)

(D) Anthrax toxin is composed of three elements: a protective antigen that serves as the toxin binding subunit that combines with an either the edema factor (EF) or a lethal factor (LF). EF is an adenylate cyclase which causes increase in cyclic AMP in affected cells while LF is a metalloprotease; cleaves mitogen-activated protein (MAP) kinases 1 and 2 short circuiting major signal transduction pathway in monocytes. *Bacillus anthracis* is an aerobic gram-positive rod with spores (see image at the end of this answer). **(A)** Hyaluronic acid is an important component of *Streptococcus pyogenes* capsule. The function of hyaluronic acid in pathogenesis of this organism is not completely understood, but it may play a role in the tissue destruction. **(B)** Lecithinase is a phospholipase that cleaves lecithin and is produced mainly by *Clostridium perfringens*. Lecithinase plays a role in tissue destruction. **(C)** Lipopolysaccharide (LPS), also referred to as endotoxin, is the extracellular component of gram-negative bacteria. It is composed of lipid A, a core polysaccharide, and O antigen. LPS is responsible for inducing endotoxic shock with gram-negative septicemia. **(E)** Plasminogen activators are produced by bacteria such as *Yersinia pestis* (plague bacillus), the staphylococci, and the streptococci. These compounds convert plasminogen to plasmin by limited proteolysis enhancing bacterial metastasis which may contribute to contribute to tissue damage.

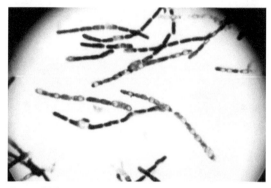

Source: CDC

17. Correct: *Acinetobacter baumannii* (A)

(A) *Acinetobacter baumannii* is an environmental organism with the capacity to survive on dry surfaces for extended periods. This gram-negative coccobacillus contaminated wounds and the hands of health care workers in the field during the Iraq war. Many wounded veterans developed pneumonia as well as wound and serious blood infections with this opportunistic pathogen. In addition to its capacity to survive in the environment, *A. baumannii* is resistant to multiple antibiotics and has become a significant source of nosocomial infections. Note: Although *A. baumannii* is classically described as a gram-negative rod or coccobacillus, in clinical isolates this pathogen is notorious for staining gram-negative and gram-positive and cocci, rods and coccobacillus forms can be seen. **(B)** *Coccidioides immitis* is a causative agent of fungal pneumonia endemic in the southwestern United States (valley fever). This agent may be seen in soldiers that are digging trenches or maneuvering (crawling) through the dirt as part of training in endemic areas. *Coccidioides* may cause respiratory infections initially and then may disseminate. However, the agent in this case is a gram-negative rod, which is not consistent with *Coccidioides*, a fungal pathogen. **(C)** *Enterococcus faecium* is a commensal intestinal colonizer that can cause opportunistic infections; it is an infrequent cause of respiratory tract infections. **(D)** *Klebsiella pneumoniae* is a source of urinary tract infections and other infections, such as antibiotic-resistant

nosocomial infections and in particular ventilator-associated pneumonia (VAP). However, it is not associated with the emerging infections seen in veterans. **(E)** Methicillin-resistant *Staphylococcus aureus* (MRSA) is a serious cause of nosocomial infections and is now considered along with *Pseudomonas aeruginosa* and *A. baumannii* in late-onset VAP. It has not been associated with veterans returning from Iraq.

18. Correct: Whooping cough (E)

(E) According to the Centers for Disease Control and Prevention (CDC), there has been a steady increase in whooping cough incidence with 32,971 cases reported in 2014; this was a 15% increase compared to 2013. An effective vaccine to *Bordetella pertussis*, the causative agent of whooping cough, has been highly successful. This vaccine was modified to an acellular form, DTaP for children and Tdap as a booster for older children and adults, in 1996 due to the postimmunization sequelae seen with the whole cell formulation. **(A)** Diphtheria is an infection of the upper respiratory tract caused by *Corynebacterium diphtheriae*. Very few cases are reported in the United States (two between the years of 2004 and 2015) due to the effective of the DTaP vaccine. This vaccine contains diphtheria toxoid which stimulates a humoral immune response to the key virulence factor. **(B)** Influenza is an infection of the respiratory tract that peaks in the winter months every year. Reimmunization of all age groups must occur on an annual basis due to the antigenic shift and drift of the major viral components. **(C)** Measles vaccine is part of the childhood immunization schedule (combined with mumps and rubella), administered as an attenuated form of the virus. Measles was declared eliminated from the United States in 2000 with reported cases originating from outside the country. **(D)** In 2000, the attenuated oral polio vaccine was no longer recommended for routine immunization in the United States and was replaced with the injectable inactive form of the vaccine. The only reported cases of polio in the United States between 1993 and 2000 were vaccine related.

19. Correct: *Actinomyces israelii* (A)

(A) This is a case of cervicofacial actinomycosis with presentation of a dental procedure and a stain showing intertwined or branching gram-positive rods (see image at the end of this answer) that may resemble fungal hyphae. Sometimes these rods are described as beaded. Both *Actinomyces* and *Nocardia* are branching gram-positive rods. *Actinomyces* is an anaerobe while *Nocardia* is an aerobe. *Actinomyces* does not stain with the modified acid-fast stain while *Nocardia* is modified acid-fast positive. Furthermore, tissue specimens with *Actinomyces* may include "sulfur" granules (which are not actually composed of sulfur but are rather a mixture of bacteria and tissue exudate). *A. israelii* is a commensal anaerobic organism that can colonize the oral cavity or large intestine. Trauma such as oral or abdominal surgery may lead to abscess formation. Due to the variety of flora in the oral cavity, infections are most likely to be polymicrobic. **(B)** *Aspergillus fumigatus* is an environmental fungus that can cause lung infections in individuals who experience chronic exposure to the spores and may be immunocompromised. It is not a typical agent of facial abscesses, such as this. **(C)** *Bacillus cereus* is a gram-positive, spore-forming rod that may be isolated from the soil. It produces a toxin that can lead to food poisoning. While food associated with *B. cereus* gastroenteritis includes meat, milk, vegetables, and fish, the vomiting-type outbreaks have generally been associated with rice products. *B. cereus* has also been implicated in causing eye infections following a penetrating eye trauma. This infection is unlikely to be caused by *B. cereus*. **(D)** *Clostridium perfringens* is a gram-positive, spore-forming rod that may cause anaerobic, necrotizing infections of wounds. It is the causative agent of gas gangrene and produces a variety of cytolysins that contribute to tissue invasion and spread. It is an unlikely agent of this infection. **(E)** *Histoplasma capsulatum* spores are associated with bird (including chicken) and bat droppings. Exposure may lead to fungal pneumonia. *H. capsulatum* grows as the mycelial (fungal) form in vitro but it is dimorphic, growing as a yeast form in tissue (in vivo). In this case, the preceding tooth extraction and the finding of sulfur granules indicate that *Actinomyces* and not *Histoplasma* is the most likely agent.

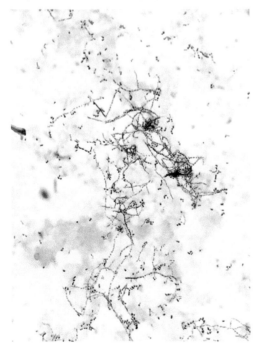

20. Correct: Polyribitol phosphate capsule (C)

(C) This child most likely has epiglottitis. The three main pathogens of epiglottitis are *Haemophilus*

influenzae type b (Hib), *Streptococcus pneumoniae,* and *Streptococcus pyogenes*. The key features of epiglottis include difficulty breathing and swallowing, drooling, and stridor. Infected individuals often assume the tripod position, in which they lean forward with their hands on their knees or another surface. Polyribitol phosphate capsule is the key virulence factor of Hib, a gram-negative coccobacillus. Hib was the most common cause of epiglottis prior to the vaccine which has reduced the incidence. **(A)** Hemagglutinin-neuraminidase produced by influenza and is responsible for attachment and entry of virus particles. Human parainfluenza viruses may cause laryngotracheitis (also known as croup). Viruses are not usual agents of epiglottis. **(B)** Pathogenic *Neisseria* including *N. meningitidis* and *N. gonorrhoeae* have pili on the surface of the cell that can vary the antigens, resulting in evasion from the host immune response. These agents are not involved in epiglottitis. **(D)** *Corynebacterium diphtheriae* produces a toxin that inhibits protein synthesis and is responsible for tissue and organ damage. This pathogen is not a typical agent of epiglottitis. *C. diphtheriae* is a gram-positive rod that may cause the formation a restrictive pseudomembrane on the pharynx. **(E)** The respiratory pathogen, *Bordetella pertussis* interacts with G inhibitory protein, leading to increase in cyclic AMP. *B. pertussis* is the agent of whooping cough and not epiglottitis.

21. Correct: *Streptococcus pneumoniae* (D)

(D) *Streptococcus pneumoniae* or pneumococcus (colloquially known as Strep pneumo) is a gram-positive coccus in chains or pairs. *S. pneumoniae* is a common cause of meningitis and community-acquired pneumonia in adults. Other infections with *S. pneumoniae* that commonly affect young children are sinusitis and acute otitis media (AOM), the most likely diagnosis in this child. *S. pneumoniae* is α-hemolytic on blood agar media, producing a green discoloration surrounding colonies. Moreover, *S. pneumoniae* is notorious for producing autolytic enzymes that cause the centers of colonies to collapse in, creating concave colony morphologies on agar. *S. pneumoniae* is optochin sensitive and like other streptococci is catalase negative. **(A)** Untypeable strains of *Haemophilus influenzae* are indeed common causes of AOM. Gram stain would show gram-negative coccobacilli. *H. influenzae* classically grows on chocolate agar, which is blood agar medium enriched with V (NAD) and X (hemin) factors that *H. influenzae* requires. **(B)** *Moraxella catarrhalis* is indeed a common cause of AOM. Gram stain would show gram-negative diplococci. Moreover, colonies classically are not concave but are said to "glide" across media plates, such as a hockey puck, when pushed with a microbiological loop. **(C)** *Staphylococcus aureus* is a gram-positive coccus in clusters or tetrads. It is an uncommon but serious cause of suppurative AOM and may be complicated by overt tympanic membrane rupture as well as mastoiditis through direct local extension of the infection out of the middle ear cavity. *S. aureus* is usually β-hemolytic (i.e., completely hemolytic), producing a clear zone around colonies on blood agar media as well as catalase and coagulase enzymes positive. **(E)** *Streptococcus pyogenes* or group A strep is a common cause of streptococcal pharyngitis and skin infection (impetigo), especially in children ages 5 to 15 years old. Group A strep is β-hemolytic and is a gram-positive coccus in chains. Although group A streptococci may occasionally cause AOM, *S. pneumoniae*, *H. influenzae*, and *M. catarrhalis* are more common agents of this infection.

22. Correct: Suffocation (E)

(E) This patient, who recently emigrated from a region of the world in which childhood vaccines may not be routine practice, is most likely affected by respiratory diphtheria caused by the gram-positive rod, *Corynebacterium diphtheriae*. This patient's clinical picture is classic for diphtheria: fever, malaise, cervical lymphadenopathy (which when severe can produce the classic "bull's neck"), and pseudomembranous pharyngitis with the characteristic "diphtheritic" membrane composed of exudate, organisms, and diphtheria toxin (DTx). The slight sinus tachycardia is probably because the child is dehydrated, stressed, and has difficulty breathing, as evidenced by the tachypnea and oxygen desaturation. The diphtheritic membrane in this case likely extends well below the level of the oropharynx and into the upper trachea, impeding the passage of air from the pharynx into the lungs. This causes stridor, respiratory distress, and, without immediate intubation, suffocation and death. **(A)** Cardiac dysfunction is a common and major complication of diphtheria. This includes myocarditis that may be accompanied by electrocardiographic and echocardiographic abnormalities, which may lead to chest pain, dyspnea, abnormal heart sounds, arrhythmia, and even congestive heart failure. Her otherwise normal electrocardiogram and unremarkable cardiac exam make myocardial dysfunction an unlikely immediate cause of death. **(B)** Endophthalmitis or ocular complication is not usually associated with diphtheria infection. **(C)** Neurological dysfunction is an uncommon but major complication of diphtheria. This includes cranial nerve neuropathies (including decreased gag reflex and palatal movement) and peripheral neuritis. Neurological complications of diphtheria are most attributable to the DTx toxin, which ADP-ribosylates eukaryotic elongation factor-2 (eEF-2), thereby inhibiting normal protein synthesis in host eukaryotic cells. Respiratory stridor suggests that upper airway obstruction is the more likely cause of impending respiratory failure rather than neurological impairment of respiration. **(D)** Skin lesions that include non-healing ulcers with an overlying gray membrane are indeed manifestations of cutaneous diphtheria infection. These are classically seen in impoverished populations in the United States including homeless alcoholic men and patients with intravenous drug use. Dermatologic complications of diphtheria are not likely to cause death in the next 24 hours.

23. Correct: Single-stranded segmented RNA genome (E)

(E) The influenza virus (i.e., "the flu"), an orthomyxovirus, is the most likely cause of this patient's symptoms. Influenza virus is an enveloped virus transmitted through direct contact, respiratory aerosol, and infected objects (fomites). The virus genome itself is composed of several individual segments of negative-sense, single-stranded RNA; this segmented genome is susceptible to genomic reassortments, or antigenic shift, which leads to the introduction of a new subtype of influenza. Antigenic shift causes large and sudden changes in the genome and contributes to pandemics. In contrast, antigenic drift is the accumulation of minor genetic changes that are gradual. These are usually due to point mutations. Antigenic drift is the primary reason the influenza vaccine must be reformulated yearly. These viruses are classified according to their specific hemagglutinin (H) and neuraminidase (N) membrane glycoproteins, which are important for virus entry into and egress out of infected cells, respectively. Other clinically significant pathogens that contain segmented RNA genomes include rotavirus and colitvirus (Colorado tick fever virus). Neither of these viruses causes respiratory infections. **(A)** The most notable organisms with circular DNA genomes that cause multisystem effects with prominent respiratory symptoms are prokaryotes (i.e., bacteria). Bacteria have a circular, single chromosome of double-stranded DNA that forms a non-membrane bound nucleoid. While bacteria such as *Streptococcus pyogenes* and *Bordetella pertussis* can cause respiratory infection, the systemic symptoms associated with these infections are less prominent. This patient's syndrome is more consistent with influenza. **(B)** Hepatitis B virus (HBV), a hepadnavirus, is a virus with a circular, partially double-stranded DNA genome. It is a major cause of viral hepatitis, including fulminant, acute, and chronic hepatitis. While hepatitis can present with multisystem symptoms, abdominal pain and jaundice would be more prominent and respiratory symptoms less so. **(C)** Rotavirus, a reovirus, does contain a segmented genome but has a double stranded RNA genome. It is a major cause of viral gastroenteritis during the winter months, especially in children under 1 year of age. Diarrhea is the most prominent symptom and unfortunately often results in severe dehydration and death if not treated promptly with oral rehydration therapy. **(D)** Organisms with segmented DNA genomes are not prominent human pathogens.

24. Correct: Respiratory syncytial virus (RSV) (D)

(D) This infant patient is likely suffering from bronchiolitis, a viral upper respiratory tract infection

205

(symptoms of nasal drainage and congestion) that usually progresses within a couple of days into a lower respiratory tract infection (symptoms of wheezing and respiratory distress). The most common cause of bronchiolitis in children less than 1 year of age is respiratory syncytial virus (RSV), a paramyxovirus. The paramyxoviruses have a nonsegmented, negative-sense, single stranded-RNA genome. Human metapneumovirus, a pneumovirus, is the second most common cause of bronchiolitis in children. **(A)** Human parainfluenza virus is a paramyxovirus. It classically causes croup, or laryngotracheobronchitis, a form of subglottic inflammation, which mainly affects young children. This can result in a "barking" cough and inspiratory stridor as edema compresses the upper airway, classically resulting in a "steeple sign" on anterior-posterior neck radiographs. Wheezing and lower respiratory tree symptoms would be unusual. **(B)** Measles virus is a paramyxovirus. It classically affects unvaccinated children in the United States or immigrant children with dubious vaccination histories. Measles classically presents with fever, sore throat, cough, conjunctivitis, and coryza (upper respiratory symptoms like nasal discharge) that eventually progress to a diffuse "morbilliform" or "measles-like" rash that is erythematous and maculopapular in nature. Koplik spots on the buccal mucosa are rare. **(C)** Mumps virus is a paramyxovirus. Like measles, mumps classically affects unvaccinated children in the United States or immigrant children with dubious vaccination histories. The MMR vaccine is protective against measles and mumps viruses, as well as the rubella togavirus. Mumps usually presents with a nonspecific viral prodrome: low-grade fever, headache, myalgias, malaise, and fatigue. These symptoms classically progress to parotitis (inflammation and infection of the parotids). Less common complications include orchitis males or oophoritis in females, pancreatitis, and aseptic meningitis. **(E)** Severe acute respiratory syndrome (SARS) virus is a coronavirus that, as the name implies, causes a severe respiratory syndrome. Patients experience a nonspecific constellation of flu-like symptoms that may culminate in a severe viral or secondary bacterial pneumonia. This patient's clinical picture of upper respiratory followed by lower respiratory tract symptoms and age are more consistent with RSV bronchiolitis.

---

25. Correct: Poliovirus (D)

(D) This patient is most likely recovering from an acute viral nasopharyngitis (i.e., infectious rhinitis, common cold). By far, the most common etiologic agent implicated is rhinovirus, a member of the picornavirus family. Picornaviruses are nonenveloped and have a small ("pico") positive-sense, single-stranded RNA genome. Unlike many of the picornaviruses, which are enteroviruses (i.e., can affect the "enteric" or GI system), rhinovirus is acid

labile and thus destroyed by the acidic gastric contents before being able to reach the distal gastrointestinal tract (GI tract) and cause enteric disease. Poliovirus is a picornavirus. It leaves the GI tract for the anterior horn of the spinal cord, destroying the α-lower motor neurons there and causing a flaccid paralysis, the hallmark of polio. Routine vaccination has eliminated polio in the United States. Following rhinovirus, the next most common cause of the common cold is coronavirus. **(A)** Hepatitis C virus (HCV) is a flavivirus. It is enveloped and transmitted parenterally. HCV causes a chronic viral hepatitis that can progress to cirrhosis and hepatocellular carcinoma. **(B)** Hepatitis E virus (HEV) is a hepevirus. It is transmitted fecal-orally and causes an acute viral hepatitis characterized by fever, right upper quadrant abdominal pain, scleral icterus, and jaundice, in addition to nonspecific viral symptoms like fatigue, malaise, and loss of appetite. HEV is associated with high mortality rates in pregnant women. **(C)** Human papillomavirus (HPV) is a papillomavirus that can be transmitted sexually or through direct contact with infected skin, mucosae, or body fluids. It predisposes to papillomas (warts) and squamous cell carcinomas of the anogenital tract and head/neck. **(E)** Respiratory syncytial virus (RSV) is a paramyxovirus and the leading cause of bronchiolitis in young children. RSV trails rhinoviruses and coronaviruses in causing the common cold.

---

26. Correct: *Burkholderia cepacia* (A)

(A) The patient most likely suffers from cystic fibrosis (CF). *Burkholderia cepacia*, a gram-negative rod, is a major cause of recurrent and chronic pulmonary infections in CF and chronic granulomatous disease patients. It has many virulence factors that make it particularly deleterious in these patient populations, including mechanisms for quorum sensing, motility, biofilm formation, siderophore expression for iron scavenging, and a type III secretion system or "injectisome." *B. cepacia* is also extremely resistant to most antimicrobials, in part because of a unique system of drug efflux pumps that actively remove antibiotics that enter these bacteria. Another gram-negative rod, *Pseudomonas aeruginosa*, is also a major pulmonary pathogen in CF patients that shares several characteristics with *B. cepacia*. Because of the poor prognosis of CF patients with *B. cepacia* following lung transplant, many transplant centers do not accept patients with *B. cepacia* pulmonary infections. The other common pathogen that is most likely to cause pulmonary infections in this patient population is the gram-positive coccus, *Staphylococcus aureus*. **(B)** *Candida albicans* is a yeast. It can certainly cause lung infection but usually in severely immunocompromised hosts. CF patients are by no means exempt from *Candida* pulmonary infection, but pulmonary candidiasis is not as common as pulmonary infections caused by *P. aeruginosa*, *B. cepacia*, and *S. aureus*. **(C)** *Klebsiella pneumoniae* is a gram-negative rod that classically causes lobar pneumonia in immunocompromised patients, especially alcoholics and those with poorly controlled diabetes mellitus. It classically yields a "red currant jelly sputum" on expectoration due its mucoid phenotype which can also be appreciated on colonized plates as mucoid, slimy colonies. *P. aeruginosa*, *B. cepacia*, and *S. aureus* are the most common agents of serious pulmonary infections in CF patients; hence, this answer choice is incorrect. **(D)** *Legionella pneumophilia* is a gram-negative rod that causes respiratory infections often following exposure to contaminated heating or cooling systems. While immunocompromised individuals are definitely at increased risk for infections with this pathogen, the typical patient is a male, older than 50 years of age, a heavy smoker and drinker, and often has a preexisting chronic lung disease. The most common causes of serious pulmonary infections in CF are *P. aeruginosa*, *B. cepacia*, and *S. aureus*. **(E)** *Streptococcus pneumoniae* is a gram-positive coccus in pairs or chains and is a common cause of lobar pneumonia in any patient population. It is α-hemolytic on blood agar media, producing a green discoloration around colonies. *P. aeruginosa*, *B. cepacia*, and *S. aureus* are the most common agents of serious pulmonary infections in CF patients; hence, this answer choice is incorrect.

27. Correct: aseptic meningitis (B)

(B) This child is most likely experiencing hand, foot, and mouth disease (HFMD), classically caused by the Coxsackie A virus, an enterovirus, a member of the picornavirus family. Enteroviruses are the most common cause of aseptic meningitis. Coxsackie A and B viruses are also implicated in other several diseases, notably herpangina (oral ulcers restricted to the mouth), viral pericarditis, and myocarditis. Note that herpes simplex virus-1 (HSV-1) may present in a similar manner with vesicular lesions, but these lesions are most often limited to the oral cavity (gingivostomatitis). Skin infections with HSV-1 in young children may include herpetic whitlow, which are usually seen on the fingers. While oral herpes infections may occur currently with herpetic whitlow in children, the findings of this case of lesions on the soles and palms indicate that HFMD is most likely. HSV cutaneous lesions in children are rarely found "all over" the body. **(A)** The spirochete *Treponema pallidum* is the causative agent of syphilis. Secondary syphilis can cause a diffuse maculopapular rash that involves glabrous skin of the palms and soles, in addition to other manifestations such as constitutional symptoms, alopecia areata (hair loss), and condyloma lata (a specific kind of genital warts). While clinicians should have a high index of suspicion for child sexual abuse and sexually transmitted infection, this patient's clinical picture is most consistent with HFMD. If untreated, the infection may progress to tertiary syphilis which can cause neurological

disease (dementia, tabes dorsalis), aortitis (answer choice A), and diffuse gummas (granulomatous lesions). Since syphilis causes a small blood vessel vasculitis, inflammation of the small vasa vasora blood vessels that supply the thick-walled aorta leads to aortic wall weakening, aneurysm, and even rupture and death. **(C)** Chronic infection with hepatitis viruses B, C, and D are associated with increased risk of liver cirrhosis. Cirrhosis and liver failure can result in jaundice from the impaired excretion of bilirubin, as well as palmar erythema and spider angiomata (vascular skin lesions) from impaired hepatic metabolism of estrogens. However, diffuse cutaneous and oropharyngeal vesicular lesions are not associated with hepatitis virus and cirrhosis. **(D)** *Chlamydia trachomatis* and *Neisseria gonorrhoeae* are major causes of pelvic inflammatory disease (PID) in women. Neither of these pathogens are agents of cutaneous infections as described in this case. If infections with *N. gonorrhoeae* or *C. trachomatis* are not appropriately treated, infections may ascend from the vagina and cervix into the upper genital tract causing inflammation (PID) and ultimately scarring of the endometrium, fallopian tubes and ovaries. **(E)** Varicella zoster virus (VZV) also called human herpes virus-3 (HHV-3) is the causative agent of varicella or "chickenpox." This presents with a prodromal viral illness that later develops into a diffuse rash that includes crops of vesicular lesions on erythematous bases in differing stages of crusting and scabbing. When patients later in life grow old or become immunocompromised, vesicular lesions (shingles) can erupt periodically in a dermatomal or "zosteriform" pattern that corresponds to the infected dorsal root ganglion (for the body) or trigeminal ganglion (for the face) harboring latent virus. Varicella immunization is part of the child vaccination schedule. This patient's clinical picture and anatomic distribution is more consistent with HFMD.

28. Correct: Parvovirus (D)

(D) This woman most likely has oral herpes (cold sore, herpes labialis) that is most often caused by herpes simplex virus-1 (HSV-1), which is a DNA virus. The only other virus that is a DNA virus among the answer choices is parvovirus (answer choice D). Herpes oral infections are most often the result of recurrent (nonprimary) infections. HSV-1 is also commonly implicated in keratoconjunctivitis, gingivostomatitis, encephalitis, pharyngitis, and herpetic whitlow. **(A)** Hepatitis A virus (HAV) is a picornavirus and thus has a small ("pico") RNA, not DNA, genome. It causes an acute viral hepatitis characterized by fever, right upper quadrant abdominal pain, scleral icterus, and jaundice, in addition to nonspecific viral symptoms such as fatigue, malaise, and loss of appetite. **(B)** Influenza virus, the agent of the "flu," is an orthomyxovirus. The genome consists of segments of negative-sense, single-stranded RNA, not

DNA. **(C)** Measles virus is a paramyxovirus and is a negative-sense, single-stranded RNA virus, not DNA. It is the agent of measles. **(E)** West Nile virus is a flavivirus arbovirus (arthropod- or mosquito-borne arboviruses). The genome is positive-sense, single-stranded RNA, not DNA. It usually causes a febrile flu-like viral syndrome but may be complicated by encephalitis and neurological abnormalities.

In children, such as this boy, the main agents of bacterial conjunctivitis are *S. pneumoniae* and *H. influenzae*. Moreover, this case is more likely to be viral conjunctivitis rather than bacterial conjunctivitis due to the serous discharge rather than mucopurulent discharge, which is typical of bacterial conjunctivitis and the presence of the preauricular lymphadenopathy, which is characteristic of viral conjunctivitis.

29. Correct: Adenovirus (A)

(A) Adenovirus is a nonenveloped, double-stranded DNA virus that affects patients of all ages. In children, adenovirus often causes pharyngoconjunctival fever, as in this case. Outbreaks of pharyngoconjunctival fever are associated with swimming in lakes or swimming pools. Adenovirus may also infect the cornea, leading to epidemic keratoconjunctivitis. Additionally, adenovirus, along with enterovirus and coxsackie viruses may be involved in acute hemorrhagic conjunctivitis. Adenovirus is not only an agent of ocular infections but may also cause other infections. It is one of the most common viral agents of pharyngitis and also causes a variety of other respiratory infections, gastrointestinal infections, and hemorrhagic cystitis. Adenovirus is highly contagious and is transmitted by respiratory droplets, fecal-orally, direct person-to-person contact, and through fomites. **(B)** *Chlamydia trachomatis* and serotypes A, B, Ba, and C are the agents of trachoma, which is the leading cause of blindness worldwide. Infections are hyperendemic in the Middle East and Africa and are transmitted by direct contact with an infected individual or fomites or from a fly which may carry the pathogen from person to person. It is unlikely, given this boy's travel history and presentation, that this infection is attributable to *C. trachomatis*. Trachoma starts as a follicular conjunctivitis. The classical finding is the roughening or follicles of the inner surface of eyelids. If the eyelids are severely irritated and inflamed, the eyelashes may turn in and rub against the cornea, which may cause scarring and eventually lead to vision loss and even blindness. **(C)** *Fusarium* is a fungal pathogen and an agent of keratitis, especially in contact lens wearers. This boy does not wear contact lenses. Additionally, manifestations of keratitis most often include eye pain and sensitivity to light. This infection is therefore more likely to be caused by adenovirus rather than *Fusarium*. **(D)** *Loa loa* is a parasite (filariarial nematode), and infections are usually limited to parts of Africa. This boy has not travelled, so loiasis is unlikely. *Loa loa* is transmitted by the bite of a deerfly, which is also called a mango fly. Infections are often asymptomatic but subcutaneous swellings, also referred to as calabar swellings, may be seen, especially on the face and the extremities. Often infections are diagnosed as the worm migrates to the eye, which may result in inflammation of the eye and surrounding area. **(E)** *Staphylococcus aureus* is a common cause of conjunctivitis, especially in adults.

30. Correct: *Neisseria gonorrhoeae* (C)

(C) At 2 days old, this patient is most likely affected by gonococcal ophthalmia neonatorum, a serious neonatal eye infection acquired through passage from a cervix and vagina infected with the sexually transmitted organism, *Neisseria gonorrhoeae*. Neonatal eye infections with this pathogen usually occur within the first 24 to 48 hours after birth. *N. gonorrhoeae* is a gram-negative diplococcus which can cause urethritis, vaginitis, cervicitis, septic arthritis, tenosynovitis, and vesiculopustular rash in adults. However, a significant percentage of infections in both males and females are asymptomatic, allowing undetected passage to not only sexual partners but also to babies delivered vaginally. The typical presentation of neonatal eye infections includes copious, thick, purulent discharge. Routine prenatal screening and treatment of gonorrhea and other sexually transmitted infections is recommended. **(A)** *Candida albicans* is a yeast that causes vaginitis in otherwise healthy females or serious infections in immunocompromised patients. Vertical transmission from mom to baby may occur but conjunctivitis is not a common finding of neonatal candidiasis. Neonatal candidiasis may be limited to the skin and mucous membranes (thrush, diaper rash) or cause serious infections such as meningitis, endophthalmitis (infection inside the globe itself), endocarditis, or urinary tract infections. **(B)** *Chlamydia trachomatis* is an obligate intracellular, sexually transmitted pathogen. Like *N. gonorrhoeae*, this pathogen can be vertically transmitted and is frequently associated with neonatal conjunctivitis. However, the key factor differentiating neonatal eye infections is that infections with *C. trachomatis* usually occur 5 to 14 days after birth, whereas infections with *N. gonorrhoeae* typically occur 24 to 48 hours after birth. Another factor that aids in differentiating these infections is that the ocular discharge associated with chlamydial neonatal conjunctivitis is less purulent and more watery than that of gonorrhea. Again, screening pregnant women for gonorrhea and chlamydia during the first prenatal care visit can facilitate appropriate management to prevent ophthalmia neonatorum. **(D)** *Streptococcus agalactiae* or β-hemolytic group B strep (GBS) is a vertically transmitted organism from mother to baby during vaginal delivery and is associated with high neonatal morbidity and mortality. However, GBS usually causes neonatal sepsis, meningitis, or pneumonia, but not typically conjunctivitis;

hence, this answer is incorrect. Women are screened for GBS using ano-vaginal swabs between 35 and 37-week gestation and if positive, they are given prophylactic penicillin hours before vaginal delivery. (E) *Trichomonas vaginalis* is a protozoan parasite that is sexually transmitted and may also be vertically transmitted to the fetus. Vertical transmission of this pathogen is mainly associated with preterm birth. Conjunctivitis is not a typical finding associated with neonatal infections.

31. Correct: Pseudounipolar primary somatosensory neurons (C)

(C) This patient is most likely affected by herpes simplex virus (HSV) keratitis. This is an inflammation and infection of the cornea that requires reactivation from latency and usually involves HSV-1 more than HSV-2. HSV keratitis is a serious and common cause of corneal blindness worldwide. The HSV itself is initially acquired through contact with infected secretions from mucous membranes (oral or genital). After episodic active lesions have resolved, the virus remains latent in the pseudounipolar primary somatosensory neuron cell bodies, which reside in the spinal dorsal root and trigeminal ganglia. Stress (which increases serum cortisol), topical or systemic corticosteroids, UV light, and trauma can lead to virus reactivation and symptoms. In the case of HSV keratitis, slit-lamp examination and fluorescein staining of the eye classically show punctate and diffusely branching "dendritic" superficial ulcers involving the corneal epithelium. Treatment usually involves antiviral topical eye drops. (A) α-Lower motor neurons of the anterior horns of the spinal cord gray matter are destroyed by polio virus, an enterovirus of the picornavirus family. Polio can cause a febrile illness that can culminate in flaccid paralysis. (B) Peripheral blood mononuclear cells, specifically B cell lymphocytes, are home to latent Epstein–Barr virus (EBV; also called HHV-4). EBV can cause infectious mononucleosis in immunocompetent patients and other diseases, including lymphoma, nasopharyngeal carcinoma, and hairy leukoplakia. (D) Segmented neutrophils may harbor several pathogens including latent cytomegalovirus (CMV) (also called HHV-5). CMV can cause infectious mononucleosis in immunocompetent patients and a variety of serious infections in immunocompromised patients, including esophagitis, hepatitis, colitis, retinitis, and pneumonia. (E) Endothelial cells are home to latent HHV-8, the causative agent of Kaposi sarcoma. Classically, Kaposi sarcoma is seen in patients with HIV/AIDS.

32. Correct: Cytomegalovirus (CMV) (B)

(B) Since this man is not currently taking his HIV drug regimen, there is a high likelihood that his CD4+ count is low. His ocular presentation of painless, monocular vision loss with blurriness, scotomata (blind spots), and photopsias (flashes or speckles of light) is classic for cytomegalovirus (CMV) retinitis.

Floaters are also common. Funduscopic examination would most likely show yellow–white, hemorrhagic, retinal lesions. CMV retinitis is a serious complication of AIDS as it can lead to rapid blindness if not treated in a timely manner. Treatment usually includes the antiviral ganciclovir. Most often CMV infections occur when the CD4+ T cell count is less than 50 cells/mL. See Appendix M for a list of the common pathogens associated with HIV/AIDS. (A) *Candida albicans* is an opportunistic yeast that is seen in AIDS patients. The most common type of infections associated with HIV and AIDS include thrush and esophagitis. While *Candida* can infect the eye, it most often causes endophthalmitis. (C) In AIDS patients, Epstein–Barr virus (EBV) is associated with primary CNS lymphoma. Additionally, EBV can cause infectious mononucleosis in immunocompetent patients and other diseases, including lymphoma, nasopharyngeal carcinoma, and hairy leukoplakia. Ocular pathology is uncommon with EBV. (D) Human herpes virus-8 (HHV-8) is the causative agent of Kaposi sarcoma. This herpes virus infects vascular endothelial cells and can lead to cutaneous or visceral purple-colored, fleshy, vascular lesions throughout the body. Eye involvement, however, is less likely. (E) *Pseudomonas aeruginosa* classically causes a severe keratitis in patients who wear contact lenses for prolonged, uninterrupted periods of time. This aerobic gram-negative rod adheres to the corneal epithelium and infiltrates, causing pain and visual changes. Retinitis would be unusual.

33. Correct: Spherule containing numerous endospores (D)

(D) This patient has coccidioidomycosis also known as "Valley Fever," caused by *Coccidioides immitis*. This is an endemic mycosis that occurs in the Southwestern United States. It is a self-limited illness in patients who do not have a cell-mediated immune deficiency. Patients are often asymptomatic but can have fever, cough, arthralgias ("desert rheumatism"), and erythema nodosum. Approximately, half of the patients with coccidioidomycoses have negative chest X-rays. This pathogen is dimorphic and can exist as both a yeast and mold. *C. immitis* will grow as fungi (hyphae with arthrospores, see image [i]) at 25°C, but appear as yeast (spherules with endospores, see image [ii]) at 37°C and in human tissue. (A) *Cryptococcus neoformans* is a heavily encapsulated yeast (image [iii]) that can grow on Sabouraud dextrose agar. It is not dimorphic and is known for causing meningitis in AIDS patients with a CD4 less than 200 cells/μL. (B) The fungus *Aspergillus fumigatus* can be described as having septate, branching hyphae (image [iv]). This pathogen is not dimorphic. They are often seen as an aspergilloma on CT in immunocompromised patients with respiratory symptoms. (C) Small yeast cells inside macrophages (image [v]) describe the yeast form of the dimorphic fungus *Histoplasma capsulatum*, which is seen in human tissue. Histoplasmosis is endemic to the Mississippi and Ohio River valleys. The fungal form that is seen at 25°C has septate hyphae with characteristic tuberculate microconidia (image [vi]). **(E)** Broad-based budding yeast describes *Blastomyces dermatitidis* (image [vii]), a dimorphic fungus. Blastomycosis is not seen in the Southwestern United States. At 25°C the fungal form appears as septate hyphae with round, pear-shaped conidia and at 37°C yeast forms are seen.

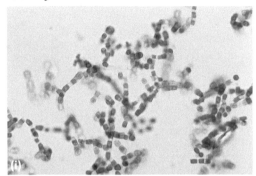

Source: CDC/Dr. Lucille K. Georg

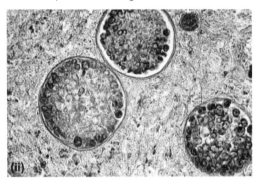

Source: CDC/Dr. Libero Ajello

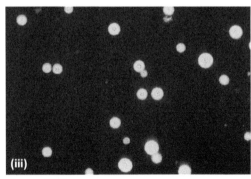

Source: CDC

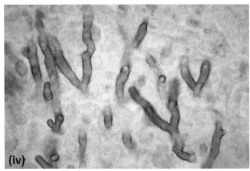

Source: CDC/Armed Forces Institute of Pathology (AFIP); Dr. Hardin

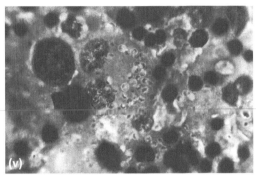

Source: CDC/Dr. Lucille K. Georg

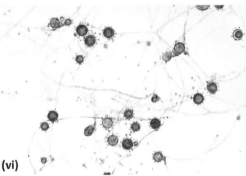

(vi)
Source: CDC/Dr. Libero Ajello

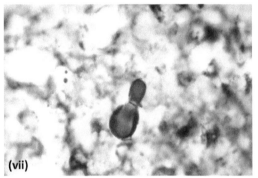

(vii)
Source: CDC/Dr. Libero Ajello

34. Correct: Enveloped, single-stranded RNA virus (D)

(D) Middle East respiratory syndrome (MERS) is caused by the MERS coronavirus and causes a syndrome like the SARS coronavirus. Coronaviruses are enveloped, single-stranded RNA viruses with positive-sense, linear RNA. **(A)** Herpesviruses, which include VZV, HSV-1, HSV-2, EBV, and CMV, are enveloped, double-stranded DNA viruses. **(B)** There are no medically significant examples of enveloped, double-stranded RNA viruses. **(C)** There are no medically significant examples of enveloped, single-stranded DNA viruses. **(E)** The adenovirus family contains double-stranded, nonenveloped DNA viruses. **(F)** Parvovirus, the smallest DNA virus, is the virus family that contains nonenveloped, single-stranded DNA virus. **(G)** The reovirus family is comprised of nonenveloped, double-stranded RNA viruses. Rotavirus is a member of this virus family. **(H)** Picornaviruses, hepevirus, and caliciviruses are all nonenveloped, single-stranded RNA viruses.

35. Correct: Inhibition of folic acid synthesis (D)

(D) This patient has a CD4 count less than 200 cells/μL, which puts him at risk for *Pneumocystis jirovecii* pneumonia. Trimethoprim–sulfamethoxazole is the treatment of choice and is an inhibitor of folic acid synthesis. The patient's medical history, fever, severe dyspnea, tachypnea, nonproductive cough, hypoxemia, positive (1-3)-β-D-glucan, low CD4 count, and a chest X-ray displaying bilateral interstitial infiltrates all strongly support a presumptive diagnosis of *Pneumocystis* pneumonia. Diagnosis is often confirmed by bronchoalveolar lavage (BAL). *Pneumocystis jirovecii* is a yeast that does not appear on Gram or KOH stains. Cysts or trophozoites can be detected by Giemsa or methenamine silver staining. Prednisone is often added when the patient demonstrates significant hypoxemia (oxygen saturation < 92%) or widened A–a gradient, so adjunctive steroids would also be indicated in this patient. Note: (1-3)-β-D-glucan is a nonspecific test diagnostic assay for fungal pathogens. (1-3)-β-D-glucan is a component of the fungal cell wall. Notable examples of fungi that are negative for this test include *Cryptococcus neoformans* and the zygomycetes. *P. jirovecii* may be positive for this test but it is not considered a typical yeast with a typical cell wall. See Appendix M for a list of common infections associated with HIV/AIDS. **(A)** Azithromycin's and ethambutol's mechanisms of action are described in answer choice A. This is the first-line therapy for nontuberculous mycobacterial infections (e.g., *Mycobacterium avium-intracellular* complex [MAC]). AIDS patients typically do not get MAC infections until their CD4 count is below 50. **(B, C)** Answer choices B and C describe antifungal agents. There is no evidence of systemic fungal infection and no aspergilloma was seen on CT scan. Answer choice B describes the mechanism of action of amphotericin B. This agent is a polyene that binds to ergosterol in the fungal cell membrane. This binding results in the formation of a pore, allowing cell contents to leak out, which eventually leads to cell death. Answer choice C describes the action of azoles, such as fluconazole, itraconazole, voriconazole, and isuvuconazole. Azoles indirectly inhibit the ergosterol synthesis pathway by inhibiting cytochrome P450 enzyme. **(E)** The four mechanisms of action being described in answer choice E are **R**ifampin, **I**soniazid, **P**yrazinamide, and **E**thambutol, respectively. These four drugs, often referred to collectively as RIPE therapy, are the drugs of choice for patients with tuberculosis. (TB). This patient did not have radiologic or laboratory (negative interferon-gamma release assay) findings consistent with TB.

36. Correct: Does not replicate well at 37°C (A)

(A) Rhinovirus replicates better at 33°C rather than 37°C, like most pathogenic organisms. This is why it primarily affects the cooler conjunctivae and nasopharyngeal mucosa. **(B)** Rhinovirus is acid labile, which means that it is destroyed when it comes into contact with stomach acid. This does not explain the rarity of lower respiratory illness. **(C)** Rhinovirus is not enveloped. Rhinoviruses belong to the picronavirus family, which are nonenveloped, single-stranded, positive-sense, RNA viruses. **(D)** Rhinovirus enters host cells by binding the cell surface receptor ICAM-1. It is present in many cells throughout the body, including lung parenchyma. It is primarily the increased temperature of the lung that leads to the decreased incidence of lower respiratory tract rhinovirus infections.

37. Correct: RNA virus (E)

(E) This child most likely has laryngotracheitis also known as croup, caused by parainfluenza virus. Parainfluenza virus is an enveloped, RNA virus belonging to the paramyxovirus family. Infections most commonly occur in children between the ages 1 and 3 and more often in boys. A barking cough and inspiratory stridor are usually mentioned in clinical scenarios of croup. The steeple sign on X-ray is diagnostic of this infection. **(A)** *Haemophilus influenzae* type b (Hib) is a gram-negative coccobacillus that causes epiglottitis. Vaccination against this capsular subtype has significantly reduced the incidence of Hib infections. Epiglottitis is a medical emergency. Children often present in distress with high fever, drooling, and dysphasia. Often the child will be described as having a muffled cry or muffled voice. A cherry red epiglottis is seen on direct visualization. The thumbprint sign is appreciated on lateral neck X-ray. **(B)** *Streptococcus pneumoniae* is an example of a gram-positive diplococcus. Although known to cause otitis media and upper and lower respiratory tract illness, it would be rare for *S. pneumoniae* to cause an isolated case of laryngotracheitis. **(C)** *Corynebacterium diphtheriae* is a gram-positive rod. Clinical features of diphtheria include pseudomembranous pharyngitis and myocarditis. Vaccination against its exotoxin prevents diphtheria and infections are rare in countries with routine childhood vaccination programs. **(D)** Adenovirus is a DNA virus that can cause laryngotracheitis and other respiratory infections, but parainfluenza is by far the most common etiology of croup.

38. Correct: Antigenically variable pili (A)

(A) This woman's infection is caused by *Neisseria gonorrhoeae*, a gram-negative diplococcus. *Neisseria* have pili that are capable of antigenic and phase variation, which assist the organism in evading the host immune response. *N. gonorrhoeae* is the causative agent of the sexually transmitted infection gonorrhea, which may affect the genital tract, oral cavity and eyes. The pathogen may also disseminate from the original site resulting in septic arthritis. In this case, the woman has pharyngitis and the organism grows on Thayer–Martin agar, which is a selective media for pathogenic *Neisseria* including *N. gonorrhoeae* and *N. meningitidis*. **(B)** *Corynebacterium diphtheriae* is the causative agent of diphtheria and produces an exotoxin that inactivates elongation factor-2 (EF-2). In this infection a greyish exudate or pseudomembrane covers the pharynx. This organism does not grow on Thayer–Martin agar. An example of selective media for *C. diphtheriae* is cysteine tellurite agar. **(C)** Herpes viruses remain latent for life and Herpes simplex virus-1 (HSV-1) may remain latent in the trigeminal ganglia. HSV-1 and HSV-2 may cause infections in the oral cavity resulting in vesicular lesions with minimal or no exudate. Viruses are obligate intercellular pathogens and do not grow on artificial media such as Thayer–Martin agar. Viruses require live cells for growth. **(D)** M protein is a characteristic of *Streptococcus pyogenes* (group A streptococci). This protein is on the cell surface of *S. pyogenes* and is an adhesion and also aids the organism in avoiding the host immune system by binding to the Fc portion of IgG. *S. pyogenes* is the main bacterial pathogen of infectious pharyngitis. This organism is β-hemolytic on Blood agar. **(E)** Many organisms have a polysaccharide capsule, including *N. meningitidis*. However, *N. gonorrhoeae* does not have a capsule.

39. Correct: Mumps (D)

(D) This girl is most likely to have mumps, especially since she is not vaccinated. Mumps is part of the paramyxovirus family (such as parainfluenza virus and measles virus) and is a single-stranded negative-sense, RNA virus. The classic sign of mumps is parotitis or inflammation of the parotid glands. Complications of mumps include orchitis, oophoritis, and aseptic meningitis. **(A)** Diphtheria is caused by the gram-positive rod, *Corynebacterium diphtheriae*. Infections may be prevented with appropriate vaccination, so this child is at risk for contracting this disease. However, the presentation of diphtheria is not consistent with the findings seen in this case. The classic presentation of diphtheria includes the formation of a pseudomembrane, a grayish-white membrane that covers the pharynx that is composed of bacteria, debris, neutrophils, and fibrin. Another telltale sign of infection with this pathogen is severe cervical lymphadenopathy that gives individuals a "bull's-neck" appearance. **(B)** Thrombophlebitis of the internal jugular vein or Lemierre's syndrome is an infection that is mainly caused by the anaerobic gram-negative rod, *Fusobacterium necrophorum*. This infection is most often preceded by pharyngitis that progresses to a peritonsillar abscess. Fever, respiratory distress, neck and throat pain, and swelling over the jugular vein and jaw are common clinical findings. There is not a vaccine to prevent this infection. The clinical findings of this case and the unvaccinated state of the patient indicate that Lemierre's syndrome is not as likely as mumps to be the diagnosis. **(C)** Ludwig's angina is an infection of the submandibular space and is most often caused by oral anaerobes including *Peptostreptococcus*, *Fusobacterium nucleatum*, and *Actinomyces*. The infection starts in the mouth and spreads to the submandibular

space. There is no abscess formation and typical clinical manifestations included drooling, dysphagia and stiff neck. The findings in the case described in the question stem are not consistent with Ludwig's angina. **(E)** Sjörgen's syndrome is an immune mediated disease that may cause enlargement of the lacrimal and salivary glands. Typical symptoms include dry eyes and mouth. The clinical manifestations and the immune status of the patient in this case indicate that Sjörgen's syndrome is unlikely to be the diagnosis.

40. Correct: Neutrophils (E)

(E) *Aspergillus* is a fungus that may cause cutaneous infections, pulmonary infections, and disseminated extrapulmonary infections. The hyphae of this organism are quite distinct (see image at the end of this answer) and are either Y-shaped or 45-degree angles as described in the question stem. Invasive infections with *Aspergillus* are associated with immunocompromised individuals, especially neutropenic patients. This is because the innate immune response to this pathogen is mediated by neutrophils. The most common species involved in clinical infections are *A. fumigatus* and *A. flavus*. Pulmonary infections include pulmonary aspergillosis in which the organism initiates cavity formation in the lungs or a fungus ball (aspergillmona) in which the fungus invades a preexisting pulmonary cavity. **(A, B, C, D)** The primary innate immune response to *Aspergillus* is neutrophils (also called polymorphonuclear cells [PMNs]); hence, basophils, eosinophils, lymphocytes, and macrophages are incorrect answer choices.

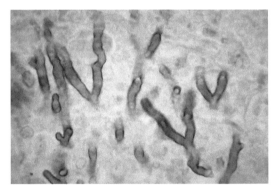

Source: CDC/Armed Forces Institute of Pathology (AFIP); Dr. Hardin

41. Correct: Capsule (A)

(A) MacConkey agar is selective media for enteric gram-negative rods. This media is also differential and shows lactose fermentation reactions. Lactose positive (fermenter) is pink on MacConkey while lactose negative (non-fermenter) is clear or colorless (see image at the end of this answer). Hence, the causative agent of this infection is a lactose-positive gram-negative rod. *Klebsiella pneumoniae* is a lactose-positive, gram-negative rod that belongs to the *Enterobacteriaceae* family. This organism causes a variety of infections including wound, urinary tract, and respiratory infections. Respiratory infections may present as consolidation or "typical" (consolidation) pneumonia, such as in this case, and a key clue is the presence of blood-tinged sputum, often described as "currant-jelly" like. One of the main pathogenesis features of this organism is the presence of a capsule that causes this organism to appear mucoid on culture media. **(B)** M protein is an important virulence factor for *Streptococcus pyogenes*. M protein plays a role in adhesion to the host cell and also in the development of the immunological sequelae of *S. pyogenes* infections. *S. pyogenes* is gram-positive coccus that does not grow on MacConkey agar. Furthermore, *S. pyogenes* is not a typical agent of pneumonia. Therefore, this answer choice is incorrect. **(C)** Pneumolysin is produced by *Streptococcus pneumoniae*, which is the most common bacterial agent of pneumonia. This pathogen is a gram-positive coccus in pairs and chains and does not grow on MacConkey agar. Pneumolysin plays a role in the lysis of host cells and evasion of the host immune system. **(D)** Pyoverdin is a green pigment produced by *Pseudomonas aeruginosa*, a gram-negative bacillus that acts as a siderophore. This organism does cause pneumonia, but is most often associated with ventilator-associated pneumonia (VAP) and respiratory infections in cystic fibrosis patients. *P. aeruginosa* is lactose negative (non-fermenter) and would be clear or colorless on MacConkey agar, not pink as seen in the image in the question stem. **(E)** Two clinically significant pathogens that produce a toxin that inhibits elongation factor-2 (EF-2) and therefore inhibit protein synthesis are *Corynebacterium diphtheriae* and *P. aeruginosa*. *C. diphtheriae* is a gram-positive rod that would not grow on MacConkey agar. The classic presentation of diphtheria includes the formation of a pseudomembrane, a grayish-white membrane that covers the pharynx that is composed of bacteria, debris, neutrophils, and fibrin. The symptoms of this case do not resemble diphtheria. *P. aeruginosa* is also incorrect as explained in the explanation for answer choice D.

Lactose positive (fermenter)   Lactose negative (non-fermenter)

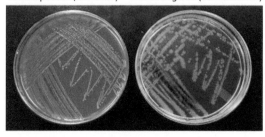

42. Correct: Doxycycline (B)

(B) This woman has pneumonia, most likely atypical pneumonia as indicated by the patchy areas of consolidation. Her work in the aviary with birds puts her at risk for pathogens associated with birds, including *Chlamydophila (Chlamydia) psittacosis*, the most likely agent of this infection. Infections

are often referred to as parrot fever or psittacosis. *Chlamydia* are obligate intracellular organisms that do not Gram stain; hence, the routine culture and Gram stain are negative. The antibiotic of choice to treat infections with *C. psittacosis* is doxycycline (answer choice B). Doxycycline is a tetracycline that has broad spectrum activity. This drug targets the 30S ribosome and inhibits bacterial translation. **(A)** Amoxicillin–clavulanate is a β-lactam antibiotic (amoxicillin) plus a β-lactmase inhibitor (clavulanate). This agent is effective against a number of respiratory pathogens including some anaerobes, streptococci, *Haemophilus influenzae*, and some *Enterobacteriaceae*. It is not effective against *Chlamydophila (Chlamydia) psittacosis*. **(C)** Itraconazole is an antifungal agent that is part of the azole family, which inhibit ergosterol synthesis. A fungal pathogen that is associated with birds and can be treated with itraconazole is *Histoplasma capsulatum*. Symptoms of acute pulmonary histoplasmosis include fever, cough, chills, chest pain, and a rash. Chest X-ray often shows pulmonary nodules. This infection is most often seen east of the Mississippi River in the Ohio and Mississippi Valley; while infections may occur in healthy individuals, immunocompromised patients are at increased risk. This woman lives in San Diego and is otherwise healthy. Chest X-ray in this case shows atypical pneumonia and not nodules; hence, this infection is more likely due to *C. psittacosis*. **(D)** Oseltamivir is used in the management of infections due to influenza virus. Some strains of influenza, mainly influenza A virus subtype H5N1 are associated with birds. This infection could possibly be due to influenza virus; however, influenza peaks in the winter months and this woman presents during the summer. Hence, this answer choice is less likely. **(E)** Penicillin G is a β-lactam antibiotic that inhibits cell wall synthesis. This agent is effective against several pathogens, including *Streptococcus pneumoniae* a common agent of pneumonia. *S. pneumoniae* grows well on bacteriology media and would also most likely be seen on Gram stain. Penicillin G is not an effective agent for *C. psittacosis*.

43. Correct: *Paragonimus westermani* (C)

(C) This man is infected with *Paragonimus westermani*, a fluke that is most often seen in East Asian countries, such as Japan and is transmitted from undercooked crustaceans such as crabs or crayfish. The image in the question stem shows an ovum of *P. westermani*. Early infections start with fever and GI symptoms. This is due to the presence of the pathogen in the GI tract. As the pathogen migrates to the lungs, pulmonary symptoms are noted including cough, dyspnea, and chest pain. Infections may then progress to late infections, in which the adult worm resides in the lungs leading inflammation and fibrosis. These late infections may closely resemble tuberculosis. Infections may be treated with praziquantel.

213

It is the eggs (ova) that are the diagnostic form of *P. westermani*. The life cycle begins in a snail which contains the miracida. This form infects crustaceans and develops into metacercaria. Humans ingest crustaceans and the metacercaria excyst in upper GI tract and enter peritoneal cavity. The metacercaria migrate to the lungs and develops into adults. The adults lay eggs and the eggs are coughed up as seen in this case. **(A)** *Ascaris lumbricoides* is a nematode that may infects humans following ingestion of contaminated food and water (contaminated with human waste containing the ova). Infections are seen worldwide. During the life cycle of this parasite, the larva migrates to the lungs and matures and there is the possibility that they may be coughed up. The patient is often symptomatic or has mild symptoms. Usually the larvae are the form seen in the sputum (not the eggs as in this case). Following maturation in the lung, the larvae are swallowed and mature into adults in the GI tract where they lay eggs (see image [i] at the end of this answer). The eggs are usually the diagnostic form. **(B)** *Echinococcus granulosus* is a tapeworm that is an accidental parasite of man. Dogs may be infected, following ingestion of larva that may be in the viscera of sheep, goats, and pigs. Humans are then infected after ingestion of food, water, or soil contaminated with infected dog feces. There is a higher incidence in Africa, Europe, Asia, and Central and South America, so this answer choice is plausible based on this man's travel history. However, the classic feature of infection with this organism is the formation of cysts within tissue, most often the liver and occasionally the lungs. The parasite is contained with the cyst and the finding of ova in the sputum would not occur. **(D)** Diagnosis of *Strongyloides stercoralis* may occur following identification of the larval (see image [ii] at the end of this answer) form in respiratory specimens. The ovum of this parasite is rarely seen clinically. The filariform larvae live in the soil and can infect humans by entering through intact skin, usually through the feet. The larva migrates to lungs for further maturation and may cause pulmonary symptoms and may also be coughed up. The larvae are then swallowed and develop into adult worms in small intestine. The adults lay eggs and eggs develop into larvae and it is the rhabditiform larva that is passed in stool and is usually the diagnostic form of this parasite. This is unlikely to be the cause of the infection described in this case because the man most likely was infected following ingestion, not skin penetration, and ova, and not larva, are seen in the sputum. **(E)** Some *Schistosoma* species, such as *S. japonicum* are mainly seen in Asia; hence, this answer choice is definitely reasonable. However, schistomsomes enter the human body via penetration, not ingestion. Once the cercariae penetrate human skin, they enter circulation and then migrate to venous plexus. While in the circulation the organisms may pass through the heart and

liver. There is the possibility that the eggs (see image [iii] at the end of this answer) may be seen in respiratory specimens during this time. Typically, respiratory symptoms are not the major features of this infection. Febrile illness (Katayama fever) or urinary or GI symptoms are typical manifestations.

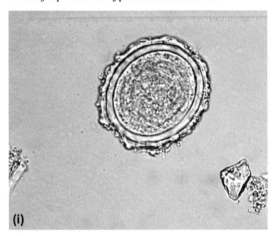

(i)

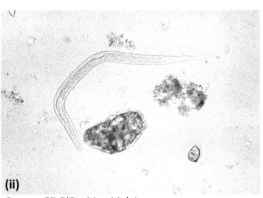

(ii)

Source: CDC/Dr. Mae Melvin

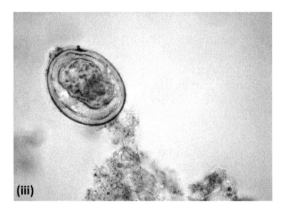

(iii)

44.   Correct: Positive heterophile antibody (D)

(D) This boy likely has infectious mononucleosis, which can be caused by Epstein–Barr virus (EBV) or cytomegalovirus (CMV). The heterophile antibody test (or monospot test) evaluates the presence of the heterophile antibody, a nonspecific antibody. EBV activates B cells and stimulates a wide repertoire of antibodies and one of these antibodies is an

IgM antibody, referred to as the heterophile antibody (reacts with something other than EBV viral proteins). This antibody does not react with EBV-specific antigens but recognizes antigenic determinants on sheep, horse, and cattle erythrocytes. In EBV mononucleosis the heterophile antibody is positive whereas in CMV mononucleosis the heterophile antibody is negative. EBV is a herpes virus and a double-stranded DNA virus. EBV may present as pharyngitis with severe lethargy as in this case. Posterior lymphadenopathy is a classic finding of EBV mononucleosis. Often atypical lymphocytes are present in the peripheral blood as seen in the figure in the question stem. EBV is also associated with nasopharyngeal carcinoma, Burkitt's lymphoma, and other malignancies. **(A)** β-Hemolytic growth on blood agar is a description of several bacterial pathogens, notably *Streptococcus pyogenes*, which is a possible causative agent of this infection. Streptococcal pharyngitis is an acute infection that may present in a similar manner. The findings of atypical lymphocytes indicate that EBV is a more likely the pathogenic agent and hence answer choice D would be a better answer. **(B)** Elek test is an immunodiffusion test that is rarely performed clinically, but is the classic test for the detection of *Corynebacterium diphtheriae* toxin. Diphtheria may present as pharyngitis with a pseudomembrane on the pharynx; however, this is an unlikely diagnosis in this case as this boy is vaccinated. **(C)** The classic organisms that grow well on chocolate agar and show little to no growth on blood agar include *Haemophilus* and *Neisseria*. *H. influenzae* is an agent of respiratory and head and neck infections, especially pneumonia, otitis media, sinusitis, epiglottitis. *N. meningitis* usually causes meningitis or septicemia and *N. gonorrhoeae* is a sexually transmitted pathogen. Based on the clinical manifestations and the CBC showing atypical lymphocytes, this infection is more likely to be due to EBV rather than *Haemophilus* or *Neisseria*. **(E)** DNase antibody is a serological test that is often utilized in the diagnosis of post *Streptococcus pyogenes* infections, especially rheumatic fever. It is not utilized for the diagnosis of *S. pyogenes* pharyngitis,

which is best diagnosed with a rapid antigen assay or culture (which remains the gold standard). DNase antibody would not aid in the diagnosis of EBV.

45. Correct: Sucrose to lactic acid (D)

(D) Cavities, also referred to as tooth decay or dental caries, are the localized destruction of dental enamel by plaque bacteria. The pathogen that is most often associated with dental caries is *Streptococcus mutans*. The pathogenic mechanism of *S. mutans* involves the conversion of sucrose to lactic acid (answer choice D). *S. mutans* and other bacteria reside within the supragingival plaque and when exposed to sucrose (usually via diet) *S. mutans* becomes cariogenic. The organism can use sucrose to produce glucans, which allows the bacteria to adhere to the tooth surface, form a biofilm and cause decay in the underlying structures. The organism can also produce lactic acid from sucrose and *S. mutans* is not only able to produce acid, but it can survive and grow in this low pH environment. Other bacteria that are also associated with dental carries include *Streptococcus sobrinus* and *Lactobacillus*. **(A)** The enzyme coagulase converts fibrinogen to fibrin. Coagulase is produced by *Staphylococcus aureus*, which is not involved in dental caries. **(B)** *Proprionibacterium* can ferment glucose to produce propionate, acetate, and carbon dioxide. *Proprionibacterium* is normal microbiota of the skin and is most often a contaminant. However, this organism can cause infections including acne and more serious infections in immunocompromised patients or infections following procedures in which skin flora may seed a normally sterile site. *Proprionibacterium* is not an agent of dental caries. **(C)** Catalase converts hydrogen peroxide to water and oxygen. Streptococci, including *Streptococcus mutans*, do not produce catalase. **(E)** Urease is an enzyme that facilitates the conversion of urea to ammonium creating an alkaline pH. Urease is produced by several pathogenic bacteria including *Proteus*, *Ureaplasma*, *Nocardia*, *Cryptococcus*, *Helicobacter pylori* (helpful mnemonic, PUNCH), and *Staphylococcus saprophyticus*. Urease is not produced by *Streptococcus mutans*.

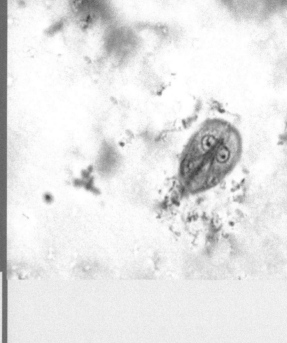

Chapter 10

Infections of the Esophagus, Stomach, Small and Large Bowel/Rectum, Liver, and Biliary Tree

Melphine M. Harriott

LEARNING OBJECTIVES

- ▶ Discuss the etiology, epidemiology, pathogenesis, clinical manifestations, complications, diagnosis, and treatment and prevention of:
    - infectious esophagitis and achalasia.
    - gastric ulcer disease.
    - infectious diarrhea and dysentery.
    - foodborne illness.
    - infectious diseases of the rectum.
    - hepatitis and other liver infections.
    - infectious of the bile duct.
    - kidney and urinary tract.
- ▶ Describe the laboratory diagnosis and antimicrobial testing methods for bacteria, viruses, fungi, yeast, and parasites.
- ▶ Discuss virulence mechanisms and correlate virulence mechanisms with specific pathogens.
- ▶ Discuss antimicrobial mechanism of action, spectrum of activity, common adverse effects, and resistance mechanisms.
- ▶ Describe the common HIV/AIDS-related opportunistic infections.
- ▶ Compare and contrast the different methods of sterilization and disinfection.
- ▶ Discuss the association between infectious agents and the development of malignancies.

10.1 Questions

Easy	Medium	Hard

1. A 40-year-old HIV-positive woman presents with heartburn and difficulty swallowing. Her temperature is 37.7°C (99.8°F). Physical examination reveals white patches in the posterior oral cavity. Endoscopy and histology show raised, white plaque-like lesions on the esophageal mucosa. Masses of hyphae and budding yeast are seen on a periodic acid–Schiff (PAS) stain. Her CD4 count is 86 cells/μL. Which of the following is the most likely mode of transmission for this infection?

A. Contact with cat feces

B. Displacement of microbiota

C. Fecal–oral

D. Oral secretions

E. Sexual

Consider the following case for questions 2 to 3:

A 38-year-old immigrant from Brazil presents with difficulty swallowing and chest pain. Her vitals and physical examination are unremarkable. Her chest X-ray shows a dilated esophagus and a barium swallow reveals narrowing of the distal esophagus. Manometry demonstrates a nonrelaxing esophageal sphincter and loss of peristaltic movement in the lower esophagus. Pertinent laboratory results include:

- *Trypanosoma cruzi* IgM: negative
- *Trypanosoma cruzi* IgG: positive

2. Which of the following findings is most likely to be in this woman's recent history?

A. Bloody stools with mucous and tenesmus

B. Circular red rash with central clearing

C. Paroxysms of fever and chills

D. Ulcerative skin lesion

E. Unilateral swelling of eyelid

3. The causative agent of this disease was most likely transmitted by a:

A. Chigger

B. Mosquito

C. Sandfly

D. Tick

E. Triatomine bug

Consider the following case for questions 4 to 5:

A 46-year-old woman presents to her primary care physician complaining of abdominal pain that has been worsening for the past 2 weeks. She states she also has frequent indigestion, nausea, vomiting, and lack of appetite. She denies diarrhea and blood in her stool. Her vitals are unremarkable. Physical examination reveals mild midepigastric tenderness. Endoscopy shows a 2 mm ulcer on the gastric antrum.

4. Detection of which of the following enzymes would best confirm the diagnosis?

A. Coagulase

B. Hyaluronidase

C. Phospholipase

D. Protease

E. Urease

5. The woman is given a 14-day regimen of lansoprazole, amoxicillin, and clarithromycin. She returns to her physician 5 weeks later for a follow-up appointment. Which of the following diagnostic tests would best confirm eradication of the pathogen?

A. Bacterial culture

B. Serum IgG testing

C. Stool Gram stain

D. Toxin analysis

E. Urea breath testing

Consider the following case for questions 6 to 8:

A 7-year-old boy is brought to the emergency department with a 3-day history of stomach ache and diarrhea. His father is concerned because the child noticed blood in his stool earlier that day. The previous weekend the family attended a picnic and consumed hamburgers. The boy's temperature is 36.1°C (97.9°F). Physical examination shows diffuse abdominal tenderness but no rebound tenderness or guarding. CBC demonstrates a leukocyte count of 14.2×10^9/L.

6. Which of the following pathogens produces a toxin with the same mechanism of action as the most likely agent of this infection?

A. *Clostridium tetani*

B. Enterotoxigenic *Escherichia coli* (ETEC)

C. *Shigella dysenteriae*

D. *Staphylococcus aureus*

E. *Vibrio cholerae*

7. One week later the boy develops complications from this infection. Which of the following conditions is most likely to be observed as a result of this complication?

A. Ascending paralysis

B. Joint pain

C. Pallor

D. Tonic–clonic seizures

E. Violaceous pretibial nodules

8. Growth on which of the following culture media would best confirm the identity of the causative agent?

A. Agar enriched with X and V factors

B. Agar supplemented with charcoal and yeast extract

C. Hektoen agar

D. MacConkey agar supplemented with sorbitol

E. Thiosulfate-citrate-bile salts-sucrose (TCBS) agar

Consider the following case for questions 9 and 10:

A 13-month-old infant in Ghana develops watery diarrhea. His mother brings him to the village clinic after she notices that he has been less active than normal. On examination, the child is restless and irritable. He is afebrile, his eyes appear slightly sunken, and skin turgor is poor. Stool from the boy grows a lactose positive (fermenter), sorbitol positive (fermenter) organism on MacConkey agar that grows best at 37°C.

9. Which of the following is the most likely causative agent?

A. *Campylobacter jejuni*

B. Enterohemorrhagic *Escherichia coli* (EHEC)

C. Enteropathogenic *Escherichia coli* (EPEC)

D. Rotavirus

E. *Shigella sonnei*

10. Which one of the following mechanisms is most likely contributing to this infection?

A. Destruction of microvilli

B. Endotoxin

C. Enterotoxin that inactivates actin polymerization

D. Exotoxin that inhibits protein synthesis

E. Invasion into host cell

11. A 19-year-old college student returns from spring break in Mexico with watery diarrhea. She claims she ate in reputable restaurants and not from street venders. She admits that she brushed her teeth with the faucet water in her hotel. Which of the following pathogens has a similar mechanism of pathogenesis as the most likely agent of this infection?

A. *Bacillus cereus*

B. *Clostridioides* (*Clostridium*) *difficile*

C. *Clostridium perfringens*

D. *Shigella dysenteriae*

E. *Staphylococcus aureus*

12. Five children (age range 2–3 years old) are sent home from a day care center with diarrhea and fever within a 2-day period. All of the children had more than 4 to 5 loose stools the day they were sent home. The next day, two of the day care workers call in sick with similar symptoms. One of the workers visits the urgent care clinic when she notices blood in her stool. Which of the following is the most likely causative agent?

A. Enteropathogenic *Escherichia coli* (EPEC)

B. Rotavirus

C. *Salmonella typhi*

D. *Shigella sonnei*

E. *Vibrio cholerae*

13. A 10-year-old boy presents with a 2-day history of bloody diarrhea, vomiting, stomach ache, and fever. On examination, his temperature is 38.8°C (101.9°F). His abdominal examination reveals right upper quadrant tenderness. A computed tomography (CT) scan rules out appendicitis. Laboratory results show elevated peripheral blood leukocytes and fecal leukocytes. After 2 days, the stool culture grows lactose negative (non-fermenter) organisms on MacConkey agar at 37°C. The unknown pathogen was later found to produce H_2S. Which of the following is the most likely to be part of his recent history?

A. Camping trip in the mountains

B. Contact with a sick dog

C. Hamburger eating contest

D. Field trip to the reptile zoo

E. Vacation to Mexico

14. A previously healthy 25-year-old woman presents with a 3-day history of fever, abdominal cramps, diarrhea, and vomiting. She denies hematochezia and has no previous medical issues. She states that about 5 days ago she ate an entire batch of uncooked cookie dough. Her temperature is 37.9°C (100.3°F). Physical examination reveals mild abdominal tenderness. Stool culture shows black colonies on Hektoen agar, and ova and parasite examination is negative. Which of the following is the most appropriate therapy for this patient?

A. Azithromycin
B. Ciprofloxacin
C. Metronidazole
D. Vancomycin
E. No antibiotic therapy should be administered

15. A previously healthy 40-year-old woman presents to the emergency department with diarrhea and severe abdominal pain. She has had 6 to 7 bowel movements per day for the past 3 days and during the last 24 hours has noticed blood in her stool. She states she had a fever and felt "flu-like" the first day of her illness but does not feel like that anymore. She attended a family picnic a week ago and ate grilled chicken. On examination, her temperature is 37.7°C (99.9°F). Physical examination reveals abdominal tenderness. The stool culture recovers curved gram-negative rods on selective media. Which of the following is a characteristic of the most likely causative agent of this infection?

A. Growth at 4°C
B. Growth at 42°C
C. Growth in strict anaerobic conditions
D. Growth in high salt concentration
E. Growth with green metallic sheen on eosin methylene blue (EMB) agar

16. A 5-year-old boy presents with a 2-day history of pronounced abdominal pain, bloody diarrhea, fever, and a sore throat. The family lives on a farm and drinks unpasteurized milk. The boy's temperature is 38.7°C (101.8°F). The boy's throat is erythematous and his tonsils are edematous. An abdominal examination reveals tenderness of the right lower quadrant and rebound with guarding. A CBC demonstrates elevated peripheral leukocytes. Fecal leukocytes are present and fecal occult blood is positive. The causative agent of this infection is most likely to infect the:

A. Duodenum
B. Gallbladder
C. Liver
D. Mesenteric lymph nodes
E. Stomach

17. A 54-year-old man presents with diarrhea of 3-day duration. He has had 8 to 9 bowel movements per day and has been periodically vomiting. The man returned 4 days ago from vacation in several South Asian countries. His temperature is 37.2°C (98.9°F) and his blood pressure is 92/63 mm Hg. On examination the man seems lethargic, his eyes are sunken, his skin feels cold and clammy, and his skin turgor is poor. Stool for culture is collected and an organism grows on selective media. A Gram stain from the colonies growing on this media is shown here:

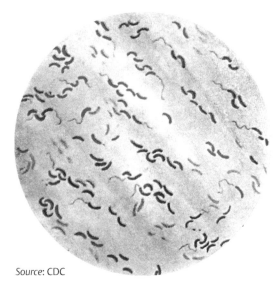

Source: CDC

Which of the following is most likely to be observed from this patient?

A. Blood in the stool
B. Clay-colored stool
C. Greasy stool
D. Mucous in the stool
E. White cells in the stool

Consider the following case for questions 18 to 19:

A 52-year-old man leaves work shortly after lunch with nausea, abdominal cramps, and vomiting. Early that morning he had consumed several chocolate éclairs at an office party. Several of his coworkers are also experiencing similar symptoms. By the next morning he is feeling fairly well and is able to return to work.

18. Which of the following is the most likely causative agent?

A. Aerobic gram-negative rods
B. Aerobic gram-positive rods with spores
C. Aerobic gram-positive cocci in clusters
D. Anaerobic gram-positive rods with spores
E. Microaerophilic curved gram-negative rods

19. Which one of the following factors is most likely mediating this infection?

A. Coagulase

B. Hyaluronidase

C. Protein A

D. Superantigen

E. Exfoliative toxin

20. A 23-year-old medical student wakes up in the middle of the night with abdominal pain, cramping, and watery diarrhea. He has had four bowel movements within 3 hours. He does not notice any blood in his stool and he does not feel feverish and is not vomiting. While he was on clerkship rotation the previous day, the hospital was celebrating Thanksgiving and he ate in the cafeteria. By early afternoon of the next day he is feeling better. Later, it is discovered that several other employees were also ill following the same meal. A toxin from an anaerobic gram-positive rod is identified from the tainted food. Which of the following foods is the most likely to be involved in the transmission of this infection?

A. Cream puffs

B. Gravy

C. Raw eggs

D. Shellfish

E. Soft cheese

21. A 46-year-old man suddenly feels ill and starts vomiting at 1:00 a.m. He continues vomiting approximately 2 to 3 times per hour for the next 4 hours. The man had leftover Chinese takeout for dinner the previous evening and consumed vegetable fried rice and beef lo mein. By the next afternoon he is feeling better. Which of the following is the most likely causative agent of this infection?

A. Aerobic gram-positive rod

B. Aerobic gram-positive cocci

C. Anaerobic gram-positive rod

D. Flagellated protozoan parasite

E. Single-stranded RNA virus

Consider the following case for questions 22 to 24:

A previously healthy 23-year-old man is admitted to the hospital following a motor vehicle collision. One week after his admission he develops watery diarrhea. He is on several medications including clindamycin. His temperature is 37.6°C (99.7°F). A CBC shows a leukocyte count of 13.8×10^9/L. Glutamate dehydrogenase (GDH) antigen and enzyme immunoassay (EIA) toxin analysis from a stool specimen are positive and confirm the diagnosis. The patient has no history of previous infection with this pathogen.

22. Which of the following is the most appropriate therapy?

A. Fecal transplant

B. Levofloxacin

C. Penicillin

D. Probiotics

E. Vancomycin

23. The most likely causative agent of this infection produces a toxin that:

A. Activates T cells

B. Depolymerizes actin

C. Hydrolyzes lecithin

D. Inhibits protein synthesis

E. Interacts with G protein

24. Which of the following would safely and effectively disinfect the surfaces of this patient's room?

A. Hypochlorite

B. Iodophor

C. Isopropanol

D. Phenol

E. Quaternary ammonium compound

25. A 61-year-old man presents with a 4-week history of watery diarrhea, weight loss and arthritic joint pain. He also reports he has noticed discoloration of his skin. He estimates he has lost 10 to 15 pounds in the past month. He has not travelled outside of the United States in 2 years. On examination, his temperature is 38.2°C (100.9°F). Hyperpigmentation of the skin on his forearm and neck are observed. Endoscopy reveals thickened mucosal folds in the small bowel, which are coated with patchy yellow plaques. A biopsy shows villous atrophy in the small bowel and PAS-positive and foamy macrophages in the lamina propria (see following image).

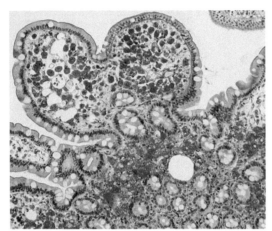

Source: Riede U, Werner M, Hrsg. Color Atlas of Pathology: Pathologic Principles · Associated Diseases · Sequela. 1st Edition. Thieme; 2004

Relevant laboratory results include:

- Stool culture: no pathogens isolated
- Ova and parasite examination: negative
- Acid-fast stains:
  - Stool specimen: negative
  - Biopsy specimen: negative
- Fecal fat: positive
- Fecal leukocyte: negative
- Fecal occult blood: negative
- HIV-1/2 antibody: negative
- HIV p24 antigen: negative
- CBC:
  - Leukocyte count: 15×10^9/L
  - Hemoglobin: 8.2 g/dL

Which of the following is the most likely diagnosis?

A. Crohn's disease

B. Histoplasmosis

C. *Mycobacterium avium-intracellulare* complex infection

D. Tropical sprue

E. Whipple's disease

26. A 48-year-old man presents with a 3-day history of abdominal pain, bloating, and fever. His history is significant for an appendectomy approximately 3 weeks prior to the onset of symptoms. His temperature is 38.8°C (101.9°F) and his heart rate is 130 beats per minute. A CBC shows elevated leukocytes. Abdominal CT scan shows fluid collection with air bubbles, suggestive of an abscess. After 2 days, blood cultures grow gram-negative rods in the anaerobic bottles but not the aerobic bottles. Which of the following is the most likely causative agent?

A. *Bacteroides fragilis*

B. *Clostridioides (Clostridium) difficile*

C. *Enterococcus faecalis*

D. *Escherichia coli*

E. *Peptostreptococcus magnus*

27. A 7-month-old infant presents to the emergency department in January with vomiting, fever and watery diarrhea of 2-day duration. The child's father states that although the baby has had more bowel movements than normal she has had fewer wet diapers. The baby attends day care 3 days a week. The infant's temperature is 39.4°C (103°F). On examination, the infant's eyes and fontanels are slightly sunken, she appears restless and her mucous membranes are dry. Which of the following would best confirm the diagnosis?

A. Culture at 42°C

B. Culture on MacConkey with sorbitol

C. Enzyme-linked immunoassay

D. Fecal leukocytes

E. Scotch tape preparation

28. An otherwise healthy 52-year-old woman presents with a 48-hour history of diarrhea and vomiting. She reports she feels more tired than usual and has a severe headache. She denies hematochezia. Three days prior to the onset of symptoms, she returned from a cruise vacation to the Bahamas. At the time of examination her temperature is 38.9°C (102°F). The next day she calls the physician's office and states that her symptoms have subsided. Which of the following is the most likely causative agent?

A. *Giardia lamblia*

B. Norwalk virus

C. Rotavirus

D. *Shigella dysenteriae*

E. *Vibrio cholerae*

29. A 56-year-old woman presents with diarrhea and fever of 6-day duration. She reports that she saw blood and mucus in her stool and she feels like she constantly has to have a bowel movement. About 2 weeks ago she returned from India. Her temperature is 38.9°C (102°F). Physical examination reveals mild abdominal tenderness. Fecal occult blood and fecal leukocytes are positive but after 2 days the stool culture is reported as normal enteric microbiota. The woman is still experiencing symptoms so further testing is performed, including an endoscopy with biopsy, which reveals the following findings:

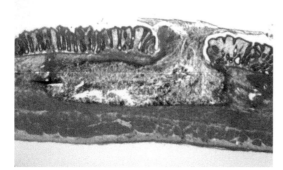

Source: Dr. Mae Melvin, USCDCP

Which of the following is the most likely causative agent of this infection?

A. Trichrome stain

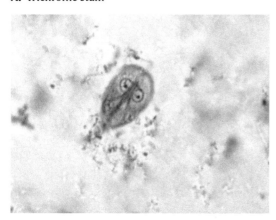

B. Gram stain

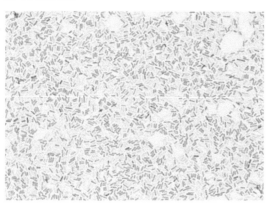

C. Trichrome stain

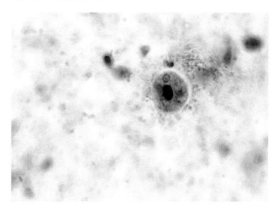

D. Gram stain

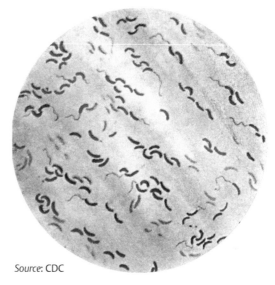

Source: CDC

E. Iodine wet mount

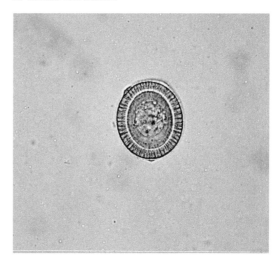

30. A 36-year-old man presents with a 4-week history of abdominal pain, frequent loose stools, and weight loss. He denies tenesmus or blood in his stool and estimates he has lost about 10 pounds in the last few weeks. He has previously been diagnosed with HIV but is not currently receiving care or taking medication for HIV. He is not currently in a relationship and admits to having unprotected sex with anonymous same-sex partners in the past. Laboratory results include:

- CD4 count: 346 cells/µL
- CBC: normal
- Stool culture: normal fecal flora; no pathogens isolated
- Ova and parasite examination: negative
- Fecal occult blood: negative
- Fecal leukocytes: negative
- Fecal fat: positive
- An immunofluorescent assay from the stool specimen is shown in the following image:

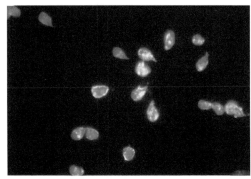

Source: CDC/Dr. Visvesvara

Which of the following is the most likely diagnosis?

A. Ascariasis
B. Enterobiasis
C. Giardiasis
D. Shigellosis
E. Whipple's disease

31. A 26-year-old man presents to his primary care physician with abdominal cramps and diarrhea of 1-week duration. He states he has been feeling more tired than normal, feels bloated and is passing an unusual amount of gas. He mentions that he went camping in the Rocky Mountains about 2 weeks ago and drank water from the stream at his campsite. At the time of examination, his temperature is 37.1°C (98.9°C). Abdominal examination reveals diffuse tenderness. Laboratory results are pending. Which of the following is the most likely causative agent?

A. *Entamoeba histolytica*
B. *Giardia lamblia*
C. *Necator americanus*
D. Norwalk virus
E. *Trichinella spiralis*

32. A 55-year-old woman presents with a 2-week history of epigastric abdominal pain and intermittent loose stools. She reports that her stool has changed colors in the last 2 weeks from brown to yellow, is oily, is difficult to flush, and has a more pungent odor than normal. Her vital signs are unremarkable. Her abdomen is soft and tender on examination with active bowel sounds. Pear-shaped trophozoites with two nuclei are recovered from a duodenal aspirate. Which of the following is the most appropriate therapy for this patient?

A. Albendazole
B. Praziquantel
C. Supportive therapy
D. Tinidazole
E. Trimethoprim–sulfamethoxazole

33. A 20-year-old college student visits the campus clinic with watery diarrhea of 3-day duration. She states that she is nauseated and also complains of severe abdominal pain and fatigue. On examination, her temperature is 37.5°C (99.5°F). She has no rebound tenderness or guarding on palpation of the abdomen. A modified acid-fast stain from the stool demonstrates the presence of the organism seen in the following image. The organism measured approximately 5 µm in diameter. The clinic physician notices that within 2 days of seeing this patient, 10 other students also presented with similar findings. It was later found that all the students drank from the same water source.

Which of the following is the most likely etiologic agent?

A. *Cryptosporidium parvum*
B. *Giardia lamblia*
C. *Naegleria fowleri*
D. *Shigella sonnei*
E. *Vibrio cholerae*

Consider the following case for questions 34 to 35:

A 61-year-old HIV-positive man presents with abdominal pain, sporadic watery diarrhea, and weight loss of 4-week duration. He denies tenesmus or blood in his stool and estimates he has lost about 15 pounds in a month. His temperature is 37.9°C (100.3°F) and his blood pressure is 118/84 mm Hg. Hyperactive bowel sounds and mild diffuse abdominal tenderness are noted on abdominal examination. His CD4 count is 70 cells/μL. A small (4 μm), round modified acid-fast oocyst is recovered from his stool.

34. Which of the following is the most likely etiologic agent?

A. *Cryptosporidium*

B. *Cystoisospora* (previously called *Isospora*)

C. Cytomegalovirus (CMV)

D. *Encephalitozoon*

E. *Mycobacterium avium-intracellulare* complex

35. Which of the following complications is most likely to be observed as a result of this infection?

A. Appendicitis

B. Cholecystitis

C. Reactive arthritis

D. Small bowel perforation

E. Toxic megacolon

36. A previously healthy 19-year-old woman presents with a 4-day history of watery diarrhea, abdominal pain, and fatigue. She denies hematochezia. She had returned from a trip to Machu Picchu (South America) 1 week prior to the onset of symptoms. A modified acid-fast organism that autofluoresces is recovered from her stool. Which of the following is the most likely causative agent?

A. Coccidian parasite

B. Flagellated protozoa

C. Fungus with spores

D. Roundworm

E. Single-stranded RNA virus

37. A 47-year-old HIV-positive woman presents with a 1-month history of weight loss, abdominal pain, and watery diarrhea. She reports that she frequently feels like she needs to empty her bowels and that she noticed blood in her stools recently. She believes she has lost about 15 pounds in the last few weeks. She has previously been diagnosed with HIV but is not currently receiving care or taking medication for the HIV infection. Her CD4 count is 38 cells/μL. An endoscopy shows inflammation of the colonic mucosa and the presence of ulcers and erosions. A biopsy is sent for histological staining and shows enlarged cells with eccentric, basophilic intranuclear inclusions. This infection was most likely transmitted via:

A. Ingestion of contaminated water

B. Ingestion of undercooked meat

C. Inhalation of conidia

D. Penetration of intact skin

E. Saliva

38. A previously healthy 33-year-old woman presents with a 1-week history of abdominal pain, nausea, and vomiting. She reports she has not had a bowel movement or passed gas in almost 5 days. She recently emigrated from Ethiopia. Her temperature is 37.8°C (100°F), heart rate is 130 beats per minute, and her blood pressure is 104/65 mm Hg. Her skin turgor is poor and her abdomen is significantly distended. An abdominal CT scan shows partial obstruction in her small bowel. Which of the following pathogens is most likely to be responsible for her current condition?

A. *Ascaris lumbricoides*

B. *Cryptosporidium parvum*

C. *Entamoeba histolytica*

D. Enterohemorrhagic *Escherichia coli* (EHEC)

E. *Yersinia enterocolitica*

39. A 6-year-old girl presents with diarrhea, vomiting and abdominal pain of 3-day duration. The girl and her mother deny seeing blood in her stool. The mother reports that the family returned from visiting relatives in Vietnam a few weeks ago. The girl's vitals are unremarkable. Examination reveals diffuse abdominal tenderness. A CBC demonstrates eosinophilia and the stool ova and parasite examination confirms an infection with *Strongyloides stercoralis*. Identification of which of the following will confirm this diagnosis?

A. Adult worm

B. Filariform larva

C. Ovum

D. Rhabditiform larva

E. Trophozoite

40. A 47-year-old woman in Thailand presents with a 3-day history of vomiting, worsening abdominal pain, lack of appetite, and generalized weakness. She has a history of eating raw meat, especially beef. During the past year she visited several clinics and had been diagnosed and treated for iron-deficiency anemia. Her physical examination shows mild abdominal tenderness. Microscopic examination of her stool reveals the organism seen in the following image:

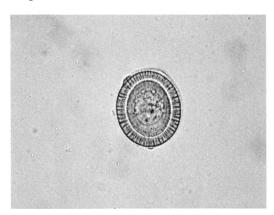

The most likely causative agent is a/an:

A. Amoeba

B. Cestode

C. Coccidia

D. Nematode

E. Trematode

41. A 28-year-old man visits his primary care physician for a routine physical examination. He reports he has occasional abdominal pain but has no other complaints and is otherwise healthy. His vitals are normal. On physical examination, he is slightly pale and his tongue is smooth, shiny, and red. During his examination, he casually mentions that he is an avid angler and frequently vacations near Lake Michigan so he can fish and he often partakes of his catch. Relevant laboratory results include:

- CBC:
    - Erythrocyte count: 3.5×10^{12}/L
    - Hemoglobin: 10.8 g/dL
    - Differential: macrocytic red blood cells observed

Which of the following organisms is most likely associated with the underlying pathogenesis of this man's illness?

A. *Clonorchis sinensis*

B. *Cryptosporidium parvum*

C. *Diphyllobothrium latum*

D. *Mycobacterium marinum*

E. *Vibrio vulnificus*

42. A 53-year-old HIV-positive man presents with a 3-week history of abdominal pain, intermittent watery diarrhea, and weight loss. He denies tenesmus or blood in his stool and estimates he has lost about 10 pounds in the month. His vitals are normal. Hyperactive bowel sounds and mild diffuse abdominal tenderness are noted on abdominal examination. His CD4 count is 82 cells/μL. The organism seen in the following image is recovered from a stool specimen.

Modified trichrome stain (100× magnification)

Which of the following is the most likely causative agent?

A. *Cryptosporidium*

B. Cytomegalovirus (CMV)

C. *Encephalitozoon*

D. *Mycobacterium*

E. Nontyphoidal *Salmonella*

43. A 3-year-old boy visits his family pediatrician with nausea and vomiting of 3-day duration. The mother states that the boy has not been sleeping well at night and has been scratching his perianal area more than normal. His vitals are unremarkable. Physical examination reveals self-inflicted perianal excoriations with intense inflammation. Which of the following would best confirm the diagnosis?

A. Enzyme immunoassay (EIA)

B. Gram stain

C. Modified acid fast stain

D. Scotch tape preparation

E. Stool ova and parasite evaluation

44. A 3-year-old girl is brought to clinic by her mother because "something" appears in the child's rectum after a bowel movement. The family recently adopted the child from Vietnam. The mother states that girl has been having intermittent diarrhea for the past few weeks. The child's vitals are normal. Protruding rings of mucosa are observed on rectal exam. The child has a bowel movement while in the clinic and protruding rectal mucosa is seen along with small white worms on the mucosa. Stool ova and parasite evaluation recover the following ovum:

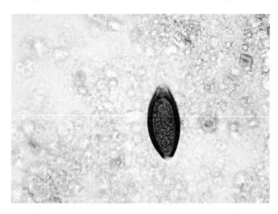

Which of the following is the most likely causative agent of this infection?

A. *Ancylostoma duodenale*

B. *Ascaris lumbricoides*

C. *Enterobius vermicularis*

D. *Taenia saginata*

E. *Trichuris trichiura*

45. A 52-year-old woman presents with rectal bleeding and blood in her stools. Her vitals are normal. On examination, a palpable mass on the rectum is detected. Endoscopy shows a large fungating mass in the rectum 8 cm from anal verge. Significant laboratory results include:

- Stool guaiac test: positive
- Hemoglobin: 7.8 g/dL
- Carcinoembriogenic antigen (CEA): 6.8 ng/mL (normal < 3 ng/mL)

This woman most likely has a current or previous infection with:

A. *Helicobacter pylori*

B. Hepatitis B virus (HBV)

C. Human papilloma virus (HPV)

D. *Schistosoma haematobium*

E. *Streptococcus bovis*

46. A 38-year-old man presents with a 3-day history of nausea, vomiting, and fatigue. His temperature is 37.6°C (99.7°F). On examination, mild jaundice of the skin and scleral icterus are noted and mild abdominal tenderness is present. Laboratory results include:

- CBC:
  - Leukocyte count: $6.2 \times 10 \times 10^9$/L
- Liver function tests:
  - AST: 384 U/L
  - ALT: 327 U/L
  - Total bilirubin: 2.9 mg/dL
- Hepatitis serology:
  - IgM anti-HA: positive
  - HBsAg: negative
  - Anti-HBs: positive
  - Anti-HCV: negative
  - IgM anti-HEV: negative

This infection was most likely transmitted via:

A. A mosquito bite

B. A blood transfusion

C. Contact with a contaminated animal

D. Ingestion of shellfish

E. Vertical transmission from his mother

47. A 24-year-old woman visits a physician for a routine pre-employment physical. She previously worked as a day care worker. She admits to previous illicit drug use but denies any use in the last year. She has no complaints except that she feels more tired than normal. On examination, her vitals are unremarkable and she appears well. Abdominal examination reveals hepatosplenomegaly. A hepatitis serology panel is ordered and results include:

- IgM anti-HAV: negative
- Total anti-HAV: positive
- HBsAg: positive
- Total anti-HBc: positive
- IgM anti-HBc: negative
- Anti-HBs: negative
- Anti-HDV: negative
- Anti-HCV: negative
- IgM anti-HEV: negative

Based on the serological profile this patient most likely has:

A. Acute hepatitis A

B. A past infection with hepatitis A

C. Acute hepatitis B

D. A coinfection with hepatitis B and D

E. Hepatitis B immunity

48. A 54-year-old woman presents to the emergency department with abdominal pain, vomiting, and diarrhea. She reports that her skin seems discolored, her urine has been darker than normal and her stools are paler than normal. She recently emigrated from El Salvador. Her temperature is 37.8°C (100.1°F). Significant jaundice of her skin and right upper quadrant tenderness are noted on physical examination. Laboratory results include:

- Liver function tests:
  - AST: 946 I/U
  - ALT: 1,678 I/U
  - Total bilirubin: 3.1 mg/dL
- Hepatitis serology:
  - IgM anti-HAV : negative
  - IgG anti-HAV: positive
  - HBsAg: positive
  - Total anti-HBc: positive
  - IgM anti-HBc: positive
  - Anti-HBs: negative
  - HBeAg: positive
  - IgM anti-HDV: positive

Based on the epidemiology and the serological profile, this patient:

A. Has a coinfection with hepatitis B and D and is highly infectious

B. Has a superinfection with hepatitis B and D and is highly infectious

C. Has an acute hepatitis B infection and is minimally infectious

D. Has a chronic hepatitis B infection and is minimally infectious

E. Is at risk for subsequent hepatitis A infections

49. A 67-year-old man presents with jaundice and distention of his abdomen. AST and ALT are grossly elevated and α-fetoprotein is increased. CT findings reveal a large liver mass which was then biopsied and confirmed as hepatocellular carcinoma (HCC). Which one of the following is most likely associated with the underlying pathogenesis of this condition?

A. Epstein–Barr virus (EBV)

B. Hepatitis B virus (HBV)

C. Human herpes virus-8 (HHV-8)

D. Human papilloma virus (HPV)

E. Human T-lymphotrophic virus (HTLV)

50. A previously healthy 29-year-old man, who has been incarcerated for the past year, presents to the prison health clinic with a 1-week history of jaundice and right upper quadrant pain. He admits to previous and current intravenous (IV) drug use. He denies any sexual activity for the past year. On examination, his vitals are normal. His skin is significantly jaundiced, his sclerae are icteric, and abdominal examination reveals hepatomegaly. The clinician also notes multiple tattoos, which the man reports he received while in prison. His AST, ALT, and bilirubin are significantly elevated. Which of the serological profiles in the following table would best confirm the most likely diagnosis?

	Profile I	Profile II	Profile III	Profile IV	Profile V
IgM anti-HAV	+	–	–	–	–
IgG anti-HAV	–	–	–	+	–
HBsAg	–	+	–	–	–
IgM anti-HBc	–	–	–	–	–
Total anti-HBc	–	+	–	–	–
Anti-HBs	–	–	–	+	–
Anti-HCV	–	–	+	–	–
HCV RNA	–	–	+	–	–
IgM anti-HEV	–	–	–	–	+
IgG anti-HEV	–	–	–	–	–

A. Profile I

B. Profile II

C. Profile III

D. Profile IV

E. Profile V

Consider the following case for questions 51 to 52:

A 30-year-old man presents with fever, vomiting, abdominal pain, and jaundice. About a month ago he returned from working in Uganda with the Peace Corp. His temperature is 38.2°C (100.9°F). On examination, significant jaundice of the skin and icterus of sclerae are noted. Abdominal tenderness is present. Laboratory results include:

- Liver function tests:
    - ALT: 2,345 U/L
    - AST: 2,789 U/L
    - Total bilirubin: 5.6 mg/dL
- Hepatitis serology:
    - IgM anti-HAV: negative
    - IgG anti-HAV: positive
    - HBsAg: negative
    - Total anti-HBc: negative
    - IgM anti-HBc: negative
    - Anti-HBs: positive
    - Anti-HCV: negative
    - Anti-HDV: negative
    - IgM anti-HEV: positive

51. Which of the following is the most likely causative agent of the current infection?

A. Delta virus

B. Flavivirus

C. Hepadnavirus

D. Hepevirus

E. Picornavirus

52. Which of the following is a characteristic of infections with this pathogen?

A. Associated with hepatocellular carcinoma (HCC)

B. Chronic infections may occur

C. High mortality in pregnant woman

D. Infections may be prevented with vaccination

E. Infections occur in conjunction with hepatitis B

53. A 71-year-old woman is brought to the urgent care clinic by her daughter with a 1-week history of abdominal pain, watery diarrhea, lack of appetite, and weight loss. The patient is from China and is visiting her family in the United States. On examination, her temperature is 37.8°C (100.1°F) and abdominal examination reveals tenderness in the right upper quadrant. Significant laboratory results include an elevated alkaline phosphatase and elevated eosinophil count. A stool sample recovers the ova shown in the following image and an endoscopic retrograde cholangiopancreatography (ERCP) shows the presence of several worms approximately 10 mm in length within the biliary tree.

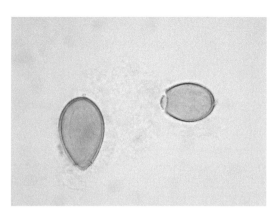

Ingestion of which of the following is most likely to be in this patient's history?

A. Escargot (snails)

B. Fecally contaminated water

C. Freshwater fish

D. Pork

E. Watercress

54. A 20-year-old woman complains of abdominal pain and fever of 1-week duration. She hasn't had an appetite for several weeks and has lost almost 10 pounds. History reveals that she returned from a semester abroad in Peru about 1 month ago. She reports she always drank bottled or filtered water and denies eating from street vendors. She does remember consuming edible flowers near a remote lake in the mountains. On examination, her temperature is 37.8°C (100.1°F). Abdominal examination reveals right upper quadrant tenderness and hepatomegaly. Her sclerae are icteric and her skin is slightly jaundiced. Pertinent laboratory results include:

- Liver function tests:
    - AST: 128 U/L
    - ALT: 224 U/L
    - Total bilirubin : 1.8 mg/dL
- Hepatitis serology:
    - IgM anti-HAV: negative
    - HBsAg: negative
    - Anti-HBs: positive
    - Anti-HCV: negative
    - IgM anti-HEV: negative

Which of the following is the most likely causative agent?

A. *Clonorchis sinensis*

B. *Giardia lamblia*

C. Hepatitis B virus (HBV)

D. *Fasciola hepatica*

E. Yellow fever virus

Consider the following case for questions 55 to 56:

A 54-year-old man from Syria presents with a 1-week history of jaundice, right upper quadrant pain, and vomiting. His medical history is unremarkable and his vitals are normal. Physical examination shows significant jaundice and scleral icterus, abdominal tenderness, and hepatosplenomegaly. AST, ALT, and total bilirubin are elevated. A CT scan shows the presence of many cysts on the liver and dilated bile ducts. The cysts were surgically removed and fluid from the cyst demonstrated the presence of the organism shown in the following image:

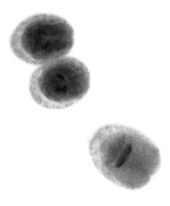

55. Which of the following is most likely causative agent of this infection?

A. *Candida albicans*

B. *Echinococcus granulosus*

C. *Entamoeba histolytica*

D. *Klebsiella pneumoniae*

E. *Staphylococcus aureus*

56. A 6-year-old boy from rural Mississippi sees the pediatrician for a well child visit. His mother says the boy seems more tired than normal, wants to sleep all the time, and does not want to play. On examination, the child's temperature is 37.1°C (98.8°F) and his heart rate is 143 beats per minute. Pallor is evident in his nail beds and conjunctiva. A CBC shows decreased hemoglobin and elevated eosinophils. A stool specimen demonstrates the presence of a thin-shelled, oval-shaped ovum shown in the following image:

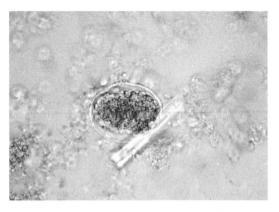

Which of the following symptoms is most likely to be in this boy's recent history?

A. Dry, nonproductive cough

B. Dysentery

C. Jaundice

D. Joint pain

E. Meningismus

57. A 5-year-old girl presents with a 2-day history of fatigue, swelling of her ankles, and blood in her urine. Her mother states that about a week ago the girl had experienced bloody diarrhea and abdominal discomfort. After a few days, the symptoms had subsided and the girl seemed to be better, so the mother did not seek medical attention at that time. On examination, the girl's temperature is 37.9°C (100.3°F) and her blood pressure is 120/85 mm Hg. Pallor of her skin and conjunctiva and significant edema of her feet are noted. Laboratory results include:

- Urinalysis–Dipstick
  - Blood: positive
  - Protein: positive
- Leukocyte esterase: negative
  - Nitrite: negative
- CBC:
  - White blood cell (WBC): 13.6×10^9/L
  - Hemoglobin: 6.8 g/dL
  - Platelets: 73×10^9/L

Which one of the following is most likely to be in this girl's history?

A. Contact with bats

B. Contact with birds

C. Contact with cows

D. Contact with pigs

E. Contact with reptiles

10.2 Answers and Explanations

Easy	Medium	Hard

1. Correct: Displacement of microbiota (B)

(B) This woman has oropharyngeal and esophageal candidiasis. *Candida* is part of the normal microbiota and colonizes the skin, vagina, and gastrointestinal tract. Infections usually arise as a result of overgrowth and/or displacement of these endogenous *Candida* strains. *Candida* is an opportunistic pathogen and infections are associated with immune deficiencies such as HIV/AIDS and hematological malignancies. *Candida* esophagitis is an AIDS-defining illness. The white patches on the buccal mucosa and white lesions on the esophagus with the presence of yeast and hyphae are classic findings of candidiasis. See Appendix M for a list of common AIDS-related opportunistic pathogens. **(A)** An infection that is transmitted by contact with cat feces is toxoplasmosis. This infection is also associated with immune deficiencies, including AIDS. In HIV-positive individuals, *Toxoplasma* most often affects the brain and eyes and not the oral cavity or esophagus as noted in this case. **(C)** HIV-positive individuals are at increased risk for more severe infections with many pathogens that are transmitted via the fecal–oral route. However, *Candida* is not transmitted by the fecal–oral route. **(D)** *Candida* is not transmitted by oral secretions. Cytomegalovirus (CMV) and herpes simplex virus-1 (HSV-1) are transmitted in this manner and both of these pathogens are AIDS-related agents of esophagitis. Histological findings would aid in differentiating *Candida*, CMV, and HSV. In CMV histology, enlarged cells with an eccentric nucleus and a clearing around the nucleus are seen. Characteristic cytology of herpes virus infections includes multinucleated giant cells and intranuclear inclusions. In this case, the masses of hyphae and yeast indicate that *Candida* is the most likely pathogen. **(E)** *Candida* is not transmitted sexually. Several sexually transmitted pathogens, including HSV-2, *Treponema pallidum* and *Neisseria gonorrhoeae* may affect the oral cavity and should be included in the differential diagnosis of pharyngitis. However, the white patches on the buccal mucosa and white lesions on the esophagus with the presence of yeast and hyphae as seen here are classic findings of candidiasis.

2. Correct: Unilateral swelling of eyelid (E)

(E) Serological analysis demonstrates that this woman has chronic Chagas disease as indicated by the positive *Trypanosoma cruzi* IgG. Infections are mainly limited to South American countries, such as Brazil, where this woman previously lived. Acute infections with *T. cruzi* begin with constitutional symptoms including fever, malaise, and anorexia. Unilateral swelling of eyelid or Romaña's sign (answer choice E) is a characteristic finding during this stage (see image at the end of this answer). Chronic Chagas disease may result in cardiomyopathy and esophageal/gastrointestinal disease, including achalasia, megaesophagus, and toxic megacolon. This woman presents with achalasia, in which there is a dilation of the esophagus because of narrowing at the lower esophageal sphincter. Symptoms of achalasia include dysphagia and chest pain. Common findings of Chagas heart disease include ventricular dysfunctions, arrhythmias, and thromboembolisms. Diagnosis of Chagas disease includes serological and molecular testing. *T. cruzi* IgM antibodies are present in acute disease whereas *T. cruzi* IgG antibodies represent recent/past exposure. **(A)** Bloody stools with mucous and tenesmus are symptoms of dysentery. Achalasia and other gastrointestinal sequelae of *T. cruzi* are not preceded by dysentery. Dysentery is most often associated with the bacterium *Shigella* and the parasite *Entamoeba histolytica*. **(B)** A circular red rash with central clearing is characteristic of the rash associated with Lyme disease. Lyme disease is caused by the spirochete *Borrelia burgdorferi*. The Lyme disease rash starts as a macule or papule and then spreads into an annular lesion with a central clearing. In Chagas disease, there may be swelling at the site of the bite, but this is different from the "bull's-eye" skin lesion characteristic of Lyme disease. **(C)** Paroxysms of fever and chills are classic findings of malaria, which, like Chagas disease, is a parasitic infection seen in tropical and subtropical countries. Paroxysms are a sudden onset of symptoms (in the case of malaria this includes fever, chills, and sweats) that are frequent or even cyclic. In acute Chagas disease, fever is present, but not paroxysms. **(D)** Several infectious diseases present with an ulcerative skin lesion. For example, with cutaneous leishmaniasis, papules develop into ulcers. This infection is also common in South America.

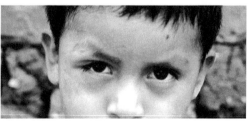

Source: CDC/Dr. Mae Melvin

3. Correct: Triatomine bug (E)

(E) *Trypanosoma cruzi* is transmitted by the bite of a triatomine bug. These bugs are also called reduviid bugs or assassin bugs. They are nicknamed "kissing bugs" because the bite is classically painless. **(A, B, C, D)** Chiggers, mosquitos, sandflies, and ticks do not transmit *Trypanosoma cruzi*. See Appendix L for a list of common insect-borne infections.

4. Correct: Urease (E)

(E) This is a case of acute gastritis. *Helicobacter pylori* is associated with acute gastritis and gastric and duodenal ulcers. *H. pylori* produces urease. The pathogen is able to survive the harsh stomach environment by the production of this enzyme. Urease splits urea into ammonia and bicarbonate and neutralizes stomach acid by increasing the pH. Diagnosis of *H. pylori* infections can be confirmed by evaluating biopsy specimens (such as antral biopsy) for the presence of urease using commercial tests, such as the CLO test (see image at the end of this answer). If present, *H. pylori* will turn the normally yellow media to a bright pink color. *H. pylori* is a curved gram-negative rod. Infections are associated with an increased risk of peptic ulcer disease, gastric adenocarcinoma, and gastric MALT lymphoma. **(A)** Coagulase is an enzyme produced by *Staphylococcus aureus*. Coagulase facilitates the conversion of fibrinogen to fibrin. This ultimately results in clot formation. The protective fibrin clot may protect the pathogen from the host immune response. *H. pylori* does not produce coagulase. **(B, C, D)** Hyaluronidase, phospholipase, and protease are produced by a number of pathogens. These enzymes aid in tissue invasion and are not produced by *H. pylori*.

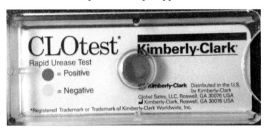

5. Correct: Urea breath testing (E)

(E) Following treatment for *H. pylori* infections, patients may be tested to confirm eradication of the pathogen. Noninvasive diagnostic tests recommended for the confirmation of eradication include the stool antigen test and the urea breath test (answer choice E). The urea breath test is thought to be more accurate. For this test, the patient drinks a solution containing ^{14}C-labeled urea. If the pathogen is present, urease will hydrolyze urea and release $^{14}CO_2$. This $^{14}CO_2$ can then be detected on the patient's breath. Treatment to eradicate *H. pylori* dramatically reduces the recurrence rate of gastric and duodenal

ulcers. Note that a test to ensure eradication (test of cure) is not warranted in all cases of *H. pylori*. It is only recommended in cases of *H. pylori*-associated ulcer (such as in this case) or *H. pylori*-associated MALT, patients with persistent symptoms of dyspepsia, or patients who have had a gastric resection due to gastric cancer. **(A)** *H. pylori* may grow in bacterial culture. However, the pathogen is difficult to grow and many clinical laboratories are unable to perform culture for *H. pylori* detection. Hence this is not the best method of diagnosis. **(B)** Serology has limited use since *H. pylori* IgG antibody is present in individuals with past infections as well as current infections. This test would not be able to confirm eradication in this case. **(C)** *H. pylori* is a curved gram-negative rod. Stool contains a plethora of normal bacterial microbiota. It would be nearly impossible to identify *H. pylori* with a Gram stain. **(D)** *H. pylori* produces VacA, which is a cytotoxin that damages epithelial cells by inducing vacuoles. However, toxin detection is not a mechanism of diagnosis for *H. pylori* eradication.

6. Correct: *Shigella dysenteriae* (C)

(C) This boy most likely has an infection with enterohemorrhagic *Escherichia coli* (EHEC). In the United States, the most common EHEC. serotype is *E. coli* O157:H7. EHEC produces the Shiga-like toxin or verotoxin, which is very similar in structure and function to the Shiga toxin of *Shigella dysenteriae* type 1 (answer choice C). These toxins cleave a single adenine nitrogenous base from the 28S rRNA of the 60S ribosome and prevent eukaryotic cell protein synthesis. Infections may arise after ingestion of undercooked ground beef (hamburgers are frequently implicated), unpasteurized milk, and other food products. Clinical manifestations include watery diarrhea that develops into bloody diarrhea as seen in this case. **(A)** *Clostridium tetani* produces an exotoxin that prevents the release of GABA and glycine inhibitory neurotransmitters in the spinal cord neurons. The EHEC toxin inhibits protein synthesis. **(B)** Enterotoxigenic *Escherichia coli* (ETEC) produces two enterotoxins. The heat-labile toxin increases cyclic AMP and the heat-stable toxin increases cyclic GMP. The EHEC toxin inhibits protein synthesis. **(D)** *Staphylococcus aureus*, a gram-positive coccus, produces an exotoxin that stimulates the vagal nerve resulting in vomiting. The EHEC toxin inhibits protein synthesis. **(E)** *Vibrio cholerae* produces the cholera toxin. This toxin ADP ribosylates Gs (G stimulatory) protein causing an increase in intracellular cyclic AMP. The EHEC toxin inhibits protein synthesis.

7. Correct: Pallor (C)

(C) This boy has an infection with the gram-negative rod enterohemorrhagic *Escherichia coli* (EHEC). Complications of EHEC infections include hemolytic uremic syndrome (HUS), which most often affects young children. Primary infections with this organism result in watery diarrhea that becomes bloody. HUS occurs 5 to 10 days after the onset of diarrhea. The typical triad of HUS includes acute renal failure, microangiopathic hemolytic anemia, and thrombocytopenia. Pallor may be observed when anemia is present. **(A)** Ascending paralysis is a classic manifestation of Guillain–Barré syndrome, which is postinfectious sequelae associated with *Campylobacter jejuni*, not EHEC. **(B)** Joint pain is a symptom of reactive arthritis, a sequela of several pathogens. Reactive arthritis is associated with infections caused by *Chlamydia*, *Salmonella*, *Shigella*, *Campylobacter*, and *Yersinia*. Certain strains of *E. coli* may also induce reactive arthritis, but not EHEC. **(D)** Tonic–clonic seizures are not seen in HUS. In encephalitis and other nervous system infections, such as *Taenia solium* and neurocysticercosis, seizures may occur. **(E)** Tender red or violet subcutaneous nodules that are found in the pretibial area are a common finding of erythema nodosum. Several pathogens are associated with erythema nodosum, including *Streptococcus pyogenes*, endemic fungi, and *Yersinia*. *Y. enterocolitica* is an agent of diarrhea and foodborne infections that occur after ingestion of undercooked pork, unpasteurized milk and other foods. The child in this case is more likely to have an infection with EHEC; hence this answer choice is incorrect.

8. Correct: MacConkey agar supplemented with sorbitol (D)

(D) One of the characteristic features of *E. coli* O157:H7 is its inability to ferment sorbitol. As a result, colonies will appear clear or colorless on MacConkey agar with sorbitol. Most other clinical isolates, including other *E. coli* strains and serotypes, are sorbitol fermenters and will appear bright pink or red on this media (see image at the end of this answer). **(A)** Chocolate agar is supplemental and enriched with X (hemin) and V (nicotinamide adenine dinucleotide/NAD) factors, which support the growth of *Haemophilus*. Although *E. coli* O157:H7 would grow on chocolate agar, it would be impossible to confirm the identity since chocolate agar is not a differential media. **(B)** Buffered charcoal yeast extract agar or BCYE is a selective medium for *Legionella pneumophila*, a gram-negative respiratory pathogen. **(C)** Hektoen agar is selective for enteric gram-negative rods. This media is also differential for lactose fermentation and hydrogen sulfide reactions. It would not differentiate between different species of *E. coli* as all strains of *E. coli* would be lactose positive (fermenter) and H_2S negative. **(E)** Thiosulfate-citrate-bile salts-sucrose (TCBS) agar is a selective and differential medium for *Vibrio* species. The high pH prevents the growth of most other enteric organisms and the sodium chloride provides a halophilic environment for *Vibrio*. The growth of *E. coli* O157:H7 is inhibited in this medium.

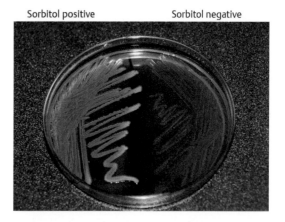

Sorbitol positive   Sorbitol negative

9. Correct: Enteropathogenic *Escherichia coli* (EPEC) (C)

(C) Any gastrointestinal pathogen may cause diarrhea in infants. However, there are several pathogens that infants are at higher risk for contracting compared to adults. These include enteropathogenic *Escherichia coli* (EPEC), enterotoxigenic *Escherichia coli* (ETEC), and rotavirus. In resource-limited countries, EPEC is a common agent of infantile diarrhea and may be so severe that dehydration occurs. Sunken eyes and poor skin turgor are often traits of dehydration, as observed in this patient. Like all *E. coli*, EPEC is lactose positive (fermenter) on MacConkey agar (see image at the end of this answer) and grows best at body temperature. Only *E. coli* O157:H7 (EHEC) is sorbitol negative. Note that the best way of differentiating the pathogenic *E. coli* is via molecular testing rather than culture. **(A)** *Campylobacter jejuni* is a leading agent of diarrhea worldwide. Diarrhea may range from watery diarrhea, bloody diarrhea, or dysentery. *C. jejuni* grows on selective media and grows best at 42°C, not 37°C; hence this answer choice is incorrect. **(B)** Enterohemorrhagic *Escherichia coli* (EHEC) is an agent of diarrhea, but often the diarrhea is bloody. Young children are at risk of developing hemolytic uremic syndrome (HUS) following diarrhea with this pathogen. In the United States, *E. coli* O157:H7 is a commonly isolated EHEC serotype and is sorbitol negative. All other *E. coli*, including strains that are part of the normal microbiota, are sorbitol positive. The pathogen in this case is unlikely to be EHEC as the clinical findings and culture characteristics are inconsistent with EHEC. **(D)** Rotavirus is a major cause of severe diarrhea in infants and young children. It is seen worldwide and is preventable by vaccination. However, this pathogen is a virus and does not grow on artificial media, including MacConkey; hence this answer choice is incorrect. Viruses are obligate intracellular pathogens and require living cells in order to replicate and will only grow in cell culture. **(E)** *Shigella* species may cause infections in children in resource-limited countries. Most often infections manifest as dysentery. *Shigella sonnei* is the main species seen in the United States. *Shigella* is a lactose negative (non-fermenter), not a lactose positive (fermenter) pathogen.

Lactose positive (fermenter)   Lactose negative (non-fermenter)

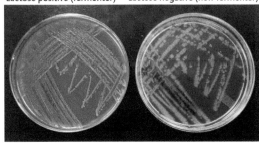

10.   Correct: Destruction of microvilli (A)

(A) Enteropathogenic *Escherichia coli* (EPEC) uses bundle-forming pili to firmly attach to enterocytes and ultimately destroys the microvilli. Once the pathogen attaches, it uses a type III secretion system to secrete its own receptor to bind to the enterocyte in a more intimate manner. The pathogen then recruits actin and causes deformation of microvilli and "pedestal" formation or effacement of the enterocyte (see image at the end of this answer). See also table at the end of this answer for a summary of the clinically significant

gastrointestinal *E. coli* strains. **(B)** Endotoxin or lipopolysaccharide (LPS) is found in virtually all gram-negative cells, including EPEC and is an integral part of the cell wall. Endotoxin plays a crucial role in eliciting an inflammatory response. LPS and inflammation are not as important as the attachment and microvilli destruction in EPEC infections. EPEC is an agent of non-inflammatory infectious diarrhea. **(C)** *Clostridioides* (previously called *Clostridium*) *difficile*, and not EPEC, produces an enterotoxin that inactivates actin polymerization. **(D)** EPEC does not produce exotoxins. *Shigella dysenteriae* and enterohemorrhagic *E. coli* (EHEC) produce toxins that inhibit protein synthesis. **(E)** EPEC firmly attaches to but does not invade the enterocyte.

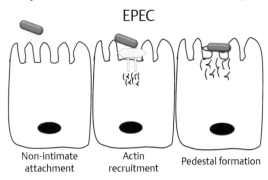

Clinically significant gastrointestinal *E. coli* strains			
	Primary infection	**Manifestation**	**Pathogenesis**
EAEC	Traveler's diarrhea	Watery diarrhea	Tight adherence Toxin—increase cyclic GMP
EPEC	Infant diarrhea in resource-limited countries	Watery diarrhea	Firm/intimate attachment to enterocyte/pedestal formation
EHEC	Diarrhea	Watery diarrhea that develops into bloody diarrhea	Shiga-like toxin that prevents protein synthesis
EIEC	Diarrhea mainly in resource-limited countries	Dysentery	Invasion of enterocyte and bowel wall
ETEC	Traveler's diarrhea Infant diarrhea in resource-limited countries	Watery diarrhea	Heat-labile toxin LT—increases cyclic AMP Heat-stable toxin ST—increases cyclic GMP

Abbreviations: EAEC, enteraggregative *E. coli*; EPEC, enteropathogenic *E. coli*; EHEC, enterohemorrhagic *E. coli*; EIEC, enteroinvasive *E. coli*; ETEC, enterotoxigenic *E. coli*.

11.   Correct: *Bacillus cereus* (A)

(A) Traveler's diarrhea may be caused by a variety of pathogens and one of the main bacterial agents is enterotoxigenic *Escherichia coli* (ETEC). ETEC produces two enterotoxins. One toxin increases cyclic AMP (heat labile toxin) and the other toxin increases cyclic GMP (heat stable toxin). Both toxins induce a diarrheal response. Several other pathogens including *Bacillus cereus* (answer choice A), *Vibrio cholerae*, and *Bacillus anthracis* also produce toxins that increase cyclic AMP. Other *E. coli* strains that may be implicated in traveler's diarrhea include entero-aggregative *E. coli*. See table presented at the end of this answer for a summary of the clinically significant gastrointestinal *E. coli* strains. **(B)** *Clostridioides* (previously called *Clostridium*) *difficile* produces two toxins, *C. difficile* toxin (CDT) A and CDT B. The mechanism of action of CDT A and CDT B are different than ETEC toxins. CDT A disrupts tight junctions which increases permeability of the intestinal wall leading to diarrhea. CDT B is a cytotoxin that destroys the cellular cytoskeleton by causing actin to depolymerize. **(C)** *Clostridium perfringens* produces an enterotoxin that disrupts selective permeability of the plasma membrane, which leads to cell death. The toxins of ETEC interfere with host cell signaling and do not cause cell death. **(D)** The Shiga toxin of *Shigella dysenteriae* type 1 cleaves the 28S rRNA of the 60S ribosome and prevents protein synthesis. In contrast, ETEC toxin intracellular increases cyclic AMP levels. **(E)** *Staphylococcus aureus* produces several toxins including a superantigen that nonspecifically activates T cells and produces a cytokine storm. ETEC does not produce a superantigen.

Clinically significant gastrointestinal *E. coli* strains			
	Primary infection	**Manifestation**	**Pathogenesis**
EAEC	Traveler's diarrhea	Watery diarrhea	Tight adherence Toxin—increase cyclic GMP
EPEC	Infant diarrhea in resource-limited countries	Watery diarrhea	Firm/intimate attachment to enterocyte/pedestal formation
EHEC	Diarrhea	Watery diarrhea that develops into bloody diarrhea	Shiga-like toxin that prevents protein synthesis
EIEC	Diarrhea mainly in resource-limited countries	Dysentery	Invasion of enterocyte and bowel wall
ETEC	Traveler's diarrhea Infant diarrhea in resource-limited countries	Watery diarrhea	Heat-labile toxin LT—increases cyclic AMP Heat-stable toxin ST—increases cyclic GMP

Abbreviations: EAEC, enteraggregative *E. coli*; EPEC, enteropathogenic *E. coli*; EHEC, enterohemorrhagic *E. coli*; EIEC, enteroinvasive *E. coli*; ETEC, enterotoxigenic *E. coli*.

12. Correct: *Shigella sonnei* (D)

(D) This is a case of shigellosis caused by the gram-negative rod *Shigella*. *Shigella* species are classified into serogroups. In the United States, *Shigella sonnei* (group D) is the most common pathogen. Shigellosis is transmitted via the fecal–oral route by contaminated food and water. *Shigella* is acid resistant and has a very low infectious dose; therefore, it is easily spread from person to person. It is a common pathogen of young children, especially those in institutionalized settings such as day care. Shigellosis may present as watery diarrhea or more serious bacillary dysentery with blood and pus in the stool. This pathogen is a facultative intracellular microbe and can invade

host cells. Some strains can also produce an enterotoxin, the Shiga toxin. **(A)** EPEC is a common agent of infant diarrhea in resource-limited countries. Moreover, infections with this pathogen usually result in watery diarrhea and not bloody diarrhea. **(B)** Rotavirus is a common agent of severe diarrhea in young children, especially during the winter. Although adults may be infected, immunocompetent adults are usually asymptomatic or have mild infections. Bloody stools are not a common finding of rotavirus infections. **(C)** *Salmonella typhi* is an agent of febrile disease, not diarrheal disease. Other nontyphoidal species of *Salmonella* are agents of bloody diarrhea. **(E)** Cholera, caused by *Vibrio cholerae*, is associated with saltwater and is transmitted following ingestion of contaminated food and water. Although direct person-to-person spread may occur, it is a less common mechanism of transmission. This pathogen is not a likely pathogen associated with diarrheal infections in day care centers.

13.   Correct: Field trip to the reptile zoo (D)

(D) This is a case of nontyphoidal salmonellosis. Nontyphoidal *Salmonella* are zoonotic and can be transmitted by direct animal contact. These pathogens are commonly associated with reptiles and amphibians, especially turtles and salamanders. Therefore, answer choice D, a field trip to the reptile zoo, is most likely to be in this boy's recent history. *Salmonella* are invasive organisms and infections may result in bloody diarrhea as described in this case. Only gram-negative rods, such as *Salmonella* grow on MacConkey. Additionally, *Salmonella* are one of few enteric pathogens that produce hydrogen sulfide (H_2S), which may assist in differentiating them from other pathogens. Some enteric bacteria induce fecal leukocytes, which are not usually present in the stool. These pathogens include *Salmonella* as well as *Campylobacter*, *Shigella*, *Yersinia enterocolitica*, and *Clostridioides* (previously called *Clostridium*) *difficile*. Human species of *Salmonella* include *Salmonella enterica* serotype Enteritidis and Typhimurium. **(A)** *Salmonella* may also be transmitted by contaminated food and water, especially water contaminated with human or animal waste. There is the possibility that freshwater from a mountain location could contain *Salmonella*. However, it is more likely that transmission occurred with reptile contact. An enteric pathogen that is commonly associated with freshwater sources and camping is the protozoan parasite, *Giardia lamblia*. **(B)** *Campylobacter jejuni* is an example of an enteric pathogen that may be transmitted via direct contact with an infected pet such as a cat or a dog. *Salmonella* is more likely to be associated with reptiles and amphibians. Furthermore, *C. jejuni* grows best on selective media in microaerophilic conditions at 42°C. **(C)** Undercooked ground beef and hamburgers are most likely to be associated with enterohemorrhagic *Escherichia coli* (also called EHEC or *E. coli* O157:H7) infections. Fecal leukocytes are not commonly seen in EHEC infections. Furthermore, EHEC like other *E. coli* strains is lactose positive (fermenter) and H_2S negative. **(E)** Many bacterial pathogens are associated with travel outside the United States. There is the possibility of contracting salmonellosis while travelling to Mexico. *Salmonella* is found worldwide and is very common in resource-rich countries, including the United States. However, traveler's diarrhea is typically associated with enterotoxigenic *Escherichia coli* (ETEC) infections. The pathogen in this case is lactose negative and produces H_2S, which is more consistent with *Salmonella*.

14.   Correct: No antibiotic therapy should be administered (E)

(E) This is a case of nontyphoidal salmonellosis. Most often infections in immune competent adults are not severe and are self-limiting; hence, antibiotic therapy is not recommended. *Salmonella* is foodborne and commonly associated foods include undercooked poultry and poultry products such as undercooked eggs, which are found in uncooked cookie dough. Some species stay in the lamina propria of the small bowel, resulting in watery diarrhea whereas other species invade the colonic mucosa, resulting in inflammatory diarrhea and bloody stools. *Salmonella* species produce hydrogen sulfide (H_2S; black colonies) on certain media including Hektoen agar (see image at the end of this answer) and xylose lysine deoxycholate (XLD) agar. XLD is selective and differential agar for *Salmonella* and *Shigella*. **(A)** Gastrointestinal infections in which macrolides, such as azithromycin, may be used include severe *Campylobacter* infections. Like *Salmonella*, *Campylobacter* is also associated with undercooked poultry. Undercooked eggs are more likely to be associated with salmonellosis. Infections with both *Salmonella* and *Campylobacter* are mostly self-limiting. **(B)** Ciprofloxacin may be used for both nontyphoidal *Salmonella* and typhoidal *Salmonella*. In the case of serious infections with nontyphoidal *Salmonella*, fluoroquinolones such as ciprofloxacin and levofloxacin are recommended. In this case, the woman was previously healthy, she does not have bloody diarrhea and is afebrile. This is most likely to be a self-limiting infection and therapy is not warranted. **(C, D)** Oral metronidazole and oral vancomycin may be used to treat nonsevere and nonrecurring *Clostridioides* (previously called *Clostridium*) *difficile* diarrhea. *C. difficile* colitis usually occurs following antibiotic use. There is no indication of prior antibiotic use in this case.

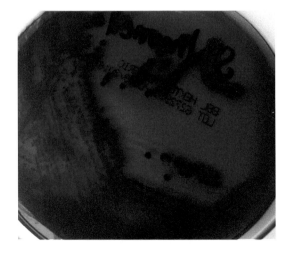

15.   Correct: Growth at 42°C (B)

(B) *Campylobacter* is a curved gram-negative rod that grows best at 42°C in microaerophilic conditions on selective media. Based on clinical presentation, it is often difficult to distinguish between the common bacterial agents of inflammatory diarrhea, which include *Campylobacter*, *Salmonella*, *Shigella*, and *Yersinia*. Infections with these pathogens are food-borne and symptoms include fever, abdominal pain, bloody diarrhea, and vomiting. Fecal leukocytes may be present. Of these agents, *Salmonella* and *Campylobacter* are most often associated with undercooked chicken. *Salmonella* is a (non-curved) gram-negative rod. With *Campylobacter* enteritis, a brief prodrome with fever, malaise, and other constitutional symptoms may be present prior to the gastrointestinal symptoms, which may aid in differentiating this infection from other gastrointestinal infections. **(A)** A stool pathogen that grows well at refrigerator temperatures is *Listeria monocytogenes*, a gram-positive rod. *Yersinia enterocolitica*, a gram-negative rod, may also grow at 4°C (refrigerator temperature), but the optimal temperature for growth is 25 to 28°C (room temperature). **(C)** An obligate anaerobe is killed by the presence of oxygen. *Campylobacter* species are microaerophilic which means that the pathogen prefers reduced oxygen levels; therefore, *Campylobacter* is not a strict (obligate) anaerobe. *Clostridioides* (previously called *Clostridium*) *difficile* is an example of a strict anaerobic gastrointestinal pathogen. **(D)** *Campylobacter* does not grow in elevated concentrations of salt (i.e., halotolerant). However, *Vibrio cholerae*, another curved gram-negative rod, is halotolerant. **(E)** *Escherichia coli*, and not *Campylobacter*, grows as green colonies with a metallic sheen on eosin methylene blue (EMB) agar.

16. Correct: Mesenteric lymph nodes (D)

(D) This is a case of enteric yersiniosis. *Yersinia enterocolitica*, a gram-negative rod, invades M cells in Peyer's patches or mesenteric lymph nodes (answer choice D) of the terminal ileum. Due to the close location to the appendix, infections may resemble appendicitis, especially in children. Because this organism has a propensity for infecting lymphoid tissue, there is the possibility that pharyngitis or tonsillitis may be present in addition to the gastrointestinal symptoms. The organism is foodborne and is commonly associated with undercooked pork and unpasteurized milk. The pathogen is also associated with contact with pigs and other animals. *Y. enterocolitica* is invasive; hence, bloody diarrhea and fecal leukocytes may be present as in this case. Cefsulodin, irgasan, novobiocin (CIN) agar is a selective and differential agar that is often used for the recovery of enteric *Yersinia*. The optimal temperature for growth is 25 to 28°C but it may also grow at 37°C and 4°C. **(A)** *Yersinia enterocolitica* is most often localized to the distal small bowel, specifically the terminal ileum, and not the duodenum. **(B, C, E)** *Yersinia enterocolitica* does not usually infect the gallbladder, liver, or stomach.

17. Correct: Mucous in the stool (D)

(D) This man most likely has cholera, caused by *Vibrio cholerae*, a curved gram-negative rod as seen in the image in the question stem. Cholera is characterized by watery diarrhea with flecks of mucus, often described as rice water stools. The man has had 8 to 9 bowel movements per day and is severely dehydrated. *V. cholerae* produces the cholera toxin that ADP ribosylates Gs (G stimulatory) protein, which in turn causes an increase in cyclic AMP. This ultimately results in an efflux of ions and water from infected enterocytes into the gut lumen. Due to the severe fluid loss, hypovolemia may occur. The organism is endemic in many parts of Africa, India and Southeast Asia and is transmitted via ingestion of fecally contaminated food and marine water. See Appendix J for a summary of bacterial virulence factors, including toxins. **(A)** Blood in the stools is not a typical characteristic of cholera. Bloody stools may be observed with non-cholera *Vibrio*, such as *V. parahaemolyticus*. Other agents of bloody diarrhea include *Salmonella*, *Shigella*, *Campylobacter*, *Yersinia enterocolitica*, and *Entamoeba histolytica*. **(B)** Clay or pale stool is indicative of decreased liver function and reduced drainage of bile into the gut lumen. This symptom is most likely to be seen with viral hepatitis and not cholera. **(C)** Greasy or oily stools are most likely to represent steatorrhea and malabsorption. Infections with several pathogens, notably the protozoan parasite *Giardia lamblia*, are associated with greasy stools. This is not a characteristic of cholera. **(E)** White cells in the stool are not normal and indicate an inflammatory response. Fecal leukocytes are usually present in infections with invasive pathogens such as *Campylobacter*, *Shigella*, and enteroinvasive *Escherichia coli*. They may also be present at times in *Salmonella* and enteric *Yersinia* infections. *Vibrio* is not an invasive pathogen and fecal leukocytes are not a common finding of cholera.

18. Correct: Aerobic gram-positive cocci in clusters (C)

(C) This man is experiencing classical food "poisoning" caused by *Staphylococcus aureus*, an aerobic gram-positive coccus in clusters. Infections are characterized by nausea and vomiting; diarrhea is rarely observed. Infections appear rapidly, within 1 to 6 hours after ingestion of food contaminated with preformed staphylococcal enterotoxin. Commonly associated foods include bakery products such as cream-filled pastries, meats, poultry and eggs, milk and other dairy products, and cold salads such as egg, potato, macaroni, and chicken salad. **(A)** There are several foodborne pathogens that are aerobic gram-negative rods, including *Escherichia coli*, *Salmonella*, and *Shigella*. Infections with these pathogens have incubation times of days and not hours and manifest as mainly diarrheal disease and not only vomiting. **(B)** *Bacillus* species, such as the food-borne pathogen *B. cereus*, are aerobic gram-positive rods with spores. *B. cereus* produces two toxins: the emetic toxin and the diarrheal toxin. Emetic disease may manifest very similar to staphylococcal food poisoning with nausea and profuse vomiting. The average incubation time is also similar to that of *S. aureus* infections. However, *B. cereus* is more likely to be associated with starchy foods such as fried rice and potatoes. Hence, in this case, *S. aureus* (aerobic gram-positive cocci in clusters) is the most likely etiological agent. Infections with the *B. cereus* diarrheal toxin are very similar to *C. perfringens* infections (see explanation for answer choice D). **(D)** *Clostridium perfringens* is an anaerobic gram-positive rod with spores. Manifestations occur approximately 8 to 24 hours after infection and include watery diarrhea, nausea, and abdominal pain. This is unlikely to be the causative agent in this case due to the short incubation observed in this patient. **(E)** Microaerophilic curved gram-negative rods best describes *Campylobacter jejuni*, another foodborne pathogen. *Campylobacter* is associated with undercooked chicken and unpasteurized milk. The average incubation period is approximately 3 days. Infections are characterized by diarrhea that is often bloody.

19. Correct: Superantigen (D)

(D) *Staphylococcus aureus* produces a number of virulence factors. Foodborne illness is toxin-mediated and the staphylococcus enterotoxin has superantigen activity. Superantigens can nonspecifically activate T cells. The toxin is heat stable and can survive both boiling and the harsh stomach acid. Once ingested, the preformed toxin stimulates the vagus nerve resulting in severe vomiting. **(A)** Coagulase is produced by *S. aureus* and facilitates the conversion of fibrinogen to fibrin, which results in clot formation. The protective fibrin clot may protect the pathogen from the host immune response. While coagulase may play a role in assisting *S. aureus* in establishing infection, it is the enterotoxin that is most important in mediating foodborne illness. **(B)** *S. aureus* may also produce hyaluronidase, an enzyme that degrades hyaluronic acid. It is thought to play an important role in the spread of *S. aureus* through tissue. **(C)** *S. aureus* produces protein A, which binds to the Fc of IgG and aids in immune system evasion. Protein A is important in establishing infection; however, it is the enterotoxin that is important in mediating foodborne illness. **(E)** *S. aureus* exfoliative toxins are proteases that split the intercellular bridges in the stratum granulosum of the epidermis. These toxins are important in the pathogenesis of *S. aureus*-mediated scalded skin syndrome.

20. Correct: Gravy (B)

(B) The etiological agent of this infection is the anaerobic gram-positive rod *Clostridium perfringens*.

This pathogen is a spore producer and the spores are heat resistant. When food is rewarmed or when food is not refrigerated, the vegetative form of the spores can multiply. Commonly associated foods include gravies (answer B) stews, soups, beef, poultry, and precooked foods. In vivo an enterotoxin, which forms pores in enterocytes, is produced. The toxin increases membrane permeability, which leads to diarrhea and loss of fluids. The incubation is approximately 8 to 24 hours after the ingestion of contaminated food. Typical symptoms include nausea, abdominal pain, and watery diarrhea as seen in this case. Infections with this pathogen may be hard to differentiate from diarrheal infections with *Bacillus cereus*, which is an aerobic gram-positive rod. **(A)** Cream puffs are commonly associated with *Staphylococcus aureus* foodborne illness. Infections with *S. aureus* have a short incubation time of 1 to 6 hours and the main symptoms are nausea and vomiting. *S. aureus* does produce an enterotoxin and is an aerobic gram-positive coccus; hence this answer choice is incorrect. **(C)** Raw eggs are commonly associated with salmonellosis, caused by nontyphoidal *Salmonella*. Certain strains of *Salmonella*, an aerobic gam-negative rod, may produce a toxin. However, the most common mechanism of *Salmonella* pathogenesis is via invasion of the host cell enterocyte, which ultimately results in inflammation. The pathogen in this case is gram positive and produces a toxin; hence *Salmonella* is unlikely the causative agent. **(D)** Contaminated shellfish is associated with several foodborne infections, including cholera, Norwalk virus (also called norovirus), and hepatitis A infections. Of these only the agent of cholera produces an exotoxin. *Vibrio cholerae* is an aerobic curved gram-negative rod. The organism in this case is gram positive. **(E)** Soft cheese is associated with *Listeria monocytogenes*, which is an aerobic, not anaerobic, gram-positive rod.

21. Correct: Aerobic gram-positive rod (A)

(A) This is an infection with *Bacillus cereus*, an aerobic gram-positive rod with spores. This pathogen causes two types of foodborne illness: diarrheal and emetic disease. In this case, the man has the emetic form of the disease. The emetic illness has a short incubation phase of less than 6 hours. Commonly associated foods include starchy foods, such as potatoes and rice. When rice is left out at room temperature, the sporulated organism germinates and produces the toxin. When the rice is reheated—such as in the case with leftover fried rice—the toxin, which is heat stable, remains functional and can then be transmitted to humans. In diarrheal disease the incubation is longer (8–24 hours) and infections are very similar to foodborne infections with *Clostridium perfringens* (see explanation for choice C). **(B)** An aerobic gram-positive coccus that is an agent of foodborne illness is *Staphylococcus aureus*. Like foodborne infections with *B. cereus*, the incubation time is about 1 to 6 hours following ingestion of contaminated food. Commonly associated foods include dairy, pastries with cream, produce, meats, and cold salads. Based on symptoms alone, this infection may be either an infection cause by *B. cereus* or *S. aureus*. However, the ingestion of leftover vegetable fried rice makes *B. cereus* a more likely agent than *S. aureus*. **(C)** *Clostridium perfringens* is an anaerobic gram-positive rod that causes foodborne illness. *C. perfringens* is commonly associated with meat, stews, soups, and gravies. The average incubation is approximately 8 to 24 hours, which is longer than the incubation with *B. cereus* emetic disease. Additionally, the main symptom of *C. perfringens* foodborne illness is watery diarrhea, not vomiting. **(D)** One of the most common flagellated protozoan parasites involved in gastrointestinal infections is *Giardia lamblia*. This pathogen is transmitted via contaminated food and water and is associated with freshwater reservoirs. With giardiasis, the average incubation time (1–2 weeks) is longer than *B. cereus* infections. Frequent symptoms include foul-smelling watery diarrhea, bloating, stomach cramps, abdominal pain, and flatulence. **(E)** Two RNA viruses that are agents of gastrointestinal infections are Norwalk virus, a single-stranded RNA virus and rotavirus, a double-stranded RNA virus. Norwalk virus is a common cause of viral gastroenteritis in the United States and infections may occur following ingestion of contaminated food and water. Frequently associated foods include shellfish. The average incubation time is approximately 24 to 48 hours, which is longer than the incubation period for *B. cereus* emetic infections. Infections with this pathogen result in watery diarrhea and vomiting.

22. Correct: Vancomycin (E)

(E) This is a case of *Clostridioides* (previously called *Clostridium*) *difficile* colitis. Initial therapy for nonserious infections includes oral vancomycin or oral metronidazole. Note that the newest guidelines for *C. difficile* treatment released in the early 2018 indicating that vancomycin or fidaxomicin (or metronidazole if vancomycin or fidaxomicin is unavailable) should be used as first-line therapy for treatment. *C. difficile* is a spore-forming anaerobic gram-positive rod. Infections may vary from asymptomatic carriage to watery diarrhea, pseudomembranous colitis and fulminant colitis with toxic megacolon. Infections are most often health care-associated and antibiotic use increases the risk of infection with this pathogen. Frequently associated antibiotics include fluoroquinolones, clindamycin, penicillins, and cephalosporins. Transmission of *C. difficile* occurs from ingestion of spores via the fecal–oral route, fomites, and less commonly, displacement of endogenous strains. Diagnosis must include detection of the toxin as

only toxin-producing strains are capable of causing infection. Glutamate dehydrogenase (GDH) is an enzyme produced by both nontoxin- and toxin-producing strains of *C. difficile*. Current diagnosis methods include detection of GDH and toxin. Recurrent infections, in which there is a relapse of infection within 8 weeks of therapy, are problematic and are treated differently than primary *C. difficile* infections (see explanation for choices A and B). **(A)** Fecal transplant is recommended for recurrent or serious infections. Antibiotic use alters the intestinal microbiota and predisposes individuals to *C. difficile* colonization. Fecal transplants assist in repopulating the beneficial bacteria and reducing the risk of recurrent infections. **(B)** Levofloxacin is a fluoroquinolone with broad spectrum activity. This drug has poor anaerobic coverage. Furthermore, use of fluoroquinolones is associated with the development of *C. difficile* infections, hence this answer choice is incorrect. **(C)** *C. difficile* diarrhea is associated with fluoroquinolones, clindamycin, penicillins, and cephalosporins. Therefore, penicillin would be inappropriate therapy in this case. **(D)** There is currently little evidence demonstrating that ingested probiotics are beneficial and effective in the treatment of *C. difficile*. However, probiotics may be effective prophylactically.

23. Correct: Depolymerizes actin (B)

(B) *Clostridioides* (previously called *Clostridium*) *difficile* produces two toxins, CDT A and CDT B. CDT A is an enterotoxin that recruits PMNs, disrupts tight junctions, increases permeability of the intestinal wall, and induces inflammation. CDT B is a cytotoxin that disrupts the cytoskeleton and depolymerizes actin (answer choice B). CDT B is essential for virulence. **(A)** Superantigens, such as the *S. aureus* toxic shock syndrome toxin-1, activate T cells resulting in cytokine storm and inflammation. *C. difficile* does not produce a superantigen. **(C)** *Clostridium perfringens* produces the α-toxin (a phospholipase) that hydrolyzes lecithin. This toxin plays a role in the pathogenesis of *C. perfringens* skin infections. *C. difficile* does not hydrolyze lecithin. **(D)** *Shigella*, *Pseudomonas aeruginosa*, and *Corynebacterium diphtheriae* produce toxins that inhibit protein synthesis. Of these, only *Shigella* is a gastrointestinal pathogen. Infections with *Shigella* most often result in bacillary dysentery and are frequently associated with either day cares or travel to endemic regions. This case is unlikely to be due to *Shigella*; hence this answer is incorrect. **(E)** Several pathogens, including the gastrointestinal pathogens *Vibrio cholerae* and enterotoxigenic *Escherichia coli* (ETEC), produce toxins that interact with G proteins and ultimately increase intracellular levels of cyclic AMP. Since the patient had been hospitalized for a week prior to symptoms, this is likely to be a nosocomial infection. Neither

239

V. cholerae nor ETEC are common nosocomial pathogens. These pathogens are more likely to be associated with travel to countries in which these pathogens are endemic.

24.   Correct: Hypochlorite (A)

(A) Disinfection is the process of eliminating most but not all pathogens found on inanimate objects. Disinfection does not necessarily eliminate bacterial spores; however, some disinfectants are sporicidal. In this case, the man has an infection with *Clostridioides* (previously called *Clostridium*) *difficile*, which has spores. Hence, a sporicidal disinfectant should be used. Currently, the Centers for Disease Control and Prevention recommends that chlorine/hypochlorite (1:10 dilution) should be used as a disinfectant in areas involving *C. difficile*. Chlorine bleach and other oxidizing agents are effective against spores, including *C. difficile* spores. **(B)** Iodophors are usually used to disinfect skin and not inanimate surfaces. Iodine can kill spores if left on a surface for a prolonged time; therefore, iodophors are not the best agent to disinfect surfaces in this patient's room. **(C)** Isopropanol and other alcohols are not sporicidal. At certain concentrations, alcohols may be effective disinfectants for HIV and hepatitis B and C. However, isopropanol would not effectively eliminate *C. difficile* spores. When working with a patient with *C. difficile*, it is important to wash hands with soap and water. Alcohol based sanitizers are not effective against *C. difficile* spores. **(D)** Phenols are not sporicidal and can be used to clean environmental surfaces and nonmedical equipment, due to their high propensity to cause skin irritation. These agents are not effective against eliminated *C. difficile* spores. **(E)** Quaternary ammonium compounds are not sporicidal, but are effective against bacterial pathogens including methicillin-resistant *Staphylococcus aureus* (MRSA), vancomycin-resistant *Enterococcus*, and *Pseudomonas aeruginosa*. They may be used to disinfect medical equipment or to sanitize floors or other surfaces in a hospital. These compounds are not effective against *C. difficile* spores.

25.   Correct: Whipple's disease (E)

(E) This man most likely has Whipple's disease caused by *Tropheryma whipplei*, a gram-positive rod. This infection may closely resemble other conditions and diagnosis often occurs after ruling out other conditions. Histological examination of the small bowel may aid in diagnosis. Findings observed in Whipple's disease include villous atrophy and foamy inclusions within macrophages that stain within lamina propria with periodic acid-Schiff (PAS). PAS is a method that stains polysaccharides purple to pink. *T. whipplei* is found in the environment and many individuals are asymptomatic carriers. Infections are rare and males are more often infected than females. Multiple organ systems are infected including the musculoskeletal system and gastrointestinal tract. Common findings include arthralgias, abdominal pain, and diarrhea that may lead to malabsorption and weight loss. Skin hyperpigmentation and anemia due to vitamin D and B12 deficiencies may be present as well. **(A)** Crohn's disease, a type of inflammatory bowel disease, may present very similarly to Whipple's disease. Crohn's disease is thought to occur as a result of an abnormal immune response to intestinal microbiota including viruses and bacteria resulting in inflammation. In Crohn's disease, endoscopy often shows ulceration, inflammation, and atrophy of villi. Histology may show giant macrophages and granulomas, but not PAS-positive macrophages. **(B)** Histoplasmosis is caused by the dimorphic endemic fungus *Histoplasma capsulatum*. Primary infections mainly affect the pulmonary system and dissemination may occur especially in HIV-positive individuals. *Histoplasma* infects macrophages and PAS-positive macrophages may be observed. The rounded 2 to 4 mm diameter pathogen may be seen within macrophages, which differentiates histoplasmosis from Whipple's disease. **(C)** *Mycobacterium avium-intracellulare* complex (MAC) is acid-fast bacilli and manifestations of infection may be similar to those in Whipple's disease. Infections are most often observed in AIDS patients, especially when CD4 T cell counts fall below 50 cells/μL. This man has a negative HIV test. PAS-positive macrophages may be observed with MAC infections. However, the key differentiation for MAC is a positive acid-fast stain, which is negative in this case. **(D)** Tropical sprue may present with abdominal pain, chronic diarrhea, steatorrhea, and malabsorption. This infection is thought to have an infectious etiology and is mainly seen in tropical regions outside of the United States. As with Whipple's disease, villous atrophy and thickening of the small bowel folds may be present; however, PAS-positive macrophages are not seen in tropical sprue.

26.   Correct: *Bacteroides fragilis* (A)

(A) Anaerobic organisms, especially *Bacteroides fragilis*, are frequently implicated as etiological agents of intra-abdominal abscesses. *B. fragilis* is a strict (obligate) anaerobe and a gram-negative rod. The presence of gram-negative rods in the blood cultures and the finding that the organisms grew anaerobically, but not aerobically, lead to *B. fragilis* as the etiological agent. Intra-abdominal abscesses are often polymicrobial and occur following perforation or trauma to the bowel, such as in the case of recent surgery. These infections may lead to sepsis; hence the positive blood cultures in this case. **(B)** *Clostridioides* (previously called *Clostridium*) *difficile* is a strict anaerobic gram-positive rod and is associated with colitis and watery diarrhea. There is a possibility that the pathogen may cause intra-abdominal abscesses following a gastrointestinal infection, but this is rare. *B. fragilis* (answer choice A) is more likely to be the causative agent. **(C)** *Enterococcus faecalis* is a facultative anaerobe that may grow in either aerobic or anaerobic conditions. This pathogen is a gram-positive coccus in chains (not a gram-negative rod as in this case) and is part of the normal microbiota, especially in the small bowel. Enterococci are frequent agents of intra-abdominal abscesses. **(D)** *Escherichia coli*, a gram-negative rod, is a normal inhabitant of the small and large intestine. *E. coli* is commonly involved in intra-abdominal infections and is a facultative anaerobe. While it is possible that this infection may be due to *E. coli*, it is more likely to be attributable to *B. fragilis* since the pathogen grew in just anaerobic conditions. If the pathogen grew in both aerobic and anaerobic conditions, the most likely etiological agent would be *E. coli*. **(E)** *Peptostreptococcus magnus* is an anaerobic gram-positive coccus. It is a normal inhabitant of the gastrointestinal tract and it is also an agent of intra-abdominal abscess. In this case, the Gram stain results indicate that *B. fragilis* is more likely to be the agent of infection.

27. Correct: Enzyme-linked immunoassay (C)

(C) This is a case of rotavirus diarrhea. The best mechanisms of diagnosing rotavirus infection include detection of virus antigens via immunoassays or detection of RNA from stool via polymerase chain reaction (PCR). Rotavirus diarrhea is caused by the double-stranded RNA virus, rotavirus. This virus is unique because of a double-layered capsid. Infections with this pathogen peak in the winter and epidemics may occur in day care centers. The organism has a low infectious dose and is transmitted via the fecal–oral route or via fomites. Rotavirus is a major cause of severe diarrhea in infants and young children (< 2 years of age). Diarrhea, vomiting, and fever are common manifestations and severe dehydration and occasionally hypernatremia may occur. Older children and adults may also be affected by this pathogen but they generally have milder infections. Immunocompromised adults may present with severe symptoms, similar to young children. It is recommended that young children be vaccinated against this virus. There are currently two vaccines available with slightly different formulations, but they are both live, oral vaccines. **(A)** *Campylobacter jejuni* grows best at 42°C. Most other clinically significant pathogens, including rotavirus, prefer growth at body temperature (35–37°C). **(B)** Culture on MacConkey agar with sorbitol would most likely assist in confirming the diagnosis of *E. coli* O157:H7. This pathogen is the only *E. coli* that is sorbitol fermentation negative and colonies would appear clear or colorless on MacConkey agar with sorbitol. Rotavirus does not grow on artificial media such as MacConkey agar. Viruses, including

rotavirus are obligate intracellular pathogens and require live cells to grow. **(D)** In rotavirus infections, fecal leukocytes are most often absent. Fecal leukocytes (see image at the end of this answer) are not normally present in the stool and may be indicative of an infection. Fecal leukocytes are most often present in infections with invasive pathogens, such as *Campylobacter*, *Shigella*, *Salmonella*, *Yersinia enterocolitica*, or enteroinvasive *E. coli*. **(E)** The scotch tape preparation is performed to aid in the diagnosis of pinworm infections caused by the nematode helminth *Enterobius vermicularis*. In this test, a piece of scotch tape is pressed against the perianal region for the evaluation and microscopic identification of ova. The scotch tape test would not aid in the diagnosis of rotavirus.

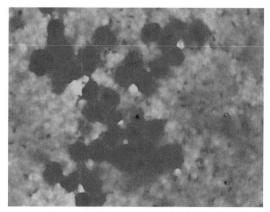

28. Correct: Norwalk virus (B)

(B) This is an infection with Norwalk virus. This virus causes a self-limiting gastroenteritis and is transmitted via contaminated food and water, aerosolization (of vomitus), or person–person from an infected individual. It is notable for causing outbreaks, especially on cruise ships, college campuses, or in other close-quarter populations. After a 24 to 48-hour incubation period, infected individuals may be either asymptomatic or present with an abrupt onset of watery diarrhea, vomiting, myalgias, malaise, and headache. Fever is present in 50% of cases. Infections are usually self-limited and resolve within 48 to 72 hours. Norwalk virus is a single-stranded, positive-sense RNA virus that is part of the Norovirus genus and calicivirus family. **(A)** *Giardia lamblia* infections occur following ingestion of contaminated food and water or via fecal–oral or anal–oral contact. This pathogen is associated with freshwater reservoirs. Watery, foul-smelling diarrhea, and greasy stools are often observed in *Giardia* infections and vomiting may or may not be present. Fever is not a common finding. This woman's recent history and clinical manifestations indicate that Norwalk virus and not *G. lamblia* is most likely the etiological agent. **(C)** Rotavirus is more likely to cause more severe manifestations in infants and young children and immunocompromised adults, especially during winter months. Immunocompetent

241

adults most often have mild infections with rota-virus. The question stem states that this woman is "otherwise healthy" and it is unlikely that rotavirus is causing her current condition. **(D)** *Shigella dysenteriae* is an agent of bacillary dysentery and bloody stools. Based on the symptoms in this case, *Shigella* is unlikely the causative agent. **(E)** Cholera infections are associated with travel to endemic regions, especially areas of Africa and South and Southeast Asia. Watery diarrhea with "rice-water stools" followed by severe fluid loss and vomiting may be present in cholera. Fever, however, is uncommon. This woman's symptoms indicate that this pathogen is not likely to be cause of her infection.

29. Correct: Trichrome stain (C)

(C) This is a case of amebic dysentery caused by the protozoan parasite *Entamoeba histolytica*. Answer choice C is an image of a trichrome stained *E. histolytica* cyst. Ulcers present on the colon and have a very classic, flask-shaped appearance as illustrated in question stem. This pathogen is found worldwide but is more common in resource-limited tropical countries. Infections are transmitted via the fecal-oral route by contaminated food and water. The cyst is the infective form. Following ingestion, cysts excyst in the small intestine and develop into a trophozoite. Most infections are asymptomatic and the organism remains in the small intestine or in the lumen of the large intestine and does not invade the mucosa. The trophozoite can invade and penetrate the mucosa of the colon resulting in ulceration, bloody stools, and amebic dysentery. In a small percentage of cases, the organism may disseminate from the intestine; common dissemination sites include the liver, brain, and lungs. The pathogen is diagnosed via recovery of cysts or trophozoites from the stool and is identified with an ova and parasite (O&P) examination. **(A)** This is an image of a *Giardia lamblia* trophozoite. This parasite stays in the lumen of the duodenum and does not invade the mucosa. Dysentery and ulcers on the mucosa would be rare; hence this answer choice is incorrect. **(B)** Many gram-negative rods, as illustrated in answer choice B, may cause bloody stools; however, *Shigella* species are the classic agents of bacillary dysentery. Like amebic dysentery infections with some strains of *Shigella* are more often found in resource-limited countries. In this case, the image of the flask-shaped ulcer indicates *E. histolytica* is more likely than *Shigella* to be the causative agent. **(D)** This image shows curved gram-negative rods, which is typical of *Campylobacter* or *Vibrio*. *Campylobacter* infections may result in watery diarrhea, bloody diarrhea, or dysentery depending on the location of the pathogen in the gastrointestinal tract. However, infections with *Campylobacter* would not result in the ulcers seen in the question stem. Cholera, caused by *V. cholerae* presents as nonfebrile, profuse watery diarrhea. **(E)** This

image shows a *Taenia* ovum (egg). *Taenia saginata* and *solium* are tapeworms, with indistinguishable ova, that may result in abdominal pain or watery diarrhea as the worm travels through the gastrointestinal tract. However, dysentery and fever are not common symptoms of infections with these pathogens.

30. Correct: Giardiasis (C)

(C) This man most likely has a case of chronic giardiasis caused by the protozoan parasite *Giardia lamblia*. Giardiasis is diagnosed via identification of the cysts or trophozoites in the stool (see images [i] and [ii] presented at the end of this answer), immunoassays including immunofluorescent assays (direct or indirect antibody tests), and nucleic acid amplification assays. The figure in the question stem shows classic pear-shaped *G. lamblia* trophozoites. It is important to note that intermittent shedding may occur; hence, multiple specimens over several days may be needed to identify this pathogen from stool specimens. Stool fecal fat is often positive and is an indication of steatorrhea. Acute infections with *Giardia* are often asymptomatic. If symptoms occur, foul-smelling watery diarrhea, abdominal cramps, bloating, flatulence, steatorrhea, nausea, anorexia, and malaise are often observed. Chronic infections may also occur as in this case. Typical findings of chronic infections include loose stools without diarrhea, steatorrhea, weight loss, and evidence of malabsorption (iron-deficiency anemia, fat-soluble vitamin deficiencies, etc.). Infections are transmitted via contaminated food and water, fecal–oral route and anal–oral sexual contact. Men who have sex with men and HIV-positive individuals are at increased risk for *Giardia* infections. See Appendix M for a list of common AIDS-related opportunistic pathogens. **(A)** Nonspecific symptoms such as abdominal pain, diarrhea, vomiting, and anorexia may be observed with *Ascaris lumbricoides* infections. Like with giardiasis, malabsorption, steatorrhea, and positive fecal fat may be present. Infections are more common following travel to endemic tropical countries. Eosinophilia is often present in infections and in this case the CBC is normal. Although men who have sex with men may be at risk for ascariasis, giardiasis is more common in this population than ascariasis. **(B)** The most common manifestation of infections with *Enterobius vermicularis* is perianal itching. Although men who have sex with men are at risk for pinworm infections, this infection is mainly seen in young children. The best way of visualizing this pathogen is via a scotch tape preparation. Like with other helminthic infections, eosinophilia is most often present. Steatorrhea is typically not observed. This infection is unlikely to be caused by *E. vermicularis*. **(D)** *Shigella* is an infrequent agent of chronic infections. However, men who have sex with men are at increased risk for shigellosis. This bacterial pathogen usually grows in culture; hence, the bacterial culture would have most likely been positive and demonstrated the growth of non-lactose fermenting organisms. Acute shigellosis may present as watery diarrhea, bloody diarrhea, or bacillary dysentery. Due to the invasive nature of this pathogen, fecal leukocytes are most often positive. (E) Chronic diarrhea, weight loss, and malabsorption may be noted in Whipple's disease. This rare infection is caused by *Tropheryma whipplei*, a gram-positive rod. Middle aged and older males are at increased risk for infection. HIV-positive individuals are not known to be at increased risk. However, this infection may mimic other gastrointestinal infections, such as *Mycobacterium avium-intracellulare* complex diarrhea, that are often seen in HIV-positive individuals. Histological findings from a small bowel biopsy would aid in confirming Whipple's disease. Villous atrophy and PAS-positive macrophages would be present. This infection does not resemble Whipple's disease.

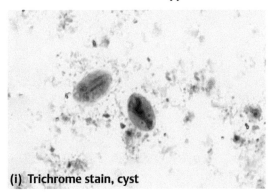

(i) Trichrome stain, cyst

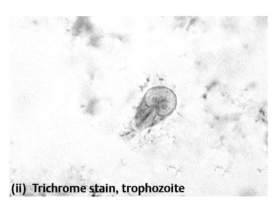

(ii) Trichrome stain, trophozoite

31. Correct: *Giardia lamblia* (B)

(B) This is a case of acute giardiasis. Classic findings of acute *Giardia* infections include foul-smelling watery diarrhea, abdominal cramps, bloating, flatulence, steatorrhea, nausea, anorexia, and malaise. Infections are transmitted via contaminated food and water and the organisms can survive in freshwater, especially mountain streams, such as described in this case. The organism is also transmitted via the fecal–oral route and anal–oral sexual contact. (A) *Entamoeba histolytica* is found worldwide but is more common in resource-limited countries. Most infections are asymptomatic; however, the classic finding of infection with *E. histolytica* is amebic dysentery with bloody stools, which is not observed in this case. (C) *Necator americanus* and the closely related *Ancylostoma duodenale* are referred to as hookworms. These pathogens enter via skin penetration by larvae, which are found in fecally contaminated soil. Most infections are asymptomatic, but nonspecific gastrointestinal symptoms such as abdominal pain and diarrhea may occur, in addition to iron-deficiency anemia from helminth-mediated blood sucking at the intestinal wall. In the United States, hookworm infections are more often seen in the South. The infection in this case most likely occurred following travel to the Rocky Mountains and symptoms do not resemble hookworm infection. (D) Norwalk virus causes a self-limiting gastroenteritis and is transmitted via contaminated food and water or person–person from an infected individual. It is notable for causing outbreaks especially on cruise ships, college campuses or in other close-quarter populations. Infected individuals may be either asymptomatic or present with an abrupt onset of watery diarrhea, vomiting, myalgias, malaise, and headache. The epidemiology and symptoms seen in this case indicate that *G. lamblia* is more likely to be the agent of infection. (E) *Trichinella spiralis* is a nematode that is transmitted via ingestion of encysted larva and is commonly associated with undercooked pork and bear meat. The initial phase of infection is mainly asymptomatic; however, nausea, vomiting, and diarrhea may be present. During the later phase, myalgias, muscle tenderness, swelling, weakness, and periorbital edema may be observed (trichinosis). The epidemiology and symptoms seen in this case indicate that *G. lamblia* is more likely to be the agent of infection.

32. Correct: Tinidazole (D)

(D) This infection is most likely due to the protozoan parasite, *Giardia lamblia* which has a characteristic pear-shaped trophozoite with two nuclei (see image at the end of this answer). Antimicrobials of choice for giardiasis include tinidazole and metronidazole. Tinidazole is resembles metronidazole in chemical structure. It is also a prodrug that is converted to the active form in vivo. The nitro group on tinidazole is reduced to toxic radicals that bind to DNA, resulting in DNA damage. In addition to giardiasis, tinidazole may also be used to treat intestinal and liver amebiasis, trichomoniasis, and bacterial vaginosis. It has a longer half-life and fewer adverse reactions compared to metronidazole. (A) Albendazole is mainly used for the treatment of nematodes and some cestodes. *Giardia* is a flagellated protozoan parasite. (B) Praziquantel is mainly used for infections with some cestodes and trematodes. *Giardia* is a flagellated protozoan. (C) Symptomatic acute and chronic *Giardia* infections should be treated. The agents of choice are tinidazole or metronidazole. (E) Trimethoprim–sulfamethoxazole is used for a number of bacterial infections and is effective against some gastrointestinal parasites as well. For example, trimethoprim–sulfamethoxazole may be used in the treatment of *Cyclospora*. Trimethoprim–sulfamethoxazole is not effective for infections with *G. lamblia*.

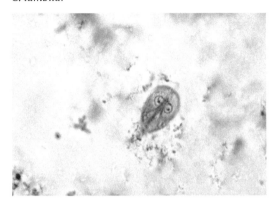

33. Correct: *Cryptosporidium parvum* (A)

(A) This infection is most likely to be caused by *Cryptosporidium*. The best stain to visualize the oocyst, the diagnostic form of the parasite, is a modified acid-fast stain. The modified acid-fast stain is similar to the traditional acid-fast stain used for *Mycobacteria* with the main difference being that a weaker decolorizer is used with the modified staining procedure. The small, round oocyst is modified acid-fast positive as shown in the image in the question stem. This organism is smaller (typically around 3–5 μm) than another closely related and similar-looking organism, *Cyclospora* (typically 5–10 μm). Polymerase chain reaction (PCR) and enzyme immunoassays (EIAs) are also available for diagnosis. Infections are often associated with contaminated water sources. In immunocompetent adults, infections are often asymptomatic. However, mild acute diarrhea with abdominal pain, malaise, and anorexia may occur. Infections are usually self-limiting. Chronic infections with this pathogen may also occur, classically in HIV/AIDS patients. In children and immunocompromised adults, infections may be more severe. Clinically significant species include *C. parvum* and *hominis*. These pathogens are protozoa and often referred to as coccidia. (B) *Giardia lamblia* is also a waterborne pathogen and, like *Cryptosporidium*, is associated with freshwater sources. Infections may present similarly with watery diarrhea, flatulence, nausea and abdominal pain. The pear-shaped flagellated *Giardia* trophozoite can be visualized with a trichrome stain, but not a modified acid-fast stain. (C) *Naegleria fowleri* is a protozoan that is associated with warm freshwater reservoirs. This pathogen enters via the cribriform plate of the ethmoid bone and migrates to the anterior part of the central nervous system resulting in a rapidly progressive and often fatal amebic encephalitis. Diarrhea is not a common manifestation of infections with this pathogen. (D) *Shigella* is a strictly human pathogen and is transmitted via the fecal–oral route and contaminated water is a common vehicle. Watery or bloody diarrhea or bacillary dysentery may be present. This pathogen is a gram-negative rod and does not stain with the modified acid-fast stain. (E) *Vibrio cholerae* is waterborne and associated with contaminated marine water. *Vibrio* is curved gram-negative rods and is not modified acid fast.

34. Correct: *Cryptosporidium* (A)

(A) The most likely etiological agent is *Cryptosporidium*. This pathogen is a small, round acid-fast oocyst that causes acute or chronic diarrhea. Chronic infections are especially common in individuals with AIDS. Manifestations of chronic cryptosporidiosis include severe weight loss, malabsorption, and steatorrhea. The oocyst is round and stains well with the modified acid-fast stain (see image [i] at the end of this answer). See Appendix M for a list of common AIDS-related opportunistic pathogens. (B) Infections with *Cystoisospora*, previously known as *Isospora*, are very similar to infections with *Cryptosporidium* and *Cyclospora* in AIDS patients. The three pathogens and their associated infections may be hard to differentiate. All of these pathogens stain well with the modified acid-fast stain. The oocyst of *Cryptosporidium* is small and round (see image [i] at the end of this answer). The oocyst of *Cyclospora* may be difficult to distinguish from *Cryptosporidium*. *Cyclospora* is larger (5–10 μm) than *Cryptosporidium* (3–5 μm) (see image [ii] at the end of this answer). *Cystoisospora* oocysts are large and oval in shape (see image [iii] at the end of this answer). The description of a small, round oocyst is more consistent with either *Cryptosporidium* or *Cyclospora* and not *Cystoisospora*, which is oval in shape. (C) Cytomegalovirus (CMV) may cause gastrointestinal infections in individuals with AIDS. This virus does not stain with the modified acid-fast stain. The enlarged CMV infected cells often contain characteristic eosinophilic inclusions that aid in diagnosis. (D) *Encephalitozoon* and the closely related species *Enterocytozoon* are the etiological agents of microsporidiosis, an opportunistic infection of AIDS patients. In the immunocompromised, severe watery diarrhea and wasting may occur. These pathogens were previously classified as protozoa but are now known to be fungi. The diagnostic forms of these organisms are the spores, which stain best with the modified trichrome stain. (E) *Mycobacterium* species are acid-fast bacilli and are rod shaped, not round. Infections with *Mycobacterium avium-intracellulare* complex may occur in AIDS and include a number of symptoms including diarrhea and weight loss. Oocysts represent a parasitic form and indicate that the pathogen is a parasite and not acid-fast bacillus.

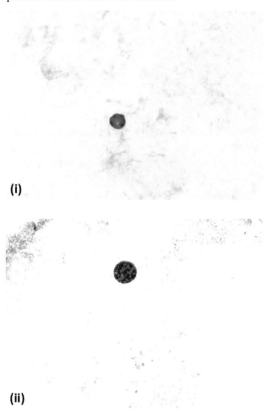

(i)

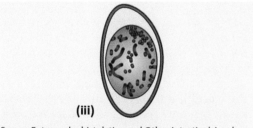

(ii)

(iii)

Source: Entamoeba histolytica and Other Intestinal Amebas. In: Kayser F, Bienz K, Eckert J et al., Hrsg. Medical Microbiology. 1st Edition. Thieme; 2004

35. Correct: Cholecystitis (B)

(B) The most likely etiological agent is *Cryptosporidium*. *Cryptosporidium* may disseminate to the biliary system resulting in hepatobiliary disease, especially cholangitis and cholecystitis. Acute cholangitis is typically a bacterial infection that occurs following common bile duct obstruction. Enteric bacteria, such as *Escherichia coli*, *Klebsiella*, and *Enterococcus*, enter the biliary tract from the duodenum following obstruction. Symptoms include fever, right upper quadrant abdominal pain, and jaundice (Charcot's triad). Acute cholecystitis involves a cystic duct obstruction, which results in constant right upper quadrant pain, fever, and leukocytosis. Murphy's sign may also be positive (patient expresses pain when clinician presses on gallbladder). See image at the

end of this answer for a comparison of cholangitis and cholecystitis. **(A)** Appendicitis may occur with several pathogens, especially worms. For example, tapeworms may cause infestations of the intestinal tract and result in mild diarrhea. However, appendicitis, although infrequent, may occur as a result of heavy infestation. *Cryptosporidium* is more likely to disseminate to the biliary system than the appendix. **(C)** Infections with many enteric bacterial pathogens including *Salmonella*, *Shigella*, and *Campylobacter* may result in reactive arthritis following gastrointestinal infection. Reactive arthritis, previously referred to as Reiter syndrome, presents classically as arthritis, urethritis, and conjunctivitis ("can't see, can't pee, can't climb a tree"). Reactive arthritis is not a typical postinfectious sequelae of *Cryptosporidium*. **(D)** Several pathogens, notably the roundworm, *Ascaris lumbricoides*, may cause small bowel perforation. Adult worms reside in the small intestine and a heavy burden of worms may result in obstruction or perforation. This is not a likely complication of cryptosporidiosis. **(E)** The gram-positive rod, *Clostridioides* (previously called *Clostridium*) *difficile* is a common agent of postantibiotic diarrhea. Complications such as toxic megacolon, colonic perforation, and peritonitis may occur. Toxic megacolon is not a complication of *Cryptosporidium*, which tends to stay in the small bowel.

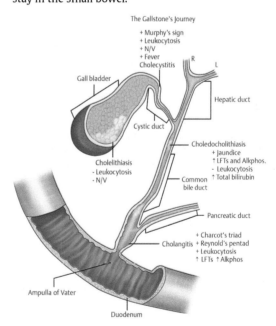

36. Correct: Coccidian parasite (A)

(A) *Cyclospora* infections are similar to infections with *Cryptosporidium*. Both are referred to as Coccidia and are classified as protozoa. The oocysts of both *Cyclospora* and *Cryptosporidium* stain with a modified acid-fast stain. However, only *Cyclospora* are autofluorescent (see image at the end of this answer), or fluorescence with ultraviolet (UV) light. Immunocompetent adults may be asymptomatic after exposure or have mild, self-limited watery diarrhea. The pathogen is found worldwide and endemic regions include several tropical and subtropical countries including Peru and Guatemala. **(B)** A flagellated protozoan parasite that should be considered in the differential diagnosis in this case is *Giardia lamblia*. This gastrointestinal pathogen is commonly associated with contaminated mountain streams, but it is not autofluorescent or acid-fast positive. **(C)** Very few fungal pathogens are agents of gastrointestinal infections. *Encephalitozoon* and *Enterocytozoon* (often referred to as microsporidia) cause mild, self-limiting watery diarrhea in immunocompetent individuals and cause severe diarrhea in the immunocompromised individuals. The best stain to visualize the spores of these pathogens is the modified trichrome stain. **(D)** The most common roundworm infection in humans is *Ascaris lumbricoides* that may cause gastrointestinal symptoms while the worm is localized to the gastrointestinal tract. Infections are more common in tropical and subtropical countries. *Ascaris* is not autofluorescent or modified acid-fast positive. **(E)** A single-stranded RNA virus that is a common agent of gastrointestinal infections is Norwalk virus. Infections are seen worldwide and commonly occur in enclosed, heavily populated settings. Norwalk virus does not autofluoresce (viruses are too small to be seen with light microscopy) and is not modified acid fast.

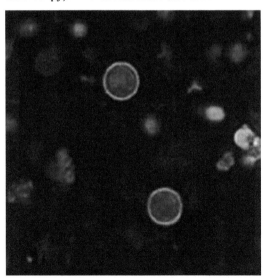

Source: CDC

37. Correct: Saliva (E)

(E) This is an infection with cytomegalovirus (CMV), a double-stranded DNA virus that is part of the herpes virus family. It is also called human herpes virus-5 (HHV-5). Infections are transmitted via saliva (answer choice E), urine, semen, and vaginal secretions. The pathogen may also be transmitted vertically and via organ transplants. All herpes viruses have the ability to establish latency following primary infections and reactivation may occur at any time; however, immunosuppression

increases the risk. CMV is frequently associated with AIDS and commonly affects the gastrointestinal tract, liver, lungs, or eyes. While any part of the gastrointestinal tract may be infected, the esophagus and colon are the most often involved. Clinical manifestations of CMV colitis may include weight loss, abdominal pain, diarrhea, and low-grade fever. Tenesmus and hematochezia may be present as well. One mechanism of identifying CMV is histological staining of biopsy specimens from the colon. Cytomegalic cells with intranuclear inclusions may be observed. These inclusions are often referred to as owl-eye inclusions (see image at the end of this answer). See Appendix M for a list of common AIDS-related opportunistic pathogens. **(A, B)** There is no evidence demonstrating that CMV is transmitted via contaminated food and water. **(C)** CMV is a virus. Conida (also called spores) are morphologic forms of fungi, not viruses. **(D)** Skin contact with contaminated secretions may be a mechanism of CMV transmission. However, there is no evidence that CMV can penetrate intact skin. An example of a pathogen that is capable of penetrating intact skin to cause infection is *Strongyloides stercoralis*.

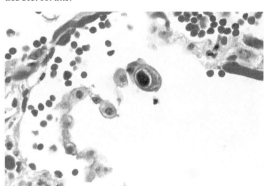

Source: CDC/Dr. Edwin P. Ewing, Jr.

38. Correct: *Ascaris lumbricoides* (A)

(A) This woman has a small bowel obstruction (see image at the end of this answer). Complications of ascariasis include mechanical small bowel obstruction due to the heavy burden and infestation of adult worms. *Ascaris lumbricoides* is a nematode that is transmitted via the fecal–oral route. The ova are the infective form and once ingested, hatch into larvae in the small intestine. The larvae penetrate the bowel wall and migrate hematogenously through the hepatic portal venous system to the lungs. Larvae then ascend the respiratory tree and enter the pharynx and then are swallowed into the gut. In the small intestine, larvae mature into adult worms. The adults reside in the small intestine and lay eggs, which are passed in the stool. Symptoms of infection will vary based on the anatomical location of the pathogen. During the gastrointestinal phase, abdominal pain, diarrhea, vomiting, and anorexia may be present. During the migration of the larva to the lungs, pulmonary symptoms (e.g., cough) and pneumonitis may be observed. Additionally, cholecystitis, acute cholangitis, acute pancreatitis, and hepatic abscess may occur due to migration of adult worms to the biliary tree. Infections are endemic in tropical and subtropical countries. **(B)** The most common site of dissemination of *Cryptosporidium* is the biliary tree, resulting in hepatobiliary disease. Small bowel obstruction with *Cryptosporidium* is not common. **(C)** Infections with *Entamoeba histolytica* are asymptomatic or may result in amebic dysentery. The trophozoites typically reside in the large bowel. In a small percentage of cases, extraintestinal infections may occur due to migration of the trophozoites to the liver, brain, lungs, and other organs. Small bowel obstruction is not complication of amebic dysentery. **(D)** Acute infections with enterohemorrhagic *Escherichia coli* (EHEC) usually present as nonfebrile, bloody diarrhea. The main complication is hemolytic uremic syndrome (HUS) wherein the kidneys are damaged due to the Shiga-like exotoxin produced by the pathogen. Infections occur worldwide following ingestion of contaminated food or contact with infected animals. Small bowel obstruction following infection with EHEC is not typically seen. **(E)** *Yersinia enterocolitica* typically invades M cells in Peyer's patches of the terminal ileum leading to pseudoappendicitis or mesenteric lymphadenitis. Small bowel obstruction is not a complication of *Yersinia* infections.

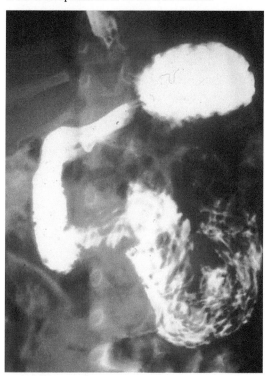

Source: Wikimedia/SuSanA Secretariat

39. Correct: Rhabditiform larva (D)

(D) Strongyloidiasis is caused by the helminthic parasite *Strongyloides stercoralis*. The filariform larvae live in the soil and can then infect humans by entering through intact skin (e.g., bare feet). The filariform larvae migrate hematogenously to the lungs for further maturation. They are then swallowed and larvae develop into adult worms in the small intestine. The adults lay eggs (ova) and eggs develop into rhabditiform larvae that are passed in the stool. The rhabditiform larvae develop into filariform larvae in the soil. The infective filariform larvae can then penetrate human skin. Hence, the diagnostic forms of the organism are the rhabditiform larvae (answer choice D). This pathogen is endemic in Southeast Asia and several other tropical countries. Infections in the immunocompetent are often asymptomatic and eosinophilia may be the only evidence of infection. Immunocompromised individuals may present with more serious hyperinfection or disseminated infections. **(A)** Adult worms reside in the intestine and are rarely passed in the stool. **(B)** The filariform larvae are found in the soil and are the infective form of the pathogen. In vivo, the rhabditiform larvae may develop into filariform larvae and can then penetrate intestinal mucosa resulting in disseminated infections. In this case there is no evidence of a disseminated infection, so the finding of a filiariform larvae is unlikely. **(C)** The ova or eggs are found in the intestines. They are rarely passed in the stool. **(E)** *S. stercoralis* is a nematode. There is no trophozoite form of the pathogen. Trophozoites are morphologic forms of some protozoan parasites.

40. Correct: Cestode (B)

(B) The image in the question stem shows an ovum of *Taenia saginata* or *solium*, which are within the phylum Platyhelminthes and the class cestodes (answer choice B). Cestodes may also be referred to as tapeworms. *Taenia saginata* is associated with ingestion of undercooked beef whereas *Taenia solium* is associated with undercooked pork. Humans ingest undercooked beef or pork and the cysticercus, a larval form, develops into an adult worm in the small intestine, which may survive for long periods of time (see image at the end of this answer). Most often infections are asymptomatic but mild gastrointestinal discomfort may be observed as well. The proglottids or segments of the adult worm may be passed in feces and adult worms produce ova or eggs that are also passed in the feces. Cows or pigs may ingest the eggs, which then develop into the cysticercus in the tissue of the animal. The cycle then begins again. In the case of *Taenia solium*, if humans ingest the ova or eggs (from fecally contaminated food or water), the eggs may develop into the cysticercus or larval forms in human tissue. *Taenia* infections are more often seen in areas of Africa, Asia, and Latin America. **(A, C)** Amoebae and coccidia are within in the phylum Protozoa. *Taenia* is cestodes. **(D)** Worms within the class nematodes, also referred to as roundworms, are part of the phylum Nemathelminthes. *Taenia* is cestodes. **(E)** Trematodes, also called flukes, are also part of the phylum Platyhelminthes but are in a different class than the cestodes. See Appendix P for a flow diagram of parasite classification.

Taenia Transmission

Cysticercus in tissue of cows *(T. saginata)* or pigs *(T. solium)* in tissue

Human ingests undercooked meat; cysticercus develops into adult worm in human intestine

Proglottids may be passed in feces

Adult worms produce eggs

Cows/pigs may ingest eggs, which develop into cysticerci

Human may ingest eggs

T. solium only

Eggs develop into cysticerci in tissue

41. Correct: *Diphyllobothrium latum* (C)

(C) One of the major features of infections with the cestode *Diphyllobothrium latum* is megaloblastic anemia secondary to vitamin B12 deficiency as presented in this case. Symptoms include those of anemia (fatigue, pallor, shortness of breath), neuropathy, and atrophic glossitis. *Diphyllobothrium latum* is associated with freshwater fish and infections are often asymptomatic. There are several larval forms of the organism and one of the larval forms lives in freshwater fish. Humans are infected after consumption of undercooked freshwater fish. Mild gastrointestinal symptoms such as diarrhea and weight loss may also occur. This is one of the longest tapeworms of man, and adult worms may reach up to 12 meters. **(A)** The trematode *Clonorchis sinensis* mainly affects the liver and is mainly seen in the Far East in countries such as China and is associated with the ingestion of raw or undercooked freshwater fish. *C. sinensis* is often referred to as the Chinese liver fluke. This man's travel history and clinical findings indicate that infections due to *C. sinensis* are highly unlikely. **(B)** *Cryptosporidium parvum* is a protozoan parasite and is associated with contaminated recreational water (fresh or saltwater), drinking water, and swimming pools but not necessarily fish; hence this is not the best answer choice. In healthy adults, such as the man in this case, infections are usually asymptomatic or manifest as mild self-limiting diarrhea. In immunocompromised individuals (e.g., HIV/AIDS), bloody diarrhea and anemia are possible findings. **(D)** *Mycobacterium marinum* is an opportunistic acid-fast bacillus. It is associated with fish tanks and causes ulcerative skin lesions that ascend proximally along lymphatics after contact of open skin with infected water (fresh or saltwater). The manifestations in this case do not resemble the findings seen with *M. marinum* infections. **(E)** Non-cholera *Vibrio* such as *Vibrio vulnificus* may cause wound infections after contact with contaminated water. Similar to *V. cholerae* these pathogens are also halotolerant and are associated with marine or estuarine environments. The organism most likely gains entry after a breach in the intact skin. Gastrointestinal infections may also occur after ingestion of contaminated food and water and infections are commonly associated with shellfish, such as oysters. *Vibrio* species are curved gram-negative rods. This man was exposed to freshwater; therefore, infections due to *Vibrio* are very unlikely.

42. Correct: *Encephalitozoon* (C)

(C) The image presented in the question stem shows several spores of *Encephalitozoon* or *Enterocytozoon*, which are also referred to as microsporidia. Microsporidia are an important cause of severe watery diarrhea in AIDS patients. These fungal pathogens are transmitted via ingestion or inhalation of spores. The best stain to visualize spores is the modified trichrome stain. In immunocompetent individuals, microsporidiosis is most often asymptomatic or causes a self-limiting watery diarrhea. The treatment of choice for these infections is albendazole, in addition to antiretroviral therapy. **(A)** *Cryptosporidium* does not stain with the trichrome or modified trichrome stains. The best stain to visualize this pathogen is the modified acid-fast stain. The manifestations of cryptosporidiosis in immunocompromised individuals may be very similar to microsporidiosis. **(B)** Cytomegalovirus (CMV) is frequently associated with AIDS and may infect the gastrointestinal tract. One mechanism of identifying CMV is histological staining of biopsy specimens from the colon. Cytomegalic cells with intranuclear inclusions may be observed. While cytological changes due to virally infected cells (i.e., CPE) can be visualized with light microscopy, visualization of actual viral particles would require higher magnification, such as the use of electron microscopy. Clinical manifestations of CMV colitis may include weight loss, abdominal pain, bloody diarrhea, and low-grade fever. The image in the question stem shows microsporidia, not CMV. **(D)** *Mycobacterium*, including *Mycobacterium avium-intracellulare* complex, are associated with AIDS. Mycobacteria are best visualized with the acid-fast stain, not with modified trichrome stain, and are rod shaped. Gastrointestinal infections with *Mycobacterium avium-intracellulare* complex may resemble the symptoms seen in this case; however, the image shows microsporidia, hence answer choice D is incorrect. **(E)** AIDS patients have a higher risk for more severe infections with *Salmonella* and may present with similar findings as described in this case. However, *Salmonella* are gram-negative rods (see image at the end of this answer), not oval-shaped spores as in the figure in the question stem. *Salmonella* is transmitted foodborne (e.g., eggs) and can also be contracted from contact with infected animals (e.g., reptiles, amphibians, and poultry). See Appendix M for a list of common AIDS-related opportunistic pathogens.

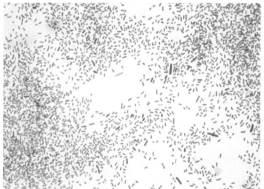

43. Correct: Scotch tape preparation (D)

(D) Perianal itching in a young child is a classic sign of pinworm. *Enterobius vermicularis* is a nematode that is commonly known as pinworm because adult worms are tiny, like a pinhead. A scotch tape preparation or a "pinworm paddle," which is a paddle-shaped stick with a sticky surface, can be used to recover eggs (see image [i] at the end of this answer), and at times, even adult worms (see image [ii] at the end of this answer). Infection begins with ingestion of the ova that hatch into larvae and mature into adults in the intestines. The females migrate to the perianal region, most often at night, leading to perianal itching and difficulty sleeping. Infections with this pathogen occur worldwide and affect all age groups, but young children are particularly prone to infections. **(A)** Enzyme immunoassays (EIAs) are often used in the diagnosis of the parasite *Giardia lamblia* but are not readily available for *E. vermicularis* detection. **(B)** The Gram stain is classically used for the identification of bacteria and not parasites such as *E. vermicularis*. Note that yeast and some fungi also may stain with the Gram stain. **(C)** Several clinically significant pathogens can be identified with the modified acid-fast stain including the gastrointestinal parasites *Cryptosporidium* and *Cyclospora*. *E. vermicularis* cannot be visualized with the acid-fast stain. **(E)** Stool ova and parasite (O&P) evaluation is not a good method of diagnosing enterobiasis. Neither the ova nor the adult worms are routinely passed in the stool.

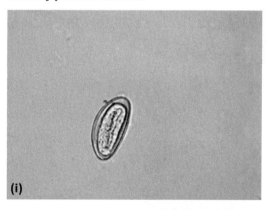

(i)

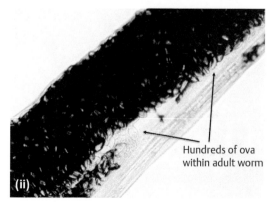

(ii)

Hundreds of ova within adult worm

44.   Correct: *Trichuris trichiura* (E)

(E) Rectal prolapse, as described in the question stem, is a common complication of heavy infections with *Trichuris trichiura*. The figure in the question stem shows an ovum of *T. trichiura*. This pathogen is also called the whipworm because the adult worms resemble a whip (see image at the end of this answer). Infections are mostly asymptomatic but in heavy infections, diarrhea may be observed. Ova are found in contaminated soil and once ingested, develop into larvae in the small intestine. The larvae mature into adult worms, which reside in the cecum and colon. The ovum, with hyaline plugs at both poles, resembles a football or barrel. Children are at increased risk for infection and complications. Infection rates are higher in sub-Saharan Africa, China, and other East Asian countries. (A) *Ancylostoma duodenale* (and *Necator americanus*) is also known as hookworm. The adult hookworm resides in the small intestine, "hooking" into the bowel wall and sucking blood. Because the adult worm mainly resides in the small bowel, rectal prolapse is not common. Common complications of hookworm infestation include nutritional impairment and iron-deficiency anemia. (B) Adult roundworms (*Ascaris lumbricoides*) mainly live in the small intestine. Heavy infections are associated with intestinal, hepatobiliary, and pancreatic obstruction. (C) *Enterobius vermicularis*, commonly known as the pinworm, most often affects young children. The adult female migrates through the colon and rectum to the perianal region to lay eggs, usually at night. There have been reports of rectal prolapse with pinworm infections; however, whipworms are more likely to be associated with this condition due to the location of adult whipworms in the cecum and colon. (D) Adult *Taenia saginata* or the beef tapeworm stays mainly in the small bowel. Complications are uncommon; however, migration to the appendix, common bile duct, and pancreas may occasionally occur.

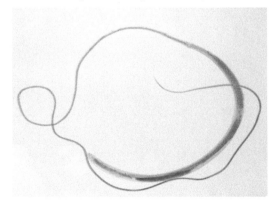

45.   Correct: *Streptococcus bovis* (E)

(E) This woman most likely has colorectal cancer as indicated by her symptoms, endoscopy, and laboratory findings. There is a strong correlation between colorectal cancer and previous infection with *Streptococcus bovis*. *S. bovis* is a gram-positive coccus in chains and is an etiological agent of infective endocarditis and bacteremia. Note that *S. bovis* has been renamed and is now called *S. gallolyticus*. (A) *Helicobacter pylori* acute gastritis increases the risk of gastric adenocarcinoma and gastric MALT lymphoma, in addition to peptic ulcer disease. *H. pylori* is not typically associated with colorectal cancer. (B) Chronic hepatitis B infections are associated with increased risk of hepatocellular carcinoma (HCC), not colon cancer. (C) Cervical cancer is linked to prior infections with human papillomavirus (HPV). The highest risk of cervical cancer is associated with HPV types 16 and 18. (D) Chronic infections with the trematode, *Schistosoma haematobium* increase the risk of bladder cancer, not colorectal cancer.

46.   Correct: Ingestion of shellfish (D)

(D) This is an acute infection with hepatitis A virus (HAV) as indicated by the positive IgM anti-HAV. HAV is transmitted by the fecal–oral route. Contaminated food and water serve as common vectors and frequently associated foods include shellfish (answer choice D), fruits, and vegetables. Hepatitis A may also be transmitted person-to-person via contact with contaminated fomites or oral-anal sex. The incubation period is about one month. HAV is a single-stranded positive sense RNA virus and is part of the picornavirus family. The initial infection is characterized by the abrupt onset of a nonspecific prodrome of symptoms. This is followed by a jaundice/icteric phase and finally full recovery. This virus does not establish chronicity. IgM anti-HAV antibodies are produced early in infection and will appear 5 to 10 days prior to symptoms. Liver enzymes are significantly elevated during viral hepatitis (sometimes > 1,000 U/L). In this case the infection is in the early stages as represented by the AST and ALT levels. The positive anti-HBs test indicates immunity to hepatitis B, a member of the hepadnavirus family. See Appendix O for a summary of the major features of hepatitis A, B, C, D, and E. (A) None of the hepatitis viruses, including hepatitis A, are transmitted via a mosquito bite. Some vector-borne infections such as yellow fever may present similarly and should be included in the differential diagnosis of viral hepatitis. (B) There is a possibility of hepatitis A transmission via contaminated blood. However, the risk is very low and this is a rare mechanism of transmission. (C) Certain genotypes of hepatitis E are zoonotic and common reservoirs include pigs and wild boars. Hepatitis A is not transmitted in this manner. (E) HAV is not transmitted vertically. Hepatitis B and C can be transmitted vertically from mom to baby. Hepatitis B is transmitted in utero, perinatally or postnatally, while hepatitis C is most often associated with in utero transmission.

47. Correct: A past infection with hepatitis A (B)

(B) This woman has had a past infection with hepatitis A and most likely a chronic infection with hepatitis B virus (HBV). In this case, the IgM anti-HAV is negative and the total anti-HAV (anti-IgM and anti-IgG) is positive, indicating a past infection with hepatitis A virus (HAV). Hepatitis A is an acute, self-limiting infection that is transmitted via the fecal–oral route. High-risk groups include day care workers and children, as well as travelers to endemic regions. Vaccination for hepatitis A is recommended for these high-risk groups. Hepatitis B may present as an acute or chronic infection. Chronic infections are characterized by symptoms lasting more than 6 months. Chronic infections may be asymptomatic or present with just fatigue. Once liver failure occurs, symptoms of chronic infections may be more apparent. Typical serology pattern of chronic hepatitis B infection includes positive HBsAg, positive total anti-HBc, and negative IgM anti-HBc. See images (i), (ii), and (iii) at the end of this answer for a summary of hepatitis B serology. Hepatitis B is transmitted percutaneously and through mucosae. This DNA virus is partially double-stranded and encodes a reverse transcriptase. See Appendix O for a summary of the major features of hepatitis A, B, C, D, and E. **(A)** The IgM-anti HAV is negative indicating that this is not likely an acute hepatitis A infection. **(C)** In an acute hepatitis B infection, the HBsAg is positive early on and then disappears with clinical improvement. The IgM anti-HBc is positive, usually with the onset of clinical symptoms and will disappear as the infection resolves (see image [iii at the end of this answer]). In the case presented here, the anti-HBs antibody and the IgM anti-HBc antibody are both negative. **(D)** A coinfection with hepatitis B and D means that an individual was infected with both hepatitis B and D at the same time. In this case, the anti-HDV is negative; hence, this woman is not infected with hepatitis D. **(E)** Recovery and natural immunity to hepatitis B would be indicated by a positive total anti-HBc and positive anti-HBs. Positive anti-HBs alone would indicate active immunity via vaccination (see image [ii]). The anti-HBs in this case are negative, so this woman is not immune to hepatitis B.

Hepatitis B virus (HBV)

- DNA/genome
  - Partially double stranded DNA
  - Encodes a reverse transcriptase
- Capsid
  - HBcAg (Hepatitis B core antigen)
- Envelope
  - HBsAg (Hepatitis B surface antigen)
- Hepatitis be antigen
  - Antigen secreted in

(i) serum during infection

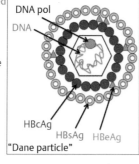

DNA pol
DNA
HBcAg
HBsAg HBeAg
"Dane particle"

HBV serology overview

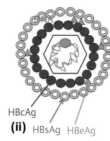

HBcAg
(ii) HBsAg HBeAg

Disease stage	Marker (positive)
Acute	HBsAg IgM anti-HBc Total anti-HBc
Chronic	HBsAg Total anti-HBc
Recovery (natural immunity)	Total anti-HBc Anti-HBs
Vaccination	Anti-HBs

HBV: serological profile

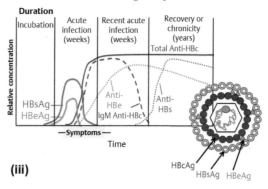

(iii)

48. Correct: Has a coinfection with hepatitis B and D and is highly infectious (A)

(A) This patient has acute hepatitis B and D or a coinfection with both viruses and is highly infectious. *Acute hepatitis B:* The positive HBsAg, total anti-HBc, and IgM anti-HBc are indicative of an acute infection with hepatitis B. HBsAg, or hepatitis B surface antigen, is positive in early acute infections prior to symptoms and during acute phase but disappears with clinical improvement (see images [i] and [ii] presented at the end of this answer). Total anti-HBc is positive in acute, chronic, and resolved infections and persists indefinitely. *Coinfection with hepatitis D:* If a patient has acute hepatitis B and is simultaneously infected with hepatitis D, this is referred to as coinfection. The positive IgM anti-HDV suggests an acute infection with hepatitis D. Hepatitis D virus is an incomplete or delta "defective" virus that requires HBV for replication. HDV core antigen is dependent upon HBsAg for replication and expression, and without HBsAg coating HDV cannot survive, multiply, or infect on its own. *Infectivity:* HBeAg is a marker of infectivity or infectiousness and a positive HBeAg indicates greater infectivity and higher viral replication activity. See Appendix O for a summary of the major features of hepatitis A, B, C, D, and E. **(B)** Superinfection with hepatitis B and D occurs when an individual has hepatitis B infection first which becomes chronic and is then infected with hepatitis D later. As indicated previously, this is an acute hepatitis B infection. A typical serological profile for a chronic infection is as follows: positive HBsAg, positive total anti-HBc, and negative

IgM anti-HBc. The positive HBeAg in this case indicates greater infectivity or that the patient is highly infectious. **(C)** This is an acute infection with both hepatitis B and hepatitis D, not just hepatitis B. The positive HBeAg indicates that this woman is highly infectious, not minimally infectious. **(D)** This is an acute infection not chronic infection with both hepatitis B and D. The positive HBeAg indicates that this woman is highly infectious, not minimally infectious. **(E)** This woman is not at subsequent risk for hepatitis A. The IgG anti-HAV provides enduring protection against reinfection with HAV and this woman has a positive IgG anti-HAV. Therefore, she has had a previous hepatitis A infection or immunization and is not at risk for reinfection. Hepatitis A infections are seen worldwide but infections are endemic in Central and South America; since this woman emigrated from El Salvador recently, there is an increased possibility that she was exposed to this virus previously.

HBV serology overview

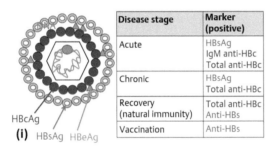

Disease stage	Marker (positive)
Acute	HBsAg IgM anti-HBc Total anti-HBc
Chronic	HBsAg Total anti-HBc
Recovery (natural immunity)	Total anti-HBc Anti-HBs
Vaccination	Anti-HBs

HBcAg

(i) HBsAg HBeAg

HBV: serological profile

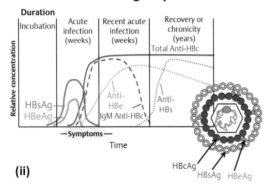

(ii)

49. Correct: Hepatitis B virus (HBV) (B)

(B) There is an established association between chronic infection with hepatitis B virus (HBV) and hepatocellular carcinoma (HCC). The HBV genome does not encode oncoproteins. However, due to the chronic hepatocyte injury and restorative hyperplasia the hepatic cells are at increased risk for subsequent damage and oncogenesis. **(A)** Epstein–Barr virus (EBV) is also called human herpes virus-4 (HHV-4) and is part of the herpes virus family. EBV infections are linked to Burkitt's lymphoma, other lymphoproliferative diseases, and nasopharyngeal cancers. More recently, evidence has shown a link between stomach cancers and prior EBV infections. EBV is not typically associated with HCC. **(C)** Human herpes virus-8 (HHV-8) is associated with Kaposi sarcoma, classically in patients with HIV/AIDS. HHV-8 is not associated with HCC. **(D)** Human papilloma virus (HPV) is associated with cervical cancer and oral/head and neck tumors and not HCC. **(E)** Human T-lymphotrophic virus (HTLV-1) is a retrovirus that is associated with adult T cell leukemia/lymphoma, not HCC.

50. Correct: Profile III (C)

(C) This man most likely has an acute hepatitis C infection. It is not possible to distinguish acute, chronic, or resolved hepatitis C infections with laboratory testing. However, if both anti-HCV and HCV RNA are positive, as in answer choice C, it is an indication of a current infection, which may be acute or chronic. The hepatitis C virus is primarily transmitted via percutaneous exposure. High-risk groups include incarcerated individuals, IV drug users, and individuals with tattoos and piercings, especially if they were obtained through unhygienic practices. Hepatitis C virus is part of the flavivirus family, which are positive-sense, single-stranded RNA viruses. One of the key features of hepatitis C virus is that the RNA-dependent RNA polymerase does not have proofreading capabilities, which leads to significant mutations and variations, making vaccine manufacturing difficult. See Appendix O for a summary of the major features of hepatitis A, B, C, D, and E. **(A)** This profile is typical of acute hepatitis A infection. The IgM-HAV is positive and all other markers are negative. Hepatitis A is transmitted mainly via the fecal–oral route. In this case, the epidemiology indicates hepatitis C is more likely to be the agent of infection. **(B)** This profile is indicative of a chronic hepatitis B infection. The HBsAg and total anti-HBc are positive, which is observed in chronic hepatitis B. Hepatitis B is transmitted percutaneously and through mucosae. There is a possibility that this infection could be due to hepatitis B; however, it is more likely based on the epidemiology that the etiological agent is hepatitis C (history of IV drug use and tattoos). **(D)** This profile shows a past infection with hepatitis A and immunity to hepatitis B. The positive IgG anti-HAV indicates a past infection with hepatitis A and immunity against subsequent exposure. The positive anti-HBs indicate immunity to hepatitis B via active immunity/vaccination. This man is more likely has an acute viral hepatitis infection as indicated by the clinical findings. **(E)** The positive IgM anti-HEV in this profile is an indication of a current infection with hepatitis E. This infection is mainly transmitted via the fecal–oral route and is not usually transmitted percutaneously. In this case, hepatitis C is more likely than hepatitis E to be the etiological agent.

51. Correct: Hepevirus (D)

(D) This man has an acute infection with hepatitis E virus as indicated by the positive IgM anti-HEV. Hepatitis E virus is a single-stranded RNA virus that is part of the hepevirus family. Hepatitis E infections are not common in the United States but are endemic in some resource-limited areas, especially in Asia, the Middle East, Africa, and Central America. The pathogen is transmitted mainly via the fecal–oral route. There are currently four known genotypes of hepatitis E. Certain genotypes are zoonotic and have been linked to undercooked pork and deer meat. Hepatitis E is self-limiting and there is not a chronic form of disease. See Appendix O for a summary of the major features of hepatitis A, B, C, D, and E. **(A)** Hepatitis D is referred to as the delta virus. In this case, the anti-HDV is negative so this is not the agent of the man's current infection. Additionally, hepatitis D infections occur only in conjunction with hepatitis B infections (as coinfection or superinfection). The negative IgM anti-HBc and negative total anti-HBc indicate that this man does not have acute hepatitis B and the negative HBsAg rules out chronic hepatitis B. This man's travel history indicates hepatitis A or E is more likely to be the etiological agent. **(B)** Hepatitis C is part of the flavivirus family. Other notable members of this family include West Nile virus, yellow fever virus, Zika virus, and dengue virus. In this case, the anti-HCV is negative indicating that this is not the current agent of infection. This man's travel history suggests that hepatitis A or E is more likely to be the etiological agent. **(C)** Hepatitis B is a hepadnavirus. The positive anti-HBs indicate that the man is immune to hepatitis B. This man's travel history indicates hepatitis A or E is more likely to be the etiological agent. **(E)** Hepatitis A is part of the picornavirus family that also includes enteroviruses, polio virus, coxsackie virus, and rhinovirus. Based on epidemiology, there is a possibility this man may have a hepatitis A infection. Infections are endemic in many resource-limited counties. However, positive IgG anti-HAV is indicative of past infection and lasting immunity to hepatitis A. Therefore, hepatitis A is not the etiological agent of the current infection.

52. Correct: High mortality in pregnant woman (C)

(C) This man has an acute infection with hepatitis E virus as indicated by the positive IgM anti-HEV. One of the characteristics of this virus is the ability to cause serious infections in pregnant females, especially during the third trimester. In this population, there is an increased risk of fulminant hepatitis and hepatic failure, and the mortality rate approaches 20%. **(A)** Chronic hepatitis B infections are associated with hepatocellular carcinoma (HCC). Hepatitis E is not associated with HCC. **(B)** Chronic infections occur with hepatitis B and C. Hepatitis A and E are acute and self-limiting. **(D)** There is currently no vaccination available for Hepatitis C, D, or E. Hepatitis A and B currently have effective vaccines that aid in preventing infections with these pathogens. **(E)** Infections with hepatitis D occur in conjunction with hepatitis B. In this case the most likely agent is hepatitis E, which does not have to occur in conjunction with hepatitis B.

53. Correct: Freshwater fish (C)

(C) The figure in the question stem shows ova of *Clonorchis sinensis*. This trematode is also referred to as the liver fluke or Chinese liver fluke. This pathogen is transmitted via ingestion of raw or undercooked freshwater fish. Humans are accidental hosts. Once ingested, the larvae excyst in the small intestine and develop into adult worms, which live in biliary ducts. Infections with this pathogen may be acute or chronic. Acute infections are most often asymptomatic or result in nonspecific findings (e.g., abdominal pain). Symptoms of chronic infections are due to the presence of the adult worms in the bile ducts. Findings include fatigue, dyspepsia, weight loss, and diarrhea. Infections with this pathogen increase the risk of cholangiocarcinoma. This fluke is mainly seen in the Far East in countries such as China, Vietnam, and Korea. Ova may be seen in the stool or bile and adult worms may be seen with ERCP. Note that infections with other flukes may present similarly (e.g., *Opisthorchis*). **(A)** Escargot is cooked snails. Snails are involved in the life cycle of *C. sinensis* and serve as the intermediate host. Once adult worms lay eggs (i.e., ova), the eggs are passed in the stool of definitive or accidental hosts. Snails ingest ova, which then develop into larvae. Freshwater fish ingest snails and human infections occur from ingestion of undercooked or raw fish. **(B)** Fecally contaminated water may contain ova of *C. sinensis*. However, ova must undergo further maturation in snails and fish prior to being transmitted to humans. **(D)** Many animals including dogs, cats, and pigs serve as the reservoir host for *C. sinensis*. Human infection does not occur from ingestion of pork but from ingestion of fish. **(E)** Watercress and freshwater plants are involved in the transmission of other trematode infections, including *Fasciola hepatica* but not *C. sinensis*.

54. Correct: *Fasciola hepatica* (D)

(D) This is an infection with *Fasciola hepatica*, a flatworm or trematode (see image at the end of this answer). This pathogen is endemic in several regions of the world, including Central and South America and is especially prevalent in Peru and Bolivia. The pathogen is transmitted to humans via ingestion of contaminated freshwater plants. The larva migrates from the small intestine to the liver and bile ducts, where adult worms reside. Infections may be acute or chronic and symptoms are often nonspecific. Specific symptoms will depend on the anatomic location of the pathogen.

253

Based on symptoms alone, this infection may be any number of pathogens. However, the travel to Peru and ingestion of edible flowers make *Fasciola hepatica* the most likely agent. **(A)** *Clonorchis sinensis* is transmitted via ingestion of raw or undercooked freshwater fish and adult worms live in biliary ducts. Infections may present very similar to the case in the stem. However, *C. sinensis* is mainly seen in the Far East and not in South America. Hence, *F. hepatica* is more likely to be the etiological agent. **(B)** *Giardia lamblia* is a protozoan parasite that is associated with contaminated freshwater. This pathogen is found worldwide and is often seen in hikers that drink contaminated freshwater. However, *Giardia* trophozoites typically remain in the lumen of the duodenum and do not usually migrate to the liver or bile ducts. **(C)** Hepatitis viruses may present with similar symptoms as seen in this patient. In most acute hepatitis infections, the liver enzymes are significantly elevated and would be higher than observed in this case. Of the hepatitis viruses, hepatitis A and E are transmitted via the fecal–oral route and travelers to endemic regions are at increased risk for infection. In this case, the serology results are negative for hepatitis A and E. Hepatitis B and C are transmitted percutaneously and through mucosae. The hepatitis C serology is negative and the hepatitis B serology indicates that she is immune to hepatitis B. **(E)** Infections with yellow fever virus, a flavivirus, typically present with more systemic signs and symptoms such as high fever (> 39°C [102.2°F]), malaise, and headache. The hepatic phase of yellow fever infection is much more severe than described in this stem and would include significantly elevated liver enzymes and bilirubin levels than those seen in this case. Yellow fever, common in tropical and subtropical regions including Central and South America, is transmitted by the bite of the *Aedes aegypti* mosquito.

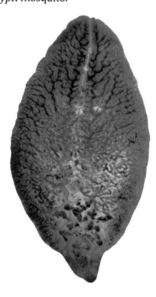

55. Correct: *Echinococcus granulosus* (B)

(B) The image in the question stem is of the cyst fluid developing scolices of the tapeworm, *Echinococcus granulosus*. The treatment of choice for these infections is albendazole. A hydatid cyst contains the developing parasite including the developing scolex (anterior end/head of tapeworm) with hooks and suckers, daughter cysts (secondary cysts), and cyst fluid (see image [i] at the end of this answer). Macroscopically the cyst fluid, containing the developing parasite, resembles grains of sand; hence the fluid material is often referred to as hydatid sand. Dogs are the definite host of *E. granulosus* and are infected with larva after ingestion of viscera of the intermediate hosts which includes sheep, goats, and pigs. Humans are accidental hosts and are infected after ingestion of food, water, or soil contaminated with infected dog feces. Infections are most often asymptomatic but the characteristic feature of infections is fluid-filled abscesses, usually in the liver or lungs. Rupture of the cyst can lead to anaphylaxis and manifestations such as urticaria, edema, and respiratory symptoms. Anaphylaxis is mediated by a type I immediate hypersensitivity reaction following exposure to *Echinococcus* antigens due to IgE-mediated granulation of mast cells. Alternative anaphylaxis may occur secondary to complement activation. There is a higher incidence of infections in Africa, the Middle East, and parts of Europe, Asia, and Central and South America. **(A)** In immunocompromised individuals, liver abscesses may be fungal in etiology. *Candida* is the most commonly and clinically isolated yeast and liver abscess may be treated with amphotericin B or fluconazole. This man's medical history is unremarkable, indicating that it is very unlikely for him to have immune deficiency. Moreover, the figure in the question stem shows hydatid sand and not *Candida*. See image (ii) at the end of this answer for an image of yeast. **(C)** The protozoan parasite *Entamoeba histolytica* is the causative agent of amebic dysentery. This pathogen may disseminate from the intestinal tract and the most common place of dissemination is to the liver, resulting in liver abscesses that may be treated with metronidazole followed by paromomycin, a luminal agent. Infections may be associated with travel to tropical countries. The figure in the question stem shows hydatid sand, not *E. histolytica* as seen in image (iii). **(D)** Many liver abscesses are polymicrobial and gram-negative enteric pathogens are frequently involved. Two of the most common agents are *Klebsiella pneumoniae* and *Escherichia coli*. Broad spectrum antimicrobials that are effective against enteric pathogens include piperacillin–tazobactam. These pathogens are most often seen when the infection originates in the biliary tract, such as in the case of acute cholangitis. See (iv) for an image of gram-negative rods. **(E)** Liver abscesses may arise as a result of hematogenous spread of microbes. In these cases, the gram-positive coccus, *Staphylococcus aureus* is the most common etiological agent. There is no indication that this infection was due to hematogenous spread and the figure in the question stem shows hydatid sand. Hence, *E. granulosus* is more likely to be the agent of infection. See (v) for an image of *S. aureus*.

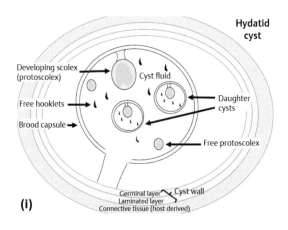

(i)

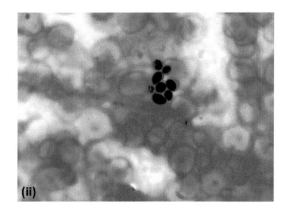

(ii)

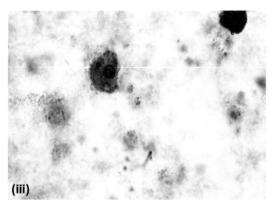

(iii)

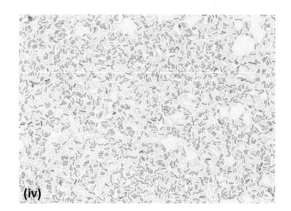

(iv)

(v)

56. Correct: Dry, nonproductive cough (A)

(A) The figure in the question stem shows a hookworm ovum. Hookworm infections are caused by *Necator americanus* and *Ancylostoma duodenale*. Infections are commonly seen in tropical and subtropical countries and in the United States infections are more common in the South. Infections occur when larvae, found in the soil contaminated with human feces, penetrate intact human skin. The larvae migrate to the lungs, ascend the respiratory tree and are then swallowed and are relocated to the gastrointestinal tract. Larvae mature into adult worms, which reside in the small intestine. The adults lay eggs that are passed in the stool. Most often infections are asymptomatic. Symptoms, if present, will depend on the anatomic location of the pathogen. Cutaneous, pulmonary, or gastrointestinal symptoms may be present. Pulmonary symptoms include a dry, nonproductive cough (answer choice A). A common complication of hookworm infection is iron-deficiency anemia from persistent blood sucking, as presented in this case. Additionally, eosinophils are often elevated in helminthic infections. (B) Hookworm infections are not associated with dysentery. The adult worms usually stay in the small intestine. Dysentery usually occurs after a pathogen invades the large bowel mucosa. With hookworm infections, mild diarrhea or abdominal pain may be observed while the pathogen is in the gastrointestinal tract. (C) Jaundice may signify that the liver or biliary tree has been affected. There is a possibility of adult hookworm migration to the liver and biliary tree; however, this is not common. **(D)** Joint pain is not a common finding of hookworm infection. Joint pain, which may be observed in reactive arthritis, is a common postinfectious sequela of several other pathogens including *Salmonella, Shigella, Campylobacter,* and *Yersinia enterocolitica.* **(E)** Meningismus suggests meningitis and hookworms rarely disseminate to the nervous system.

57.   Correct: Contact with cows (C)

(C) This is a case of hemolytic uremic syndrome (HUS). Enterohemorrhagic *Escherichia coli* (EHEC), a gram-negative rod, is an agent of bloody diarrhea that may progress to HUS. EHEC is most often transmitted via contaminated food, especially undercooked ground beef. However, the pathogen may also be transmitted from person to person via the fecal–oral route or via contact with infected animals, especially cattle (answer choice C), deer, and elk. HUS is characterized by a triad of acute renal failure, microangiopathic hemolytic anemia, and nonimmune thrombocytopenia. HUS typically presents 5 to 10 days following diarrhea. **(A)** Bats are associated with a number of infections including rabies, which targets the nervous system. Infections with viruses such as Marburg, Ebola, Nipah, and Hendra and the fungal pathogen *Histoplasma capsulatum* are also associated with bats. However, infections with these pathogens are not associated with HUS. **(B)** Several pathogens are associated with contact with contaminated birds or their waste, including *Chlamydophila psittaci, Cryptococcus neoformans, Histoplasma capsulatum,* and *Mycobacterium avium-intracellulare* complex. Infections with these pathogens are not associated with HUS. **(D)** Yersiniosis, caused by the enteric pathogen *Yersinia enterocolitica,* is associated with ingestion of contaminated pork and rarely following contact with infected pigs. Like EHEC, bloody diarrhea may be present. In children, this pathogen often presents as mesenteric lymphadenitis or pseudoappendicitis. HUS is not associated with *Y. enterocolitica* infections. Other pathogens also associated with undercooked pork including *Taenia solium* and *Trichinella spiralis,* which are both parasites. **(E)** An infection that is associated with reptile contact is salmonellosis, caused by nontyphoidal *Salmonella.* Depending on the species, bloody diarrhea may be present; however, HUS is not associated with *Salmonella* diarrhea.

Chapter 11

Renal and Urinary Tract Infections

Melphine M. Harriott

LEARNING OBJECTIVES

▶ Discuss the etiology, epidemiology, pathogenesis, clinical manifestations, complications, diagnosis, and treatment and prevention of:

- urinary tract infections.
- infectious diarrhea and dysentery.

▶ Describe the laboratory diagnosis and antimicrobial testing methods for bacteria, viruses, fungi, yeast, and parasites.

▶ Discuss virulence mechanisms and correlate virulence mechanisms with specific pathogens.

▶ Discuss antimicrobial mechanism of action, spectrum of activity, common adverse effects, and resistance mechanisms.

▶ List the normal microbiota for each organ system and explain the roles played in health and disease by the normal microbiota.

11.1 Questions

Easy	Medium	Hard

1. A 28-year-old primigravida woman at 10-week gestation visits her obstetrician for an initial prenatal appointment. Pregnancy is uncomplicated and she has no complaints. Her physical examination is normal. A routine urine dipstick is negative for ketones, glucose, and proteins but is positive for nitrites. Clean-catch midstream urine is obtained for culture and reveals $\geq 10^5$ CFU/mL of *Escherichia coli*. An additional urine culture 2 days later demonstrates $\geq 10^5$ CFU/mL of *E. coli*. Which of the following is the most appropriate management for this patient?

A. Administration of cephalexin

B. Administration of ciprofloxacin

C. Administration of tetracycline

D. Administration of trimethoprim/sulfamethoxazole

E. No antibiotic therapy should be administered

Consider the following case for questions 2 to 3:

A 35-year-old man is in the hospital following a motor vehicle accident. Three days after admission, he develops dysuria and increased frequency of urination. His temperature is 37.7°C (99.9°F). CBC demonstrates elevated white blood cells (WBCs). Clean-catch midstream urine is collected and the urinalysis is positive for leukocyte esterase and nitrites and the urine culture grows 10^3 CFU/mL of *Escherichia coli*. Antimicrobial susceptibility results demonstrate that the organism is an extended-spectrum beta-lactamase producer (ESBL).

2. The most appropriate management for this patient is to:

A. Collect a catheterized urine specimen to confirm the results

B. Do nothing further; this probably indicates contamination

C. Start antimicrobial therapy with ceftriaxone

D. Start antimicrobial therapy with fluconazole

E. Start antimicrobial therapy with nitrofurantoin

3. The most likely virulence mechanism mediating this infection is:

A. Enterotoxin

B. M protein

C. Mycolic acid

D. P-fimbriae

E. Urease

4. A 19-year-old woman visits her physician for a routine physical examination. She has no complaints and her vital signs and physical examination are unremarkable. Blood and urine are collected for routine laboratory tests. The urine culture grows 10^3 CFU/mL coagulase-negative staphylococci, 10^3 CFU/mL lactobacilli, and 10^3 CFU/mL of diphtheroids (*Corynebacterium* species). Which of the following is the most appropriate management for this patient?

A. Collect a catheterized urine specimen to confirm the results

B. Do nothing further; this probably indicates contamination

C. Start antimicrobial therapy with fluconazole

D. Start antimicrobial therapy with metronidazole

E. Start antimicrobial therapy with trimethoprim/sulfamethoxazole

5. A 23-year-old woman visits her physician with burning and pain upon urination, and increased frequency and urgency of urination. She states she recently returned from her honeymoon. Her vital signs are normal and mild suprapubic tenderness is noted on physical examination. A urinalysis is positive for leukocyte esterase and all other urinalysis values including nitrite are within normal limits. Clean-catch midstream urine demonstrates the presence of $\geq 10^5$ CFU/mL of a catalase-positive, coagulase-negative organism that grew on blood agar but not on MacConkey agar. Which of the following is the most likely etiological agent of this infection?

A. *Pseudomonas aeruginosa*

B. *Streptococcus agalactiae*

C. *Staphylococcus aureus*

D. *Staphylococcus saprophyticus*

E. *Trichomonas vaginalis*

Consider the following case for questions 6 to 8:

A 56-year-old man presents to the emergency department with severe back pain, blood in his urine, fever, and nausea of 3-day duration. On examination his temperature is 38.4°C (101.1°F) and he has costovertebral angle tenderness on the right side. No penile drainage is observed and no rebound tenderness or guarding on palpation of his abdomen is noted. An abdominal computed tomography (CT) scan demonstrates the presence of calculi in the right ureter. Laboratory results are shown below:

- CBC:
  - Leukocyte count: 15×10^9/L
  - Segmented neutrophils: 82%
  - Bands: 3%
  - Eosinophils: 1%
  - Basophils: 0%
  - Lymphocytes: 27%
- Monocytes: 5%
- Urinalysis–Dipstick:
  - pH: 9
  - Blood: positive
  - Leukocyte esterase: positive
  - Nitrite: positive
  - Protein: positive
- Urine culture:
  - $\geq 10^5$ CFU/mL lactose-negative bacteria on MacConkey agar

6. The most likely diagnosis is:

A. Appendicitis

B. Cholecystitis

C. Cystitis

D. Pyelonephritis

E. Urethritis

7. The most likely etiological agent of this infection is:

A. *Chlamydia trachomatis*

B. *Escherichia coli*

C. *Proteus mirabilis*

D. *Staphylococcus aureus*

E. *Streptococcus pyogenes*

8. Based on the etiological agent, which of the following is the most likely mechanism mediating the pathogenesis and contributing to the altered pH of the urine?

A. Exotoxin

B. Lipopolysaccharide (LPS)

C. P-fimbriae

D. Superantigen

E. Urease

Consider the following case for questions 9 to 10:

An 81-year-old man, who lives in a nursing home, is transferred to the hospital with fever and chills. The nurse notes that his Foley catheter bag contains cloudy urine. On examination, his temperature is 39.0°C (102.3°F). Urine from the catheter is collected for urinalysis and culture and results are shown below:

- Urinalysis–Dipstick:
  - pH: 6.4
  - Blood: positive
  - Leukocyte esterase: positive
  - Nitrite: negative
- Urine culture:
  - $\geq 10^5$ CFU/mL *Enterococcus faecium*
- Antimicrobial susceptibility:
  - Resistant to gentamicin, penicillin, and vancomycin

9. Which of the following findings is most likely to be observed in this patient's urine sediment?

A. Gram-negative rods

B. Gram-negative diplococci

C. Gram-positive cocci in chains

D. Gram-positive cocci in clusters

E. Gram-positive rods, pleomorphic

10. Which of the following is the most appropriate management for this patient?

A. Do nothing further; this probably indicates contamination

B. Removal of catheter; no antimicrobial treatment is needed

C. Start antimicrobial therapy with ampicillin

D. Start antimicrobial therapy with daptomycin

E. Start antimicrobial therapy with gentamicin

11. A 73-year-old woman is hospitalized, following a hip fraction and subsequent surgery. On day 3, following surgery, the patient develops a fever up to 38.4°C (101.2°F). The nurse notes that the urine drainage bag from the patient's Foley catheter contains cloudy, foul smelling urine. Urine is sterilely collected and sent to the laboratory for analysis. A microscopic image of the urine sediment shows many neutrophils and the following organism:

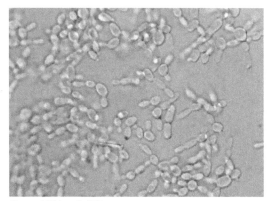

Source: Wikimedia/Microrao

Which of the additional conditions is this pathogen most likely cause?

A. Atypical pneumonia

B. Dysentery

C. Pelvic inflammatory disease

D. Toxic shock syndrome (TSS)

E. Vaginitis

12. A 63-year-old man visits his physician complaining of pain when urinating. He denies increased frequency or urgency of urination. His vitals and physical examination are unremarkable. The urine is positive for leukocyte esterase and negative for nitrites. Which of the following is the most likely etiological agent of this infection?

A. *Enterococcus faecalis*

B. *Enterobacter cloacae*

C. *Escherichia coli*

D. *Klebsiella pneumoniae*

E. *Proteus mirabilis*

Consider the following case for questions 13 to 14:

An 8-year-old boy is brought to the pediatrician by his father with a 2-day history of swelling in his hands and ankles and blood in his urine. The father states that about 2 weeks ago the boy had been sick with fever and complaining of a sore throat. They didn't visit the doctor at that time because the boy felt better after 2 days without antimicrobial treatment. The boy's temperature is 37.1°C (98.8°F) and his blood pressure is 210/140 mm Hg. Physical demonstrates significant edema of the hands, wrists, feet, and ankles. A urine specimen is collected and results are given below:

- Urinalysis–Dipstick
  - Blood: positive
  - Protein: positive
  - Leukocyte esterase: negative
  - Nitrite: negative

13. Which of the following is most likely directly involved in the development of the boy's current condition?

A. Antigen-antibody complex

B. β-Hemolysin

C. M protein

D. Polysaccharide capsule

E. Superantigen

14. Which of the following is the most appropriate diagnostic test?

A. Throat culture

B. PCR for group A antigen

C. Rapid EIA for group A antigen from throat

D. Serology for antibodies to streptolysin O

E. Urine culture

15. A 40-year-old woman presents with painful urination, increased urge to urinate, abdominal pain, and fever. Her temperature is 38.2°C (100.8°F). Physical examination reveals costovertebral tenderness. The urinalysis is positive for nitrites and leukocyte esterase. Her culture grows the following organism on MacConkey agar:

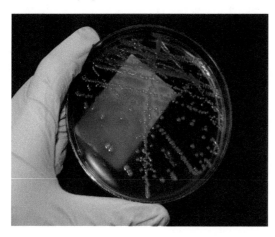

Which of the following is most likely mediating this infection?

A. Capsule

B. Exotoxin that blocks protein synthesis

C. Hyaluronidase

D. Lipooligosaccharide (LOS)

E. Pili

16. A 3-year-old boy is brought to the emergency department with blood in his urine and a stomach ache. His mother states the boy has been more tired than normal and seems to look really pale. Further questioning reveals the boy had diarrhea a week ago. The boy attends daycare. His temperature is 37.9°C (101.2°F) and his blood pressure is 117/80 mm Hg. On examination, pallor of the skin and mucous membranes and edema of the hands and feet are noted. Abdominal exam shows no rebound tenderness. Urinalysis and CBC results are shown below:

- Urinalysis–Dipstick
  - Blood: positive
  - Protein: positive
  - Leukocyte esterase: negative
  - Nitrite: negative
- CBC:
  - WBC: 12×10^9/L
  - Hemoglobin: 6 g/dL
  - Platelets: 85×10^9/L

See following image for blood smear.

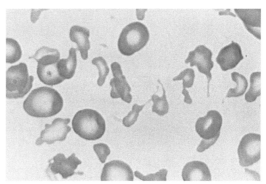

Source: Differential Diagnosis of Nephrologic Syndromes. In: Siegenthaler W, Hrsg. Siegenthaler's Differential Diagnosis in Internal Medicine: From Symptom to Diagnosis. 1st Edition. Thieme; 2007

The most likely mechanism involved is an exotoxin that:

A. Activates T cell MHC

B. Inactivates elongation factor-2 (EF-2)

C. Inactivates ribosomes

D. Increases cAMP

E. Increases cGMP

11.2 Answers and Explanations

Easy	Medium	Hard

1. Correct: Administration of cephalexin (A)

(A) This patient does not have symptoms of cystitis or pyelonephritis but the urine dipstick and urine culture demonstrates bacteriuria. Hence this woman has asymptomatic bacteriuria. Asymptomatic bacteriuria is defined as having no signs and symptoms of a urinary tract infection (UTI), and according to the Infectious Disease Society of America (IDSA), the following quantities of bacteria: women, $\geq 10^5$ CFU/mL of the same bacteria in two consecutive clean-catch midstream urine specimens; men, $\geq 10^5$ CFU/mL of bacteria in a single clean-catch midstream urine specimen; and women and men, catheterized specimens, $\geq 10^5$ CFU/mL of bacteria in a single specimen. Treatment is recommended only for pregnant women and individuals undergoing urological procedures that may result in mucosal bleeding. Hence, in this case antimicrobial treatment is warranted. Several antibiotics are effective, safe, and recommended for treatment of pregnant women with asymptomatic bacteriuria. These include cephalosporins, such as cephalexin (answer choice A), or other agents, including amoxicillin–clavulanate, nitrofurantoin, and fosfomycin. Cephalexin inhibits bacterial cell wall synthesis. See Appendix I for a summary of antimicrobials spectrum of activity and mechanism of action. While cephalexin does have activity against some *Enterobacteriaceae*, including *Escherichia coli*, other agents may have better activity; however, in this case, it is the best answer choice. Normally, urine is a sterile fluid. However, it's difficult to collect a sterile clean-catch midstream voided urine specimen (and even catheter specimens) due to contamination with urethral, vaginal, or skin flora. Therefore, quantitative cultures are performed on urine specimens and the number of organisms per milliliter of urine is determined and expressed as colony forming unit per milliliter (CFU/mL). The organism count allows differentiation of contamination (normal flora) from pathogens (infection). Briefly, a calibrated loop delivers 0.001 mL or 0.01 mL of urine. Each culture plate is inoculated with one loopful of urine and the plates are incubated for 24 to 48 hours at 35 to 37°C. The colony count is then determined by multiplying the number of colonies by the dilution factor. For example, if a 0.001 mL loop is used and 10 colonies are observed, the colony count would be 10 × 10,000 or 10,000 CFU/mL (10^4 CFU/mL). If a 0.01 mL loop is used and 10 colonies are observed, the colony count would be 10 × 100 or 1,000 CFU/mL (10^3 CFU/mL). Patients with UTIs usually have at least $\geq 10^5$ CFU/mL of bacteria per milliliter of urine and this is often reported by the clinical microbiology laboratory as > 100,000 CFU/mL. This concentration of 10^5 CFU/mL is referred to as significant bacteriuria and these patients may be symptomatic. However, some patients may present with asymptomatic bacteriuria. It is important to note that < 10^4 CFU/mL may be significant when there is strong clinical evidence of a UTI. Moreover, fastidious bacteria and fungi have slower growth and may be significant at <10^4 CFU/mL. Lastly, catheterized urine specimens and suprapubic specimens are far less likely to be contaminated with normal flora compared to clean-catch midstream urine specimens and bacteriuria may significant at < 10^5 CFU/mL. **(B)** Fluoroquinolones, such as ciprofloxacin and levofloxacin, are assigned category C by the FDA (animal studies show some risk, evidence in human and animal studies is inadequate, but clinical benefit sometimes exceeds risk) and are not recommended for pregnant women. Fluoroquinolones block DNA synthesis by inhibiting DNA gyrase. **(C)** Tetracycline may have adverse effects on fetal bone and teeth development and should be avoided during pregnancy. Tetracyclines inhibit protein synthesis. **(D)** There is the possibility that trimethoprim/sulfamethoxazole may interfere with folic acid and decrease folic acid levels during the first trimester of pregnancy. Furthermore, sulfonamides may displace bilirubin resulting in kernicterus, which especially affects preterm infants; therefore, these agents should be avoided toward the end of the third trimester as well. **(E)** Bacteriuria in pregnant women should be treated because of the increased risk of developing pyelonephritis and delivering preterm, low-weight infants.

2. Correct: Start antimicrobial therapy with nitrofurantoin (E)

(E) This patient has clinical manifestations of cystitis and laboratory results support this finding; although, the quantity of *Escherichia coli* recovered from the culture is lower than the customary $\geq 10^5$ CFU/mL of organisms. However, since he is symptomatic, he should be treated with antimicrobials. The antimicrobial susceptibility demonstrates that the *E. coli* is an extended spectrum beta-lactamase (ESBL) producer. Several organisms can produce ESBLs but *Enterobacteriaceae*, particularly *E. coli* and *Klebsiella* are notorious for this. ESBLs have a plasmid-mediated point mutation in the β-lactamase gene that confers resistance to penicillins and extended-spectrum cephalosporins (including third generation). They are generally susceptible to nitrofurantoin (answer choice E), fosfomycin, cephamycins, and carbapenems. In cases of uncomplicated UTIs, fosfomycin or nitrofurantoin is recommended. In more serious infections, carbapenems may be warranted. **(A)** There is no need to repeat the culture, especially with an invasive catheterization, since the patient is demonstrating symptoms. **(B)** Because this patient is exhibiting signs and symptoms of a UTI, he should be treated, even with the lower colony count. This is most likely not a contaminant, but rather a true pathogen in this case. **(C)** The *E. coli* in this case is an ESBL, which is resistant to third generation cephalosporins, such as ceftriaxone. Therefore, this is not a good choice for treatment.

(D) The etiological agent of this infection is a gram-negative pathogen and fluconazole is an antifungal agent and would not be effective.

(D) The etiological agent of this infection is *Escherichia coli*. An important virulence factor of uropathogenic *E. coli* is fimbriae, which allow the organism to adhere to the uroepithelium and colonize the urinary tract. Fimbriae may also stimulate local inflammation leading to the clinical manifestations of cystitis. **(A)** Enterotoxins are secreted toxins (exotoxins) that target the enteric (gastrointestinal) tract. Although some strains of *E. coli* (enterotoxigenic *E. coli* [ETEC] and enterohemorrhagic *E. coli* [EHEC]) do produce enterotoxins, this is not a usual mechanism of virulence for uropathogenic *E. coli*. **(B)** M protein is an important virulence mechanism of the gram-positive pathogen *Streptococcus pyogenes* (group A streptococcus). It aids the pathogen in avoiding the immune system. **(C)** Mycolic acid is an important component of the mycobacteria (acid-fast bacilli) cell wall and is not found in *E. coli*. **(D)** *E. coli* does not produce urease. Gram-negative organisms that produce urease include *Proteus, Klebsiella, Morganella, Providencia,* and *Helicobacter pylori*.

4. Correct: Do nothing further; this probably indicates contamination (B)

(B) The patient has no clinical symptoms of infection and all the organisms are in quantities $\geq 10^5$ CFU/mL. All three organisms are normal microbiota of the skin, vagina, and rectum and most likely represent contamination from an inappropriately collected urine specimen. Therefore, it is not necessary to treat this patient with antimicrobials. **(A)** There is no need to repeat the culture, especially with an invasive catheterization since the patient is not demonstrating symptoms. **(C)** Fluconazole, an antifungal agent, may be used to treat yeast; however, yeast is not present. **(D)** Metronidazole is not an antimicrobial agent routinely used to treat UTIs. **(E)** Trimethoprim/sulfamethoxazole, an antibacterial agent, is commonly used to treat uncomplicated UTIs; however, treatment is not needed in this case.

5. Correct: *Staphylococcus saprophyticus* (D)

(D) Dysuria, increased frequency and urgency of urination, and suprapubic pain are classic symptoms of cystitis. Women, especially sexually active women, are more prone to urinary tract infections (UTIs) than men. The urinalysis is positive for leukocyte esterase, which is an enzyme produced by white blood cells and may indicate pyuria and a potential urinary tract infections (UTIs). Nitrites are negative and are usually positive in the presence of certain gram-negative organisms, which can reduce nitrate to nitrites. The causative organism in this case grew on blood agar, which grows both gram-positive and gram-negative organisms, but did not grow on

MacConkey agar, which is selective for gram-negative organisms. This indicates the organism is most likely gram positive. *Staphylococcus saprophyticus* (answer choice D), a gram-positive, catalase positive, coagulase negative organism, is the most likely cause of this infection. Another biochemical test that is often performed to identify *S. saprophyticus* is the novobiocin test. *S. saprophyticus* is novobiocin resistant while other staphylococci species are novobiocin sensitive. Women are more frequently affected by *S. saprophyticus* than men and infections are often referred to as "honeymooners cystitis." **(A)** *Pseudomonas aeruginosa* may also cause UTIs, especially nosocomial-associated UTIs, however, *P. aeruginosa* is a gram-negative rod, not gram-positive cocci as in this case. **(B)** *Streptococcus agalactiae* (also called group B *Streptococcus* or GBS) is an infrequent agent of UTIs and is a gram-positive coccus in chains. GBS is most commonly associated with neonatal meningitis and sepsis and is part of the streptococci family. Streptococci are catalase negative. **(C)** *Staphylococcus aureus* is a gram-positive coccus and like all staphylococci species is catalase positive. *S. aureus* is coagulase positive, which differentiates it from other staphylococci. While it is possible that *S. aureus* may cause UTIs, it is not a typical agent of UTIs. **(E)** *Trichomonas vaginalis* is a protozoan parasite and therefore does not grow on blood agar. It causes the sexually transmitted infection trichomoniasis. Women may be asymptomatic or present with dysuria as in this case or vaginal discharge and pruritus. Wet preparations or molecular assays (preferred and recommended) may be used to identify *T. vaginalis* trophozoite.

6. Correct: Pyelonephritis (D)

(D) This is most likely to be pyelonephritis. Clinical manifestations of pyelonephritis include dysuria, increased frequency and urgency of urination, a temperature of >38°C, chills, flank pain, costovertebral tenderness, nausea, and vomiting. Hematuria may or may not be present. In this case, the patient's blood demonstrates elevated WBCs and the urine is positive for leukocyte esterase and nitrites, which indicate an infection may be present. The urine culture with $\geq 10^5$ CFU/mL confirms a UTI. The fever and costovertebral tenderness indicate that this is likely to be pyelonephritis rather than cystitis. Additionally, the presence of renal calculi may be contributing to the symptoms, especially the hematuria. **(A, B)** Appendicitis and cholecystitis should be included in the differential diagnosis of pyelonephritis. Both may present with upper right abdominal pain, nausea, vomiting, and fever. However, the CT scan doesn't support these conditions. Since the urine culture is positive, this is most likely a UTI. **(C)** The clinical manifestations of cystitis and pyelonephritis are often similar. However, fever, chills, flank pain, costovertebral tenderness, nausea, and vomiting are usually absent in cases of cystitis and are indicative of pyelonephritis. **(E)** Urethritis should also be considered in the differential diagnosis of pyelonephritis and cystitis. The clinical manifestations of urethritis include dysuria and similar to UTIs the leukocyte esterase may be positive. However, penile or vaginal discharge is often present with urethritis. This case is more likely to be pyelonephritis.

7.   Correct: *Proteus mirabilis* (C)

(C) The gram-negative rod, *Proteus mirabilis*, is the most likely pathogen of this infection. The organism produces clear colonies and is lactose negative on Mac-Conkey agar (see image [i] at the end of this answer) and due to the motility of this organism, swarming is often noted on blood agar (see image [ii] at the end of this answer). This pathogen may cause a variety of infections including wound infections, respiratory infections, bloodstream infections, and UTIs. UTIs with this organism may involve renal calculi as in this case. **(A)** *Chlamydia trachomatis* is a sexually transmitted pathogen that may cause urethritis, cervicitis, proctitis, and epididymitis. This is most likely not urethritis. Additionally, *C. trachomatis* is an obligate intracellular pathogen and will not grow on artificial media and in this case the etiological agent grew on routine urine culture media (blood and MacConkey agars). **(B)** *Escherichia coli*, the most common agent of UTIs, is a gram-negative rod; however, it is produces lactose on MacConkey agar and is bright pink (see image [i]). This organism is not usually associated with kidney stones. **(D, E)** *Staphylococcus aureus* and *Streptococcus pyogenes* are both gram-positive cocci. Neither pathogen is a common agent of UTIs. Moreover, neither of these gram-positive organisms grows on MacConkey agar, since MacConkey agar is selective for gram-negative enteric organisms.

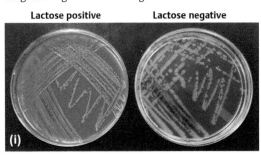

Lactose positive   **Lactose negative**

(i)

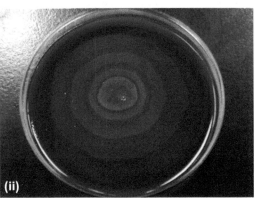

(ii)

8.   Correct: Urease (E)

(E) *Proteus* produces urease, which breaks down urea into carbon dioxide and ammonia, resulting in elevated urinary pH levels. Increases in urine pH can contribute to renal toxicity and urinary stone formation. Urinary stones can result in further renal damage by obstructing urine flow. Often struvite crystals (also called triple phosphate; see image at the end of this answer) are observed in the urine of patients with UTIs caused by *Proteus*. Other urinary tract pathogens that also produce urease include *Klebsiella pneumoniae*, *Morganella*, *Providencia*, *Staphylococcus saprophyticus*, and *Corynebacterium urealyticum*. **(A)** Exotoxins (secreted toxins) do not contribute to the pathogenesis of *P. mirabilis* and other *Proteus* species. **(B)** LPS or endotoxin is part of the gram negative cell wall and contributes to the virulence of gram-negative organisms, such as *Proteus*. However, this does not contribute to the pathogenesis or altered pH or urinary stones as seen in this case. **(C)** P-fimbriae and other types of fimbriae are important virulence factors for uropathogenic *Escherichia coli* and allow the organism to adhere to the uroepithelium, resulting in inflammation and infection. However, this does not contribute to the altered pH or urinary stones as seen in this case. **(D)** *Proteus* does not produce a superantigen, which nonspecifically activates T cells. One notable superantigen is the toxic shock syndrome toxin (TSST) of *Staphylococcus aureus*.

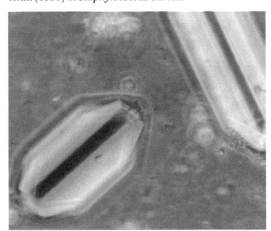

Source: Differential Diagnosis of Pathologic Urine Findings. In: Siegenthaler W, Hrsg. Siegenthaler's Differential Diagnosis in Internal Medicine: From Symptom to Diagnosis. 1st Edition. Thieme; 2007

9.   Correct: Gram-positive cocci in chains (C)

(C) The organism isolated from the urine culture is *Enterococcus faecalis*, which is a frequent pathogen of UTIs. Enterococci are gram-positive cocci in chains and were previously called group D streptococci. Most often the nitrite is negative with gram-positive pathogens such as *Enterococcus*. This patient most likely has a catheter related pyelonephritis. **(A)** Common gram-negative rods implicated in UTIs include *Escherichia coli*, *Klebsiella* and other *Enterobacteriaceae*, and *Pseudomonas aeruginosa*. Enterococci are gram positive. **(B)** *Neisseria gonorrhoeae*, a gram-negative diplococcus, causes the sexually transmitted infection gonorrhea and may be isolated from urine. The patient presentation and Gram stain is not consistent with gonorrhea. **(D)** Gram-positive cocci in clusters describes staphylococci, not enterococci. **(E)** *Corynebacterium* is pleomorphic gram-positive rods. Several *Corynebacterium* species are normal microbiota of the urogenital tract and may be isolated from improperly collected urine specimens. *Corynebacterium urealyticum* is rarely isolated, but is associated with cystitis.

10. Correct: Start antimicrobial therapy with daptomycin (D)

(D) The *Enterococcus* isolate in this case is a vancomycin-resistant enterococci (VRE) and is also resistant to aminoglycosides and penicillins. It is not uncommon for enterococci to demonstrate such resistance clinically. Antibiotics that are effective against VRE include daptomycin (answer choice D), linezolid, tigecycline, quinupristin-dalfopristin, teicoplanin, and telavancin. Daptomycin is a cyclin lipopeptide that destroys the bacterial cell membrane. Note that daptomycin binds to pulmonary surfactant; hence it should not be used to treat pulmonary infections. **(A)** This culture is from a catheterized specimen and has ≥ 10⁵ CFU/mL of *Enterococcus*. Moreover, the patient is exhibiting signs and symptoms of infection. Therefore, this is most likely not contamination from periurethral flora, but rather a true infection that should be treated with antimicrobials. **(B)** If possible the catheter should be removed and if needed be replaced intermittently. However, because the patient is exhibiting signs of a UTI, antimicrobial therapy is warranted. **(C)** Ampicillin is an aminopenicillin that inhibits cell wall synthesis. Since this isolate is penicillin resistant it is likely also ampicillin resistant; therefore, daptomycin is a better answer choice. **(E)** In vitro susceptibility demonstrates that this organism is resistant to the aminoglycoside gentamicin, which is an aminoglycoside that inhibits protein synthesis. See Appendix I for a summary of antimicrobials spectrum of activity and mechanism of action.

11. Correct: Vaginitis (E)

(E) The unstained image presented in the question stem shows budding yeast. The most common clinically isolated yeast is *Candida*. *Candida* and other yeast typically cause mucocutaneous infections, such as vaginitis (answer choice E), esophagitis and thrush, or more serious systemic/invasive infections, such as bloodstream infections. This patient has a catheter-related urinary tract infection (UTI). Several organisms are associated with catheter-related UTIs. The most common pathogens include enteric gram-negative organisms, such as *Escherichia coli* or gram-positives organisms, such as *Staphylococcus aureus* and *Enterococcus*. Yeast, including *Candida*

may also be implicated in catheter-related infections. **(A)** Bacterial pathogens that are implicated in atypical pneumonia include *Mycoplasma pneumoniae* and *Chlamydophila pneumoniae*. These agents are not typically seen by traditional light microscopy. Furthermore, these organisms are not typical agents of UTIs. **(B)** Several pathogens are associated with dysentery, notably *Shigella*, a gram-negative rod. However, yeast such as *Candida* are typically normal microbiota of the gastrointestinal tract and are not typically agents of gastroenteritis. The agents of dysentery typically are not agents of UTIs. **(C)** Pelvic inflammatory disease (PID) occurs following a genital tract infection with *Neisseria gonorrhoeae* or *Chlamydia trachomatis* D-K. *N. gonorrhoeae* are small diplococci and are obligate intracellular organisms that cannot be visualized by a wet preparation as in this case. *Candida* is not associated with PID. **(D)** Toxic shock syndrome (TSS) is most often caused by *Staphylococcus aureus* or *Streptococcus pyogenes*, which are small cocci and not a large oval shaped budding organism as seen in the image. Neither *S. aureus* or *S. pyogenes* are typical agents of UTIs.

12. Correct: *Enterococcus faecalis* (A)

(A) In this case the urine is positive for leukocyte esterase and negative for nitrites so the most likely pathogen is *Enterococcus faecalis*, a gram-positive coccus. There are several urinalysis indicators that may assist in diagnosing urinary tract infections (UTIs), including nitrite and leukocyte esterase. Some gram-negative bacteria, notably the *Enterobacteriaceae*, can reduce nitrate to nitrites by producing nitrate reductase. Hence, a positive nitrate reduction test suggests that *Enterobacteriaceae*, such as *Citrobacter*, *Enterobacter*, *Escherichia*, *Klebsiella*, *Morganella*, and *Proteus* may be causative agents. Gram-positive pathogens, such as *E. faecalis* and other non-*Enterobacteriaceae* gram-negative pathogens such as *Pseudomonas aeruginosa* do not reduce nitrates. Leukocyte esterase is produced by white blood cellsand may indicate pyuria and a potential UTI. Note all the answer choices are common agents of UTIs. **(B-E)** *Enterobacter cloacae*, *Escherichia coli*, *Klebsiella pneumoniae*, and *Proteus mirabilis* are all gram-negative rods and members of the family *Enterobacteriaceae*. Hence, they would most likely produce a positive nitrite result.

13. Correct: Antigen-antibody complex (A)

(A) This is a case of poststreptococcal glomerulonephritis. *Streptococcus pyogenes* (also called group A streptococci or GAS), a gram-positive coccus in chains, is a causative agent of pharyngitis. If untreated, pharyngitis lasts about 1 week or less. However, postinfectious conditions such as glomerulonephritis or rheumatic fever may occur approximately 1 to 3 weeks after the pharyngitis. Antibodies to GAS are made during pharyngitis and these antigen-antibody immune complexes are then deposited in the glomerular basement membrane. Complement is activated, which induces inflammation. Typical symptoms of poststreptococcus glomerulonephritis in children include edema, hematuria, and hypertension. Glomerulonephritis and rheumatic fever may also arise, following untreated GAS skin infections. Note that the mechanism of rheumatic fever is due to cross-reactive antibodies rather than antibody-antigen complex deposition. **(B)** *S. pyogenes* produces a β-hemolysin (streptolysin) and is therefore β-hemolytic on blood agar. This does not play a role in the development of glomerulonephritis. **(C)** M protein is an important virulence factor found in the cell wall of *S. pyogenes*. It plays a role in helping the organism evade the host immune response. This does not play a role in the development of glomerulonephritis. **(D)** *S. pyogenes* is surrounded by a polysaccharide capsule, which aids the organism in evading the host immune response. This does not play a role in the development of glomerulonephritis. **(E)** *S. pyogenes* does produce an exotoxin that acts as a superantigen and nonspecifically activates T cells. But this is important for the pathogenesis of toxic shock like syndrome, not glomerulonephritis.

14.   Correct: Serology for antibodies to streptolysin O (D)

(D) The best diagnostic test in this case would be serology to detect antibodies to streptococcal proteins. This commonly includes antistreptolysin (ASO), but other determinants are also useful, such as anti-DNAase B antibodies, anti-streptokinase (ASKase), anti-hyaluronidase (AHase), and anti-nicotinamide-adenine dinucleotidase (anti-NAD). **(A)** The throat culture would most likely be negative because the organisms have been cleared from the respiratory tract. **(B)** Although some diagnostic PCR tests for *Streptococcus pyogenes* do exist, this is not a common mechanism for identifying this pathogen. **(C)** The rapid EIA or rapid "strep" screen is often performed on throat specimens to quickly diagnose group A streptococci pharyngitis. This test would not be helpful in this case. **(E)** The urine will most likely not grow group A streptococci because the infection has cleared and the resulting glomerulonephritis is antibody-antigen mediated.

15.   Correct: Pili (E)

(E) This woman has pyelonephritis with *Escherichia coli*. The positive nitrites indicate that the pathogen is most likely gram negative. MacConkey agar is selective for enteric gram-negative rods. This media is also differential for lactose. *E. coli* is lactose positive (*Klebsiella* is also lactose positive whereas *Proteus* and *Pseudomonas* are lactose negative). The most important virulence mechanism mediating uropathogenic *E. coli* are pili, which aid in adhesion to the mucosal epithelium. **(A)** Some strains of *E. coli*, such as *E. coli* K1, do produce a capsule. *E. coli* K1 is an important cause of meningitis in neonates but is not a typical agent of UTIs. **(B)** Enterohemorrhagic *Escherichia coli* (EHEC) produces an exotoxin that blocks protein synthesis. The most notable EHEC is *E. coli* O157:H7. Uropathogenic *E. coli* does not produce this particular exotoxin. **(C)** Hyaluronidase is produced by *Streptococcus pyogenes*, a gram-positive coccus in chains, but not *E. coli*. **(D)** Lipooligosaccharide (LOS) is part of the cell wall of *Neisseria* and *Campylobacter*. LOS is similar to lipopolysaccharide (LPS), which is found in the cell wall of gram-negative organisms.

16.   Correct: Inactivates ribosomes (C)

(C) This is a case of hemolytic uremic syndrome (HUS), which is associated with enterohemorrhagic *Escherichia coli* (EHEC). The most notable EHEC serotype is *E. coli* O157:H7. Less commonly, infections with *Shigella dysenteriae* type 1 also result in HUS. EHEC is transmitted via contaminated food and water, contact with contaminated animals or from oral–fecal transmission from an infected individual. Infections begin as diarrhea, usually with blood. Children less than 5 years of age are prone to developing HUS after an EHEC infection. *Shigella dysenteriae* type 1 produces the Shiga toxin (stx) and EHEC produces a very similar toxin, the Shiga-like toxin, also called verotoxin. The receptor for the toxin is found on a number of cells, including renal epithelial cells. These toxins bind to and inactivate the 28S ribosome (answer choice C), resulting in inhibition of protein synthesis. As a result of the protein synthesis inhibition the cells die. This leads to platelet and fibrin deposition in the microcapillaries of the kidney leading to decreased blood flow and shearing of the red cells. **(A)** Superantigens are capable of activating the T cell MHC resulting in a cytokine flood. *Staphylococcus aureus* produces the toxic shock syndrome toxin-1 (TSST-1) and *Streptococcus pyogenes* produces exotoxin A that act as superantigens. Infections with these pathogens do not progress to HUS. **(B)** *Corynebacterium diphtheriae* and *Pseudomonas aeruginosa* both produce exotoxins that inactivate elongation factor-2 (EF-2). Infections with these pathogens do not progress to HUS. **(D)** Several pathogens produce toxins that increase cyclic AMP including enterotoxigenic *Escherichia coli* (ETEC), *Bacillus anthracis*, and *Vibrio cholerae*. Infections with these pathogens do not progress to HUS. **(E)** Enterotoxigenic *Escherichia coli* (ETEC) produces a heat-stable toxin that increases cyclic GMP. It does not result in HUS.

Chapter 12

Reproductive and Sexually Transmitted Infections

Melphine M. Harriott

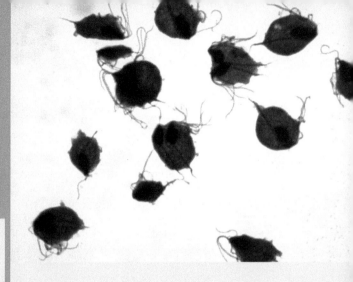

LEARNING OBJECTIVES

- ▶ Discuss the etiology, epidemiology, pathogenesis, clinical manifestations, complications, diagnosis, and treatment and prevention of:
  - – genital tract infections.
  - – congenital and neonatal infections.
  - – upper and lower respiratory tract infections.
- ▶ Describe the laboratory diagnosis and antimicrobial testing methods for bacteria, viruses, fungi, yeast, and parasites.
- ▶ Discuss virulence mechanisms and correlate virulence mechanisms with specific pathogens.
- ▶ Discuss antimicrobial mechanism of action, spectrum of activity, common adverse effects, and resistance mechanisms.
- ▶ Compare and contrast the structure and function of bacterial, viral, fungal, yeast, and parasitic cells.

12.1 Questions

Easy	Medium	Hard

1. A 54-year-old woman visits the urgent care clinic with vaginal itchiness, discharge, and pelvic discomfort of 3-day duration. She mentions that a few days ago she completed a course of azithromycin for an upper respiratory infection. She denies any sexual activity for the past 2 months. A pelvic examination reveals significant vulvar erythema and mild edema and thick, white vaginal discharge. No genital lesions are present. Which of the following is most likely to be observed from the discharge?

A. Gram-negative diplococci

B. Gram-positive rods

C. Hyphae

D. Pear-shaped protozoa

E. Spirochetes

Consider the following case for questions 2 to 3:

A previously healthy 23-year-old woman complains of vaginal irritation, painful urination, and pain during sexual intercourse. Her symptoms seemed to have worsened over the past week. She denies the use of oral contraceptives and states her menstrual period began 4 days ago. A pelvic examination reveals significant vaginal, vulvar, and cervical erythema. Additionally, punctate hemorrhages are noted on the vagina and cervix. No vesicular or ulcerative lesions or cervical motion tenderness is observed. A small amount of thin, yellow–green vaginal discharge is collected for testing.

2. Which of the following diagnostic tests would best aid in determining the causative agent of this infection?

A. Gram stain

B. KOH preparation

C. Pap smear

D. Tzanck smear

E. Wet mount

3. Which of the following is the best treatment for this infection?

A. Acyclovir

B. Azithromycin

C. Fluconazole

D. Metronidazole

E. Penicillin

4. A 23-year-old woman visits her OB-GYN for an annual gynecologic exam. She has no complaints and is healthy. She is sexually active and has several partners. Her physical examination is unremarkable other than the presence of thin, white vaginal discharge. The discharge is collected for culture and Gram stain and is shown as follows.

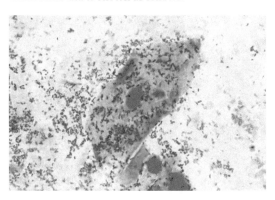

What is the most likely diagnosis?

A. Bacterial vaginosis

B. Candida vulvovaginitis

C. Chlamydia

D. Gonorrhea

E. Trichomoniasis

5. A sexually active 40-year-old woman presents to her primary care physician with vaginal discharge of 1-week duration. She denies vaginal pruritus or irritation and pelvic or abdominal pain. Physical exam is normal except for the discharge, which appears thin and cream-like and has a foul smell. A vaginal swab is collected and sent to the laboratory for further testing. The whiff test performed on the vaginal discharge is positive and the vaginal pH is 4.9. No white blood cells (WBCs) are present in the wet preparation from the discharge. Which of the following are the most likely causative agents of this infection?

A. *Candida* and *Mobiluncus*

B. *Chlamydia* and *Neisseria*

C. *Gardnerella* and *Mobiluncus*

D. *Gardnerella* and *Trichomonas*

E. *Neisseria* and *Trichomonas*

6. A 33-year-old woman presents with vaginal itchiness and dysuria. She takes oral contraceptives. Her physical examination reveals vulvar edema and erythema, and a small amount of vaginal discharge is present. No vaginal lesions are observed. A wet preparation from the discharge demonstrates the presence of budding yeast and hyphae. Which of the following would best confirm the identity of the most likely causative agent?

A. Coagulase

B. Germ tube

C. Oxidase

D. Whiff test

E. VDRL

7. A 20-year-old woman presents to her OB-GYN with vaginal discharge, abdominal pain, and fever. She states she missed her last menstrual period, and although she has an intrauterine device (IUD) she took a home pregnancy test just in case, and it was negative. Her temperature is 38.4°C (101.2°F) and her pulse is 106 beats per minute. Physical examination reveals abdominal tenderness in the left lower quadrant. A complete blood count (CBC) shows a white blood cell (WBC) count of 18.2 × 109/L. The IUD is removed, and small, yellow granules are observed covering the device. Which of the following is the most likely causative agent of this infection?

A. Acid-fast bacilli

B. Budding yeast and hyphae

C. Gram-positive rods

D. Pear-shaped protozoa

E. Spirochete

Consider the following case for questions 8 to 10:

A 23-year-old man visits his physician because of a sore on his penis. He states the sore does not hurt, but he is concerned because it has been present for about 2 weeks. He has not travelled outside of the United States recently. His temperature is 37.1°C (98.8°F) and his pulse is 85 beats per minute. Physical examination reveals a single, indurated ulcer with well-demarcated edges on the penile shaft. No urethral discharge is noted. Mild inguinal lymphadenopathy is observed, and the lymph nodes are firm and nontender.

8. Which of the following is most likely to be found in scrapings from the genital ulcer?

A. Gram-negative rods

B. Gram-negative diplococci

C. Intraepithelial cell inclusions

D. Multinucleated giant cells

E. Spirochetes

9. Which of the following tests is the best next step in diagnosing this patient's infection?

A. Chlamydia PCR

B. Fluorescent treponemal antibody-absorbed assay (FTA-ABS)

C. Routine bacterial culture

D. Rapid plasma regain (RPR)

E. Viral culture

10. After the diagnosis is confirmed the man is treated with penicillin. Twenty-four hours after starting the antibiotic he develops an abrupt onset of headache, fever, chills, and myalgia. His temperature is 38.9°C (102°F) and his pulse is 154 beats per minute. Which other pathogen is also associated with this antibiotic reaction?

A. *Bacillus anthracis*

B. *Borrelia burgdorferi*

C. *Escherichia coli*

D. *Staphylococcus aureus*

E. *Vibrio cholerae*

11. A 46-year-old woman complains of a 1-week history of extreme exhaustion, headache, fever, sore throat, and loss of appetite. She states she was concerned when she noticed a rash on her body, which she claims is not itchy. She is sexually active and in a monogamous relationship. At the time of exam, her temperature is 38.1°C (100.6°F). Her pharynx is erythematous and no exudate is seen. Her cervical lymph nodes are enlarged, firm, and nontender. A diffuse maculopapular rash is present on her trunk, back, palms, and soles. The physician decides to do a pelvic exam. Which additional finding is most likely to be observed during the pelvic exam?

A. Cervical motion tenderness

B. Mucopurulent vaginal discharge

C. Painful, vesicular vaginal ulcer

D. Smooth, hypopigmented perianal papule

E. Verrucous, cauliflower-like perianal mass

Consider the following case for questions 12 to 14:

An 18-year-old college student visits her physician because of painful blisters in her vagina, vaginal itching, and painful urination. She does not own a thermometer, but she thinks she also has a fever and complains of a headache. She recently had her first sexual encounter with someone she met on campus. Her temperature is 38.7°C (101.8°F). On examination, two small ulcers with raised edges are noted on the labia. Bilateral inguinal lymphadenopathy is present and the lymph nodes are firm and tender.

12. The most likely causative agent of this infection lies latent in:

A. B-lymphocytes

B. Mucoepithelial cells

C. T-lymphocytes

D. The sacral ganglia

E. The dorsal root ganglia

13. Which of the following microscopic findings from the ulcer is expected?

A.

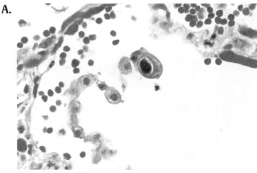

Source: CDC/Dr. Edwin P. Ewing, Jr.

B.

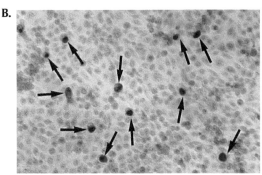

Source: CDC/Dr. E. Arum, Dr. N. Jacobs

C.

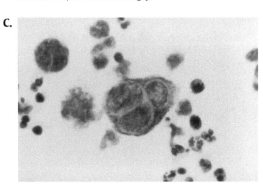

Source: CDC

D.

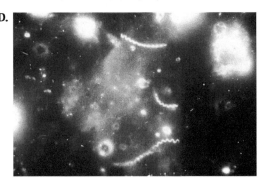

Source: CDC/Susan Lindsley

E.

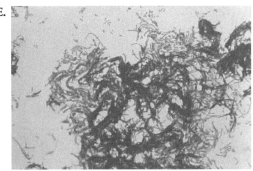

Source: CDC/Dr. Mike Miller

14. Which of the following is the most appropriate first line antimicrobial agent for this patient's infection?

A. Azithromycin

B. Foscarnet

C. Ganciclovir

D. Penicillin

E. Valacyclovir

15. A 44-year-old man presents with a painful sore on his penis. He recently returned from a trip to South Sudan and indicates that he participated in unprotected sexual activity while abroad. His temperature is 37.1°C (98.8°F). Physical examination reveals four ulcers on the glans penis and prepuce. The base of the ulcers contains purulent material. Inguinal lymphadenopathy is pronounced and can be seen in the following image.

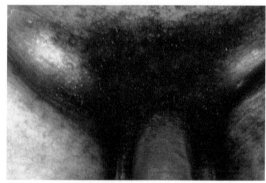

Source: CDC/Susan Lindsley

Which of the following is the most likely causative agent of this infection?

A. *Haemophilus ducreyi*

B. Herpes simplex virus-2 (HSV-2)

C. *Chlamydia trachomatis* serovars A, B, Ba, or C

D. *Chlamydia trachomatis* serovars D-K

E. *Chlamydia trachomatis* serovars L1, L2, or L3

F. *Klebsiella granulomatis*

G. *Treponema pallidum*

16. A 57-year-old Nigerian man visits the village clinic with a sore on his penis. He claims it does not hurt, but his partner wanted him to have a doctor look at it prior to engaging in sexual activity. Vitals are normal, and physical examination shows the presence of two ulcers on the penis, one of which is shown in the following image. Inguinal lymphadenopathy is not present.

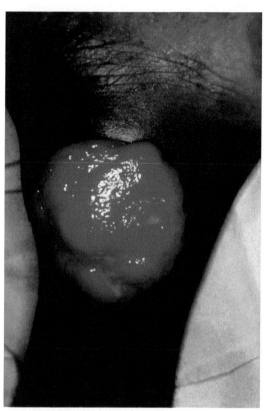

Source: CDC/ Joe Miller; Slides provided by Dr. Tabua, Chief Medical officer from Port Moresby, Papua, New Guinea

Which of the following microscopic findings from the ulcer is expected?

A. Donovan bodies

B. Multinucleated giant cells

C. Inclusions surrounded by a clear halo

D. Iodine staining inclusions

E. Negri bodies

17. A 24-year-old man in Bangkok, Thailand, visits his physician with fever and painful swelling in his groin. He states that about 1 month ago he had a small sore on his penis, but it went away within a few days so he did not seek medical attention. He mentions he feels tired and achy all the time. He is sexually active and has several male partners. His temperature is 38.2°C (100.8°F). No genital ulcers are present, but a bubo is seen on his right groin. Which of the following is a characteristic of the most likely causative agent?

A. Antigenically variable pili

B. Inability to synthesize ATP

C. Mycolic acid in the cell wall

D. Lack of a cell wall

E. Latency in sacral ganglia

18. A 41-year-old man presents to his physician with urethral discharge and painful urination of 4-day duration. He travelled to Miami a few weeks ago, and while there he engaged in a one-time sexual encounter with a woman he met at the club, he did not use a condom. His temperature is 37.1°C (98.8°F) and his blood pressure is 102/80 mm Hg. Physical exam reveals mucopurulent urethral discharge. No inguinal lymphadenopathy, genital, or rectal lesions are noted. A culture and Gram stain from the urethral discharge are sent to the microbiology laboratory and the Gram stain is shown as follows.

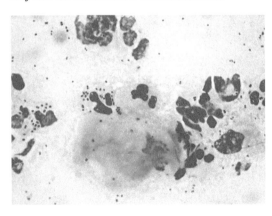

Which of the following is the most likely causative agent of this infection?

A. *Chlamydia trachomatis*

B. *Klebsiella granulomatis*

C. *Neisseria gonorrhoeae*

D. *Treponema pallidum*

E. *Ureaplasma urealyticum*

19. A 24-year-old woman presents with abdominal pain and pain when urinating. She states the symptoms started about 4 days ago. She denies vaginal discharge and hematuria. Her temperature is 37.2°C (98.9°F) and her pulse is 104 beats per minute. Abdominal tenderness of the lower right quadrant is noted on examination and rebound tenderness is absent. A bimanual exam reveals cervical motion and uterine tenderness. Urinalysis shows negative nitrites and leukocyte esterase. Urine hCG is negative. Which of the following organisms was this patient most likely recently infected with?

A. Double-stranded DNA virus

B. Gram-negative rods

C. Gram-negative diplococci

D. Spirochete

E. Yeast

20. A 30-year-old woman comes to the emergency department with a 1-week history of mild vaginal bleeding and abdominal pain. The first day of her last menstrual period was approximately 7 weeks ago. She assumed she now has her menstrual period, but the cramping is more severe than she normally experiences. Her temperature is 37°C (98.6°F) and her pulse 120 beats per minute. Physical examination reveals lower right quadrant abdominal tenderness. An ultrasound shows an empty uterus and adnexal mass. Urine hCG is positive, and serum hCG results are pending. With which of the following organisms has this patient most likely been infected in the past?

A. *Actinomyces israelii*

B. *Chlamydia trachomatis*

C. *Escherichia coli*

D. *Listeria monocytogenes*

E. *Treponema pallidum*

21. A 26-year-old man sees his physician with pain in his knees, ankles and hips, red painful eyes and pain when urinating. He states the symptoms seemed to suddenly appear about 2 weeks ago. His temperature is 37°C (98.6°F) and his pulse is 94 beats per minute. On examination, his left knee and both ankles are significantly swollen, tender, erythematous, and warm. There is also remarkable tenderness of the left sacroiliac joint. His eyes appear red, but no discharge is noted. No genital ulcers are present, but clear urethral discharge is observed. A Gram stain from urethral discharge shows no organisms are present, and the bacterial culture from the discharge is reported as no growth. Which of the following organisms was this patient most likely recently infected with?

A. *Chlamydia trachomatis*

B. *Neisseria gonorrhoeae*

C. *Staphylococcus aureus*

D. *Treponema pallidum*

E. *Vibrio cholerae*

22. A 46-year-old man complains of a 4-day history of pain and burning when urinating. His temperature is 37.1°C (98.7°F) and his pulse is 111 beats per minute. Examination reveals clear urethral discharge after penile stripping. No genital ulcers are observed. Urinalysis shows negative nitrates and positive leukocyte esterase. A Gram stain from urethral discharge shows no organisms are present and the bacterial culture from the discharge is reported as no growth. Which of the following is a characteristic of the most likely causative agent?

A. Chitin in the cell wall

B. Lack of the cell wall

C. Lipooligosaccharide (LOS) in the cell wall

D. Mycolic acid in the cell wall

E. Thick peptidoglycan layer in the cell wall

23. A 54-year-old man who has sex with men presents with a mass on his perianal region. He states the mass is itchy, tender, and burns but does not hurt. His vials are unremarkable. Physical examination of the anus reveals the findings seen in the following image. The rest of his physical exam is unremarkable. The MHA-TPA (a treponemal antibody test) is negative.

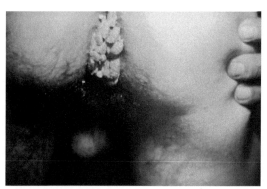

Source: CDC/Dr. Wiesner

The most likely diagnosis is:

A. Chancroid

B. Condyloma acuminata

C. Genital herpes

D. Lymphogranuloma venereum (LGV)

E. Secondary syphilis

24. A 30-year-old woman presents to her physician with a sore throat of 4-day duration. One week ago she visited Las Vegas and while there she engaged in a one-time sexual encounter with a man she met at the casino. She denies vaginal intercourse but admits to participating in oral sex. Her temperature is 37.1°C (98.8°F). Examination reveals an erythematous pharynx, yellowish exudate covering the tonsillar pillars and cervical lymphadenopathy. A throat swab was sent to the laboratory for culture and the resulting pathogen grows well on Thayer–Martin agar, but not on blood agar. Which of the following is a characteristic of the most likely agent causing this infection?

A. Antigenically variable pili

B. Exotoxin that inactivates elongation factor-2 (EF-2)

C. Latency in trigeminal ganglia

D. M protein

E. Polysaccharide capsule

25. Pregnant women are screened during the last trimester for group B streptococcus (GBS). If the screen is positive for GBS, what is the most appropriate next step?

A. Administer aztreonam during delivery

B. Administer penicillin G during delivery

C. Administer trimethoprim–sulfamethoxazole (TMP–SMX) during delivery

D. GBS is normal flora and no further treatment is needed

E. Treat the woman as soon as possible with penicillin

12.2 Answers and Explanations

Easy	Medium	Hard

1. Correct: Hyphae (C)

(C) This is a case of *Candida* vulvovaginitis. Although several species of *Candida* are implicated in vaginitis, *C. albicans* is the most common clinically isolated species. *C. albicans* is unique among the *Candida* because it exists as a yeast and fungus and produces budding yeast as well as pseudohyphae and true hyphae (see image at the end of this answer). *Candida* colonizes the vagina of healthy women and infections arise due to an imbalance of normal vaginal flora. Vaginal pH remains within the normal range. Risk factors for infection include antibiotic use (especially broad spectrum agents, such as azithromycin), increased estrogen levels, contraceptive use, diabetes mellitus, and immunosuppression. Perivaginal and vulvar pruritus and irritation are common. Most often there is little or no vaginal discharge, but if discharge is present it is classically described as thick, white, and cottage cheese like. Vaginal and mucosal erythema and edema is often observed. See table at the end of this answer to review the major features of vaginitis and vaginosis. **(A)** *Gardnerella vaginalis* is a gram-positive or gram-variable rod and an agent of bacterial vaginosis, which is due to an imbalance in normal vaginal flora. Vaginal pH is often greater than 4.5. Most women are asymptomatic; however, when discharge is present it is described as thin, off-white and malodorous (fishy smell). There is also copious shedding of vaginal epithelial cells. When these epithelial cells are covered in bacteria, they are called clue cells and are suggestive of a diagnosis of bacterial vaginosis if seen on wet mount. Neutrophils are most often absent in bacterial vaginosis. Risk factors for infection include new or increased numbers of sexual partners, douching, and women who have sex with women. Antibiotic use is not a major risk factor. **(B)** *Neisseria gonorrhoeae*, a gram-negative diplococcus is the causative agent of gonorrhea, a sexually transmitted infection. Females may present with vaginal pruritus, discomfort, and discharge; however, the discharge is most often purulent, rather than thick and white as in this case. Antibiotic use is not a major risk factor. **(D)** A common agent of vaginitis is the sexually transmitted, pear-shaped protozoan parasite, *Trichomonas vaginalis*. Vaginal irritation, pruritus, and erythema are common manifestations. The discharge associated with infections is described as thin, purulent, or green-frothy and malodorous. Antibiotic use is not a major risk factor. **(E)** A spirochete that is commonly involved in urogenital infections is *Treponema palladium*, the causative agent of syphilis, a sexually transmitted infection. Primary syphilis is often asymptomatic or presents with a painless chancre. Most often there is no exudate present. Antibiotic use is not a major risk factor. If untreated, the disease can progress to secondary, latent, or late syphilis.

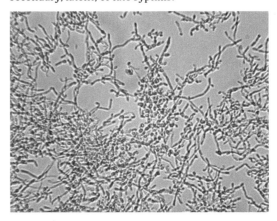

Vaginitis and vaginosis differentiation				
	Normal	**Bacterial vaginosis**	**Candidiasis**	**Trichomoniasis**
Symptom presentation		Odor, discharge	Itch, discomfort, dysuria, thick discharge	Itch, discharge, 70% asymptomatic
Vaginal discharge	Clear to white	Homogenous, adherent, thin, milky white; malodorous "foul fishy"	Thick, clumpy, white "cottage cheese"	Frothy, gray, or yellow–green; malodorous
Clinical findings			Inflammation and erythema	Cervical petechiae "strawberry cervix"
Vaginal pH	3.8–4.2	> 4.5	Usually ≤ 4.5	> 4.5
KOH "whiff" test	Negative	Positive	Negative	Often positive
NaCl wet mount	Lactobacilli	Clue cells (≥ 20%), no/few WBCs	Few to many WBCs	Motile flagellated protozoa, many WBCs
KOH wet mount			Pseudohyphae or spores if non-albicans species	

Abbreviations: NaCl, sodium chloride; KOH, potassium hydroxide; WBC, white blood cell.

Source: CDC.

2. Correct: Wet mount (E)

(E) This woman most likely has trichomoniasis caused by *Trichomonas vaginalis. T. vaginalis* is a pear-shaped flagellated protozoan parasite (see images [i] and [ii] at the end of this answer) that exhibits jerky motility. The motility can be visualized with a wet mount (also referred to as wet preparation). *T. vaginalis* is the number one agent of vaginitis and is also the most common nonviral sexually transmitted infection worldwide. Many females are asymptomatic; however, clinical manifestations in females include purulent thin, green-frothy discharge, vulvar irritation, pruritus, dysuria, and dyspareunia. Erythema is often pronounced, and the cervix is described as "strawberry cervix" (punctate hemorrhage) due to mucosal capillary dilation. Symptoms of infection are often worse during menstrual period. In the past, the wet prep was utilized for diagnosis. But due to poor sensitivity, this test has now been replaced with molecular assays. However, many OB-GYN outpatient clinics still use the wet mount. (See table at the end of this answer to review the major features of vaginitis and vaginosis.) (A) A Gram stain is used to visualize bacterial pathogens and is not the best method to observe *T. vaginalis* or other parasites. (B) A potassium hydroxide (KOH) preparation is useful for the diagnosis of fungi or yeast. *Candida* and other yeast may be implicated in vaginitis and 10% KOH is often used to dissolve cellular debris and better visualize hyphae. Like trichomoniasis, *Candida* vulvovaginitis is often worse around menstrual period. However, the strawberry cervix and thin vaginal discharge is more likely with *Trichomonas vaginalis* infections. (C) Pap smears aid in the diagnosis of human papillomavirus (HPV). Rounded and clumped koilocytotic squamous epithelial cells may be noted on smears when HPV is present. (D) A Tzanck smear, which is not widely utilized anymore, may aid in the diagnosis. This is performed by scraping the base of a lesion. If herpes virus is present, multinucleated giant cells and/or intranuclear inclusions will be seen. Most often with HSV infections, a painful genital ulcer is present.

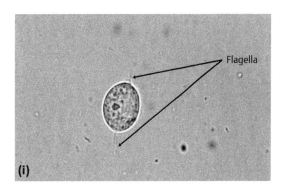

(i)

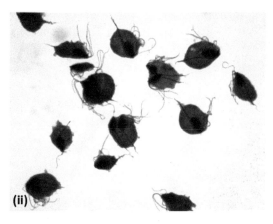

(ii)

Vaginitis and vaginosis differentiation

	Normal	Bacterial vaginosis	Candidiasis	Trichomoniasis
Symptom presentation		Odor, discharge	Itch, discomfort, dysuria, thick discharge	Itch, discharge, 70% asymptomatic
Vaginal discharge	Clear to white	Homogenous, adherent, thin, milky white; malodorous "foul fishy"	Thick, clumpy, white "cottage cheese"	Frothy, gray, or yellow-green; malodorous
Clinical findings			Inflammation and erythema	Cervical petechiae "strawberry cervix"
Vaginal pH	3.8–4.2	> 4.5	Usually ≤ 4.5	> 4.5
KOH "whiff" test	Negative	Positive	Negative	Often positive
NaCl wet mount	Lactobacilli	Clue cells (≥ 20%), no/few WBCs	Few to many WBCs	Motile flagellated protozoa, many WBCs
KOH wet mount			Pseudohyphae or spores if non-albicans species	

Abbreviations: NaCl, sodium chloride; KOH, potassium hydroxide; WBC, white blood cell.

Source: CDC.

3. Correct: Metronidazole (D)

(D) This infection is due to *Trichomonas vaginalis*. The antimicrobial agents of choice for trichomoniasis are metronidazole and tinidazole. Metronidazole must be reduced in vivo for the drug to be activated. Once activated metronidazole creates toxic intermediates that damages the pathogen DNA. The spectrum of activity includes obligate anaerobes, select microaerophilic bacteria, and some protozoa. Tinidazole also damages DNA and is effective against protozoa. See Appendix I for a summary of antimicrobials spectrum of activity and mechanism of action. *T. vaginalis* is a pear-shaped, flagellated protozoan parasite that exhibits jerky motility. Many females are asymptomatic; however, clinical manifestations in females include purulent, thin, green-frothy discharge, vulvar irritation, pruritus, dysuria, and dyspareunia. Erythema is often pronounced and the cervix is described as "strawberry cervix" (punctate hemorrhage) due to mucosal capillary dilation. Symptoms of infection are often worse during menstrual period. **(A)** Acyclovir is an antiviral agent that may be used to manage herpes simplex and varicella zoster virus infections. Acyclovir is a nucleoside analog that inhibits viral DNA polymerase. This agent must first be converted to the active form by the virally encoded

enzyme thymidine kinase. However, in this case herpes is unlikely due to the lack of the typical painful genital lesions seen in herpes infection. **(B)** Azithromycin is the antibiotic of choice for *Chlamydia trachomatis* urogenital infections. This agent is a macrolide that binds to the bacterial ribosome (50S subunit) and blocks protein synthesis. Azithromycin is considered a broad-spectrum agent and can be used for select gram-positive and gram-negative pathogens as well as *Chlamydia* and *Mycoplasma*. Most often females are asymptomatic when infected with *C. trachomatis* but mucopurulent discharge, dysuria and increased urinary frequency may be present. In this case the "strawberry cervix" is indicative of vaginitis due to *T. vaginalis*. **(C)** Fluconazole is an antifungal agent used to treat fungal vaginitis. Fluconazole works by inhibiting lanosterol 14-α-demethylase, a cytochrome P450 dependent enzyme. Without this enzyme the fungal cell is unable to convert lanosterol to ergosterol, which is a necessary part of the fungal cell membrane. Fluconazole is active against most *Candida* species (note that *C. krusei* is resistant and *C. glabrata* can be resistant) and is also active against *Blastomyces*, *Coccidiodes*, and *Histoplasma* (endemic fungi). Like trichomoniasis, candida vulvovaginitis is often worse around menstrual period. The strawberry cervix and thin vaginal discharge is more likely with *Trichomonas vaginalis* infections. **(E)** Penicillin is used for many types of infections and is the antimicrobial of choice for early syphilis infections. Penicillin inhibits bacterial cell wall synthesis. Penicillin is also active against gram-positive cocci (that do not produce penicillinase), anaerobes and select gram-positive rods and *Neisseria*. In this case the patient does not have genital lesions so syphilis is unlikely.

4. Correct: Bacterial vaginosis (A)

(A) The Gram stained image presented in the question stem shows a clue cell, which is indicative of bacterial vaginosis. Clue cells are vaginal epithelial cells with bacteria attached to the cells. There are several etiological agents that may be involved in bacterial vaginosis, most notably the facultative anaerobe *Gardnerella vaginosis* (gram-positive or gram-variable rods) and gram-positive anaerobes such as *Mobiluncus* and *Atopbium* (gram-negative or gram-variable rods). Bacterial vaginosis is an infection with limited to no inflammation and arises due to an imbalance of the local microbiota. *Lactobacilllus* is an inhabitant of a healthy vagina and aids in keeping the vaginal pH acidic. In bacterial vaginosis, levels of lactobacilli are decreased leading to alterations in pH and overgrowth of *Gardnerella* and other pathogens. It is estimated that 75% of women with bacterial vaginosis are asymptomatic. Symptoms, if present, include thin, off-white homogenous vaginal discharge that has a "fishy" odor. Little to no vaginal edema or pruritus is present. Coinfections with *Candida* and *Trichomonas* are common so patients may exhibit symptoms of both vaginosis and vaginitis. See table at the end of this answer to review the major features of vaginitis and vaginosis. **(B)** In *Candida* vulvovaginitis, perivaginal, and vulvar pruritus and irritation are common. Most often there is little or no vaginal discharge, but if discharge is present it is classically described as thick, white, and cottage cheese like. Vaginal and mucosal erythema and edema is often observed. None of these findings are present in this case; hence *Candida* is not the likely agent of this infection. **(C, D)** Many times, chlamydia and gonorrhea infections are asymptomatic. Mucopurulent discharge may be present with both infections and a concurrent urethritis may be present resulting in abdominal pain, dysuria, and dyspareunia. Clue cells are not associated with either of these infections. *Chlamydia* is considered Gram negative since it has lipopolysaccharide (LPS) in its cell wall. However, *Chlamydia* Gram stains poorly or not at all, in part due to the small size and lack of muramic acid in the cell wall. **(E)** Trichomoniasis is caused by the protozoan parasite *Trichomonas vaginalis*. Most infections are asymptomatic and clinical manifestations, if present, include purulent thin, green-frothy discharge, vulvar irritation, pruritus, dysuria, and dyspareunia. Erythema is often pronounced and the cervix is described as "strawberry cervix" due to mucosal capillary dilation. None of these findings are present in this case; hence *T. vaginalis* is not the likely agent of this infection.

Vaginitis and vaginosis differentiation				
	Normal	**Bacterial vaginosis**	**Candidiasis**	**Trichomoniasis**
Symptom presentation		Odor, discharge	Itch, discomfort, dysuria, thick discharge	Itch, discharge, 70% asymptomatic
Vaginal discharge	Clear to white	Homogenous, adherent, thin, milky white; malodorous "foul fishy"	Thick, clumpy, white "cottage cheese"	Frothy, gray, or yellow–green; malodorous
Clinical findings			Inflammation and erythema	Cervical petechiae "strawberry cervix"
Vaginal pH	3.8–4.2	> 4.5	Usually ≤ 4.5	> 4.5
KOH "whiff" test	Negative	Positive	Negative	Often positive
NaCl wet mount	Lactobacilli	Clue cells (≥ 20%), no/few WBCs	Few to many WBCs	Motile flagellated protozoa, many WBCs
KOH wet mount			Pseudohyphae or spores if non-albicans species	

Abbreviations: NaCl, sodium chloride; KOH, potassium hydroxide; WBC, white blood cell.

Source: CDC.

5. Correct: *Gardnerella and Mobiluncus* (C)

(C) Several pathogens are implicated in bacterial vaginosis, including *Gardnerella vaginalis* and *Mobiluncus*. *Gardnerella vaginalis* are gram-positive or gram-variable rods. *Mobiluncus* is strict anaerobe, while *Gardnerella* is a facultative anaerobe. In bacterial vaginosis the vaginal pH is elevated and the discharge, if present, is malodorous, thin and white. This is due to anaerobes, which break peptides into amines, which characteristically have a distinct odor. In the whiff test, 10% KOH is added to the vaginal discharge and if positive, a fishy odor is detected. Additionally, in vaginosis there is little to no inflammation and therefore few to no white blood cells (WBCs) present on microscopy. The Amsel criteria are used to diagnose bacterial vaginosis, and three of the following must be present: (1) thin, off-white discharge; (2) vaginal pH greater than 4.5; (3) positive whiff test; and (4) clue cells. See table at the end of this answer to review the major features of vaginitis and vaginosis. **(A)** *Candida* is a yeast and an agent of vaginitis.

In vulvovaginal candidiasis, pruritus and inflammation may be present, the vaginal pH is usually normal (pH < 4.5), and WBCs are most often present on saline wet mount. *Mobiluncus*, however, is an agent of vaginosis. **(B)** In *Chlamydia* and *Neisseria* infections, mucopurulent discharge may be present. A concurrent urethritis may be also present resulting in abdominal pain, dysuria, and dyspareunia. A positive whiff test is not associated with either of these infections. **(D)** *Trichomonas* is a protozoan parasite and an agent of vaginitis. Although coinfections with agents of vaginitis and bacterial vaginosis are common, this patient does not exhibit symptoms of vaginitis, nor are the results from the vaginal specimen indicative of vaginitis. In vaginitis, pruritus and inflammation are common, and WBCs would most likely be seen on a wet preparation. *Gardnerella*, however, is an agent of vaginosis. **(E)** *Neisseria gonorrhoeae* causes gonorrhea. Infections are often asymptomatic or may result in cervicitis or urethritis with the presence of purulent vaginal discharge. *Trichomonas* is an agent of vaginitis and not vaginosis.

Vaginitis and vaginosis differentiation				
	Normal	**Bacterial vaginosis**	**Candidiasis**	**Trichomoniasis**
Symptom presentation		Odor, discharge	Itch, discomfort, dysuria, thick discharge	Itch, discharge, 70% asymptomatic
Vaginal discharge	Clear to white	Homogenous, adherent, thin, milky white; malodorous "foul fishy"	Thick, clumpy, white "cottage cheese"	Frothy, gray, or yellow–green; malodorous
Clinical findings			Inflammation and erythema	Cervical petechiae "strawberry cervix"
Vaginal pH	3.8–4.2	> 4.5	Usually ≤ 4.5	> 4.5
KOH "whiff" test	Negative	Positive	Negative	Often positive
NaCl wet mount	Lactobacilli	Clue cells (≥ 20%), no/few WBCs	Few to many WBCs	Motile flagellated protozoa, many WBCs
KOH wet mount			Pseudohyphae or spores if non-albicans species	

Abbreviations: NaCl, sodium chloride; KOH, potassium hydroxide; WBC, white blood cell.

Source: CDC.

6. Correct: Germ tube (B)

(B) This woman has vulvovaginitis and the wet preparation shows budding yeast and hyphae. *Candida* is most often implicated in vulvovaginitis, and *C. albicans* is the most common species. *C. albicans* is unique because it exists as a yeast and fungus and produces budding yeast as well as pseudohyphae and true hyphae. The germ tube test is used to identify *C. albicans*. In the germ tube test, a well-isolated colony of the unknown organism, growing on media, is incubated in serum for 2 hours and then viewed microscopically for the presence of germ tubes. *C. albicans* produces germ tubes, which are short outgrowths of nonseptate hyphae. While the germ tube test is the classic test utilized for the diagnosis of *Candida*, it is not very sensitive. Risk factors for vulvovaginal candidiasis include antibiotic use (especially broad-spectrum agents), increased estrogen levels, contraceptive use, diabetes mellitus, and immunosuppression. Perivaginal and vulvar pruritus and irritation are common. Most often there is little or no vaginal discharge, but if discharge is present it is classically described as thick, white, and cottage cheese like. Vaginal and mucosal erythema and edema is often observed. See table at the end of this answer to review the major features of vaginitis and vaginosis. **(A)** The coagulase test is most often used to identify *Staphylococcus aureus*, which is the only clinically significant staphylococci that is coagulase positive. *S. aureus* is not a common agent of vaginitis or vaginosis. **(C)** The oxidase test can be used to identify several organisms including the urogenital pathogen *Neisseria gonorrhoeae*, which is oxidase positive. **(D)** The whiff test is used to detect odor associated with a predominance of anaerobic bacteria during bacterial vaginosis. In bacterial vaginosis, little to no inflammation is present, and in this case, vaginal erythema is present. **(E)** Venereal disease research laboratory (VDRL) test is used to screen for the sexually transmitted infection, syphilis, caused by *Treponema palladium*. Primary syphilis is often asymptomatic or presents with a painless chancre. If untreated, the disease can progress to secondary, latent, or late syphilis. There is no evidence of any lesions/chancre in this case.

Vaginitis and vaginosis differentiation				
	Normal	**Bacterial vaginosis**	**Candidiasis**	**Trichomoniasis**
Symptom presentation		Odor, discharge	Itch, discomfort, dysuria, thick discharge	Itch, discharge, 70% asymptomatic
Vaginal discharge	Clear to white	Homogenous, adherent, thin, milky white; malodorous "foul fishy"	Thick, clumpy, white "cottage cheese"	Frothy, gray, or yellow–green; malodorous
Clinical findings			Inflammation and erythema	Cervical petechiae "strawberry cervix"
Vaginal pH	3.8–4.2	> 4.5	Usually ≤ 4.5	> 4.5
KOH "whiff" test	Negative	Positive	Negative	Often positive
NaCl wet mount	Lactobacilli	Clue cells (≥ 20%), no/few WBCs	Few to many WBCs	Motile flagellated protozoa, many WBCs
KOH wet mount			Pseudohyphae or spores if non-albicans species	

Abbreviations: NaCl, sodium chloride; KOH, potassium hydroxide; WBC, white blood cell.

Source: CDC.

7. Correct: Gram-positive rods (C)

(C) This describes pelvic actinomycosis caused by *Actinomyces israelii*. *Actinomyces* are anaerobic, branching gram-positive rods. Clinical specimens may contain sulfur granules. While these granules are called sulfur granules, note that they are not composed of sulfur. These yellow granules are composed of *Actinomyces* filaments surrounded by PMNs. *Actinomyces* may also cause cervicofacial, thoracic, and abdominal infections. Clinical manifestations of IUD infections include flu-like symptoms, nausea and vomiting, fever and chills, late menstrual period, vaginal discharge, abdominal pain, and dyspareunia. Microscopically *Actinomyces* may resemble *Nocardia*. Both are branching gram-positive rods. However, *Actinomyces* is anaerobic while *Nocardia* is aerobic. *Actinomyces* is negative for the modified acid-fast stain and *Nocardia* stains positive with the modified-acid fast stain. Lastly, sulfur granules are pathognomonic for *Actinomyces*. **(A)** Bacteria that are acid-fast bacilli include *Mycobacteria* and *Nocardia* (modified acid-fast). Neither pathogen is a usual agent of IUD infections. Like *Actinomyces*, *Nocardia* is a branching gram-positive rod, but it is modified acid-fast, is an aerobe and is not associated with sulfur granules. **(B)** Yeast with hyphae describes *Candida*, an agent of vaginitis. *Candida* is not associated with sulfur granules. **(D)** A pear-shaped trophozoite is a description of *Trichomonas vaginalis*, which causes vaginitis. This pathogen is not associated with sulfur granules. **(E)** The spirochete *Treponema pallidum* is an agent of urogenital infections but is not associated with sulfur granules.

8.   Correct: Spirochetes (E)

(E) This is most likely a case of primary syphilis, a sexually transmitted infection caused by *Treponema pallidum*, a spirochete shaped bacterium. Spirochetes can be visualized with dark-field microscopy; however, this technique is no longer utilized routinely in the clinical laboratory. The chancre or ulcer of primary syphilis may go unnoticed because it is painless and is self-resolving. The chancre is usually indurated (hard) with well-defined edges. With primary syphilis genital exudate is usually absent, but mild to moderate inguinal lymphadenopathy is present. Syphilis can be treated with a single intramuscular injection of penicillin G. See table at the end of this answer for a comparison of the major types of genital ulcer disease. **(A)** *Haemophilus ducreyi* and *Klebsiella*

granulomatis are gram-negative rods that may cause sexually transmitted infections with genital ulcers. Both are more common in tropical climates outside of the United States. The ulcers of chancroid, caused by *H. ducreyi* are painful, soft and have ragged edges. In granuloma inguinale, caused by *K. granulomatis*, the ulcer is painless, and lymphadenopathy is usually absent. **(B)** A gram-negative diplococcus that causes genital infections is *Neisseria gonorrhoeae*. Gonorrhea may be asymptomatic or manifest as urethritis or cervicitis with mucopurulent genital discharge. There is typically no genital lesion present. **(C)** *Chlamydia* is obligate intracellular pathogens and infected cells contain inclusions. *C. trachomatis*, serotypes D-K infect epithelial cells and cause the sexually transmitted infection chlamydia. Infections may be asymptomatic or result in genital discharge with the absence of a genital lesion. *C. trachomatis*, serotypes L1, L2, and L3 infect macrophages and are the agents of lymphogranuloma venereum (LGV). This infection is more common in tropical countries and similar to syphilis, the genital ulcer in primary LGV is painless. **(D)** Multinucleated giant cells are seen with herpes infections. Herpes simplex virus-2 (HSV-2) and less commonly HSV-1 cause genital herpes. In genital herpes, a vesicular lesion or painful ulcer is seen on the genitals. Additionally, constitutional or "flu-like" symptoms, including a fever, are sometimes present along with the lesion.

Comparison of clinically significant genital ulcer diseases					
Feature	**Genital herpes**	**Chancroid**	**Syphilis**	**LGV**	**Granuloma inguinale (donovanosis)**
Causative agent	HSV (most often type 2)	*H. ducreyi*	*T. pallidum*	*C. trachomatis* L1, L2, and L3	*K. granulomatis*
Typical lesion	Early on—vesicles • Erythematous Later—ulcer • Shallow • Raised edges	Ulcer • Purulent base • Nonindurated • Ragged edges	Ulcer/chancre • Indurated • Demarcated edges	Early on—papule Later—ulcer • Small • Shallow	Ulcer • Highly vascular "beefy red"
Painful or painless	Painful	Painful	Painless	Painless	Painless
Number of lesions	Multiple	Usually multiple	Usually singular	Usually singular	Variable
Inguinal lymphadenopathy	Yes	Yes Buboes	Yes In late primary syphilis	Yes—painful In secondary LGV Buboes	Not usually Pseudobuboes
Constitutional symptoms	Yes	No	Yes In secondary syphilis	Yes In secondary LGV	No

Abbreviations: HSV, herpes simplex virus; LGV, lymphogranuloma venereum.

9. Correct: Rapid plasma regain (RPR) (D)

(D) This patient has primary syphilis caused by the spirochete *Treponema pallidum*. Diagnosis includes microscopic evaluation of clinical specimens or serological assays. Serological tests may be classified as nontreponemal or treponemal tests. Traditionally, nontreponemal tests such as the RPR (answer choice D) are performed first prior to performing treponemal tests. Nontreponemal tests include RPR (rapid plasma reagin), VDRL (venereal disease research laboratory), and TRUST (toluidine red unheated serum test). These tests detect antibodies to cardiolipin antigen and evaluate damaged host cells. They must be used in conjunction with specific treponemal tests because these tests are not specific for *T. pallidum*. Nontreponema tests may be positive in other *Treponema* infections including yaws and pinta and other non-infectious conditions such as rheumatoid arthritis. *Treponema*-specific tests include fluorescent *Treponema* antibody-absorption (FTA-ABS), *Treponema pallidum* hemagglutination (TPHA), *Treponema pallidum* particle agglutination assay (TP-PA), and microhemagglutination *Treponema pallidum* (MHA-TP). These confirmatory tests detect anti-*Treponema* antibody. If both the nontreponema test and the treponemal-specific tests are positive, the individual is likely to have a current or past infection with syphilis. Current recommendations for syphilis diagnosis include the reverse sequence algorithm which would aid in the detection of early primary and treated infections (which may be missed using the traditional algorithm). In the reverse sequence algorithm, a screening treponemal specific test (immunoglobulin G [IgG] antibody) is performed first and if positive, then the RPR, a nontreponemal test is used. If the patient is positive for both the IgG and the RPR, the patient either has a past or present infection with syphilis. If the RPR is negative this is reflexed to another treponmal test such as the TP-PA. Clinical specimens, especially lesions of primary or secondary syphilis can be evaluated microscopically for the presence of spirochetes. In the past dark-field microscopy was frequently used. Now, very few clinical laboratories use dark-field microscopy. **(A)** This infection is due to syphilis and not chlamydia; hence chlamydia PCR is incorrect. **(B)** Classically, nontreponemal tests are usually performed prior to the treponemal tests, such as the FTA-ABS. **(C)** This man has syphilis and the causative agent of the infection *T. pallidum*, does not grow on routine microbiological media. **(E)** This infection is not due to a virus, such as herpes, hence viral culture is incorrect.

10. Correct: *Borrelia burgdorferi* (B)

(B) This is a case of primary syphilis, a sexually transmitted infection, caused by *Treponema pallidum*, a spirochete shaped bacterium. Primary syphilis may be treated with penicillin; however, there is a possibility of developing a Jarisch–Herxheimer reaction. The Jarisch–Herxheimer reaction is an acute febrile reaction that is usually seen during the first 24 hours of treatment with penicillin. It is thought to be due to an exaggerated proinflammatory immune response to the dying spirochetes. This reaction is also seen with other spirochete diseases including Lyme disease (*Borrelia burgdorferi*) (answer choice B), relapsing fever (*Borrelia recurrentis*), and leptospirosis (*Leptospira*). Nonspirochetes including the bacteria *Brucella*, *Bartonella*, *Salmonella*, and the parasite *Trichinella* may also induce this reaction.. **(A, C, D, E)** *Bacillus anthracis*, *Escherichia coli*, *Staphylococcus aureus*, and *Vibrio cholerae* are not associated with the Jarisch–Herxheimer reaction.

11. Correct: Smooth, hypopigmented perianal papule (D)

(D) This woman most likely has secondary syphilis caused by the spirochete *Treponema pallidum*. The stages of syphilis are primary syphilis, secondary syphilis, and tertiary syphilis. Syphilis may be latent as well. Typical findings of secondary syphilis include a nonpruritic, bilaterally symmetrical, maculopapular rash on the trunk, back and extremities, including the palms and soles, generalized lymphadenopathy, "flu-like" symptoms, alopecia and condylomata lata (answer choice D). Condylomata lata are smooth, flat papules that are generally painless (see image at the end of this answer). They are usually found on the genitals, perianal region and other areas that are moist. Other findings of secondary syphilis include central nervous system (CNS) abnormalities and ocular abnormalities. **(A)** Cervical motion tenderness is most likely indicative of pelvic inflammatory disease (PID). PID is usually preceded by the sexually transmitted infections gonorrhea and chlamydia. **(B)** Mucopurulent vaginal discharge may indicate cervicitis or vaginitis but is not typically a manifestation of secondary syphilis. *Neisseria gonorrhoeae* and *Chlamydia trachomatis* are causative agents of cervicitis. Vaginitis is usually caused by yeast (*Candida*) and the parasite, *Trichomonas vaginalis*. **(C)** Painful, vesicular genital ulcers are highly indicative of genital herpes, caused by herpes simplex virus-2 (HSV-2) and to a lesser extent HSV-1. **(E)** Verrucous, cauliflower-like masses are seen with human papillomavirus (HPV). Genital warts are sexually transmitted and can be found on the genitalia and anogenital region. Genital warts are also referred to as condyloma acuminata.

(i) Condylomata lata: syphilis

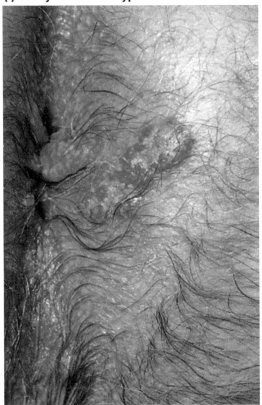

Source: Secondary Syphilis. In: Sterry W, Paus R, Burgdorf W, Hrsg. Thieme Clinical Companions - Dermatology. 1st Edition. Thieme; 2006

(ii) Condyloma acuminata: HPV

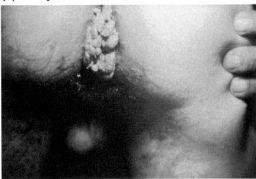

Source: CDC/Dr. Wiesner

12. Correct: The sacral ganglia (D)

(D) This woman most likely has genital herpes. Genital herpes is usually caused by herpes simplex virus-2 (HSV-2) but HSV-1 may also cause genital infections. All herpes viruses establish life-long latency and may be reactivated later, resulting in recurring infections. HSV-1 establishes latency in the trigeminal ganglia and HSV-2 establishes latency in the sacral ganglia (answer choice D). In genital herpes, vesicles evolve into pustules then painful shallow ulcers with a raised edge. There are often multiple lesions present. The vesicles may crust over and scab but most often resolve within 3 weeks. Local tingling and itching, dysuria and systemic manifestations ("flu-like" symptoms) may also be present. See table at the end of this answer for a comparison of the major types of genital ulcer disease. **(A)** Another member of the herpes virus family, Epstein–Barr (EBV) virus targets and remains latent in B-lymphocytes. **(B)** Herpes simplex viruses (HSVs) initially infect muco-epithelial cells. The virus then disseminates from the initial infection site and is transported to the sensory ganglia in a retrograde fashion. **(C)** An example of a pathogen that establishes latency in T-lymphocytes is human immunodeficiency virus (HIV). **(E)** Varicella zoster virus (VZV), which is also a member of the herpes virus family, remains latent in the dorsal root ganglia.

Comparison of clinically significant genital ulcer diseases

Feature	Genital herpes	Chancroid	Syphilis	LGV	Granuloma inguinale (donovanosis)
Causative agent	HSV (most often type 2)	*H. ducreyi*	*T. pallidum*	*C. trachomatis* L1, L2, and L3	*K. granulomatis*
Typical lesion	Early on—vesicles • Erythematous Later—ulcer • Shallow • Raised edges	Ulcer • Purulent base • Nonindurated • Ragged edges	Ulcer/chancre • Indurated • Demarcated edges	Early on—papule Later—ulcer • Small • Shallow	Ulcer • Highly vascular "beefy red"
Painful or painless	Painful	Painful	Painless	Painless	Painless
Number of lesions	Multiple	Usually multiple	Usually singular	Usually singular	Variable
Inguinal lymphadenopathy	Yes	Yes Buboes	Yes In late primary syphilis	Yes—painful In secondary LGV Buboes	Not usually Pseudobuboes
Constitutional symptoms	Yes	No	Yes In secondary syphilis	Yes In secondary LGV	No

Abbreviations: HSV, herpes simplex virus; LGV, lymphogranuloma venereum.

---

13. Correct: (C)

(C) This is a case of genital herpes caused by herpes simplex virus (HSV). A Tzank smear is can be used in the diagnosis of herpes and scrapings from the base of the lesion will demonstrate multinucleated giant cells as seen in answer choice C. Currently, Tzanck smears are not performed clinically. This test has largely been replaced by other methods of diagnosis including direct fluorescent antibody (DFA) tests and PCR from the lesion fluid. (A) Image A shows owl-eye inclusions (inclusions surrounded with a clear halo), which are typical of cytomegalovirus (CMV). CMV is not an agent of genital ulcer disease. (B) Image B shows intranuclear inclusions stained with iodine, which are characteristic of *Chlamydia*. Females with chlamydia are either asymptomatic or present with cervicitis or urethritis. This woman has a genital ulcer so *Chlamydia* is unlikely. (D) This is a dark-field image of spirochetes. Syphilis is caused by the spirochete, *Treponema pallidum*. In syphilis, the genital ulcer is most often painless (not painful as in this case), indurated and has well-demarcated edges. (E) Gram-negative rods such as those seen in this image that may be involved in genital infections include *Haemophilus ducreyi* (chancroid) and *Klebsiella granulomatis* (granuloma inguinale). The ulcers of chancroid are painful and the ulcers of granuloma inguinale are usually painless. In both infections, constitutional symptoms as seen in this case are absent.

14. Correct: Valacyclovir (E)

(E) Primary herpes infections should be treated with antiviral therapy. Active agents include the nucleoside analogues, acyclovir, famciclovir, and valacyclovir (answer choice E), which inhibit viral DNA polymerase. All of these agents are prodrugs which must be converted to the active form in vivo by viral thymidine kinase. (A) Azithromycin, a macrolide that inhibits protein synthesis, is typically used for the treatment of chlamydia. This woman most likely has herpes, not chlamydia; hence, valacyclovir is a better agent for treatment. (B) Foscarnet is primarily used in the treatment of ganciclovir-resistant cytomegalovirus (CMV) in immunocompromised patients. It may also be used in the management of acyclovir-resistant herpes simplex virus (HSV) and varicella zoster virus (VZV) infections. However, first-line therapy for herpes should include acyclovir, famciclovir or valacyclovir. Foscarnet inhibits viral DNA polymerase by binding near the pyrophosphate-binding site of the DNA polymerase. (C) Ganciclovir, a nucleoside analogue, is utilized for cytomegalovirus (CMV) infections, especially in immunocompromised patients. Ganciclovir must first be converted to an active form. CMV viral kinase phosphorylates ganciclovir and activates it. (D) Penicillin, which inhibits bacterial cell wall synthesis, is the antimicrobial of choice for syphilis caused by the spirochete *Treponema pallidum*. This woman has painful genital lesions, which is typical of genital herpes and not primary syphilis.

15.   Correct: *Haemophilus ducreyi* (A)

(A) This man most likely has chancroid caused by the gram-negative rod, *Haemophilus ducreyi*. Chancroid starts as an erythematous papule that develops into a pustule and then soft, painful ulcer/chancre with ragged edges. Often multiple lesions are present and inguinal lymphadenopathy and buboes may be seen. Chancroid is more common in sub-Saharan Africa and Southeast Asia than in the United States. *H. ducreyi* is a gram-negative bacillus that often clump together resulting in a "school-of-fish" appearance on Gram stain. *Haemophilus* species are fastidious, meaning they have complex nutritional requirements. *H. ducreyi* needs hemin, also known as X factor to grow. See table at the end of this answer for a comparison of the major types of genital ulcer disease. (B) HSV-2 is an agent of genital herpes. In genital herpes, vesicles evolve into pustules then painful ulcers. There are often multiple lesions present. The vesicles may crust over and scab but most often resolve within 3 weeks. Constitutional symptoms are usually present, although are not present in this man. The marked inguinal lymphadenopathy indicates that *H. ducreyi* is most likely to be the causative agent of this infection. (C) *Chlamydia trachomatis* serovars A, B, Ba, and C are agents of trachoma, a serious ocular infection that may result in blindness. These strains are not agents of urogenital infections. (D) *Chlamydia trachomatis* serovars D-K are agents of the sexually transmitted infection chlamydia. Males may be asymptomatic or present with urethritis, dysuria, epididymitis, and proctitis. Genital ulcers are not present as seen in this case. (E) *Chlamydia* serovars L1, L2, and L3 are agents of the sexual transmitted infection, lymphogranuloma venereum (LGV). The ulcer associated with the primary stage of this infection is most often a painless papule that may ulcerate. During the secondary stage, which is usually 2 to 6 weeks after the initial infection, painful lymphadenopathy with bubo formation may occur. The concurrent findings of the ulcer and the inguinal lymphadenopathy indicate that this is most likely chancroid. (F) *Klebsiella granulomatis* is the agent of granuloma inguinale. The lesions are firm, painless nodules or papules that eventually ulcerate. Inguinal lymphadenopathy is generally not present as seen in the image in this case. (G) *Treponema pallidum* is the causative agent of syphilis. The chancre seen in primary syphilis is generally painless, hard, and has sharply demarcated edges with minimal discharge present. The ulcer in this case is painful and contains purulent material. This infection is unlikely syphilis.

Comparison of clinically significant genital ulcer diseases					
Feature	Genital herpes	Chancroid	Syphilis	LGV	Granuloma inguinale (donovanosis)
Causative agent	HSV (most often type 2)	*H. ducreyi*	*T. pallidum*	*C. trachomatis* L1, L2, and L3	*K. granulomatis*
Typical lesion	Early on—vesicles • Erythematous Later—ulcer • Shallow • Raised edges	Ulcer • Purulent base • Nonindurated • Ragged edges	Ulcer/chancre • Indurated • Demarcated edges	Early on—papule Later—ulcer • Small • Shallow	Ulcer • Highly vascular "beefy red"
Painful or painless	Painful	Painful	Painless	Painless	Painless
Number of lesions	Multiple	Usually multiple	Usually singular	Usually singular	Variable
Inguinal lymphadenopathy	Yes	Yes Buboes	Yes In late primary syphilis	Yes—painful In secondary LGV Buboes	Not usually Pseudobuboes
Constitutional symptoms	Yes	No	Yes In secondary syphilis	Yes In secondary LGV	No

Abbreviations: HSV, herpes simplex virus; LGV, lymphogranuloma venereum.

16. Correct: Donovan bodies (A)

(A) The image presented in the question stem shows a typical genital ulcer of granuloma inguinale caused by the gram-negative pathogen, *Klebsiella granulomatis*. Identification of Donovan bodies (see image [i] at the end of this answer) from the ulcer will aid in diagnosis. Donovan bodies are rod-shaped bacteria within the cytoplasm of monocytes, macrophages and histiocytes that can be visualized with Giemsa or other histological stains. Other organisms that also may be seen in macrophages include *Histoplasma capsulatum* (fungi), *Talaromyces (Penicillum) marneffei* (fungi), and *Leishmania* (parasite). In granuloma inguinale, firm, painless nodules or papules form at the site of inoculation. These eventually ulcerate. The ulcers are highly vascular and bleed easily giving them a "beefy" red appearance. While lymphadenopathy is not usually present, pseudobuboes (subcutaneous granulomas) may be present. See table at the end of this answer for a comparison of the major types of genital ulcer disease. (B) A Tzank smear is often used in the diagnosis of herpes. Scrapings from the base of the lesion will demonstrate multinucleated giant cells (see image [ii] at the end of this answer). In genital herpes, vesicles evolve into pustules then painful ulcers with an erythematous base. This man has painless ulcer; hence genital herpes is unlikely. (C) Inclusions surrounded by a clear halo or "owl-eye" inclusions are typical of CMV (see image [iii] at the end of this answer). CMV is does not cause genital ulcer disease. (D) *Chlamydia* species are intracellular and demonstrate intranuclear inclusions when stained with iodine (see image [iv] at the end of this answer). Genital ulcers are not typically present in *Chlamydia*. (E) Negri bodies are characteristic of rabies virus, a CNS infection. Most often the diagnosis is made postmortem by histological analysis of brain tissue in which eosinophilic inclusions (Negri bodies) may be seen (see image [v] at the end of this answer).

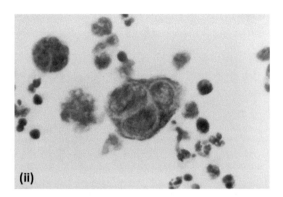

(ii)

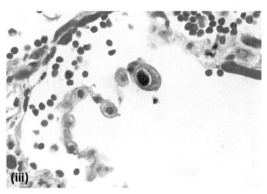

(iii)

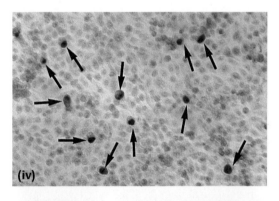

(iv)

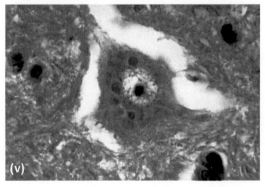

(v)

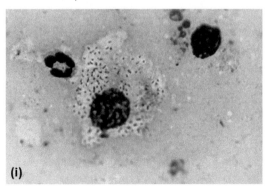

(i)

Comparison of clinically significant genital ulcer diseases					
Feature	Genital herpes	Chancroid	Syphilis	LGV	Granuloma inguinale (donovanosis)
Causative agent	HSV (most often type 2)	H. ducreyi	T. pallidum	C. trachomatis L1, L2, and L3	K. granulomatis
Typical lesion	Early on—vesicles • Erythematous Later—ulcer • Shallow • Raised edges	Ulcer • Purulent base • Nonindurated • Ragged edges	Ulcer/chancre • Indurated • Demarcated edges	Early on—papule Later—ulcer • Small • Shallow	Ulcer • Highly vascular "beefy red"
Painful or painless	Painful	Painful	Painless	Painless	Painless
Number of lesions	Multiple	Usually multiple	Usually singular	Usually singular	Variable
Inguinal lymphadenopathy	Yes	Yes Buboes	Yes In late primary syphilis	Yes—painful In secondary LGV Buboes	Not usually Pseudobuboes
Constitutional symptoms	Yes	No	Yes In secondary syphilis	Yes In secondary LGV	No

Abbreviations: HSV, herpes simplex virus; LGV, lymphogranuloma venereum.

17. Correct: Inability to synthesize ATP (B)

(B) This patient likely has lymphogranuloma venereum (LGV) caused by *Chlamydia trachomatis* serovars L1, L2, or L3. These strains infect macrophages while other *C. trachomatis* strains infect epithelial cells. Like all *Chlamydia*, L1 to L3 are intracellular and unable to synthesize ATP, relying on the host cell to do so (answer choice B). LGV is a sexually transmitted infection that is mainly found in tropical and subtropical climates including West and East Africa, India, South East Asia, South America, and some Caribbean Islands. Men who have sex with men and HIV-positive individuals are at increased risk for infection. LGV typically has three stages, the primary, secondary and tertiary stages. In the primary stage, a small painless ulcer on the genitals or rectum may be seen. This heals spontaneously and about a month later secondary LGV characterized by painful regional lymphadenopathy occurs. In men, the inguinal lymph nodes are usually affected, and a positive groove sign may be noted. This is due to the separation of the inguinal and femoral lymph nodes by Poupart's ligament. This is not pathognomonic for LVG since a positive groove sign may occur with other conditions but can aid in the diagnosis. Painful buboes may form and rupture. During the tertiary stage, a chronic inflammatory response occurs in which there is scarring and fibrosis, which may cause lymphatic obstruction. Diagnosis includes serology and molecular testing from lesion material. Infections can be treated with a macrolide, such as azithromycin or doxycycline. (A) Pathogenic *Neisseria* can vary the antigens on their pili, which aids in evading the host immune response. *N. gonorrhoeae* is a gram-negative diplococcus that causes the sexually transmitted infection gonorrhea. In men, manifestations include urethritis, epididymitis, and proctitis. The presence of a genital lesion in this case indicates gonorrhea is less likely to be the agent of infection. (C) *Mycobacteria* have mycolic acid, a fatty acid in the cell wall. Mycobacteria are rare agents of urogenital infections. The presence of the bubo in this case, indicates that LGV is a more likely diagnosis. (D) *Mycoplasma* and *Ureaplasma* both lack a cell wall. *Ureaplasma* may cause nongonococcal urethritis (NGU), but the symptoms seen in this case are not consistent with urethritis. (E) Herpes simplex virus-2 (HSV-2) causes genital herpes. In genital herpes, vesicles evolve into pustules then painful ulcers with erythematous bases. There are often multiple lesions present. The vesicles may crust over and scab, but most often resolve within 3 weeks. Local tingling and itching, dysuria, and "flu-like" symptoms may also be present. The presence of the bubo in this case indicates LGV is more likely to be the agent of this infection.

18. Correct: *Neisseria gonorrhoeae* (C)

(C) The Gram stain shows intracellular and extracellular gram-negative diplococci, which are characteristic of *Neisseria gonorrhoeae*. This sexually transmitted infection may be asymptomatic or manifest as cervicitis, urethritis, epididymitis, proctitis, or pharyngitis. **(A)** *Chlamydia trachomatis* may present in a similar manner as gonorrhea. *Chlamydia* has a gram-negative cell wall but Gram stains very poorly. This may be due to multiple factors, including the organism's small size and the lack of muramic acid (a component of peptidoglycan) in the cell wall. The gram-negative diplococci seen in this case indicate that *N. gonorrhoeae* is more likely. **(B)** *Klebsiella granulomatis*, a gram-negative rod, causes granuloma inguinale. This infection is typically seen in tropical countries, and a painless genital ulcer is usually present. **(D)** *Treponema pallidum* causes syphilis. This spirochete can be visualized with dark-field microscopy, not Gram stain as in this case. Painless genital ulcers are usually present in primary syphilis. Urethral discharge as seen in this case is not common. **(E)** *Ureaplasma urealyticum* causes non-gonococcal urethritis (NGU). This organism does not have a cell wall, and hence it does not Gram stain. Therefore, Gram stain, as seen in this case, would not aid in the diagnosis.

19. Correct: Gram-negative diplococci (C)

(C) This woman has pelvic inflammatory disease (PID), which may occur weeks or months following a genital infection with *Chlamydia trachomatis* or *Neisseria gonorrhoeae*. Other pathogens that are less frequently associated with PID include *Gardnerella*, *Mycoplasma*, and *Ureaplasma*. *N. gonorrhoeae* is a gram-negative diplococcus. *C. trachomatis*, while technically Gram negative, are not well-visualized by Gram stain and, therefore, are not diagnosed by this method. These two pathogens infect the lower genital tract but may gain access to the upper genital tract resulting in salpingitis, oophoritis, or other conditions. Additionally, perihepatitis (Fitz-Hugh–Curtis syndrome) is associated with PID. Manifestations of PID include pelvic/abdominal pain, abnormal vaginal bleeding, and dyspareunia. Uterine tenderness, adnexal, or cervical motion tenderness may be present. **(A)** Double-stranded DNA viruses that affect the urogenital tract include herpes simplex virus (HSV) and human papillomavirus (HPV). Neither organism is associated with PID. **(B)** *Haemophilus ducreyi* and *Klebsiella granulomatis* are gram-negative rods that affect the urogenital tract. Both are sexually transmitted and are agents of genital ulcer disease. Neither pathogen is associated with PID. **(D)** A spirochete that is associated with urogenital infections is *Treponema pallidum*, the causative agent of syphilis. This pathogen is not associated with PID. **(E)** *Candida* and other yeast cause vaginitis but are not associated with PID.

20. Correct: *Chlamydia trachomatis* (B)

(B) The positive hCG indicates that this woman is pregnant, and the adnexal mass suggests an ectopic pregnancy. Pelvic inflammatory disease (PID) can

cause ectopic pregnancy. PID is most often associated with *Chlamydia trachomatis* (answer choice B) and *Neisseria gonorrhoeae*. *C. trachomatis* and *N. gonorrhoeae* typically infect the lower genital tract, but the pathogens may gain access to the upper genital tract resulting in inflammation (salpingitis or oophoritis), which can then lead to scarring and subsequent ectopic pregnancy as in this case. **(A)** *Actinomyces israelii* is a branching gram-positive rod that is associated with infected intrauterine devices (IUDs). It is not typically associated with PID. **(C)** The gram-negative rod, *Escherichia coli* is not a usual pathogen of the genital tract and is not associated with PID. **(D)** *Listeria monocytogenes* may cause mild febrile illness in healthy pregnant women. This subsequently may affect the fetus or neonate resulting stillbirth, granulomatosis infantiseptica, and meningitis. *L. monocytogenes* is not associated with PID. **(E)** *Treponema pallidum*, the causative agent of syphilis, is not associated with PID.

21. Correct: *Chlamydia trachomatis* (A)

(A) This man has the classic triad of reactive arthritis (Reiter syndrome), which includes arthritis, conjunctivitis, and urethritis ("can't pee, can't see, can't climb a tree"). Reactive arthritis is associated with several pathogens including *Chlamydia trachomatis* (answer choice A). Reactive arthritis typically occurs about one month following a genital infection with *Chlamydia*. Reactive arthritis is also associated with other pathogens including *Escherichia coli*, *Salmonella*, *Shigella*, *Campylobacter*, *Clostridium difficile*, *Chlamydia pneumoniae*, and less commonly *Ureaplasma* and *Mycoplasma*. There is an association between reactive arthritis and human leukocyte antigen (HLA) B27. *C. trachomatis* is not visible with Gram stain and is an intracellular pathogen, hence does not grow on artificial media as in this case. **(B)** *Neisseria gonorrhoeae*, a gram-negative diplococcus, is associated with septic arthritis following a genital infection. Manifestations include swollen, painful joints; however, uveitis is not typically present. *N. gonorrhoeae* grows well on chocolate agar and Thayer–Martin agar. **(C)** The gram-positive coccus, *Staphylococcus aureus* is the agent of many infections including septic arthritis. An *S. aureus* infection would not explain this patient's urethral discharge. The manifestations described in this case are more consistent with reactive arthritis. **(D)** *Treponema pallidum*, a spirochete, is the agent of the sexually transmitted infection syphilis. The organism does not Gram stain or grow well on artificial media. For this question, it is important to notice the triad of arthritis, conjunctivitis, and urethritis, as this presentation is most consistent with reactive arthritis. *T. pallidum* is not associated with reactive arthritis. **(E)** Several enteric pathogens including *Escherichia coli*, *Salmonella*, *Shigella*, and *Campylobacter* are associated with reactive arthritis. *Vibrio cholerae* is not typically associated with this condition.

22.　Correct: Lack of the cell wall (B)

(B) This man most likely has urethritis and which is most commonly associated with chlamydia and gonorrhea. Infections with gonorrhea are referred to as gonococcal urethritis and urethritis caused by other pathogens is referred to as non-gonococcal urethritis (NGU). In addition to *Chlamydia*, *Mycoplasma genitalium* and *Ureaplasma urealyticum* are agents of NGU. *Mycoplasma* and *Ureaplasma* are unique among the bacteria because they lack a cell wall (answer choice B); hence they do not Gram stain. Additionally, these pathogens do not grow on routine culture (bacterial) media. **(A)** Yeast and fungi have chitin in their cell wall and are not common agents of urethritis. These organisms would also grow well on artificial media and should be seen on a Gram stain, if present. **(C)** *N. gonorrhoeae*, a common agent of urethritis, contains LOS in the cell wall. *N. gonorrhoeae* is a gram-negative diplococcus that grows well on chocolate and Thayer–Martin media and is a gram-negative diplococcus, which should be seen on a Gram stain. **(D)** *Mycobacteria* have mycolic acid, a fatty acid, in their cell wall. *Mycobacteria* are not common agents of urethritis. **(E)** Gram-positive bacteria have a thick layer of peptidoglycan in the cell wall. None of the common pathogens implicated in NGU are gram-positive organisms.

23.　Correct: Condyloma acuminata (B)

(B) The image in the question stem depicts genital warts or condyloma acuminata, which is caused by human papillomavirus (HPV), a double-stranded DNA virus. While there are many types of HPV, type 6 and type 11 are most commonly associated with developing condyloma acuminata. The skin colored or pink warts are often described as verrucous or cauliflower-like. Condyloma acuminata is a sexually transmitted infection and men who have sex with men are at risk for perianal warts. Other strains of HPV, most notably types 16 and 18, increase the risk of squamous cell carcinoma. **(A)** The gram-negative rod, *Haemophilus ducreyi*, causes chancroid. The characteristic feature of chancroid is a painful genital ulcer. The warts in the image in the question stem are characteristic of HPV and not chancroid. **(C)** In genital herpes, vesicular lesions or painful ulcers may be present on the genitals. Often this is accompanied by flu-like symptoms, such as fever and malaise. The clinical manifestations and findings in this case are not consistent with herpes. **(D)** Lymphogranuloma venereum (LGV) is caused by *Chlamydia trachomatis* serovars L1, L2, and L3. In this infection, a painless genital ulcer may be present. The lesion is generally a small papule or shallow ulcer and does not resemble the warts seen in this case. **(E)** One of the manifestations of secondary syphilis is condylomata lata (see image at the end of this answer), which are grey, flat-topped papules. These may be confused with genital warts caused by HPV. However, the MHA-TPA, a treponemal test for syphilis, is negative. In the past, RPR and VRDL, which are nonspecific for *T. pallidum*, were used as screening tests for syphilis. More recently, the reverse algorithm for syphilis has been introduced wherein treponemal tests are performed first and if positive, nontreponemal tests are performed. In this case, the patient does not have a rash or any other findings commonly seen in secondary syphilis. Hence, this infection is more likely to be caused by HPV.

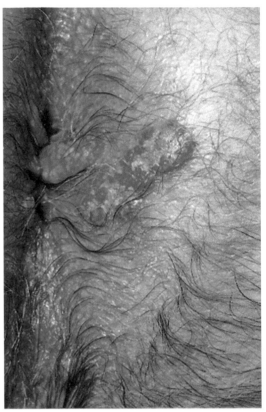

Source: Secondary Syphilis. In: Sterry W, Paus R, Burgdorf W, Hrsg. Thieme Clinical Companions - Dermatology. 1st Edition. Thieme; 2006

24.　Correct: Antigenically variable pili (A)

(A) This woman is most likely to have pharyngitis caused by *Neisseria gonorrhoeae*. Thayer–Martin agar is a selective media for pathogenic *Neisseria* including *N. gonorrhoeae*. This pathogen has pili that are capable of antigenic and phase variation, which assist the organism in evading the host immune response. *N. gonorrhoeae* is a gram-negative diplococcus that causes infections of the genital tract, oral cavity, and eyes and may also disseminate from the original site resulting in septic arthritis. While not mentioned in this vignette, *N. gonorrhoeae* would also grow well on chocolate agar. **(B)** *Corynebacterium diphtheriae*, the causative agent of diphtheria, produces an exotoxin that inactivates elongation factor-2 (EF-2). In diphtheria infection a greyish exudate or pseudomembrane covers the pharynx. This organism does not grow on Thayer–Martin media. An example of selective media for *C. diphtheriae* is cysteine tellurite agar. **(C)** Herpes simplex virus-1 (HSV-1) remains latent in the trigeminal ganglia. HSV-1 and HSV-2 may cause infections in the oral cavity, resulting in vesicular lesions with minimal or no exudate. However, HSV is not likely to be the agent of this infection since viruses are obligate intercellular pathogens and do not grow on artificial media such as Thayer–Martin media. **(D)** M protein is a characteristic of *Streptococcus pyogenes* (group A streptococci). M protein is an adhesin on the cell surface of *S. pyogenes* that aids the bacterium in avoiding phagocytosis within the host. *S. pyogenes* is the main bacterial pathogen of infectious pharyngitis and grows well on blood agar as β-hemolytic colonies. **(E)** Many pathogenic organisms have a polysaccharide capsule, including *N. meningitidis*. However, *N. gonorrhoeae* does not have a capsule.

25. Correct: Administer penicillin G during delivery (B)

(B) GBS may be part of the microbiota of the female gastrointestinal and genital tract and can then be transmitted to neonates during vaginal delivery. Hence all pregnant women are screened at 35 to 37 weeks and if positive, intravenous (IV) antimicrobials are administered during delivery. The antimicrobial of choice is penicillin G (answer choice B). Penicillin is a β-lactam agent that inhibits bacterial cell wall synthesis. If the patient is allergic to penicillin, erythromycin or clindamycin may be used instead. See Appendix I for a summary of antimicrobials spectrum of activity and mechanism of action. **(A)** Aztreonam is a β-lactam agent that has poor coverage for streptococcal species and has better coverage of gram-negative bacilli. **(C)** Sulfonamides such as trimethoprim–sulfamethoxazole (TMP–SMX) may displace bilirubin resulting in kernicterus, which especially affects preterm infants. Sulfa drugs should be avoided, especially toward the end of the third trimester and during the neonatal period. TMP–SMX inhibits folate synthesis. **(D)** Although GBS is normal flora of the female vaginal tract it may cause pneumonia, meningitis or sepsis in neonates. Therefore, it is recommended that if the GBS screen is positive, IV antimicrobials should be administered during delivery. **(E)** Since GBS is not causing harm and is a colonizer in the mother, immediate treatment is not warranted. Intrapartum antimicrobial prophylaxis is the recommended protocol for women with GBS positive vaginal or rectal screens at 35 to 37 weeks.

Chapter 13

Congenital and Neonatal Infections

Melphine M. Harriott

LEARNING OBJECTIVES

▶ Discuss the etiology, epidemiology, pathogenesis, clinical manifestations, complications, diagnosis, and treatment and prevention of congenital and neonatal infections.

▶ Describe the laboratory diagnosis and antimicrobial testing methods for bacteria, viruses, fungi, yeast, and parasites.

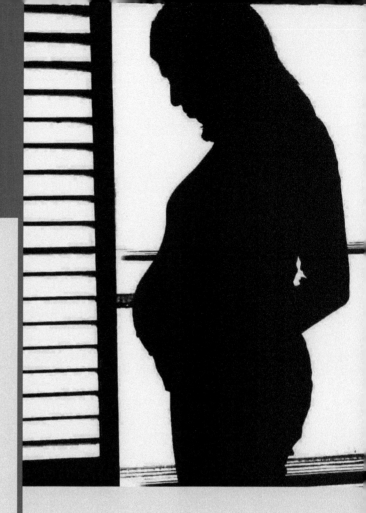

13.1 Questions

Easy	Medium	Hard

1. A 9-year-old girl visits the dentist for the first time for a routine dental cleaning. The dentist notices the girl's teeth (as shown in the following image) and refers the girl to a pediatrician. The girl has normal intelligence but an audiogram shows sensory neural deafness. A slit-lamp examination shows evidence of interstitial keratitis.

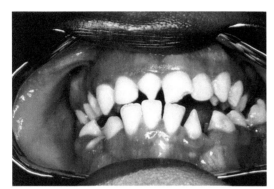

Source: CDC/Robert E. Sumpter

The most likely cause of this girl's condition is:

A. Cytomegalovirus (CMV)

B. Herpes simplex virus-2 (HSV-2)

C. Rubella virus

D. *Toxoplasma gondii*

E. *Treponema pallidum*

Consider the following case for questions 2 to 3:

A 38-year-old woman, gravida 2, para 2, 15 weeks pregnant, presents to her obstetrician with fever, malaise, lethargy, and headache. Her pregnancy has been uneventful and the woman is otherwise healthy. She is up to date on her vaccinations. She has two cats. No one else in her family is ill. Her temperature is 38.4°C (101.2°F). Physical examination reveals significant posterior cervical lymphadenopathy.

2. Which of the following is the most likely involved in the transmission of this infection?

A. Contact with contaminated cat litter

B. Contaminated soft cheese

C. Infected body fluids

D. Respiratory droplets

E. Sexual contact

3. Which of the following findings is most likely to be present in her newborn?

A. Chorioretinitis

B. Conjunctivitis

C. Pneumonia

D. Saddle nose

E. Vesicular lesions on the skin

4. A pediatrician examines a newborn in the hospital 12 hours after birth. The baby was born full term via a vaginal delivery. The baby's respiratory rate is elevated and physical examination reveals a continuous heart murmur heard best along the upper left sternal border. A chest radiograph demonstrates left atrial and left ventricular enlargement. The ascending aorta is also enlarged and there is increased pulmonary blood flow. The mother states the pregnancy was uneventful and her first trimester screen for chromosomal abnormalities was negative. She does not have a history of sexually transmitted infections. The mother has never been vaccinated. Which of the additional findings is most likely to be present in this baby?

A. Anemia

B. Cleft lip and palate

C. Granulomatous skin lesions

D. Spina bifida

E. Petechial rash

5. A 31-year-old pregnant woman, 8 weeks gestation, works as a nanny and takes care of a 5-year-old boy. The boy has a slight fever and is more tired than normal. A few days later, the woman notices a pinpoint, flat, red rash on the boy's face and seems to be more prevalent on his cheeks. She returns to work 3 days later and notices the boy now has a rash on his stomach, arms, and legs. The woman's baby is at greatest risk for developing:

A. Ascites

B. Hearing loss

C. Pulmonary artery hypoplasia

D. Osteochondritis

E. Retinitis

6. A 5-day-old infant is brought to her pediatrician with a yellowish discharge from her eyes and swollen eyelids. The mother is 17 years old and did not have any prenatal care. The baby was born at 39 weeks by vaginal delivery. Other than the mucopurulent eye discharge from both eyes, the baby's physical examination is unremarkable. A Gram stain from the discharge reveals no organisms. The pathogen grows only in cell culture and a Giemsa stain of the organism reveals intracellular inclusion bodies. Which of the following is the most likely etiologic agent of infection?

A. *Chlamydia trachomatis*

B. *Listeria monocytogenes*

C. *Neisseria gonorrhoeae*

D. *Streptococcus agalactiae*

E. *Treponema pallidum*

7. A 9-day-old infant is brought to the emergency room with blisters in his mouth and on his feet, as seen in the following image. The mother states the pregnancy was uneventful and the infant was born full term via a vaginal delivery at home. She did not see a clinician regularly during her pregnancy.

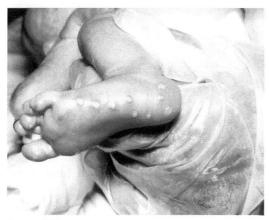

Source: CDC

The most likely etiologic agent of this infection is a:

A. Double-stranded DNA virus

B. Gram-negative diplococcus

C. Protozoan parasite

D. Single-stranded RNA virus

E. Spirochete

8. A 35-year-old woman, gravida 3, para 3, 28 weeks pregnant, develops fever, chills, and backache. Her husband is also ill and has fever and mild stomach cramps. They both ate a salami sandwich at the corner delicatessen a few days ago. Three weeks later, the woman goes into preterm labor and delivers a stillborn baby. Which of the following is the most likely etiologic agent that caused this fetal demise?

A. Cytomegalovirus (CMV)

B. *Listeria monocytogenes*

C. Parvovirus B19

D. *Streptococcus agalactiae*

E. *Toxoplasma gondii*

13.2 Answers and Explanations

Easy	Medium	Hard

1. Correct: *Treponema pallidum* (E)

(E) This is most likely a case of congenital syphilis caused by the spirochete *Treponema pallidum*. This pathogen may be passed to the fetus in utero and result in stillbirth, neonatal death, and neonatal disorders. Classic features of congenital syphilis in older children include deafness (eighth cranial nerve), Hutchinson's teeth (as shown in the image in the question stem; notched incisors that are more widely spaced than normal), saddle nose, and interstitial keratitis. This pathogen is part of the TORCH group, which is an acronym for perinatal/congenital pathogens (**T**oxoplasma gondii; **O**ther [*Treponema pallidum*; varicella zoster virus; Parvovirus B19, HIV; **R**ubella virus; **C**ytomegalovirus; **H**erpes simplex virus). **(A)** Manifestations of congenital CMV include hearing loss, neurological issues such as microcephaly and developmental delays. Hutchinson's teeth are not a characteristic of congenital CMV. **(B)** HSV-2 may be transmitted vertically either in utero or more commonly perinatally. The most common manifestations of perinatal infections include vesicular lesions on the skin or mucous membranes, eye infections, and central nervous system infections. **(C)** Rubella is relatively rare in countries that routinely immunize for rubella. Features of congenital rubella include hearing loss, cataracts and cardiac abnormalities such as patent ductus arteriosus and pulmonary artery hypoplasia and a distinct petechial rash, often described as a blueberry muffin rash. **(D)** The classic triad of congenital toxoplasmosis includes chorioretinitis, hydrocephalus and intracranial calcifications. Hutchinson's teeth are not a characteristic of congenital toxoplasmosis.

2. Correct: Contact with contaminated cat litter (A)

(A) This woman most likely has toxoplasmosis, caused by the protozoan parasite, *Toxoplasma gondii*. In pregnant women, infections are most often asymptomatic but if symptoms do occur, manifestations are often nonspecific "flu-like" symptoms. Lymphadenopathy, often posterior cervical lymphadenopathy, may be present. *T. gondii* is transmitted to humans via ingestion of undercooked meat or ingestion of contaminated soil or water. The organism is associated with cat feces. This woman has pet cats so it is likely that she came in contact with the pathogen via her cats. Pregnant woman may then transmit the pathogen to their fetus, resulting in congenital toxoplasmosis; hence they are advised not to change cat litter. This pathogen is part of the TORCH group, which is an acronym for perinatal/congenital pathogens (*Toxoplasma gondii*; **O**ther [*Treponema pallidum*; varicella zoster virus; Parvovirus B19, HIV; **R**ubella virus; **C**ytomegalovirus; **H**erpes simplex virus). **(B)** *Listeria monocytogenes*, a gram-positive bacillus, is transmitted via ingestion of contaminated food such as soft cheese and cold cut deli meat. Pregnant woman can transmit *L. monocytogenes* in utero resulting in abortions, stillbirth, and neonatal infections such as meningitis and granulomatosis infantiseptica. Most often pregnant women with listeriosis present with a febrile illness, however, posterior lymphadenopathy is not classic finding. **(C)** Cytomegalovirus (CMV), HIV, and hepatitis B are viruses that can be transmitted via infected body fluids and can then be transmitted from pregnant women to the fetus. Symptoms of CMV and early HIV may resemble the symptoms seen in this case; however, since the woman has contact with cats, it is more likely that *T. gondii* is the causative agent. She is up to date with vaccinations so she most likely has been vaccinated for hepatitis B as well. **(D)** Parvovirus B19 and rubella are viruses that may be transmitted via respiratory droplets. Infections with these pathogens can then be vertically transmitted and may cause serious congenital infections. This woman is up to date with vaccinations, so it's unlikely she has a rubella infection. Because this woman has cats, toxoplasmosis is more likely than a parvovirus infection. **(E)** There are many pathogens that are sexually transmitted and may then be vertically transmitted including chlamydia, gonorrhea, syphilis, herpes, HIV, and hepatitis. However, sexual transmission is not a mechanism of *T. gondii* transmission.

3. Correct: Chorioretinitis (A)

(A) This woman most likely has toxoplasmosis, caused by the protozoan parasite, *Toxoplasma gondii*. The classic triad of congenital toxoplasmosis includes chorioretinitis, hydrocephalus, and intracranial calcifications. **(B)** Chlamydia, gonorrhea, and HSV infections are the most common causes of neonatal conjunctivitis which is typically transmitted perinatally, especially during vaginal birth. This woman does not have manifestations of any of these infections, so conjunctivitis is not a finding expected to be present in her newborn. **(C)** There are several pathogens that are common agents of neonatal pneumonia, most notably *Streptococcus agalactiae* and *Chlamydia trachomatis*. There is some evidence in literature to suggest that neonatal pneumonia may occur with congenital toxoplasmosis but it is not the most likely finding. **(D)** One of the characteristics of congenital syphilis is saddle nose. This is not generally seen in congenital toxoplasmosis. **(E)** Herpes simplex virus (HSV) may be transmitted vertically and result in vesicular lesions on the skin or mucous membranes, eye infections, and meningoencephalitis. This is not typically seen in congenital toxoplasmosis.

4. Correct: Petechial rash (E)

(E) Because this mother has never been vaccinated, the most likely pathogen in this case is rubella virus. Features of congenital rubella include a petechial rash ("blueberry muffin" rash). Other characteristics are intrauterine growth restriction, hearing loss, cataracts, cardiac abnormalities (such as patent ductus arteriosus and pulmonary artery hypoplasia), and neurological issues. Rubella is part of the TORCH group, which is an acronym for perinatal/congenital pathogens (*Toxoplasma gondii*; **O**ther [*Treponema pallidum*; varicella zoster virus; Parvovirus B19, HIV; **R**ubella virus; **C**ytomegalovirus; **H**erpes simplex virus). **(A)** Anemia is associated with congenital parvovirus B19 infections. **(B)** Craniofacial malformations such as cleft lip and palate are not typically associated with congenital infections, such as rubella. Most often these malformations are associated with environmental factors, chromosomal abnormalities, and gene mutations. **(C)** Granulomatous skin lesions are a characteristic of early neonatal infections with *Listeria monocytogenes*. **(D)** The etiology of neural tube defects, such as spina bifida, is multifactorial and is most often due to environmental factors or chromosomal abnormalities. The screen for chromosomal abnormalities was negative, which does not rule out chromosomal abnormalities completely, but makes this answer choice less likely.

5. Correct: Ascites (A)

(A) The boy in this case most likely has erythema infectiosum (also called fifth disease or slapped cheek syndrome), which is caused by a DNA virus, parvovirus B19. This pathogen is transmitted via respiratory droplets and can then be transmitted in utero causing fetal death and/or nonimmune hydrops fetalis. Hydrops fetalis is characterized by abnormal collection of fluid in fetal soft tissue and serous cavities and may involve ascites (answer choice A), edema, pericardial, or pleural effusion. Parvovirus B19 affects red blood cells and can result in aplastic crisis in individuals with underlying issues. **(B)** Hearing loss is a feature of several congenital infections including congenital cytomegalovirus (CMV), congenital rubella, and congenital syphilis. This is not a classic finding of congenital parvovirus B19 infections. (C) Pulmonary artery hypoplasia is a characteristic of congenital rubella, not parvovirus. (D) Congenital syphilis may result in osteochondritis, especially of the long bones and ribs. This is not typically seen in congenital parvovirus. (E) Retinitis is a feature congenital toxoplasmosis, not congenital parvovirus.

---

6. Correct: *Chlamydia trachomatis* (A)

(A) *Chlamydia trachomatis*, serovars D-K are sexually transmitted and cause infections in both adults and neonates. Neonatal eye infection or ophthalmia neonatorum is usually a result of transmission from an infected mother during birth and occur 5 to 14 days after birth. *C. trachomatis* is intracellular and a key microscopic clue is the presence of intracellular inclusions. In addition to conjunctivitis, infants born to mothers with chlamydia are likely to have pneumonia, which usually occurs at around 4 to 12 weeks after birth. (B) *Listeria monocytogenes* is a facultative intracellular gram-positive bacillus that grows well on artificial media. It may be transmitted vertically and result in stillbirth, meningitis, or granulomatous lesions in the newborn. Eye infections are not a typical characteristic of neonatal infections. (C) *Neisseria gonorrhoeae* is an important agent of neonatal eye infections. In contrast to chlamydia conjunctivitis, infections with this pathogen usually occur within the first 24 to 48 hours after birth. The discharge from *Neisseria* also tends to be purulent while *Chlamydia* is mucopurulent. *Neisseria* is a gram-negative diplococcus and would most likely be seen on a Gram stain. (D) *Streptococcus agalactiae* or group B streptococcus is a gram-positive coccus in chains that may be transmitted vertically during parturition. Infections in neonates typically manifest as pneumonia or meningitis. This organism grows well on artificial media, such as blood agar. (E) *Treponema pallidum* is the causative agent of syphilis. Conjunctivitis is not a typical feature of congenital infections. This organism does not grow in culture and is best diagnosed with serological tests.

---

7. Correct: Double-stranded DNA virus (A)

(A) This infant has neonatal herpes, caused by herpes simplex virus (HSV). Herpes viruses are double-stranded DNA viruses. HSV-2, and less commonly HSV-1, is sexually transmitted and results in painful genital ulcers that may be on the genitalia or on the buttocks, inner thighs, or anus. The virus may then be transmitted vertically in utero or more commonly perinatally. Neonatal infections include skin and mucous membrane lesions, which usually occur within 2 weeks after birth and meningitis or meningoencephalitis, which occur approximately 3 weeks after birth. Herpes is part of the TORCH group, which

is an acronym for perinatal/congenital pathogens (*Toxoplasma gondii*; **O**ther [*Treponema pallidum*; varicella zoster virus; Parvovirus B19, HIV; **R**ubella virus; **C**ytomegalovirus; **H**erpes simplex virus). HSV belongs to the herpes virus family that also includes Epstein–Barr virus (EBV), cytomegalovirus (CMV), varicella zoster virus (VZV). (B) *Neisseria gonorrhoeae* is a gram-negative diplococcus that causes neonatal conjunctivitis. Usually, infections occur 24 to 48 hours after birth. Vesicular skin lesions are not characteristic of this pathogen. (C) A protozoan parasite that causes congenital infections is *Toxoplasma gondii*. This pathogen is transmitted in utero and classic manifestations of congenital infections include chorioretinitis, hydrocephalus, and intracranial calcifications. (D) A single-stranded RNA virus capable of causing congenital infections is rubella virus. Manifestations of congenital rubella include hearing loss, cataracts, and cardiac abnormalities, such as patent ductus arteriosus and pulmonary artery hypoplasia. (E) *Treponema pallidum* is a spirochete that may be transmitted vertically, in utero or perinatally. Classic features of congenital syphilis in older children include deafness (eighth cranial nerve), Hutchinson's teeth (notched incisors that are more widely spaced than normal), saddle nose, and interstitial keratitis.

---

8. Correct: *Listeria monocytogenes* (B)

(B) This woman most likely has listeriosis caused by the facultative intracellular gram-positive bacillus, *Listeria monocytogenes*. *L. monocytogenes* is capable of surviving in cold temperatures and can grow at refrigerator temperature (4°C). The pathogen is transmitted via contaminated food and water and is associated with cold cut deli meat, soft cheese, and unpasteurized milk. In pregnant women, infections manifest as a febrile illness. Infections can then be *transmitted* in utero resulting in fetal abortion and granulomatosis infantiseptica in newborns. In children and nonpregnant adults, infections with *L. monocytogenes* are largely asymptomatic but can also result in mild gastroenteritis. Immunocompromised individuals, neonates, and the elderly are at risk of severe infections, such as meningitis. (A) Cytomegalovirus (CMV) is transmitted via close contact, infected body fluids, and organ transplants. Immunocompetent adults are rarely symptomatic. In pregnant women, manifestations are often nonspecific and include fever, malaise, and myalgia. The virus may then be transmitted in utero resulting in hearing loss, jaundice, hepatosplenomegaly, thrombocytopenia, petechiae, pneumonia, chorioretinitis, microcephaly, and motor disability. (C) Parvovirus B19 infections start with a prodrome phase of nonspecific symptoms and are then followed by a red, maculopapular rash on the face that moves to the trunk and extremities. Parvovirus B19 is transmitted via respiratory droplets and can be transmitted in utero resulting in stillbirth, as seen in this case. However, the woman and her husband are both ill and ate a salami sandwich prior to the symptoms. Therefore, the causative agent is more likely to be *L. monocytogenes*. **(D)** Many women are asymptomatic carriers of *Streptococcus agalactiae* (group B streptococcus or GBS) in their GI tract and/or vagina. The pathogen may be transmitted to the baby perinatally, resulting in meningitis, pneumonia, and bloodstream infections. This pathogen is not foodborne. **(E)** In pregnant woman, *Toxoplasma gondii* infections are most often asymptomatic but if symptoms do occur, manifestations are often nonspecific "flu-like" symptoms. Posterior lymphadenopathy is usually present. *T. gondii* is transmitted to humans via ingestion of undercooked meat or contaminated soil or water. This organism is associated with cat feces.

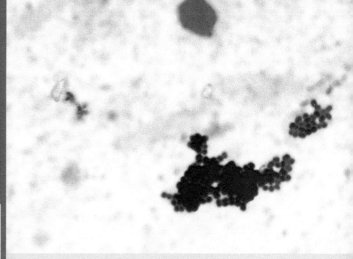

Chapter 14

Skin, Soft Tissue, and Musculoskeletal Infections

Matthew P. Jackson and Melphine M. Harriott

LEARNING OBJECTIVES

▶ Discuss the etiology, epidemiology, pathogenesis, clinical manifestations, complications, diagnosis, and treatment and prevention of:

– skin, soft tissue, joint, muscle, and bone infections.

– infectious diarrhea and dysentery.

– foodborne illness.

– genital tract infections.

▶ Describe the laboratory diagnosis and antimicrobial testing methods for bacteria, viruses, fungi, yeast, and parasites.

▶ Discuss virulence mechanisms and correlate virulence mechanisms with specific pathogens.

▶ Discuss antimicrobial mechanism of action, spectrum of activity, common adverse effects, and resistance mechanisms.

▶ Discuss bacterial metabolism, growth, and genetics.

14.1 Questions

Easy	Medium	Hard

1. The parents of a 2-day-old infant are shocked by their child's condition when they are ready to take him home. He has peeling skin and fluid-filled blisters over most of his body as seen in the following image. An infection control investigation reveals an outbreak of this condition in the newborn nursery.

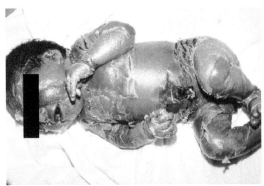

Source: Laskaris G, Hrsg. Color Atlas of Oral Diseases. Diagnosis and Treatment. 4th Edition. Thieme; 2017

A virulence factor most likely produced by the causative agent of this outbreak is:

A. α-Toxin
B. Exfoliative toxin (ET)
C. Streptolysin O (SLO)
D. Streptococcal pyrogenic exotoxin (SPE)
E. Toxic shock syndrome toxin (TSST)

2. A 5-year-old boy presents to his pediatrician in June with lesions on his legs and arms. Some of the lesions are pustules that have ruptured presenting with a yellow–brown colored crust as seen in the following image. The physician notices that the child is vigorously scratching the sores when she enters the examination room.

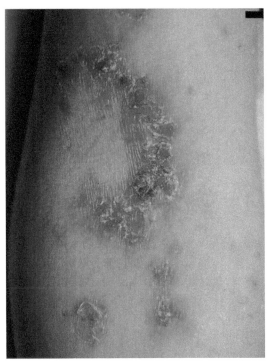

Source: Evanherk at Dutch Wikipedia [CC-BY-SA-3.0 (http://creativecommons.org/licenses/by-sa/3.0/)], via Wikimedia Commons

Which of the following is the most likely diagnosis?

A. Scalded skin syndrome
B. Carbuncle
C. Erysipelas
D. Impetigo
E. Necrotizing fasciitis

3. A 68-year-old man presents to an urgent care clinic with bilateral bright red erythema on the face as seen in the following image. The patient had a temperature of 38.5°C (101.3°F) and regional lymphadenopathy on presentation to the clinic.

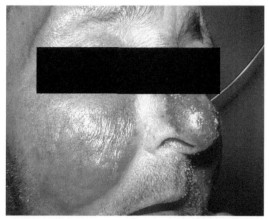

Source: CDC/Dr. Thomas F. Sellers, Emory University

Which of the following is the most likely diagnosis?

A. Erysipelas

B. Fifth disease

C. Impetigo

D. Lupus erythematosus

E. Necrotizing fasciitis

4. A 13-year-old boy receives multiple bite wounds to his left hand and forearm by a neighbor's dog. The boy was delivering promotional flyers for a local grocery store to neighborhood mailboxes when a dog pushed open the front door and attacked the boy. The dog was impounded and placed in quarantine for rabies monitoring. His mother cleaned and dressed her son's wounds, some of which penetrated to 1-cm depth, but she did not seek medical treatment for the boy. Two days following the attack, the boy developed a low-grade fever 38°C (100.4°F), redness, pain, and a purulent exudate at the several of the bite wounds. A sample of the pus was collected in the emergency department of the local hospital and a Gram stain is shown as follows.

Which of the following is the most likely causative agent?

A. *Acinetobacter baumannii*

B. *Corynebacterium pseudotuberculosis*

C. *Pasteurella multocida*

D. *Staphylococcus aureus*

E. *Streptococcus pyogenes*

5. A 15-year-old boy presents to his primary care physician with multiple small skin-colored papules on his forehead and chin. He also has several whiteheads on his nose, but no inflammation is noted on the infected regions of skin. He is concerned because he has a school dance in a week and sought medical care for possible treatment. The physician explains to the boy that his condition is most likely caused by a facultative gram-positive rod and prescribes topical clindamycin. Which of the following byproducts of metabolism is produced by the bacterium associated with this infection?

A. Butyric acid

B. Cytochrome c oxidase

C. Lactic acid

D. Propionic acid

E. Pyocyanin

6. A 37-year-old aid worker returns to the United States after spending 15 months in a Tanzanian health care facility. While out of the country he observed numerous cases of patients with thickened skin growths on various parts of their body. Many of his patients had foot ulcers that seemed to be insensitive to pressure or pain. The man is at risk for developing:

A. Hansen's disease

B. Impetigo

C. Plantar warts

D. Tertiary syphilis

E. Tinea corporis

7. A 24-year-old man presents with palmar lesions and plantar lesions as seen in the following images. He also complains that his hair has been falling out. He is not an "outdoors person" and has no known tick exposure. He is sexually active and is currently in a monogamous relationship with a female partner. His vital signs are normal. On physical examination, the rash is noted to be nonerythematous, maculo-papular, and diffuse and located on his trunk, both extremities, and his palms and soles. When asked, the man says the rash is nonpruritic. There are several bald spots of missing hair on his head. The rest of his physical examination is normal.

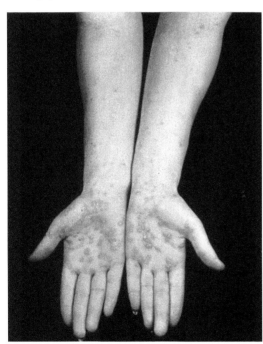

Source: CDC/Robert Sumpter

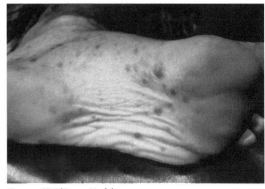

Source: CDC/Susan Lindsley

The most likely diagnosis is:

A. Chicken pox

B. Gonorrhea

C. Rocky Mountain spotted fever (RMSF)

D. Scarlet fever

E. Secondary syphilis

F. Smallpox

8. A 23-year-old man living in Vermont wakes up one night with severe pain in his left knee. He is shocked to discover significant swelling and the inability to bear his body weight on that side. An answering service for his primary care physician suggested that he report to the local emergency department. A history revealed that the patient belongs to a club that takes regular cross-country biking and camping trips in rural areas. The attending physician found no abnormalities on a neurologic assessment. However, the patient reported experiencing intermittent headaches and muscle pains over the past month, which he attributed to hitting the bike trail too hard. Enzyme-linked immunosorbent analysis (ELISA) from a blood sample is most likely to confirm which of the following diagnoses?

A. *Borrelia burgdorferi*

B. *Chlamydia trachomatis*

C. *Rickettsia rickettsii*

D. *Salmonella enteritidis*

E. *Staphylococcus aureus*

9. A 12-year-old boy living in Arkansas became ill with a fever of 40°C (104°F) and a mild sore throat for 2 days. His illness appeared in January so the parents suspected the flu and failed to seek medical attention. On the third morning of symptoms the boy remained bedridden with coughing and severe muscular pain. When his parents noticed dark macular skin eruption on his stomach the boy was rushed to the local emergency department. No antibiotics were administered during a 6-day hospitalization because the diagnosis was fever of undetermined origin. On day 7 of hospitalization, the boy died of multiple organ system failure. Arkansas state and Center for Diseases Control and Prevention investigators visited the boy's residence and found a colony of eastern flying squirrels in the attic near his bedroom. Blood specimens would most likely show antibodies against which of the following?

A. *Coxiella burnetii*

B. *Orientia tsutsugamushi*

C. *Rickettsia prowazekii*

D. *Rickettsia rickettsii*

E. *Rickettsia typhi*

10. The father of a 5-year-old boy is alarmed by the appearance of a large (5 cm) bald spot on his son's scalp. Several days prior to this finding, the father noticed that the boy was scratching his head excessively but had not noticed the hair loss because his son wears a cap to school. The only notable history was that the boy was selected to appear in an after-school production of Robin Hood with the appropriate costumes.

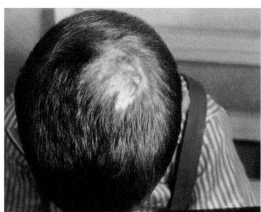

Source: CDC

What is the most likely diagnosis?

A. Candidiasis

B. Chicken pox

C. Folliculitis

D. Ringworm

E. Tinea versicolor

11. While working as part of a medical relief team in Belize, a medical student observes a 35-year-old man with a lesion seen on his hand. A skin scraping is taken from the lesion and stained with Giemsa (see following images).

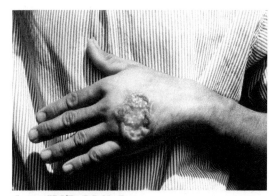

Source: CDC/Dr. D.S. Martin

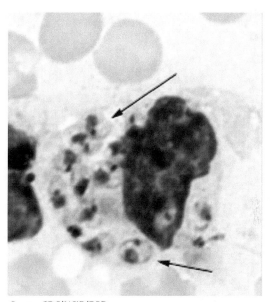

Source: CDC/NCID/DPDx

Which of the following arthropod vectors transmitted this infection?

A. Mosquito

B. Sandfly

C. Tick

D. Tsetse fly

E. Triatominae bug

301

12. A 23-year-old woman fell from her bicycle and sustained a 10-cm abrasion injury to her right knee. She rode home, showered and placed a gauze bandage over the wound. The woman experienced pain, erythema, and pus formation at the site of injury. Two days later she is awakened at 2:00 a.m. with a fever and noticed that redness at the wound site had spread to her right calf. There were areas on her thigh that appeared to be bruised with two blisters. In the emergency department, work-up included a CT scan of her leg which is shown in the following image. She is given intravenous cefazolin and sent to the operating room for surgical debridement. The tissue from the debridement was sent to the microbiology lab and Gram stain showed gram-positive cocci in chains.

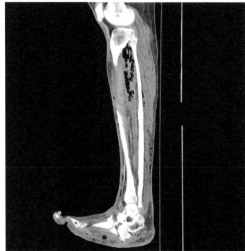

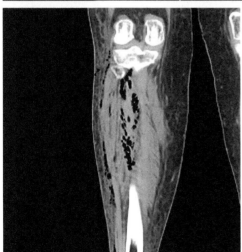

Source: Cellulitis and Necrotizing Fasciitis. In: Baxter A, ed. Emergency Imaging. A Practical Guide. 1st Edition. Thieme; 2015

Postsurgery, the patient was monitored for multi-system organ failure due to which of the following virulence factors?

A. α-Toxin
B. β-Toxin
C. Lipopolysaccharide (LPS) endotoxin
D. Pneumolysin O
E. Streptococcal pyrogenic exotoxin (SPE)

13. A 32-year-old man had surgery to repair a fractured tibia following a biking accident. The patient developed erythema (redness), fever, swelling, and a slight amount of discharge from the surgical site 48 hours following the operation. The pus is Gram stained and clusters of gram-positive cocci were seen. Subsequently, the patient had an additional surgery to remove metal pins. Which of the following is the most likely cause of this infection?

A. Enterococcus faecalis
B. Haemophilus influenzae
C. Staphylococcus aureus
D. Staphylococcus epidermidis
E. Pseudomonas aeruginosa

14. A 71-year-old retired woman presented to the urgent care clinic with severe pain in her left knee. Examination of the knee discloses a small puncture wound, swelling of the joint, and some discoloration. The woman explains that while gardening she sustained a puncture wound from a splinter. Her knee is painful at rest and more so upon movement. Synovial fluid is most likely to reveal which of the following organisms?

A. Escherichia coli
B. Chlamydia trachomatis
C. Neisseria meningitidis
D. Salmonella enteritidis
E. Staphylococcus aureus

15. A 42-year-old agriculture worker in South Carolina presents to a regional health care facility with a 3-cm lesion on his chin. The clinic staff refers him to the local hospital where a skin biopsy fails to reveal a diagnosis. A chest X-ray reveals a left lower lobe granuloma. The lung and lymph node biopsies reveal the organism seen in the following image.

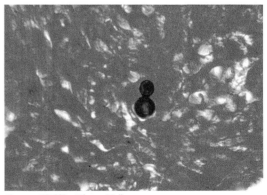

Source: CDC/Dr. Libero Ajello

What is the most likely diagnosis?

A. Blastomyces dermatitis
B. Histoplasma capsulatum
C. Sporothrix schenckii
D. Streptococcus pyogenes
E. Trichophyton rubrum

16. A soldier who sustains a penetrating wound to the left foot and is admitted to the hospital. Approximately 24 hours following admission, he experiences severe pain in his leg. The skin of the affected leg appears purple. Later that evening overlying bullae are apparent on the leg. Physical examination reveals crepitus and radiographic imaging demonstrates the presence of gas within the soft tissue. Which of the following caused the tissue destruction?

A. α-Toxin produced by *Clostridium perfringens*

B. α-Toxin produced by *Staphylococcus aureus*

C. β-Toxin produced by *Clostridium perfringens*

D. Exfoliative toxin produced by *Staphylococcus aureus*

E. Streptolysin O produced by *Streptococcus pyogenes*

17. A 54-year-old woman with diabetes and chronic deep vein thromboses in her lower extremities is diagnosed with bacterial cellulitis in her right foot. A few days later, she notes that skin surrounding the affected area has changed from red to a slightly blue color. The foot is extremely painful and by the time she seeks medical treatment, bullae and frank gangrene are observed on the affected foot. Surgical debridement and antimicrobial therapy are not successful, resulting in the decision to amputate the foot. Isolation of the most likely infecting organism would require:

A. Anaerobic culture

B. Bordet–Gengou agar at 35°C

C. Capnophilic culture on blood agar plates

D. Sabouraud dextrose agar (SDA)

E. Thayer–Martin media

18. A 35-year-old man presented with multiple discharging sinuses on his arm for 2 years (see the following image). The patient had been in a motor vehicle collision 9 months prior to the clinic visit when he had experienced multiple lacerations to the face and arms. A few weeks after the accident, the patient noticed pimple-like lesions at the site of wound which did not respond to oral ciprofloxacin. The pimples eventually spread up his arm and when they failed to heal on their own, he sought medical care.

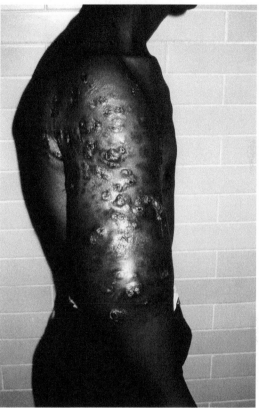

Source: CDC/Dr. Libero Ajello

An infectious disease specialist orders Gram stain and cultures of the lesions. What is the most likely microscopic observation?

A. Branching gram-positive rods

B. Broad-based budding yeast cells

C. Septate hyphae

D. Gram-negative coccobacilli

E. Spirochetes by fluorescent staining

19. While on a medical relief trip in Belize, a fourth-year medical student performs a physical exam on a 9-year-old boy who presents with the skin lesions as shown in the following image. The student recognizes this disease and although the health facility lacks the capacity for sophisticated microscopy but they can perform serologic assays.

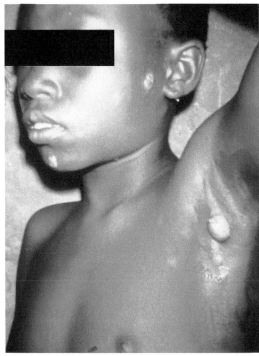

Source: CDC/Dr. Peter Perine

Which of the following is the most appropriate assay for diagnosis?

A. Anti–streptolysin O titers

B. Complement fixation for antibody to fungal antigens

C. Herpes simplex virus (HSV) serology

D. Rapid plasma reagin (RPR)

E. Subcutaneous injection of purified protein derivative (PPD)

20. A 25-year-old man who works as a deep-sea fisherman develops pruritic and painful lesion on his fingers and the backs of both hands. He states that the lesion was a bright red but now turned into a purplish color. On examination, his vital signs are normal. A violaceous lesion with a central clearing and raised borders is noted on both arms and hands. There is no inflammation of the infected areas. The most likely diagnosis is:

A. Anthrax

B. Bullous impetigo

C. Dermatophytosis

D. Erysipeloid

E. Erysipelas

21. A 10-year-old girl is brought to her pediatrician for removal of rough, 3-mm growth resembling a cauliflower from the dorsal surface left ring finger. Liquid nitrogen is used to successfully remove the growth. Which of the following is most likely responsible for this infection?

A. Double-stranded DNA virus

B. Double-stranded RNA virus

C. Single-stranded RNA virus

D. Gram-positive cocci in clusters

E. Gram-positive bacilli with spores

22. A 4-year-old boy is seen by his pediatrician for a painful rash on his finger (see the following image). The child's mother states the boy recently had a cold and cough and a cold sore on his lip. During the examination, the physician notices that the boy sucks his thumb.

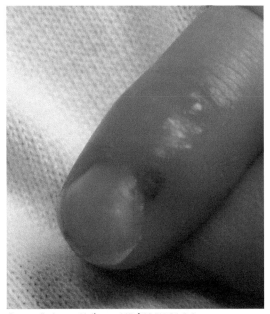

Source: By James Heilman, MD [CC BY-SA 3.0 (https://creativecommons.org/licenses/by-sa/3.0) from Wikimedia Commons

The organism most likely responsible for this infection is also associated with:

A. Erythema multiforme

B. Rheumatic fever

C. Guillain–Barré syndrome

D. Reactive arthritis

E. Shingles

23. A 72-year-old woman presents to the emergency department experiencing a painful vesicular and ulcerative rash on her right side at waist level. The patient has been experiencing this condition for the past 48 hours. Vaccination against which of the following would have prevented this condition?

A. Hepatitis B

B. Human papillomavirus (HPV)

C. Polio

D. Rubella

E. Varicella and herpes zoster

24. A 12-year-old girl from a Northern California community with a significant portion of the population expressing personal belief exemptions to childhood immunization presents with fever, tiredness, loss of appetite, headache, and rash as shown in the following image.

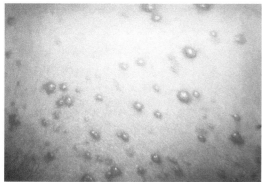

Source: CDC/Joe Miller

What is the most likely diagnosis?

A. Herpes simplex virus-1 (HSV-1)

B. Measles

C. Varicella

D. Variola

E. Rubella

25. In January 2015, the California Department of Public Health was notified that an 11-year-old girl presented to her pediatrician with fever, a maculopapular rash, cough, conjunctivitis, and coryza (inflammation of the mucus membranes of the nose). Her only significant travel history was a visit to a Disney theme park located in Orange County, California. Immunization against which of the following would have presented her disease?

A. Conjugated polysaccharide capsule

B. Double-stranded, enveloped, DNA virus

C. Recombinant surface antigen

D. Single-stranded, enveloped, RNA virus

E. Toxoid

26. A 4-year-old boy is brought to his pediatrician with a rash on his face as seen in the following image. He had a 24-hour history of fever and malaise prior to the appearance of the rash. The child attends day care. The pediatrician explained that this condition was typically self-limiting but expressed concern that the patient may expose other children at day care.

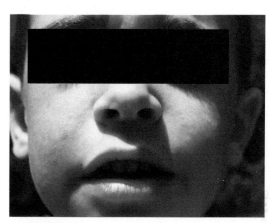

Source: CDC

Depending on the health status of the other children at day care there might be a risk for causing which of the following conditions?

A. Subacute sclerosing panencephalitis (SSPE)

B. Guillain–Barré syndrome

C. Transient aplastic crisis

D. Seizures

E. Secondary bacterial infection

27. A 32-year-old woman visited an outpatient clinic reporting a 3-day history of fever, myalgia, a severe headache, and arthralgia. She described recent travel to Haiti for a 1-week missionary trip and indicated that her illness began 3 days after her return. Physical examination revealed a blanching rash on her chest. Which of the following is the most likely diagnosis?

A. Dengue

B. Malaria

C. Typhoid fever

D. Trypanosomiasis

E. Yellow fever

28. A 5-year-old boy is seen at a mobile clinic in a rural part of Florida. He has been experiencing intense itching on his right foot with raised red tracks over a 7-cm surface. Abrasions on the soles of his feet reveal that the boy spends a great deal of time outdoors without shoes. He tells the nurse that the family pets include four dogs as well as a number of feral cats. The boy was prescribed topical thiabendazole and instructed to wear shoes. What is the most likely diagnosis?

A. Cercarial dermatitis

B. Chagas disease

C. Impetigo

D. Tinea pedis

E. Cutaneous larva migrans

29. A fourth-year medical student on an international elective in Nigeria observes that a significant number of the adults from rural areas suffer from blindness. Children are responsible for elder care. In addition, many young adults have patchy areas of discolored and thickened skin, especially in the inguinal regions. A local health care provider explains that these individuals are infected with a parasite that is transmitted by an arthropod vector. What is the etiologic agent?

A. *Loa loa*

B. *Onchocerca volvulus*

C. *Schistosoma japonicum*

D. *Trypanosoma cruzi*

E. *Wuchereria bancrofti*

30. An otherwise healthy 33-year-old woman who works on a ranch in western Arizona presents to her physician with a cluster of painful nodules on her left calf. She has also been overwhelmed with fatigue and experiences stiff joints, especially in the morning. Her vital signs indicate a temperature of 38.4°C (101.1°F). She mentions that she has had a bit of a cough for a few weeks, but her lung examination is unremarkable. Which of the following is the most likely causative agent?

A. *Aspergillus fumigatus*

B. *Blastomyces dermatitidis*

C. *Coccidioides immitis*

D. *Cryptococcus neoformans*

E. *Histoplasma capsulatum*

31. In the fall of 2001, 12 United States mail handlers were infected with following exposure to letters purposefully contaminated with anthrax spores. Which of the following best describes the dermatologic manifestation of this disease?

A. Carbuncle

B. Chancre

C. Eschar

D. Papilloma

E. Papule

32. A 47-year-old man presents with a 1-week history of muscle pain and muscle weakness, fever, headache, and swelling in the face. He reports that he recently had a stomach ache and diarrhea but is no longer experiencing those symptoms. He denies blood in the stool. About one month prior to the onset of symptoms he had traveled to Germany and toured a sausage factory and had consumed samples of pork and beef sausages. On examination, his temperature is 39.1°C (102.4°F) and significant facial edema is noted, predominantly around his eyelids. Laboratory results are shown below:

- Complete blood count (CBC):
  - White blood cells (WBCs): 15.1×10^9/L
  - Eosinophils: 5.2%
- Serum chemistry:
  - Creatine phosphokinase (CPK): 150 U/L
  - Lactate dehydrogenase (LDH): 134 U/L
- Microbiology:
  - Stool ova and parasite (O&P) examination: negative
- Which of the following is the most likely diagnosis?

A. Chagas disease

B. Cystercercosis

C. Trichinellosis

D. Visceral larva migrans

E. Yersiniosis

33. A 23-year-old man presents to the emergency department with a "sore" on his right leg. He had recently gone surfing with friends in southern California and reports that his leg had been injured in the water. His vitals are normal. On examination, an approximately 4-cm circular wound is seen on his right leg. The wound is shallow and red in color, and a small amount of pus is evident. Gram stain from the purulent material reveals curved gram-negative rods. Which of the following is the most likely causative agent?

A. *Aeromonas hydrophila*

B. *Campylobacter coli*

C. *Erysipelothrix rhusiopathiae*

D. *Mycobacterium marinum*

E. *Vibrio vulnificus*

Consider the following case for questions 34 to 35:

A 6-year-old girl with sickle cell disease presents with a 2-day history of fever and 4-day history of worsening leg pain. Her mother reports that prior to the leg pain, the girl had missed several days of school due to the "stomach flu." The mother was worried because the girl refused to walk on her affected leg. The girl's temperature is 38.8°C (101.9°F). On examination, the upper right leg is tender on palpation and warm to the touch. The girl is reluctant to ambulate. X-ray shows marked soft tissue edema along the femur. Significant laboratory results are shown below:

- CBC:
  - Leukocyte count: 15.7×10^9/L
- Erythrocyte sedimentation rate (ESR): 25 mm/h
- Blood cultures: gram-negative rods isolated, identification pending

34. Which of the following is most likely the causative agent of this condition?

A. *Salmonella*

B. *Shigella*

C. *Staphylococcus aureus*

D. *Staphylococcus epidermidis*

E. *Pseudomonas aeruginosa*

35. Which one of the following bacterial mechanisms is most important in mediating the girl's primary infection?

A. Mucosal invasion

B. Toxin that inhibits protein synthesis

C. Coagulase

D. Biofilm formation

E. M protein

36. A previously healthy 22-year-old woman is experiencing pain and swelling of her right knee. Her temperature is 37°C (98.6°F). On examination, the knee is significantly swollen, tender, erythematous, and warm. The infected knee exhibits a decreased range of motion. Synovial fluid is obtained and a Gram stain from the fluid is shown as follows:

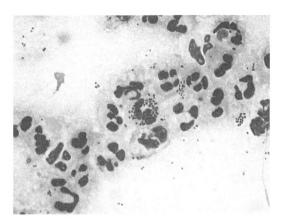

Which of the following is the most likely involved in the transmission of this infection?

A. Contaminated food or water

B. Contaminated medical device

C. Overgrowth of normal microbiota

D. Respiratory droplets

E. Sexual encounter

37. An otherwise healthy 10-year-old girl visits her pediatrician for a routine examination. Overall the child is well appearing and has no significant past medical history. The child's vital signs are normal. On physical examination, six small waxy appearing papules, clumped together, are noted on her face (see following image). The examination is otherwise unremarkable. The girl's mother states the papules appeared a couple of weeks ago and the girl did not complain of pain at the site. She thought they were warts, so she did not seek medical care at the time. All routine laboratory tests are within normal limits.

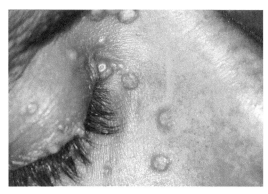

Which of the following is the most likely diagnosis?

A. Molluscum contagiosum

B. Herpes gladiatorum

C. Common wart

D. Chicken pox

E. Ringworm

38. During a relief trip to Guatemala, a medical student participates in the establishment of a mobile clinic for local residents who have very limited access to health care. She sees a patient with an indurated lesion on his right ankle that appears like craters with raised edges. She is not provided with any diagnosis on site so she looks up the case back home. Which of the following a likely causative agent of this infection?

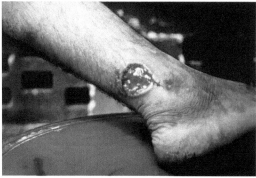

Source: CDC/Dr. Mae Melvin

A. Herpes simplex virus-2

B. *Histoplasma capsulatum*

C. *Leishmania donovani*

D. *Plasmodium vivax*

E. *Trypanosoma cruzi*

14.2 Answers and Explanations

Easy	Medium	Hard

1. Correct: Exfoliative toxin (ET) (B)

(B) Exfoliative toxin (ET) is produced by some strains of *Staphylococcus aureus*, the causative agent of staphylococcal scalded skin syndrome (SSSS, also called Ritter's disease). ET is produced by the bacterium at a locus of infection and spreads causing bullous impetigo. ET is a protease that cleaves desmoglein. ET functions by causing a cleavage plane between the stratum spinosum and stratum granulosum of the epidermis (see image at the end of this answer). The toxin causes exfoliation or peeling of the skin as described in the case and seen in the image in the question stem. If the isolate is a methicillin-sensitive *S. aureus* (MSSA), then nafcillin may be used to treat infections. Treatment of methicillin-resistant *S. aureus* (MRSA) may include vancomycin. Infections may be passed from person to person via health care personal and epidemics in nurseries, such as in this case, may occur. **(A)** A variety of bacteria produce cytolysins referred to as α-toxin: *S. aureus*, *Escherichia coli*, and *Clostridium perfringens*. *S. aureus* and *E. coli* α-toxin are pore-forming cytolysins while the α-toxin produced by *C. perfringens* is a phospholipase that contributes to deep-tissue infections and gangrene. The peeling skin and fluid-filled blisters are classic findings of SSS; hence α-toxin is the incorrect answer. **(C)** Streptolysin O (SLO) is a thiol-activated membrane-damaging cytolysin produced by β-hemolytic *S. pyogenes*. SLO binds to cholesterol in the target membrane of erythrocytes and forms a pore up to 30 nm in diameter. Anti-SLO (ASO) antibody is produced to circulating cytolysin in the bloodstream of infected individuals. ASO titers are used as an indicator of infection and scarlet fever and can aid in the diagnosis of poststreptococcal sequelae rheumatic fever and glomerulonephritis. **(D)** Streptococcal pyrogenic exotoxins (SPEs) or erythrogenic toxins are a group of exotoxins secreted by *Streptococcus pyogenes*. SpeA and SpeC are superantigens produced and as with TSST, cross-link T cell receptor and major histocompatibility complex (MHC) II of antigen-presenting cells causing indiscriminate proliferation of T cells and massive cytokine release. SpeB is a cysteine protease. SpeA and SpeC are the causative agents of scarlet fever and streptococcal toxic shock-like syndrome. **(E)** TSST is a superantigen produced by some strains of *S. aureus* and *S. pyogenes*. Toxic shock syndrome toxin (TSST) cross-links T cell receptor and the major histocompatibility complex (MHCII) of antigen-presenting cells causing indiscriminate proliferation of T cells and massive cytokine release. Symptoms of toxic shock seen most commonly in menstruating women using tampons include fever, rash, and hypotension. The skin infection in this case is unlikely to be caused by TSST producing *S. aureus*.

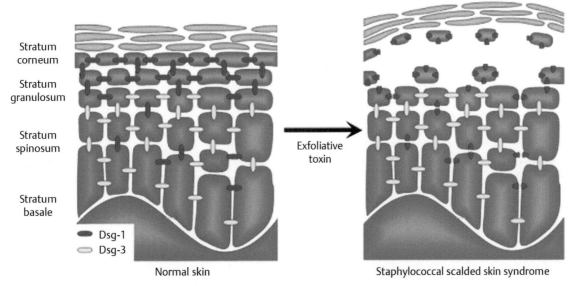

| Stratum corneum |
| Stratum granulosum |
| Stratum spinosum |
| Stratum basale |

Dsg-1
Dsg-3

Exfoliative toxin

Normal skin

Staphylococcal scalded skin syndrome

Source: Bukowski M, Wladyka B, Dubin G. Exfoliative Toxins of Staphylococcus aureus. Toxins 2010;2(5):1148-1165

2. Correct: Impetigo (D)

(D) The yellow–brown crust (sometimes referred to as honey-colored) around the skin lesions is indicative of nonbullous impetigo. In nonbullous impetigo, lesions are located mainly on the face and extremities. Lesions typically begin as papules that turn into vesicles that crust over. Impetigo may be primary and caused by direct pathogen invasion of skin or secondary, which occurs after another skin infection. There are three main types of impetigo, nonbullous (also referred to as impetigo contagiosa), bullous and ecthyma. *Staphylococcus aureus* is the main agent of nonbullous and bullous impetigo whereas *Streptococcus pyogenes* (group A streptococci) is the main agent of ecthyma. These infections are highly contagious and occur more commonly during the warmer summer months. **(A)** Scalded skin syndrome is caused by *S. aureus*. This bacterial skin infection presents in infants and may occur as a hospital-acquired infection. Exfoliative toxin is the virulence factor that cleaves the stratum spinosum and stratum granulosum of the epidermis. The skin lesion in this case does not resemble the typical peeling skin seen in scalded skin syndrome (see image [i] at the end of this answer). **(B)** A carbuncle is a focal suppuration or abscess caused by *S. aureus*. A carbuncle is a cluster of boils (see image [ii] at the end of this answer) most commonly on the back or nape of the neck. The bacterial infection may start as folliculitis (hair follicle) and can be seen in patients with weakened immune systems. An example would be infection of the foot or lower leg in a diabetic patient. The clinical findings in this case do not indicate a carbuncle. **(C)** Erysipelas is an infection of the dermis caused by *S. pyogenes* which appears on the face. Typically, the source of infection is the upper respiratory tract. Erysipelas (see image [iii] at the end of this answer) may also present on the extremities and can be distinguished from impetigo by the lack of pus formation and a rash with sharp margins. **(E)** Necrotizing fasciitis (see image [iv] at the end of this answer) is a potentially life-threatening infection of deep tissue layers (fascia) caused by invasive strains of *S. pyogenes* (group A streptococci). Also referred to as the flesh-eating infection, this is a rare disease that follows trauma to the skin. Exotoxins contribute to bacterial spread by causing cell death and possibly the breakdown of connective tissue. In addition to group A streptococci, other bacterial etiologies of necrotizing fasciitis include *S. aureus*, anaerobes including *Clostridium* species, and *Enterobacteriaceae*, including *Klebsiella pneumoniae*, *Escherichia coli*, and *Aeromonas hydrophila*. The findings of this case indicate that necrotizing fasciitis is unlikely.

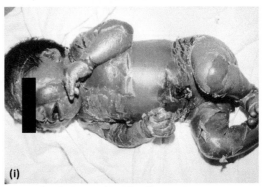

(i)

Source: Staphylococcal Scalded Skin Syndrome. In: Laskaris G, Hrsg. Color Atlas of Oral Diseases. Diagnosis and Treatment. 4th Edition. Thieme; 2017

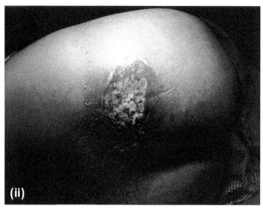

Source: By Drvgaikwad [CC BY 3.0 (https://creativecommons.org/licenses/by/3.0)], from Wikimedia Commons

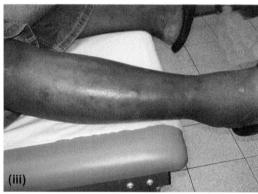

Source: By Grook Da Oger [CC BY-SA 3.0 (https://creativecommons.org/licenses/by-sa/3.0)], from Wikimedia Commons

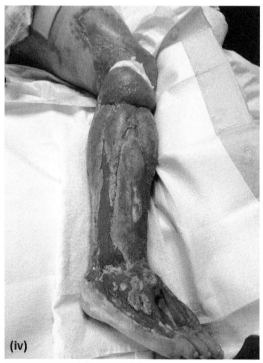

Source: By Doetsch [CC BY-SA 4.0 (https://creativecommons. org/licenses/by-sa/4.0)], from Wikimedia Commons

3.   Correct: Erysipelas (A)

(A) This is a presentation of erysipelas caused by *Streptococcus pyogenes*. Erysipelas mainly affects the upper dermis and superficial lymphatics of infants, young children, and adults. Infections typically arise following skin trauma or from a previous superficial infection with *S. pyogenes*. The onset of symptoms is often acute and includes a bright red, painful indurated lesion with a raised border as seen in the image in the question stem. Although infections may affect the face, most infections occur in the lower extremities. **(B)** Fifth disease or erythema infectiosum is a childhood syndrome caused by parvovirus B19. The disease is more common in child than adults and causes a slapped cheek appearance of mild erythema (see image [i] at the end of this answer). Typically, the symptoms are mild and include fever, runny nose, and headache. **(C)** While impetigo (or pyoderma) (see image [ii] at the end of this answer) is also caused by *S. pyogenes* it has a distinct presentation when compared to erysipelas. Impetigo presents as epidermal lesions with a honey-colored crust. While any *S. pyogenes* infection carries the risk of progressing to cellulitis and erysipelas, impetigo is typically limited to the epidermis. It may appear on the limbs or face. Lesions on the face are usually not bilateral. **(D)** Lupus erythematosus is an autoimmune disease characterized by inflammation in different regions of the body. Systemic lupus erythematosus (SLE) is the most common form of the disease. SLE affects multiple sites including internal organs. A characteristic butterfly rash may appear on the cheeks and bridge of the nose. While the rash has a bilateral appearance as with erysipelas it does not affect deeper tissue layers. **(E)** Necrotizing fasciitis (see image [iii] at the end of this answer) is a potentially life-threatening infection of the fascia caused by invasive strains of *S. pyogenes*, *Klebsiella pneumoniae*, *Clostridium perfringens*, *Escherichia coli*, *Staphylococcus aureus*, and *Aeromonas hydrophila*. Also referred to as the flesh-eating infection, this is a rare disease that follows trauma to the skin. Any skin infection with group A streptococcus has the potential to progress to deep tissues depending on the virulence of the strain.

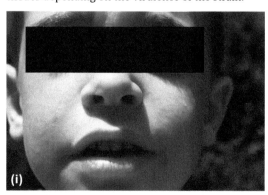

Source: CDC

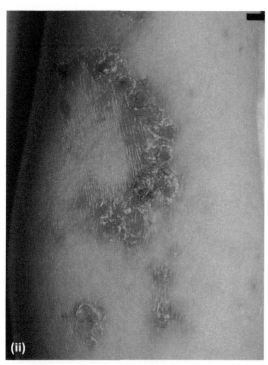

(ii)

Source: Evanherk at Dutch Wikipedia [CC-BY-SA-3.0 (http://creativecommons.org/licenses/by-sa/3.0/)], via Wikimedia Commons

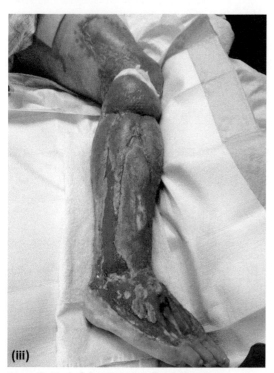

(iii)

Source: By Doetsch [CC BY-SA 4.0 (https://creativecommons. org/licenses/by-sa/4.0/)], from Wikimedia Commons

4. Correct: *Pasteurella multocida* (C)

(C) *Pasteurella multocida* is a gram-negative coccobacillus that is capable of causing cellulitis and antimicrobial therapy is warranted to prevent serious complications. Cellulitis is an infection of the deeper dermis and subcutaneous fat and many organisms may be involved in causing cellulitis, commonly *Streptococcus pyogenes* and *Staphylococcus aureus*. In this case, because of the dog bite and the Gram stain showing gram-negative coccobacilli, *P. multocida* is the most likely causative agent. *P. multocida* is normal oral microbiota of dogs and cats and infections most often arise following an animal bite or scratch. Amoxicillin-clavulanate is effective against this organism. (A) The morphology of *Acinetobacter baumannii* resembles the isolate shown in the Gram stain (gram-negative coccobacilli) or it can frequently be gram-variable with pleomorphic morphology. However, the case presentation is not indicative of this opportunistic bacterium. *A. baumannii* is an environmental organism found in soil and water with preponderance of infections in hospitals and among immunocompromised individuals. A significant incidence of *A. baumannii* infections was associated with injured veterans serving in Iraq and Afghanistan. These infections were acquired during care at one of the medical facilities used by the military. (B) *Corynebacterium pseudotuberculosis* is a gram-positive rod that causes caseous lymphadenitis in Australian sheep. Lymphadenopathy may occur in people who work with sheep, the meat, hides, or wool, with entry of the bacterium following trauma to the extremities. (D) While *S. aureus* is a reasonable choice for skin infections, its etiology and Gram stain are not consistent with this case. *S. aureus* colonizes the skin and nares of some individuals and skin infections are via autoinoculation. (E) *S. pyogenes* is a cause of impetigo, erysipelas, and cellulitis following trauma to the skin. It can also be a resident of the upper respiratory tract so infection is through autoinoculation. While it can invade tissue the etiology and Gram stain seen with this case are not consistent with an *S. pyogenes* infection.

5. Correct: Propionic acid (D)

(D) *Cutibacterium* (formerly called *Propionibacterium*) *acnes* is a gram-positive rod that can be isolated from the skin of healthy adults, but can also cause acne, as in this case. This bacterium is an aerotolerant anaerobe. Ordinarily existing as a commensal it metabolizes the fatty acids in sebum secreted by sebaceous glands producing propionic acid. Because it is aerotolerant, metronidazole is ineffective against this organism. Clindamycin and vancomycin may be used to treat infections. *C. acnes* is a prolific biofilm producer and as a result this organism often seeds medical devices such as cerebrospinal shunts and orthopedic hardware. (A) Butyric acid is a carboxylic acid with that is a product of anaerobic fermentation. It is not produced as a byproduct of the skin colonizer *C. acnes*. Butyric acid is produces the distinctive odor of human vomit. (B) Cytochrome c oxidase is a large transmembrane complex and is the terminal enzyme in the electron transport chain of bacteria and

311

eukaryotic mitochondria. It is a component that is used for the rapid identification of several pathogenic bacteria including *Pseudomonas*, *Neisseria*, *Moraxella*, *Vibrio*, *Campylobacter*, and *Helicobacter*. (C) Lactic acid is produced from pyruvate by the enzyme lactate dehydrogenase. Lactic acid bacteria such as the Lactobacilli convert simple carbohydrates such as glucose, sucrose, or galactose to lactic acid. (E) *Pseudomonas aeruginosa* is the only organism known to produce pyocyanin, a blue-pigmented metabolite that provides the bacterium with a growth advantage over other bacteria. It has a negative impact on the cystic fibrosis (CF) lung by causing epithelial cell dysfunction and impaired ciliary action. Pyocyanin also impairs the immune system and depletes ATP, which damages the cystic fibrosis transmembrane conductance regulator (CFTR). A mutation in the ABC transporter CFTR results in cystic fibrosis.

6. Correct: Hansen's disease (A)

(A) Also known as leprosy, this is a bacterial infection caused by the acid-fast bacilli *Mycobacterium leprae*. Recent statistics show approximately 175 annual cases in the United States with the majority reported in Arkansas, California, Florida, Hawaii, Louisiana, New York, and Texas. Zoonotic infections were associated with armadillos that have been shown to carry *M. leprae* although the risk infection is low. Hansen's disease presents as discolored skin lesions, thick skin growths (see images [i] and [ii] at the end of this answer), severe pain, or numbness depending on the duration of infection and ultimately muscle weakness or paralysis in the hands and feet. The two main forms of leprosy are paucibacillary (tuberculoid), which is the milder form, and lepromatous. In the paucibacillary form, patients will have less than five lesions and peripheral nerve enlargement may be present. In the multibacillary or lepromatous form, patients will have more than five lesions, nerve endings are affected, and cartilage damage may occur. Although the disease presents as skin and nerve manifestations, it can be transmitted from person to person by aerosol. (B) *Streptococcus pyogenes* (with possible superinfection *Staphylococcus aureus*) is the etiologic agent of impetigo (see image [iii] at the end of this answer). It presents as skin lesions with a yellow–brown crust. A characteristic presentation would be autoinoculation of insect bites with a respiratory colonizer. (C) Plantar warts are caused by HPV and occur on the sole of the foot and toes. They typically appear as focal calloused lesions and can be painful. It can spread to other parts of the body and from person to person through fomites. (D) Syphilis is a sexually transmitted infection caused by the spirochete bacterium *Treponema pallidum*. Primary stage syphilis presents as a painless chancre in the genital region and without treatment may progress to secondary syphilis in 2 to 10 weeks. Secondary syphilis presents as distributed skin lesions on the hands, palms, and soles of the feet.

Tertiary syphilis is a disfiguring disease of the skin that may spread to the peripheral and central nervous system (CNS), resulting in systemic effects such as paralytic dementia and demyelination of the spinal cord. (E) Tinea corporis and ringworm are terms used to describe infection with the dermatophytic fungi, including *Trichophyton mentagrophytes*. This is an infection of the superficial skin layers that may spread from person to person by direct contact with fomites. Zoonotic infection is possible through contact with an infected pet. The infection presents as a scaly, circular lesion on various parts of the body (see image [iv] at the end of this answer) with infection of the scalp referred to as tinea capitis, of the feet as tinea pedis, and of the groin as tinea cruris. Regardless of body site, ringworm is a pruritic (itchy) self-limited infection in immunocompetent individuals. T cell deficiencies may lead to chronic infections with the fungus.

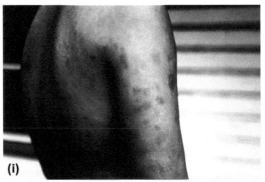

(i)

Source: CDC/Arthur E. Kaye

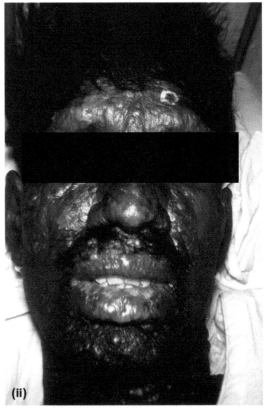

(ii)

Source: CDC/Dr. Andre J. Lebrun

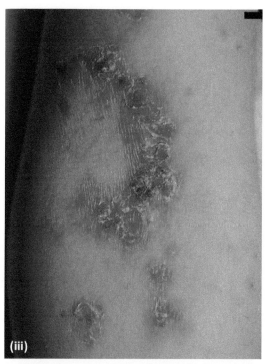

(iii)

Source: Evanherk at Dutch Wikipedia [CC-BY-SA-3.0 (http://creativecommons.org/licenses/by-sa/3.0/)], via Wikimedia Commons

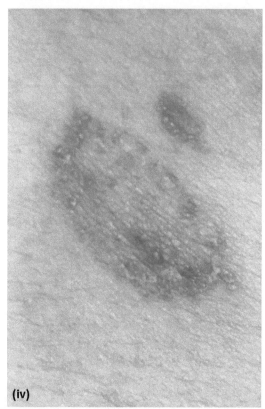

(iv)

Source: CDC/Dr. Lucille K. Georg

7. Correct: Secondary syphilis (E)

(E) This man has secondary syphilis caused by the spirochete *Treponema pallidum*. If left untreated, secondary syphilis develops 2 to 10 weeks after the primary lesion (chancre) has healed or symptoms of primary syphilis may overlap. Distribution of the rash on the soles and palms is a unique presentation for this stage of the disease. Typically, the rash is nonpruritic, diffuse, and bilaterally symmetrical as presented in this case. Other findings of secondary syphilis may include constitutional symptoms, such as fever and headache, alopecia, and condylomata lata (flat-topped papules on moist areas of the body; see image [i] at the end of this answer). Approximately 30% of secondary syphilis cases are resolved by the host immune response with the remainder becoming latent infections with the potential for neurologic complications. (A) Chicken pox is caused by the varicella zoster virus (VZV), an enveloped single-stranded DNA virus of the herpes virus family. Chicken pox appears as rash with pruritic (itchy), fluid-filled blisters that turn into scabs (see image [ii] at the end of this answer). The rash first appears on the face and trunk and may spread to other parts of the body. Blisters are at various stages of development and do not appear on the palms or soles of the feet. (B) Similar to syphilis, gonorrhea is a sexually transmitted bacterial infection. Gonorrhea is caused by the gram-negative diplococcus *Neisseria gonorrhoeae*. In women, the disease presents as vaginal discharge, urinary frequency, dysuria, and chronic pelvic pain. However, it can be asymptomatic in women. Men infected with *N. gonorrhoeae* present with urethritis including a discharge of pus from the meatus. The infection rarely disseminates to other body sites. (C) Rocky Mountain spotted fever (RMSF) is caused by *Rickettsia rickettsii*, a gram-negative coccobacillus that lives inside cells of the vascular endothelium. It is transmitted to humans by the bite of the *Dermacentor* tick with a variety of animal reservoirs. The disease presents as a petechial (minute, nonblanching) or maculopapular (flat, papule) rash on the extremities including the palms and soles of the feet. See image [iii] at the end of this answer shows the later-stage rash of a RMSF patient. RMSF can be difficult to differentiate from secondary syphilis. In this case, the findings of alopecia make syphilis a better answer choice than RMSF. (D) Scarlet fever, caused by the gram-positive coccus *Streptococcus pyogenes*, derives its name from the red rash with a sandpaper feel. The infection initiates in the pharynx and initially presents as a sore throat with fever and swollen cervical lymph nodes. A patient may also have a strawberry tongue. If untreated then the disease may progress to scarlet fever caused by the streptococcal pyrogenic exotoxins, which are superantigens. In this case, the rash was nonerythematous and the patient did not have any other findings associated with scarlet fever. (F) The World Health Organization declared that smallpox had been eradicated worldwide in 1980. Therefore, any case would be caused by a bioterrorism attack. Smallpox is caused by two variants of Variola virus which are members of the poxvirus family. These are double-stranded DNA viruses. Smallpox is transmitted from person to person by droplet and presents as fluid-filled blisters that may cover all parts of the body including the palms and soles of the feet (see image [iv] at the end of this answer).

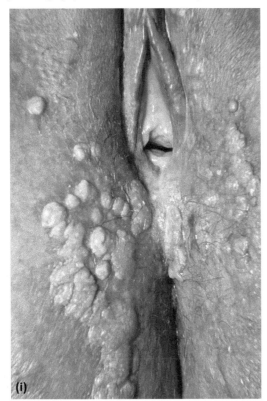

(i)

Source: CDC/Joyce Ayers

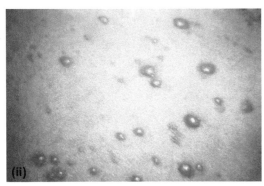

(ii)

Source: CDC/Dr. K.L. Hermann

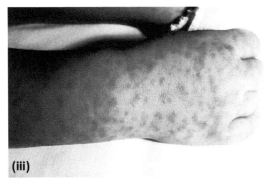

(iii)

Source: CDC

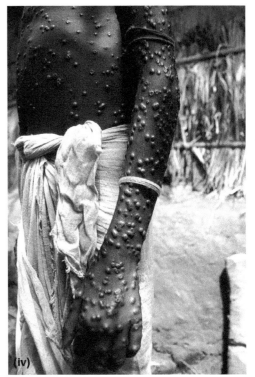

(iv)

Source: CDC/Jean Roy

8.   Correct: *Borrelia burgdorferi* (A)

(A) *Borrelia burgdorferi* is the causative agent of Lyme disease, a vector-born infection transmitted by the *Ixodes* tick. See Appendix L for a list of vector-borne infections and associated vectors. Lyme disease incidence is highest in the northeastern United States and parts of Midwest, including Wisconsin. A characteristic bulls-eyes rash (see image [i] at the end of this answer) is typically seen upon initial infection although as in this case it may not be present at the time other symptoms appear. Arthritis, particularly in large, weight-bearing joints, may occur after several months postinfection. Patients may also experience neurologic signs of infection such as facial or Bell's palsy (droop on one side of the face). Lyme carditis, or infection of heart muscle, is another potential complication. Lyme disease is diagnosed by serological testing, which may include ELISA. **(B)** *Chlamydia trachomatis* is a pleomorphic intracellular bacterium that lacks a cell wall. It is the primary sexually transmitted pathogen in the United States. Reactive arthritis is sequelae of *C. trachomatis* infection presenting as asymmetrical, additive, and oligoarticular. Infection with this pathogen would have to be ruled out in this case. **(C)** *Rickettsia rickettsii* is the causative agent of Rocky Mountain spotted fever (RMSF). Similar to Lyme disease, RMSF is a vector-borne bacterial infection transmitted to humans by the *Dermacentor* tick. It presents with a characteristic rash that involves the palms and soles of the feet (see image [ii] at the end of this answer) as well as malaise, myalgia, fever, and headache. RMSF predominates in the Midwestern part of the United States. Similar to Lyme disease, RMSF is also diagnosed with serological testing. In this case, the lack of a rash and the more indolent nature of the arthralgia and the geographic location of the patient indicate RMSF is less likely to be the diagnosis. **(D)** Similar to *C. trachomatis, Salmonella enteritidis* can lead to a reactive arthritis following a gastrointestinal infection. A relatively recent history of gastroenteritis would lead to the suspicion that this is a case of reactive arthritis. Additionally, the classic triad seen in reactive arthritis—uveitis, conjunctivitis, and arthritis—is not present, making this a less likely diagnosis. **(E)** As a colonizer of the human upper respiratory tract and occasional colonizer of the skin, *Staphylococcus aureus* is a potential cause of osteomyelitis and septic arthritis. A case matching this diagnosis would present a patient who sustained a recent penetrating injury to the affected knee and would include fever and pus formation.

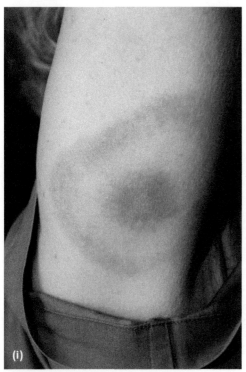

(i)

Source: CDC/James Gathany

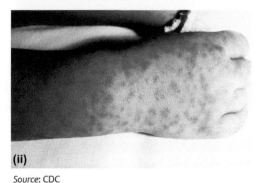

(ii)

Source: CDC

9. Correct: *Rickettsia prowazekii* (C)

(C) *Rickettsia prowazekii* is the causative agent of epidemic typhus, typically a louse-borne disease associated with poverty, overcrowding, and poor sanitation that may occur in refugee camps. Flying squirrels are an animal reservoir in the United States. In this case the lice probably lived on the flying squirrels and then transmitted the infection to the boy. Epidemic typhus presents with symptoms similar to Rocky Mountain spotted fever (RMSF): headache, chills, high fever, prostration, coughing, and severe muscular pain. A macular skin eruption (dark spots) develops first on the upper trunk and spreads to the rest of the body but usually not to the face, palms of the hands, or soles of the feet. Unlike RMSF, the mortality rate for untreated cases can be as high as 40%. Doxycycline is the antibiotic of choice to treat epidemic typhus and RMSF. See table presented at the end of this answer for a summary of clinically significant Rickettsial infections and Appendix L for a list of vector-borne infections. **(A)** *Coxiella burnetii* is the causative agent of Q (query) fever which is a zoonotic disease with worldwide distribution having both acute and chronic stages. Cattle, sheep, and goats are the primary reservoirs and the pathogen is transmitted via aerosols. Humans may become infected during birthing since the pathogen is shed in high numbers within the amniotic fluids and the placenta of these animals; hence veterinarians and farmers are at high risk. Symptoms include high fever, headache, malaise, myalgia (muscle pain), and chest pain. Chronic infections are possible and clinical findings include endocarditis and chronic hepatitis. Doxycycline is the treatment of choice. In this case, the exposure to flying squirrels makes *R. prowazekii* a more likely agent of this infection. **(B)** *Orientia tsutsugamushi* is the causative agent of scrub typhus transmitted to humans from a rodent reservoir by the larvae of a mite (chigger). It is endemic in northern Japan, Southeast Asia, the western Pacific Islands, eastern Australia, China, maritime areas, and several parts of south-central Russia, India, and Sri Lanka. It can be transmitted to humans who are walking through high grass (scrub) while hunting or camping. It appears as a nonspecific febrile illness. A lesion that develops into an eschar may occur at the site of the bite and a rash, if present generally spares the extremities. **(D)** *Rickettsia rickettsii* is the causative agent of Rocky Mountain spotted fever (RMSF). *R. rickettsii* is a gram-negative coccobacillus that lives inside cells of the vascular endothelium. This pathogen cannot be detected by Gram stain. It is transmitted to humans by the bite of the *Dermacentor* tick with a variety of animal reservoirs. The disease presents as a petechial (minute, nonblanching) or maculopapular (flat, papule) rash on the extremities including the palms and soles of the feet. The image at the end of this answer shows the later-stage rash of a RMSF patient. The clinical findings in this case are not consistent with RMSF. **(E)** *Rickettsia typhi* is the causative agent of murine or endemic typhus, which is transmitted to humans by fleas with rats and mice as animal reservoirs. This is an uncommon disease in mainland United States and Hawaii reports on average five or six cases annually. Symptoms are similar to RMSF with fever, headache, joint and muscle pain, and a discrete rash in approximately half of human cases.

Features of clinically significant Rickettsial infections			
Organism	**Disease**	**Signs and symptoms**	**Vector**
R. rickettsii	RMSF	Constitutional symptoms	Tick
		Rash: maculopapular or petechial; starts at ankles/wrist and spreads to trunk; includes palms and soles	
R. typhi	Murine (endemic typhus)	Constitutional symptoms	Flea
		Rash: maculopapular; starts at trunk and spreads; spares palms and soles	
R. prowazekii	Epidemic typhus	Constitutional symptoms	Louse
		Rash: maculopapular; starts at trunk and spreads to extremities; spares palms and soles	
		Brill–Zinsser disease—recurrence of infection years after initial episode; milder disease	
R. akari	Rickettsialpox	Lesion: papule that develops into vesicle then eschar that crusts	Mite
		Constitutional symptoms	
		Rash: generalized papular or vesicular rash	
O. tsutsugamushi	Scrub typhus	Lesion at bite site: papule that develops into ulcer; then eschar that crusts	Mite
		Constitutional symptoms	
		Rash: macular starts on trunk and spreads to extremities; lymphadenopathy	

Abbreviation: RMSF, Rocky Mountain spotted fever.

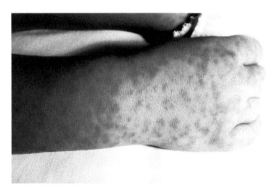

Source: CDC

10. Correct: Ringworm (D)

(D) There are three genera of dermatophytic fungi that infect different parts of the body: *Trichophyton*, *Epidermophyton*, and *Microsporum*. *Trichophyton* usually infects the skin, hair and nails. *Epidermophyton* infects the skin and nails. On the contrary, *Microsporum* infects the skin and hair. Lateral spread of the infection gives the appearance of tunneling worms; hence the terms tinea (Latin for worm) or ringworm. The disease has been designated by descriptive names such as tinea corporis (body site), tinea pedis (feet), and tinea capitis (scalp). Ringworm is a pruritic (itchy) and highly contagious fungal infection of the keratin layers that can spread from person to person or from animals to humans, by close physical contact, or from fomites such as contaminated floors in public showers (athlete's foot). The boy in the case most likely contracted the infection by sharing a contaminated hat. Ringworm of the scalp is treated with prescription oral antifungal medications, typically terbinafine, but griseofulvin, terbinafine, itraconazole, or fluconazole can alternatively be used as well. **(A)** Candidiasis is caused by *Candida albicans*, a colonizer of the skin and mucosal surfaces. Candidiasis is associated with chronically moist skin surfaces such as crural folds. For example, diaper rash may be caused by *C. albicans*. Chronic candidiasis of mucosal surfaces is associated with immunocompromised individuals. Genital/vulvovaginal candidiasis (yeast infection) occurs when there is overgrowth of the commensal *C. albicans* in the vagina. This infection affects nearly 75% of all adult women. The infection in this case is unlikely to be cause by *Candida*. **(B)** Chicken pox is caused by the varicella zoster virus, an enveloped single-stranded DNA virus of the herpes virus family. Chicken pox appears as a rash with pruritic (itchy), fluid-filled blisters that turn into scabs (see image [i] at the end of this answer). The rash first appears on the face and trunk and may spread to other parts of the body. Blisters are at various stages of development and do not appear on the palms or soles of the feet. This boy does not have the characteristic vesicles of chicken pox; hence this answer choice is incorrect. **(C)** By definition folliculitis is an infection of the hair follicles (see image [ii] at the end of this answer). While the hair loss seen with ringworm of the scalp is caused by invasion of the hair shaft by fungal arthroconidia, the term folliculitis typically refers to bacterial skin infections with *Staphylococcus aureus* and *Pseudomonas aeruginosa*. *S. aureus* is a skin colonizer that can cause folliculitis following mild trauma such as shaving. *P. aeruginosa* which colonizes water can cause hot tub folliculitis. Note that tinea barbae is a ringworm folliculitis of the beard area caused by *Trichophyton* species following mild trauma such as shaving. **(E)** Tinea versicolor (also referred to as pityriasis versicolor) is caused by two species: *Malassezia furfur* and *Malassezia globosa*. This is a superficial mycosis that causes patchy discoloration of the skin (see image [iii] at the end of this answer). It is a common disease of the skin in tropical and subtropical areas of the world and organism growth is enhanced by humidity, sweat, and oily skin. The scalp of this child does not resemble the typical skin discoloration of tinea versicolor.

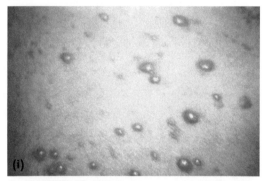

Source: CDC/Dr. K.L. Hermann

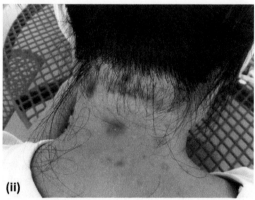

Source: By Lforlav [CC BY-SA 3.0 (https://creativecommons.org/licenses/by-sa/3.0)], via Wikimedia Commons

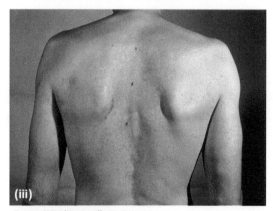

Source: CDC/Dr. Lucille K. Georg

11. Correct: Sandfly (B)

(B) The image of the cutaneous skin lesion (shown in the question stem) is the classic finding seen in cutaneous leishmaniasis, which is transmitted by the sandfly. See Appendix L for a list of vector-borne infections and associated vectors. Sandflies are small (approximately one third the size of a mosquito) insects that take blood meals most commonly at dawn and dusk. Cutaneous leishmaniasis endemic to the Middle East, Asia, tropical regions in North Africa, southern Europe, Mexico, Central America, and South America. Specific species of *Leishmania* are endemic to select geographic regions. *Leishmania* is a protozoan parasite and is an obligate intracellular organism that lives within macrophages. Although *Leishmania* is considered a flagellated organism, the flagellated form is not seen in clinical specimens. The diagnostic form of this pathogen is the amastigote which can be seen in clinical specimens, such as skin scrapings. In the image in the question stem, the amastigotes can be seen within the macrophage and the kinetoplast is clearly visible. Note that other intracellular pathogens that also infect macrophages, including *Histoplasma capsulatum*, may closely resemble *Leishmania* microscopically. Clinical history, including travel history and the presence of a kinetoplast, will aid in differentiating *Leishmania* from *Histoplasma*. The kinetoplast is thought to be a source of energy for movement of the flagellated form of the organism. See image at the end of this answer for an overview of the amastigote anatomy. Other forms of Leishmaniasis include mucocutaneous and visceral leishmaniasis. **(A)** Mosquitoes transmit a significant number of parasitic and viral human diseases including yellow fever, dengue, chikungunya, Zika, West Nile, malaria, and filariasis. Mosquitos are not involved in the transmission of leishmaniasis. **(C)** Ticks are vectors that transmit the following bacterial diseases: anaplasmosis, ehrlichiosis, Lyme disease, Rocky Mountain spotted fever (RMSF), tularemia, and epidemic typhus. Ticks also transmit the parasitic disease babesiosis. Ticks do not transmit *Leishmania*. **(D)** Tsetse flies are responsible for transmitting or African trypanosomiasis or sleeping sickness (*Trypanosoma brucei gambiense* or *T. b. rhodesiense*). An early sign of disease is a chancre at the site of infection. However, trypanosomiasis is a systemic infection that induces a host cytokine response ultimately leading to cachexia (wasting) and neurologic symptoms. The clinical findings in this case are not consistent with African trypanosomiasis. **(E)** Triatomine bugs transmit American trypanosomiasis or Chagas disease (*Trypanosoma cruzi*). Members of the triatomine subfamily (reduviid family) are also known as kissing bugs because they take their blood meal from around the mouth and eyes. Classic findings include swelling at the site of the bite, which may include a chagoma or Romaña's sign around the eye. At times, a chagoma may possibly resemble the lesion of cutaneous leishmaniasis. However, Chagas disease is mainly limited to Brazil and South America and usually it is the flagellated form of the pathogen that is diagnostic.

Amastigote

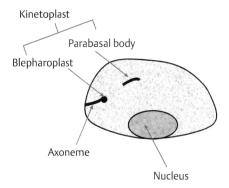

Kinetoplast

Parabasal body

Blepharoplast

Axoneme

Nucleus

Amastigotes are round or oval in shaped. Within the cell is a large oval eccentric nucleus and a kinetoplast. The kinetoplast consists of the blepharoplast and the adjacent parabasal body. The blepharoplast is attached to the axoneme. The average size of amastigotes is 5 by 3 μm.

12.   Correct: Streptococcal pyrogenic exotoxin (SPE) (E)

(E) Streptococcal pyrogenic exotoxin (SPE) is a superantigen produced by *Streptococcus pyogenes*, a gram-positive coccus in chains. It is also referred to as group A streptococcus and β-hemolytic streptococcus. This is a case of necrotizing fasciitis following contamination of a wound with the transient skin colonizer *S. pyogenes*. It is referred to as the "flesh-eating" bacterium. Necrotizing fasciitis is a rapidly progressing and a serious infection. Imaging studies may show gas (as seen in the image in the question stem) and crepitation may be present. Circulating SPE can result in cross-linking of the major histocompatibility complex (MHC) class II and T cell receptor inducing the release of high cytokine levels. A systemic response including fever, vasodilation, disseminated intravascular coagulation, and multiorgan system failure may ensue. Necrotizing fasciitis can be polymicrobial with the presence of at least one anaerobe and other aerobic or facultative anaerobic organisms. However, group A streptococci is capable of causing monomicrobic necrotizing infections as seen in this case. (A) α-Toxin produced by *Staphylococcus aureus* is a pore-forming cytolysin that contributes to localized tissue damage at the site of infection. *S. aureus* can be a source of cellulitis following trauma. However, it would not be the most likely organism causing fulminant necrotizing fasciitis. (B) β-Toxin is a pore-forming cytolysin produced by *Clostridium perfringens*, a gram-positive anaerobic rod that can cause necrotizing fasciitis and gas gangrene following a traumatic wound or surgical procedure with contaminated instruments. Ingested β-toxin can cause a necrotizing disease of the jejunum referred to as enteritis necroticans or pigbel. The Gram stain in this case showed gram-positive cocci; hence *S. pyogenes* is the most likely agent. (C) Lipopolysaccharide (LPS) endotoxin is produced by all gram-negative bacteria; it is a component of the cell envelope. Gram-negative LPS induces a cytokine response potentially leading to endotoxic shock.

Streptococcus pyogenes is a gram-positive organism. (D) Pneumolysin O is a pore-forming cytolysin produced by *Streptococcus pneumoniae*. It may contribute to tissue damage and inflammation associated with bacterial pneumonia. *S. pyogenes* produces a related cytolysin referred to as SLO. *S. pneumoniae* is not a typical agent of necrotizing fasciitis.

13.   Correct: *Staphylococcus aureus* (C)

(C) *Staphylococcus aureus* is a gram-positive coccus in clusters. This organism colonizes the human host and can cause pyogenic (pus-forming) infections of the bone and joint. In this case, the source of contamination was most likely the patient's skin or the hands of a health care worker. (A) *Enterococcus faecalis* is a gram-positive coccus related to the genus *Streptococcus*. *E. faecalis* is an intestinal colonizer that may be the source of urinary tract infections or infections following abdominal surgery. (B) *Haemophilus influenzae* is a gram-negative coccobacillus that inhabits the upper respiratory tract. It may cause otitis media and sinusitis. It is not a common agent of wound infections. (D) *Staphylococcus epidermidis* is a gram-positive coccus that colonizes the skin and is the potential source of postsurgical infections. The rapid onset of symptoms including fever and pus formation indicates the more virulent *Staphylococcus aureus* is responsible for the infection. *S. aureus* is coagulase positive while *S. epidermidis* is coagulase negative. (E) *Pseudomonas aeruginosa* is a gram-negative rod that is found in the environment. It is a leading cause of nosocomial skin infections. It may cause endocarditis in intravenous drug misusers, keratoconjunctivitis due to contaminated contact lenses, pneumonia in cystic fibrosis patients, and folliculitis due to improperly sanitized hot tubs. It is not typically an agent of postsurgical infections.

14.   Correct: *Staphylococcus aureus* (E)

(E) This woman has septic arthritis and the most common agent is *Staphylococcus aureus*. *S. aureus* is a gram-positive coccus and is catalase and coagulase positive. It may colonize the human anterior nares and skin. Skin infections, such as in this case, can predispose individuals to septic arthritis. Additionally, the elderly are at increased risk for septic arthritis. Other frequent agents of septic arthritis include streptococci. **(A)** *Escherichia coli* is a gram-negative rod that colonizes the intestine. Different serotypes are responsible for causing urinary tract infections and gastroenteritis. It is not typically an agent of septic arthritis. **(B)** *Chlamydia trachomatis* is a common sexually transmitted infection that may cause reactive arthritis, not septic arthritis. Reactive arthritis differs from septic arthritis and usually occurs postinfection with a particular pathogen. Additionally, reactive arthritis is usually culture negative because it is due to the reaction to the pathogen rather than the presence of the pathogen itself. Classic findings of reactive arthritis include conjunctivitis, urethritis, and arthritis. **(C)** *Neisseria meningitidis* is a gram-negative diplococcus that can be passed from person to person by droplet. A typical case presentation would be an outbreak of meningitis in a closed community such as a college dormitory. This infection is not associated with septic arthritis. However, another species of *Neisseria*, *N. gonorrhoeae* is an agent of septic arthritis, especially in otherwise healthy, sexually active young people. **(D)** *Salmonella enteritidis* is a cause of gastroenteritis most commonly associated with the consumption of poultry or eggs. Postinfection sequelae of *Salmonella* and other enteric pathogens including *Campylobacter*, *Shigella*, and *Yersina* may include reactive arthritis, not septic arthritis. However, the etiology and rapid onset of symptoms in this case argue against reactive arthritis.

15. Correct: *Blastomyces dermatitis* (A)

(A) The image in the question stem shows broad-based budding yeast, which is classic of *Blastomyces dermatitidis*. *B. dermatitidis* is an environmental, dimorphic fungus capable of causing deep-tissue mycoses. Dimorphic means the organism exists both as a yeast (at 37°C [98.6°F]) and a mold (at 25°C [77°F]). In tissue (i.e., clinical specimens), the organism appears as a broad-based budding yeast. In culture at 25°C (77°F), the organism appears as hyphae with spores (also called condia). The organism is associated with rotting wood and infections occur following inhalation of spores. Dissemination to secondary sites is possible, especially in immunocompromised individuals. The most common sites of dissemination are the skin (see image [i] at the end of this answer) and bone. The organism is endemic in the central and southeastern regions of the United States, especially in states that border the Ohio River and Mississippi River valleys. **(B)** *Histoplasma capsulatum* is an environmental, dimorphic fungus capable of causing deep-tissue mycoses. *H. capsulatum* is also dimorphic and endemic in a similar region as

Blastomyces. However, it is most commonly associated with exposure to chickens, starlings, and other birds and bats because the fungi are enriched by the droppings. It would be characterized as intracellular yeast cells within macrophages (see image [ii] at the end of this answer) isolated from lung or lymph node biopsy, not broad-based budding yeast. **(C)** *Sporothrix schenckii* is an environmental dimorphic fungus found in soil that may cause lesions with draining lymph channels (see image [iii] at the end of this answer) following traumatic inoculation. Note that infections with *Mycobacterium marinum*, *Nocardia brasiliensis*, and *Franciscella tularensis* may also present similarly with lymphocutaneous infections or "marching" lymph nodes. *S. schenckii* is often associated with prick from a thorn and infections may be referred to as rose gardener's disease. This organism primarily infects the skin rather than the lung as seen in this case. Budding yeast cells that may be elongated, giving a "cigar body" appearance (see image [iv] at the end of this answer) would be seen on biopsy of the infected tissue. **(D)** *Streptococcus pyogenes* is a gram-positive coccus that may cause impetigo or other skin infections. This organism rarely causes lung granulomas. **(E)** *Trichophyton* (see image [v] at the end of this answer) is one of the fungi that cause ringworm. This fungus infects the superficial layers of skin. Case presentation is a pruritic (itchy) rash on various parts of the body. Transmission is typically through fomites (contaminated objects). This organism does not cause lung infections.

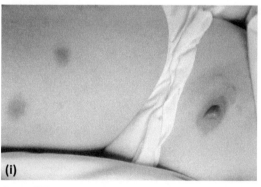

(i)

Source: CDC

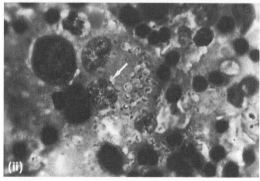

(ii)

Source: CDC/Dr. Lucille K. Georg

319

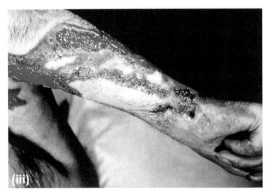

(iii)

Source: CDC/Dr. Lucille K. Georg

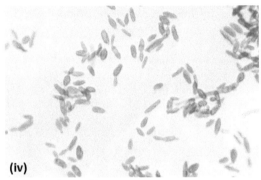

(iv)

Source: CDC/Dr. Lucille K. Georg

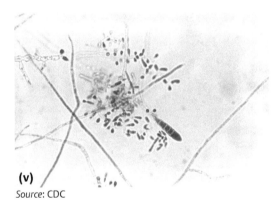

(v)

Source: CDC

16. Correct: α-Toxin produced by *Clostridium perfringens* (A)

(A) α-Toxin is a phospholipase C that affects a variety of cell types. This toxin is also called lecithinase and it is phospholipase that hydrolyzes lecithin, resulting in the disruption of RBCs, WBCs, and other cell membranes. It is the principal virulence factor produced by *Clostridium perfringens* causing tissue destruction leading to gas gangrene. *C. perfringens*, an obligate anaerobe, is a gram-positive bacillus. **(B)** *Staphylococcus aureus* produces a pore-forming α-cytolysin that contributes to tissue damage, principally carbuncles and furuncles. **(C)** *Clostridium perfringens* β-toxin causes necrotizing enteritis also referred to as enteritis necroticans or pigbel. This is a disease that results from a diet

consisting of large quantities of sweet potatoes that produce a trypsin inhibitor; gastric trypsin being responsible for proteolysis of β-toxin. **(D)** Exfoliative toxin (ET) is produced by some strains of *Staphylococcus aureus*, the causative agent of staphylococcal scalded skin syndrome (SSSS) in newborns. ET functions by causing a cleavage plane between the stratum spinosum and stratum granulosum of the epidermis. The disease is self-limiting and does not result in scarring. **(E)** Streptolysin O (SLO) is an oxygen-labile, pore-forming cytolysin produced by *Streptococcus pyogenes*. This exotoxin contributes to the tissue damage and spread of streptococcal cellulitis and may have a role in the heart damage associated with rheumatic heart disease. Circulating anti-SLO antibodies (ASO or ASLO) are a diagnostic indicator for *S. pyogenes* infection and may be a marker for rheumatic fever.

17. Correct: Anaerobic culture (A)

(A) Necrotizing fasciitis is often polymicrobial with the presence of at least one anaerobe and other aerobic or facultative aerobic organisms. Hence, anaerobic culture would aid in identification of the likely pathogen. **(B)** Bordet–Gengou agar is a selective media used for the growth of *Bordetella pertussis*, the causative agent of whooping cough. Deep nasopharyngeal swabs are used and diagnosis is by the polymerase chain reaction. **(C)** Capnophilic culture is reduced oxygen with approximately 2 to 10% CO_2. This is typically used for *Campylobacter jejuni*, a causative agent of gastroenteritis. **(D)** Sabouraud dextrose agar (SDA) is used to cultivate yeast and fungi. For example, *Histoplasma capsulatum* or *Coccidioides immitis* may be cultured using SDA. Cultivation of pathogenic fungi presents a significant health risk to laboratory personnel due to the infectious nature of the conidia shed by mycelial forms. **(E)** Thayer–Martin media is chocolate agar with antibiotics and is selective for pathogenic *Neisseria*, especially *Neisseria gonorrhoeae* and *Neisseria meningitidis*. It contains the antibiotics vancomycin, colistin, trimethoprim, and nystatin that inhibit the growth of other gram-negative bacteria, gram-positive bacteria, and fungi.

18. Correct: Branching gram-positive rods (A)

(A) This is an infection with *Nocardia*, likely *Nocardia brasiliensis*. These pathogens are normally found in soil and infections may occur following traumatic inoculation such as in the case of motor vehicle collision. They have a characteristic appearance and are filamentous, branching gram-positive rods (see image at the end of this answer). Cutaneous infections with *Nocardia* often result in draining sinus tracts along the lymphatic channel. Other organisms that may also present in a similar way include *Mycobacterium marinum*, *Sporothrix schenckii*, and

Francisella tularensis. Nocardia most often causes respiratory infections and disseminated infections, especially of the nervous system and cutaneous infections may occur, such as in this case. Immunocompromised patients are at higher risk for infections with this organism. Another organism to keep in mind, when branching gram-positive bacilli are observed, is *Actinomyces. Actinomyces* is normal microbiota of various areas of the body including the gingival crevices and tonsillar crypts of the oral cavity and infections usually occur due to displacement of endogenous strains after breach in mucosa. Risk factors for oral infections include dental manipulation, and the classical findings of *Actinomyces* are that the abscess may drain yellow exudate referred to as sulfur granules. The major difference between these organisms is that *Nocardia* is aerobic and stains with the modified acid-fast stain whereas *Actinomyces* is an anaerobic gram-positive branching bacillus that is not partially acid fast. The drug of choice to treat *Nocardia* infections is trimethoprim–sulfamethoxazole. **(B)** Broad budding yeast cells refer to *Blastomyces dermatitis*, a dimorphic fungus that can disseminate from the lung to various sites, especially the skin and bone, in the human host. Draining sinus tracts along the lymphatic channel indicate that *Nocardia* is the most likely agent in this case. **(C)** Septate hyphae refer to fungal pathogens. Hyphae may be septate or nonseptate. For example, *Aspergillus fumigatus* may produce septate hyphae. However, the draining sinus tracts along the lymphatic channel indicate that *Nocardia* is the most likely agent in this case. **(D)** Gram-negative coccobacilli refer to several organisms including *Haemophilus influenzae* (the cause of upper respiratory tract infections), *Haemophilus ducreyi* (the cause of chancroid), and *Francisella tularensis* (the cause of tularemia). While *F. tularensis* can possibly be the agent of this infection, tularensis is transmitted either from contact with an infected animal or from a bite of a tick. This man was in an accident and more likely to be traumatically inoculated with a pathogen. Furthermore, patients with tularensis may have draining sinus tracts; however, they are classically "sicker" with constitutional symptoms. The more indolent progression of this infection makes *Nocardia* more likely the causative agent. **(E)** There are several pathogenic spirochetes, all of which cannot be visualized microscopically by Gram stain: *Treponema pallidum* (the cause of syphilis), *Borrelia burgdorferi* (the cause of Lyme disease), *Borrelia recurrentis* (the cause of relapsing fever), and *Leptospira* species (the cause of leptospirosis). Infections with these pathogens would not present with draining sinus tracts.

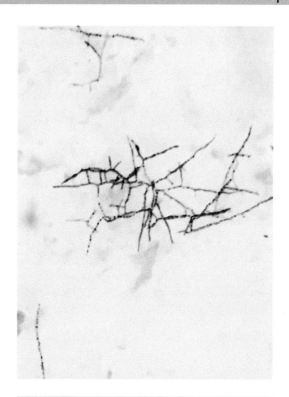

19. Correct: Rapid plasma reagin (RPR) (D)

(D) This is a case of yaws caused by the spirochete *Treponema pallidum* subspecies *pertenue* seen most commonly in children less than 15 years of age. Yaws predominates in humid climates of Latin American, Asia, and Africa. It is passed from person to person by nonsexual contact. Infections begin with papules that eventually develop into a nodule then ulcerate. Similar to *T. pallidum*, the causative agent of syphilis, it can be diagnoses using the rapid plasma reagin (RPR) assay. This assay is a nontreponema screening test and detects reagin antibodies to cardiolipin antigen. **(A)** Streptolysin O (SLO) is a pore-forming cytolysin produced by *Streptococcus pyogenes*, the causative agent of pharyngitis, impetigo, and erysipelas. Anti-SLO titers can be used to track the potential for poststreptococcal sequelae. This infection is not likely to be due to *S. pyogenes*. **(B)** Respiratory mycoses such as histoplasmosis, coccidioidomycosis, and, in particular, blastomycosis can disseminate to the skin. Serology is of limited value due to the ubiquitous exposure to the fungi. The presentation, age, geographic region, and lack of pulmonary involvement argue against a deep-tissue mycosis in this case. **(C)** Lesions of herpes simplex virus (HSV) type 1 and 2 present as small painful blisters or ulcers typically on the mouth or in the genital region. Therefore, HSV can be ruled out by the presentation in this case. **(E)** Purified protein derivative (PPD) is used for the tuberculin skin test, a delayed-type hypersensitivity reaction indicating exposure to *Mycobacterium tuberculosis*. Leprosy, caused by *Mycobacterium leprae*, is a disfiguring diseased of the skin that also impacts peripheral sensory nerves. The presentation in this case is not consistent with leprosy. Furthermore, PPD is not used to diagnose leprosy.

20.   Correct: Erysipeloid (D)

(D) Erysipeloid, caused by the gram-positive rod *Erysipelothrix rhusiopathiae*, is an infection of individuals who work with fish or animals, in particular pigs. The condition is typically seen on the hands of fisherman, animal breeders, veterinarians, slaughterhouse workers, cooks, and grocers. Typical lesions begin as bright red papules that become violaceous (purplish). Lesions may be asymptomatic or accompanied with pain, pruritus, and fever. **(A)** Cutaneous anthrax presents as a painless black ulcer referred to as an eschar. It may be seen in individuals who work with animal carcasses due to the potential exposure to the spores of *Bacillus anthracis*. A bioterrorism attack in 2001 resulted in cutaneous anthrax in United States postal workers. The lack of an eschar in this case makes cutaneous anthrax an unlikely diagnosis. **(B)** Bullous impetigo is caused by the exfoliative toxin of *Staphylococcus aureus*. This infection is primary see in children and is characterized by vesicles that develop into fluid-filled bullae. This is unlikely to bullous impetigo. **(C)** Dermatophytosis is also referred to as ringworm, a contagious and highly pruritic infection of the keratin layer. Ringworm presents as circular scaly patches on the feet, groin, or body. Infection of the scalp results in bald patches because the fungal arthroconidia invade the hair shaft. The main pathogens involved in dermatophytosis are *Microsporum*, *Epidermophyton*, and *Trichophyton*. The presentation in this case is not consistent with dermatophytosis. **(E)** Erysipelas is an infection of the dermis caused by *Streptococcus pyogenes*, which appears on the face. Erysipelas may also present on the extremities and can be distinguished from impetigo by the lack of pus formation and a rash with sharp margins. Lymphangitis and inflammation of regional lymph nodes are commonly seen in association with these infections. In this case, the man's occupation as a fisherman and the lack of inflammation indicate that erysipeloid is the best answer.

21.   Correct: Double-stranded DNA virus (A)

(A) This infection is likely to be caused by human papilloma virus (HPV), a double-stranded DNA virus. There are more than 100 serotypes of HPV. Several serotypes including 1, 2, 3, 4, 7, and 10 are implicated in warts, such as in this case. **(B)** Human papilloma virus (HPV) is a double-stranded DNA virus. Rotavirus is a double-stranded RNA virus and a leading cause of severe acute gastroenteritis in children. **(C)** There are many clinically significant viruses that are single-stranded RNA viruses including paramyxoviruses and orthomyxoviruses. See Appendix N for a summary of the major characteristic, including genomic features of clinically significant viruses. Human papilloma virus (HPV) is a double-stranded DNA virus. **(D)** Staphylococci are gram-positive cocci and *Staphylococcus aureus* is commonly implicated in cutaneous infections. However, warts, such as described in this case, are caused by HPV. **(E)** *Bacillus* and *Clostridium* species are the only clinically significant gram-positive bacilli with spores and both species may cause infections of the skin. *B. anthracis* is an agent of cutaneous anthrax and the classic findings include an eschar. Clostridia are anaerobic pathogens and infections usually affect deep tissue and not the superficial layers of the skin. The infection in this case is unlikely to be cause by either *Bacillus* or *Clostridium*.

22.   Correct: Erythema multiforme (A)

(A) This boy most likely has herpetic whitlow, which is caused by herpes simplex virus-1 (HSV-1). Erythema multiforme is a self-limiting, immune mediated disease that is associated with herpes simplex virus infections. The classic finding is a target-shaped, raised lesion. Deposition of immune complexes is thought to play a role in the pathogenesis. Other pathogens have also been implicated with erythema multiforme, but HSV is the classic pathogen associated with this condition. Children who suck their thumb are prone to herpetic whitlow. In this case the boy had a preceding oral herpes infection and sucking his thumb probably led to the herpetic whitlow. Dentist and dental hygienists are also at risk for herpetic whitlow. Another type of skin infection caused by HSV-1 is herpes gladiatorum, in which lesions are mainly seen on the trunk and extremities. This infection is classically associated with wrestlers. **(B)** Rheumatic fever is postinfectious sequelae of *Streptococcus pyogenes*, not herpes simplex virus. Molecular mimicry plays an important role in the pathogenesis of rheumatic fever. Antibodies for *S. pyogenes* cross-react with host antigens in cardiac tissue. **(C)** Guillain–Barré syndrome is an ascending paralysis that occurs following *Campylobacter* gastroenteritis. During *C. jejuni* infection, antibodies are produced that target *C. jejuni* lipopolysaccharide (LPS). These antibodies are cross-reactive because of the sharing of cross-reactive epitopes (molecular mimicry). As a result, antibodies unintentionally target host nerve tissue. **(D)** Reactive arthritis is most often associated following infections with *Chlamydia* or enteric pathogens including *Salmonella*, *Shigella*, *Campylobacter*, and *Yersina*. The exact pathogenesis is unclear but it may involve cross-reactive antibodies that eventually lead to joint damage. **(E)** Shingles is caused by varicella zoster virus (VZV). VZV may also cause chicken pox with vesicular lesions. This is usually seen in young children and usually starts on the face and moves to the extremities. However, the infection in this case is caused by HSV, which is not associated with shingles.

23. Correct: Varicella and herpes zoster (E)

(E) Vaccination is recommended for anyone over 60 years of age to prevent shingles, also known as zoster or herpes zoster. Currently there are two FDA-approved shingles vaccines, a live attenuated vaccine and a recombinant, adjuvanted vaccine. Shingles is a result of reactivation of a latent varicella zoster virus (chicken pox) infection. Immunosuppression including age can lead to reactivation of the latent virus. **(A)** Hepatitis B is currently provided as part of the pediatric immunization schedule recommended at birth and 2 months of age. High-risk adults including medical staff, immunocompromised patients, and men who have sex with men are included in the recommended hepatitis B immunization schedule. The hepatitis B vaccine is a recombinant vaccine. **(B)** Human papillomavirus (HPV) is the causative agent of genital warts that have been linked to cervical cancer. Immunization is recommended for 11- to 12-year-old girls, 13- to 26-year-old teenagers/young women not previously vaccinated, and 9- to 26-year-old boys/men. Currently, there are three HPV vaccines that cover various HPV types. However, all the vaccines are recombinant vaccines. **(C)** Poliovirus is a neurotropic enterovirus that can be transported to the central nervous system resulting in paralytic disease in 1% of infections. There are two types of vaccine attenuated that is administered orally and the inactivated with is administrated parenterally. The inactivated poliovirus vaccine is part of the pediatric immunization schedule in the United States. **(D)** Rubella is administered as a live attenuated vaccine in combination with the measles and mumps vaccine beginning at 1 year of age in the United States. In developing countries where these diseases are still widespread, vaccination begins at 6 months of age.

24. Correct: Varicella (C)

(C) This is a case of chicken pox (varicella) caused by varicella zoster virus (VZV) in an unimmunized adolescent. Unimmunized children are at increased risk for infection. A goal of the pediatric immunization program is to create herd immunity with a significant population of protected individuals reducing infectious disease incidence. Chicken pox is mainly an infection of children younger than 13 years old. Infections tend to peak in the late winter and early spring. Transmission occurs via respiratory droplets and individuals are most infective 48 prior to the onset of the rash and remain infective until the lesions crust over. Following an initial prodrome phase, the typical exanthem develops. The rash starts as macules that progress into papules and vesicles. The rash typically starts on the face and moves to the trunk and extremities. A key feature of the vesicles is that they are all in different stages of development. VZV is part of the herpes virus family and is a double-stranded, enveloped, DNA virus. **(A)** Herpes simplex virus (HSV) infections may manifest as cutaneous infections such as herpes gladiatorum or herpetic whitlow. Herpes viruses are double-stranded DNA viruses. The typical lesion of HSV is vesicular and may be similar to chicken pox. However, to date there is no HSV vaccine. Hence, this answer choice is incorrect. **(B)** Measles is another vaccine-preventable disease. It would present with generalized respiratory symptoms (conjunctivitis, coryza, and cough) with a maculopapular rash that starts on the face and spreads over the body (see image [i] at the end of this answer). The vesicular rash seen in the question stem does not resemble the maculopapular rash of measles. Measles is also called the first disease or rubeola and is caused by the measles virus, a single-stranded, negative-sense RNA virus. **(D)** Smallpox, caused by two virus variants Variola major and Variola minor, was declared eradicated by the World Health Assembly in 1980; there have been no cases of naturally occurring smallpox since then due to effective vaccination. Smallpox presents as a pustular rash (see image [ii] at the end of this answer) over the body. In contrast to chicken pox that has lesions at various stages of development, the rash of smallpox presents with all pustules at the same stage of development. Variola virus is a double-stranded DNA virus. This is unlikely to be a case of smallpox. **(E)** Infections with rubella being with a general prodrome followed by a rash that starts on the face and moves down the body. The typical rash is pinpoint, pink, and maculopapular (see image [iii] at the end of this answer). Infections are also called the third disease or German measles. Like chicken pox, rubella may be prevented with vaccination. However, the image in the question stem shows the typical vesicular lesion of chicken pox.

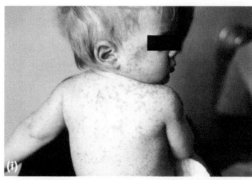

Source: CDC

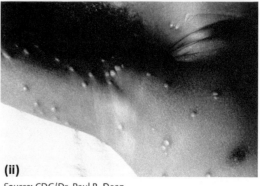

(ii)
Source: CDC/Dr. Paul B. Dean

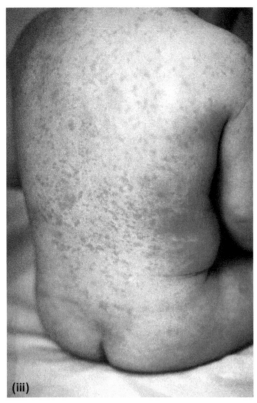

(iii)

Source: CDC

25.   Correct: Single-stranded, enveloped, RNA virus (D)

(D) This was a case of measles during an outbreak among visitors to the Disney theme park in California. Clusters of underimmunized individuals are observed in some regions of the country. In addition to a rash, note that this patient presented with the "three Cs" of measles: cough, conjunctivitis, and coryza. **(A)** Examples of conjugated polysaccharide capsular vaccines are for protection against meningitis caused by *Streptococcus pneumoniae, Haemophilus influenzae* type b, and *Neisseria meningitidis*. **(B)** Examples of double-stranded, enveloped, DNA viruses are the herpes family of viruses including herpes simplex virus (HSV), varicella zoster virus (VZV), Epstein–Barr virus (EBV), and cytomegalovirus (CMV). **(C)** Recombinant hepatitis B surface antigen (HBsAg) is administered at birth and at 2 months of age. Infants born to HBsAg-positive mothers are simultaneously immunized at birth with HBsAg and hepatitis B immune globulin. **(E)** Toxoid vaccines protect against tetanus and diphtheria. They are composed of inactivated forms of the tetanus toxin and diphtheria toxin.

26.   Correct: Transient aplastic crisis (C)

(C) This is a case of erythema infectiosum, or fifth disease, caused by parvovirus B19, a DNA virus. Patients with chronic hemolytic anemia, immunodeficiency, or sickle cell disease may experience a transient aplastic crisis (answer choice C) caused by

viral suppression of bone marrow activity. This virus infects red blood cells and replication of the virus requires that the host cell is undergoing DNA replication. The virus cannot initiate cell DNA synthesis. As a result, parvoviruses are restricted to dividing cells such as red cell precursors. Infections are transmitted by respiratory droplets or may be vertically transmitted. Postnatal infections start with a prodrome followed by the class exanthem that resembles "slapped cheeks." The rash is erythematous and maculopapular. The rash eventually spread to the trunk and limbs. **(A)** Subacute sclerosing panencephalitis (SSPE) is a rare complication of the measles virus. This condition occurs 5 to 6 years after the initial measles infection. Children who have had measles while under the age of 2 years are at increased risk for developing SSPE. In this infection, the virus remains in the brain resulting in a progressive brain infection that eventually leads to death. Findings include personality changes, seizures, and physical disabilities. **(B)** Guillain–Barré syndrome is an autoimmune disorder affecting the peripheral nervous system following a viral or bacterial infection of the gastrointestinal or respiratory tracts. Classically *Campylobacter* infections are associated with Guillain–Barré syndrome. **(D)** Seizures may be associated with several infections including exanthem subitum (also called roseola), which is caused by human herpes virus-6 (HHV-6). In this infection, there is an abrupt onset of high fever followed by a blanching maculopapular, nonpruritic rash, which starts at the neck and trunk and moves to the face and extremities. Because of the high fever, seizures may be seen. The clinical presentation and the exanthem in the case presented in the question stem do not resemble an infection with HHV-6. **(E)** Secondary bacterial infections are not associated with erythema infectiosum. Chicken pox is an example of an infection with a rash in which secondary bacterial infections are a complication. This is because the rash is typically pruritic and the scratching may lead to the introduction of bacteria and therefore infection.

27.   Correct: Dengue (A)

(A) The blanching rash combined with the fever, headache, arthralgia, and travel history indicates that dengue is the most likely diagnosis. Other symptoms associated with dengue fever include retro-orbital pain. Dengue may also present as hemorrhagic fever characterized by bleeding from mucosa or other sites. Dengue is caused by a flavivirus, which is transmitted to humans by mosquitoes. Dengue is a disease of the tropics and subtropics affecting as many as 400 million people yearly. Flaviviruses are positive-sense, single-stranded RNA viruses. Other important flaviviruses include West Nile virus, Zika virus, and yellow fever virus, which are also transmitted by mosquitos. See Appendix L for a list of common vector-borne infections. **(B)** Malaria is caused by *Plasmodium* parasites and is transmitted by mosquitoes.

Symptoms would include cyclical bouts of fever and anemia. Malaria may be seen in Haiti; however, the clinical manifestations in this case indicate malaria is an unlikely diagnosis. **(C)** *Salmonella typhi* is the agent of typhoid fever. Infections typically present as a sudden onset of fever, headache, and nausea. Gastrointestinal symptoms and a transient, macular rash (rose-colored spots) on the trunk may also be present. Infections with this pathogen are possible with this woman's travel history, but her clinical manifestations are more consistent with dengue. **(D)** Trypanosomiasis, particularly African sleeping sickness caused by subspecies of *Trypanosoma brucei* initially presents as a lesion at the site of the tsetse fly bite followed by fever, headache, myalgia, and dark urine due to red blood cell–induced hemolysis. A blanching rash is characteristic of early disease and neurologic symptoms appear with progression. However, trypanosomiasis is largely limited to Africa; hence this answer choice is incorrect. **(E)** Yellow fever is caused by a flavivirus and transmitted to humans by the bite of a mosquito. The disease is endemic to the tropical and subtropical areas in South America and Africa. Symptoms include fever, severe headache, myalgia, nausea, and 15% of cases may involve the liver resulting in jaundice. The blanching rash and arthralgia, in this case, indicate dengue is the most likely diagnosis.

28. Correct: Cutaneous larva migrans (E)

(E) Also known as zoonotic hookworm, cutaneous larva migrans is an infection in which humans are the accidental host. It is caused by the dog and cat hookworm with *Ancylostoma braziliense* and *A. caninum* the most common in the United States. Infections are usually seen in tropical countries, and in the United States, infections are mainly limited to the coastal areas of the Southeast and West. Animal waste with the larva may be found in sand. Humans present with skin manifestations caused by the larval form of the parasite burrowing under the skin, usually the feet. As the larvae migrate, tracks appear due to the larval movement which is accompanied by pruritis (see image at the end of this answer). Diagnosis is usually made on clinical findings and infections are self-limiting with symptoms disappearing within 5 to 6 weeks following the initial infection. Treatment is not usually indicated; however, topical thiabendazole or albendazole may be effective. Other members of the hookworm family for which humans are definitive hosts are *A. duodenale* and *Necator americanus*. **(A)** Cercarial dermatitis (swimmer's itch) is caused by an allergic reaction to the cercariae of a schistosome parasite with birds and nonhuman mammals as their definitive host. Snails are an intermediate host for the schistosomes. The cercariae burrow into the skin causing a diffuse dermatitis. This is caused by *Schistosoma* species and occurs following contact with contaminated water. The rash occurs on parts of the body that were contact with water and is typically pruritic, red, and becomes vesicular within a day. While it is possible this infection could be cercarial dermatitis, the raised tracks indicate that cutaneous larva migrans is more likely the causative agent. **(B)** Chagas disease, caused by the parasite *Trypanosoma cruzi*, is transmitted to humans through the bite of the triatomine bug. Infected individuals present with local swelling at the site of infection (Romaña's sign) in the acute phase. Systemic parasitemia including cardiac complications occur during the chronic phase of infection. *T. cruzi* infections are mainly limited to South America. The clinical findings and the lack of travel history to a Chagas disease endemic area indicate that Chagas disease is an unlikely diagnosis. **(C)** Impetigo is a superficial infection of the skin caused by *Streptococcus pyogenes* and *Staphylococcus aureus*. Superinfection of lesions may occur. Infections may occur following direct pathogen invasion of the skin or following another skin condition or skin trauma, such as in this case. However nonbullous impetigo, the most common form, begins as papules that turn into vesicles that crust over with a honey-colored crust. In bullous impetigo, the vesicles turn into bullae with clear fluid that will then crust over. The clinical findings of the case described in the question stem are not consistent with impetigo. **(D)** Tinea pedis (also ringworm of the feet and athletes foot) is caused by a dermatophytic infection of the stratum corneum. It is typically passed from human to human through contaminated surfaces or fomites. Less common forms of ringworm can be contracted from animals. Dry, itchy, scaly red feet are the typical findings of this fungal infection. The raised red tracts described in the question stem are characteristic findings of cutaneous larval migrans and not tinea pedis.

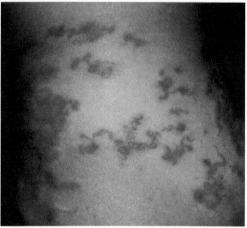

Source: WeisSagung [Public domain], from Wikimedia Commons

29. Correct: *Onchocerca volvulus* (B)

(B) Humans are infected with the larva of the *Onchocerca volvulus* nematode through the bite of the blackfly. The microfilariae mainly affect the eye and inflammation in the cornea and optic nerve results in blindness. However, the larvae can migrate systemically causing cutaneous lesions and a "leopard skin" appearance in infected individuals as described in the question stem. The disease is referred to as river blindness because the blackfly vector reproduces near flowing water and the infection is mainly limited to sub-Saharan Africa. (A) *Loa loa*, also referred to as the African eye worm, is a nematode that may be seen in the region presented in this case. Infections are transmitted by the bite of a deer fly and both skin manifestations and ocular manifestations may be seen. Typical skin manifestations are subcutaneous swellings (Calabar swellings), which are due to the migration of the worm through the skin. The skin manifestations described in the question stem are not consistent with Calabar swellings. The worm can also migrate to the eye, but is typically limited to the conjunctiva and does not cause severe inflammation or usually lead to blindness. Hence, this answer choice is incorrect. (C) *Schistosoma japonicum* is a digenetic blood trematode that is transmitted to humans exposed to contaminated water containing the skin-penetrating cercariae. Paired adult worms migrate to the mesenteric venules of the human host and produces eggs through sexual reproduction. The complete life cycle involves freshwater snails that shed infectious cercariae. A rash may develop in the early stage of infection with chronic infection of the liver, intestines, spleen, lungs, and bladder. This parasite is mainly seen in Southeast Asia and infections do not result in blindness. (D) *Trypanosoma cruzi* is the protozoan parasite that causes Chagas disease. It is transmitted to humans through the bite of the triatomine bug. Infected individuals present with local swelling at the site of infection (Romaña's sign) in the acute phase. Systemic parasitemia including cardiac complications occur during the chronic phase of infection. This infection is limited to South America and does not cause blindness. (E) *Wuchereria bancrofti* causes lymphatic filariasis in humans. It is a nematode transmitted by mosquitoes. Larvae migrate through the lymphatic system and adults may remain in lymph vessels and lymph nodes for years. Lymphedema particularly in the legs, groin, and breasts is a symptom of lymphatic filariasis. Hardening and thickening of the skin commonly referred to as elephantiasis is another characteristic of the chronic disease. *Wuchereria* infections do occur in Africa; however, the manifestations described in this case are not consistent with lymphatic filariasis.

30. Correct: *Coccidioides immitis* (C)

(C) This patient is suffering from valley fever (also called dessert fever, dessert rheumatism, San Joaquin Valley fever), which is a systemic mycosis caused by the dimorphic fungi *Coccidioides immitis* and *Coccidioides posadasii*. Infections with *C. immitis* are limited to mainly California, particularly the San Joaquin Valley while *C. posadasii* is seen in areas of Arizona, Texas, and New Mexico. Inhalation of spores results in a pulmonary infection. Primary pulmonary infections may reveal infiltrates, hilar adenopathy, and pleural effusions. Lung cavities may occur in a small percentage of cases. Pulmonary symptoms may or may not be present. However, the classic triad of findings of infection include fever, erythema nodosum, and joint pain as described in this case. The organism may cause disseminated infections, especially in immunocompromised patients and most commonly disseminates to the skin, joints, and bone. (A) *Aspergillus fumigatus* is an environmental mold that can cause pulmonary infections in immunocompromised individuals. *Aspergillus* may disseminate from the lung to other sites including the CNS; however, this organism rarely disseminates to the skin. When skin infections with *Aspergillus* are seen, infections are most likely due to direct skin inoculation of the fungal spores. (B) *Blastomyces dermatitidis* is an environmental fungus capable of causing deep-tissue mycoses. It occurs most commonly in the southeastern regions of the United States. Dissemination to secondary sites is possible with the most common skin and bone. The geographic location and symptoms of this make this answer choice less likely. (D) *Cryptococcus neoformans* is a ubiquitous fungus that typically causes asymptomatic lung infections. Cryptococcal meningitis may occur in immunocompromised individuals such as AIDS patients. Skin lesions with this organism may be seen in disseminated *Cryptococcus* infections but the patient presentation is not consistent with *C. neoformans*; hence this is unlikely to be the etiological agent in this case. (E) *Histoplasma capsulatum* is a dimorphic fungus capable of causing deep-tissue mycosis in the lungs. Exposure to the infectious spores is associated with bird and bat droppings and typically seen in the central and eastern part of the United States. Pulmonary and systemic symptoms may mimic tuberculosis. This organism may disseminate to the bone and joints and in these cases erythema nodosum may also be present. However, the geographic location makes this pathogen a less likely agent of this infection.

31. Correct: Eschar (C)

(C) Cutaneous anthrax presents as a lesion of necrotic tissue with a coal black center referred to as an eschar. (A) A carbuncle or boil is a skin abscess caused by *Staphylococcus aureus*. They appear as pustules with necrotic tissue and pus. A cluster of carbuncles is referred to as a furuncle. (B) A chancre is seen during primary syphilis, caused by *Treponema pallidum* or in chancroid caused by *Haemophilus ducreyi*. Chancre is also the term used to describe the skin lesion at the initial stage of African sleeping sickness, which is caused by *Trypanosoma brucei*. **(D)** Human papillomavirus (HPV) is a cause of common skin and genital warts. Sexually transmitted HPV has been linked to cervical cancer. **(E)** Papules are small, raised, solid pimples that may be caused by the bacterium *Cutibacterium* (formerly *Propionibacterium*) *acnes*.

32. Correct: Trichinellosis (C)

(C) This is a case of trichinellosis (also called trichinosis) caused by the nematode *Trichinella spiralis*. The pathogen is most often transmitted via ingestion of undercooked pork or bear meat. Initial diarrhea and other symptoms such as nausea and vomiting are due to the intestinal invasion by the larva. The pathogen then encysts in skeletal muscle, leading to myalgia, weakness, headache, and periorbital edema. Eosinophilia is often present after the worm leaves the intestine. Once the worm migrates from the bowel, stool ova and parasite (O&P) results may be negative but the larvae may be observed encysted within skeletal muscle. The encysted larvae within the skeletal muscle are referred to as nurse cells (see image at the end of this answer). **(A)** The etiological agent of Chagas disease is the flagellated protozoan *Trypanosoma cruzi*. This pathogen is mainly seen in Central and South America and is transmitted via the reduviid, triatomine (kissing) bug. One of the characteristic features of Chagas disease is the Romaña's sign, which involves periorbital swelling. *T. cruzi* normally does not infect muscles. **(B)** Cystercercosis, caused by the cestode (tapeworm) *Taenia solium*, is associated with pigs but is transmitted via the ingestion of fecally contaminated material containing ova. The larval form of the pathogen can embed in human tissue. Most often, *T. solium* migrates to the brain leading to neurocysticercosis. While not common, the pathogen can also encyst in muscles. There is higher prevalence of infections in Central and South America and parts of Africa and Asia. In this case, it is more likely that the etiological agent is *T. spiralis*. **(D)** Visceral larva migrans is an infection caused by the nematode *Toxocara* (*cati* or *canis*). This pathogen can also induce eosinophilia but does not commonly affect muscles. *Toxocara* is transmitted to humans via ingestion of material contaminated with cat or dog feces containing ova. This infection occurs more often in children. **(E)** Yersiniosis is caused by the gram-negative enteric pathogen *Yersinia enterocolitica*. This pathogen is transmitted via ingestion of contaminated food and is often associated with undercooked pork. *Y. enterocolitica* infections generally present as diarrhea. Postinfectious sequelae such as reactive arthritis may occur. However, muscle involvement is not generally observed.

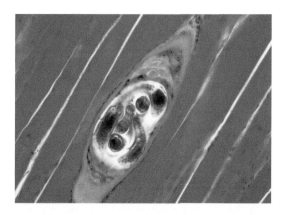

33. Correct: *Vibrio vulnificus* (E)

(E) This wound was most likely to be infected with a non-cholera strain of *Vibrio*, which are curved gram-negative rods. Non-cholera *Vibrio*, such as *Vibrio vulnificus*, may cause wound infections after contact with contaminated water. Individuals with underlying liver disease and hemochromatosis or iron overload are at greater risk for developing more serious infections. Similar to *V. cholerae*, these pathogens are also halotolerant and are associated with marine or estuarine environments. The organisms most likely gain entry after a breach in the intact skin. While this organism may cause a mild cellulitis, it may progress to cause a serious necrotizing fasciitis or myositis. Gastrointestinal infections may also occur after ingestion of contaminated food and water and infections are commonly associated with shellfish, such as oysters. **(A)** *Aeromonas hydrophila* is a gram-negative rod and is associated with fresh and estuarine, and less commonly marine, water. This pathogen may cause wound infections or diarrheal disease. Cellulitis, especially of the extremities, is the most common presentation. Like *V. vulnificus*, this organism can also cause necrotizing fasciitis. In this case, the Gram stain of a curved gram-negative rod indicates *Vibrio* is more likely to be the causative agent. **(B)** Like *Vibrio*, *Campylobacter* are curved gram-negative rods. *C. coli* is zoonotic and associated with pigs. Humans may shed *C. coli* in feces and there is a possibility that this pathogen could be found in water environments. However, most infections with this pathogen result in gastroenteritis or colitis and possibly sepsis. Wound infections are not a common manifestation of *C. coli* infection. **(C)** The gram-positive rod, *Erysipelothrix rhusiopathiae*, is zoonotic and is commonly associated with pigs, sheep, cows, and horses. This organism also affects marine life, including fish, and can contaminate water. Typically, infections are localized to the skin and are referred to as erysipeloid. The Gram stain indicates *Vibrio*, which is more likely to be the causative agent. **(D)** *Mycobacterium marinum* is an opportunistic acid-fast bacillus. It is associated with fish and may contaminate water, resulting in skin lesions, usually on the nonintact skin of the extremities. Infections are typically lymphocutaneous. Mycobacteria are rod-shaped but and do not typically Gram stain, but if they do stain they appear as gram-positive rods.

34. Correct: *Salmonella* (A)

(A) Sickle cell disease patients are prone to invasive infections with nontyphoidal *Salmonella*, which are gram-negative rods. Post-gastrointestinal sequelae may include osteomyelitis, as described in this case, and infective endocarditis. *Salmonella* are primarily foodborne pathogens and diarrhea and other gastrointestinal symptoms occur following ingestion of contaminated food or contact with contaminated animals. In sickle cell disease, there is capillary occlusion due to sickling of the red blood cells, which leads to the more invasive sequelae. **(B)** *Shigella*, an enteric gram-negative rod, is a cause of diarrhea and bacillary dysentery. Postinfectious sequelae include reactive arthritis, which is often seen in middle-aged men. Leading agents of osteomyelitis in sickle cell disease include gram-negative enteric pathogens. However, the most frequently associated pathogens are *Salmonella* and *Escherichia coli*, not *Shigella*. **(C, D)** Common agents of osteomyelitis include *Staphylococcus aureus*, a gram-positive coccus in clusters, and *Staphylococcus epidermidis*, a coagulase-negative staphylococcus. Coagulase-negative staphylococci are often involved in orthopedic hardware-related infections. In this case, the blood culture reveals gram-negative rods; hence, the etiological agent in this case is not *S. aureus* or *S. epidermidis*. **(E)** *Pseudomonas aeruginosa* is a gram-negative rod and an agent of osteomyelitis. However, *P. aeruginosa* osteomyelitis is more likely to be associated with injection drug use.

35. Correct: Mucosal invasion (A)

(A) Sickle cell disease patients are prone to invasive infections with nontyphoidal *Salmonella*, which are gram-negative rods. The main mechanism of virulence of nontyphoidal *Salmonella* is mucosal invasion. In osteomyelitis, pathogens may enter the bone directly via trauma or other means, from direct contiguous spread from another site or via hematogenous spread. In the case of *Salmonella*, the pathogen first causes gastroenteritis, enters the bloodstream (hence the positive blood cultures), and then disseminates to the bone. The primary infection in this case is gastroenteritis ("stomach flu"). **(B)** Several pathogens produce toxins that inhibit protein synthesis, including *Shigella* and *Pseudomonas aeruginosa*. *Salmonella* does not produce a toxin that inhibits protein synthesis. **(C)** Coagulase is an enzyme produced by *Staphylococcus aureus* that facilitates the conversion of fibrinogen to fibrin. This ultimately results in clot formation. The protective fibrin clot may protect the pathogen from the host immune response. *Salmonella* does not produce coagulase. **(D)** *Salmonella* may form a biofilm on the mucosa; however, the most important factor mediating gastrointestinal disease is invasion of the mucosa. **(E)** M protein is found in the cell wall of *Streptococcus*

pyogenes (group A streptococci). M protein binds collagen, fibrinogen, and other extracellular matrix proteins. It also assists the pathogen in evading the host immune response by binding to the Fc portion of IgG.

36. Correct: Sexual encounter (E)

(E) The Gram stain image (presented in the question stem) shows intracellular and extracellular gram-negative diplococci. This is characteristic of *Neisseria gonorrhoeae*, which is sexually transmitted. This organism causes primary infections of the genital tract, oral cavity, and eye and can disseminate resulting in septic arthritis, such as in this case. It is important to note that infections of the genital tract may be asymptomatic. Septic or purulent arthritis in otherwise healthy young adults is most likely due to *N. gonorrhoeae*. Days to weeks after a genital infection, infections of the joints may occur. **(A)** There are many pathogens that are transmitted via contaminated food and water. However, *N. gonorrhoeae* is solely a human pathogen and is not transmitted in this manner. **(B)** *Staphylococcus*, *Candida*, *Pseudomonas*, and other pathogens are common nosocomial pathogens and often cause device-related infections. However, *N. gonorrhoeae* is typically implicated in device-related infections. **(C)** Overgrowth of normal flora leads to infections such as *Candida* vulvovaginitis but not gonorrhea. **(D)** *Neisseria meningitidis* and many other pathogens are transmitted via respiratory droplets. This is not a mechanism of transmission of *N. gonorrhoeae*.

37. Correct: Molluscum contagiosum (A)

(A) The figure in the question stem shows the classic dome-shaped papules with central umbilication of molluscum contagiosum, a viral infection. Molluscum contagiosum virus is a double-stranded DNA virus that infections and replications in epithelial cells. The papules are often described as waxy—may be located anywhere on body excluding the palms and soles. Transmission occurs from direct contact with an infected individuals or fomites and from sexual contact. Infections may be associated with contact sports and is mostly seen in children ages 1 to 10 years of age. Most infections are self-limiting and nonlife threatening; however, HIV-positive individuals may have more serious infections. The classic histopathogic findings are molluscum bodies, which are intracytoplasmic inclusions in epithelial cells. **(B)** Herpes gladiatorum is also caused by a viral pathogen, herpes simplex virus-1 (HSV-1). This infection manifests as vesicular lesions and is classically with wrestlers. The lesions may be painful and local tingling or constitutional symptoms may occur. Infections are often secondary and occur following a primary oral infection. Recurrence of herpes gladiatorum may occur. Lesions are often on the face, neck, or arms. Herpes lesions are also vesicular; however, in this case, the dome-shaped papules with the central umbilication and the lack of any other clinical symptoms indicate that molluscum contagiosum is more likely than herpes gladiatorum.

(C) Common warts are caused by the human papilloma virus (HPV), a DNA virus. Warts usually lack a central depression and are more wrinkled or "wart-like" (see image [i] at the end of this answer). (D) Chicken pox is caused by the varicella zoster virus (VZV), an enveloped single-stranded DNA virus of the herpes virus family. Chicken pox appears as rash with pruritic (itchy), fluid-filled blisters that turn into scabs (see image [ii] at the end of this answer). The rash first appears on the face and trunk and may spread to other parts of the body. This is unlikely to be chicken pox. (E) Ringworm (also called dermatophytosis and cutaneous mycosis) is a fungal infection of the superficial skin layers of the skin. Infections may spread from person to person by direct contact with fomites. The infection presents as a scaly, circular lesion on various parts of the body (see image [iii] at the end of this answer). The clinical findings in this case indicate that ringworm is not the most likely diagnosis.

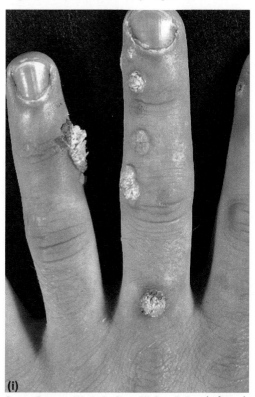

(i)

Source: Common Warts. In: Sterry W, Paus R, Burgdorf W, ed. Thieme Clinical Companions - Dermatology. 1st Edition. Thieme; 2006

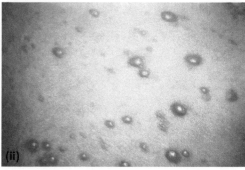

(ii)

Source: CDC/Dr. K.L. Hermann

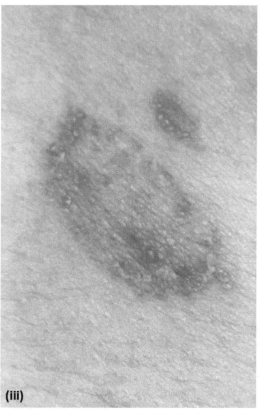

(iii)

Source: CDC/ Dr. Lucille K. Georg

38. Correct: *Leishmania donovani* (C)

(C) This infection is most likely caused by *Leishmania donovani*. *L. donovani* is transmitted by the bite of a sandfly and is endemic in Central America, South America, and Mexico. The parasite may cause cutaneous or visceral leishmaniasis. Cutaneous leishmaniasis may in rare cases spread to the mucosal surfaces of the mouth and nose. The cutaneous presentation is an ulcerative skin lesion with a raised outer border resembling a volcano. (A) Herpes simplex virus-2 is a sexually transmitted virus that usually presents as small painful lesions on the genitalia. (B) *Histoplasma capsulatum* is a fungal pathogen that may infect the lungs. It is transmitted to the human lung via conidia (spores) and in rare cases may disseminate to other body sites such as the eye and may disseminate to the skin. (D) *Plasmodium vivax* causes malaria, a blood-borne parasitic disease that causes recurrent cycles of fever and chills. It may result in profound anemia and a skin lesion is not typically present. (E) *Trypanosoma cruzi* is the parasitic pathogen that causes Chagas disease in Mexico, Central America, and South America. It is transmitted to humans through the bite of the triatomine bug (also known as the kissing or reduviid bug). Chagas disease initially presents as a chagoma at the site of infection and then progresses to a chronic infection with 20 to 30% of infected individuals progressing to serious debilitating disease with cardiac involvement.

Chapter 15

Cardiovascular, Systemic, Lymph Nodes, and Multisystem Infections

Melphine M. Harriott, Matthew P. Jackson, and Michelle Swanson-Mungerson

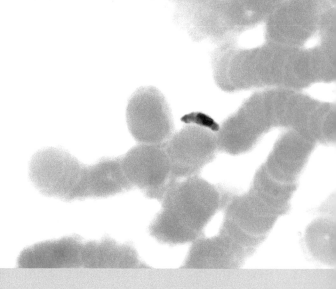

LEARNING OBJECTIVES

▶ Discuss the etiology, epidemiology, pathogenesis, clinical manifestations, complications, diagnosis, and treatment and prevention of:
  - infective endocarditis.
  - bloodstream and lymphatic infections.
  - meningitis, meningoencephalitis, encephalitis, myelitis, and brain lesions.
  - infectious hepatitis and
  - other liver infections and infections of the bile duct.

▶ Describe the laboratory diagnosis and antimicrobial testing methods for bacteria, viruses, fungi, yeast, and parasites.

▶ Discuss virulence mechanisms and correlate virulence mechanisms with specific pathogens.

▶ Discuss antimicrobial mechanism of action, spectrum of activity, common adverse effects, and resistance mechanisms.

▶ Discuss the production methods and advantages and disadvantages of a live attenuated vaccine.

15.1 Questions

Easy	Medium	Hard

1. A 28-year-old woman presents with fever, lethargy, and shortness of breath, especially upon physical exertion. She has a history of intravenous drug use (IVDU). Her temperature is 101.5°F (38.6°C) and a systolic murmur is heard on examination. An echocardiogram demonstrates vegetations on the native tricuspid valve leaflets. After 2 days, blood cultures grow gram-positive cocci. Which of the following is a characteristic of the most likely causative agent of this infection?

A. Catalase positive, coagulase negative

B. Catalase positive, coagulase positive

C. Catalase negative, α-hemolytic

D. Lactose positive (fermenter), oxidase negative

E. Lactose negative (non-fermenter), oxidase positive

2. A 62-year-old man presents to his primary care physician with a 2-week history of fever, muscle aches, and night sweats. He is otherwise healthy and active. History reveals a recent dental root canal procedure 5 weeks prior to the physician visit. On examination, his temperature is 38.6°C (100.4°F). Physical examination shows petechiae on his finger pads and hemorrhages under several fingernails. What other clinical or laboratory findings are most likely to be observed?

A. Headache and stiff neck

B. Heart murmur

C. Myocardial abscess

D. Antibody titers to streptolysin O

E. Positive tuberculin skin test

3. HACEK refers to a group of gram-negative bacteria that are an infrequent cause of native valve endocarditis. These organisms are considered culture negative because they:

A. Are strict anaerobes

B. Have fastidious growth requirements

C. Lack a cell wall

D. Require culture on Bordet–Gengou agar

E. Require culture on Thayer–Martin agar

4. A previously healthy 67-year-old woman presents with a 2-week history of generalized weakness, myalgia, fever, and headache. She recently travelled to Tennessee to see her grandchildren and reports that she removed a tick from her leg while there. She has no other significant travel or medical history. At the time of examination, her temperature is 38.7°C (101.8°C). Physical examination is unremarkable. Significant laboratory results are shown below:

- CBC:
  - WBC: 5.7×10^9/L
  - Platelets: 45×10^9/L
- Liver function tests:
  - AST: 679 U/L
  - ALT: 589 U/L
- Blood cultures:
  - No growth after 5 days

Which of the following is most likely to be observed from this patient's blood?

A. Peripheral blood, Giemsa stain

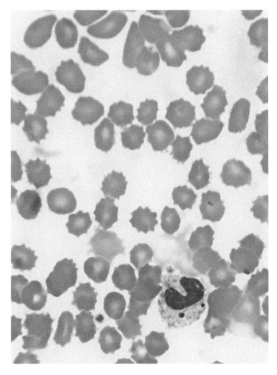

B. Bone marrow, Giemsa stain

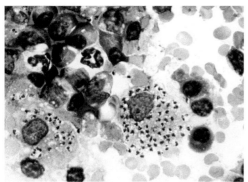

Source: Harriott M. Microbiology in Your Pocket. New York, NY: Thieme; 2017

C. Peripheral blood, Giemsa stain

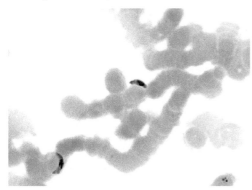

Source: Harriott M. Microbiology in Your Pocket. New York, NY: Thieme; 2017

D. Peripheral blood, Giemsa stain

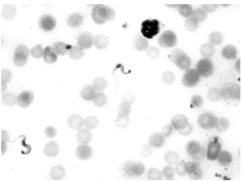

Source: Harriott M. Microbiology in Your Pocket. New York, NY: Thieme; 2017

E. Peripheral blood, Giemsa stain

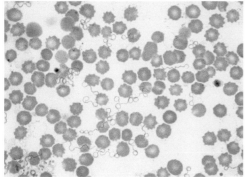

Source: Harriott M. Microbiology in Your Pocket. New York, NY: Thieme; 2017

5. A 34-year-old man presents with fever, chills, and headache of 3-day duration. He is an avid hunter and in the past several months he has skinned rabbits. On examination, his temperature is 38.8°C (101.9°F) and a small ulcer with a raised border and black base is seen on his right index finger. The epitrochlear lymph nodes on his right arm are swollen. Scrapings from the ulcer show gram-negative coccobacilli. Which of the following is the most likely causative agent of this infection?

A. *Bacillus anthracis*

B. *Corynebacterium diphtheriae*

C. *Coxiella burnetii*

D. *Francisella tularensis*

E. *Orientia tsutsugamushi*

6. A previously healthy 51-year-old woman, who works as a meat packer, complains of a 1-month history of fatigue, myalgia, and intermittent fever, which seems to get better during the night. In the last week she has also been experiencing arthralgia, especially in her hips. Her temperature is 38.4°C (101.1°F) and her physical examination is unremarkable. Blood cultures are obtained and after 2 days the Gram stain shows small gram-negative coccobacilli. Which of the following pathogens is most likely responsible for her symptoms?

A. *Bacillus anthracis*

B. *Bartonella henselae*

C. *Brucella abortus*

D. *Pasturella multocida*

E. *Streptobacillus moniliformis*

7. A previously healthy 28-year-old man has a 4-day history of fever, headache, and myalgia. He subsequently develops jaundice and seeks medical attention. He has a recent history of canoeing down a river while on a camping trip and states that his canoe tipped over, exposing him to the water. On examination, his temperature is 38.9°C (102°F) and his skin and eyes are icteric. Hepatomegaly is also observed.

- CBC:
  - Leukocyte count: 18.4×10^9/L
  - Bands: 8.2%
- Erythrocyte sedimentation rate (ESR): 40 mm/h
- ALT: 120 U/L
- AST: 189 U/L
- Total bilirubin: 4.3 mg/dL
- Microscopic agglutination test (MAT): positive

A liver biopsy is performed. Which of the following is the best stain to visualize the most likely agent of this infection from the liver biopsy?

A. Gram stain

B. Periodic-acid Schiff (PAS)

C. Trichrome

D. Warthin–Starry stain

E. Kinyoun

333

8. A previously healthy 55-year-old man presents with a 4-day history of fever and painful swelling of his thigh. He lives alone in a wooded mountain area in Eastern California. His temperature is 38.5°C (101.3°F). On examination, a bubo is noted over his right groin. The fluid from the bubo is aspirated and shows small gram-negative rods with a bipolar staining pattern. Which other infection is transmitted by the same vector as the most likely agent of this infection?

A. Babesiosis

B. Murine typhus

C. Rickettsialpox

D. Trench fever

E. Yellow fever

9. A 21-year-old man in Tanzania presents to the clinic with severe swelling of his leg. The swelling started approximately a year ago but has progressively become worse in the last several months and he is now having difficulty walking. On examination, extreme lymphedema of his right leg is noted and the skin on the affected leg is hardened. Two separate blood samples were obtained from the patient, one during the day and the other during the night. A blood smear from the specimen collected during the night shows the following organism.

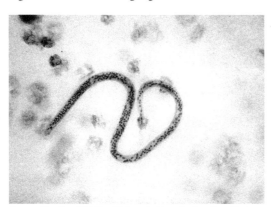

Source: Harriott M. Microbiology in Your Pocket. New York, NY: Thieme; 2017

Which of the following is the most likely causative agent of this infection?

A. *Dracunculus medinensis*

B. *Loa loa*

C. *Strongyloides stercoralis*

D. *Onchocerca volvulus*

E. *Wuchereria bancrofti*

10. A 45-year-old man presents to the emergency department with fever and chills of 4-day duration. He states that he has also been extremely tired and weak. He mentions that about 2 months ago he had vacationed in Martha's Vineyard in Massachusetts. On examination, his temperature is 39.9°C (103.8°F). His physical examination is unremarkable. A blood smear demonstrates the presence of a ring-shaped structure within red blood cells (RBCs). Which of the following agents would best manage this patient's infection?

A. Albendazole

B. Atovaquone plus azithromycin

C. Doxycycline

D. Nifurtimox

E. Miltefosine

11. A 37-year-old man in Ethiopia presents with a 2-day history of fever, chills, headache, myalgia, nausea, and vomiting. He reports that approximately a week and a half ago he had experienced fever but felt better within a few days. However, similar symptoms returned, which concerned him. His temperature is 38.9°C (102°F) and he is ill appearing. Blood smears demonstrate the presence of a spirochete. Which of the following is most likely to be directly contributing to the pathogenesis of this infection?

A. Antigen variation

B. Endotoxin

C. Erythrocyte invasion

D. Exotoxin

E. Molecular mimicry

12. A 4-year-old girl, who recently emigrated from Uganda, presents with a 5-day history of fever, chills, abdominal discomfort, nausea, and vomiting. Her parents state that the fever "seems to come and go." The parents mention that she had a similar illness in Uganda. On examination, her temperature is 39.3°C (102.7°F) and her blood pressure is 85/60 mm Hg. Her physical examination is unremarkable. A CBC shows a hemoglobin value of 10.2 g/dL. A blood smear from the patient is shown as follows:

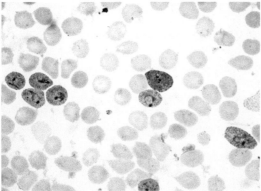

Source: Harriott M. Microbiology in Your Pocket. New York, NY: Thieme; 2017

Which of the following morphologic forms of the pathogen is most likely responsible for the relapse of this infection?

A. Gametocyte

B. Hypnozoite

C. Merozoite

D. Schizont

E. Trophozoite

13. A 23-year-old student who travelled to Ghana on a medical relief trip experiences periodic bouts of fever and chills 3 months after returning to the United States. She was provided prophylaxis medication prior to the trip but had not been consistently taking her dosage during the trip. Initially, the fever and chills occurred on a daily basis but became synchronized occurring every third day. Which molecular mechanism is responsible for the recurrent bouts of illness?

A. ADP-ribosylation

B. Antigenic variation

C. Molecular mimicry

D. Signal transduction

E. Type III secretion

14. A 28-year-old man presents with a 4-day history of fever, headache, myalgia, and right eye swelling. His symptoms started approximately 2 weeks following a trip to Rio de Janeiro, Brazil. On examination, his temperature is 37.5°C (99.5°F) and there is significant periorbital edema of his right eye. No drainage from the eye is noted, his sclerae are anicteric, and his conjunctivae appear normal without injection. The rest of his examination is normal. Which of the following laboratory tests would best confirm the diagnosis?

A. Culture on blood agar

B. Culture on Lowenstein–Jenson agar

C. KOH preparation

D. The stool ova and parasite examination

E. Thick and thin blood films

Consider the following case for questions 15 to 16:

A 60-year-old man presents with a 2-week history of fever, headache, and malaise. He is a dairy farmer and has daily exposure to many farm animals, especially cattle. He mentions that one of his female cows recently birthed a calf. His temperature is 38.4°C (101.2°F), his pulse is 93 beats per minute, and his blood pressure is 118/80 mm Hg. His physical examination is unremarkable. Pertinent laboratory results are shown below:

Laboratory tests from time of presentation:
• Brucella IgG antibody: <1:20
• Q fever IgG antibody: 1:64

The patient is seen in the clinic 3 weeks later for follow up, and laboratory results reveal the following:
• Brucella IgG antibody: <1:20
• Q fever IgG antibody: 1:256

15. Which of the following is the best treatment for this infection?

A. Ceftriaxone

B. Doxycycline

C. Nafcillin

D. Nitrofurantoin

E. Penicillin

16. Which of the following conditions is most likely to be observed in chronic infections with the causative agent of this infection?

A. Cellulitis

B. Endocarditis

C. Megacolon

D. Meningitis

E. Pneumonia

17. An 11-year-old boy presents with fever, chills, headache, and malaise of 4-day duration. His mother states that he recently returned from a camping trip with the Boy Scouts. His past medical history is unremarkable. His temperature is 38.4°C (101.7°F). Physical examination reveals conjunctival injection and a maculopapular rash on his trunk but not on his face or palms and soles. Routine laboratory tests including a CBC are ordered. While reviewing the Giemsa stained peripheral blood smear, a technologist notices inclusion bodies within monocytes. Which of the following is the most likely causative agent of this infection?

A. *Anaplasma phagocytophilum*

B. *Babesia microti*

C. *Borrelia burgdorferi*

D. *Ehrlichia chaffeensis*

E. *Rickettsia rickettsii*

Consider the following case for questions 18 to 20:

A 28-year-old man presents to the local clinic with hives, fever, chills, malaise, and headache of 2-day duration. He currently lives in Malawi and works with the Peace Corps. He states that the previous weekend he visited Lake Malawi and had gone kayaking and waterskiing. His temperature is 38.8°C (101.8°F). Physical examination is unremarkable. Laboratory results are shown below:

- CBC:
  - Leukocyte count: 8.9 × 10⁹/L
  - Segmented neutrophils: 58%
  - Bands:, 3%
  - Eosinophils: 7%
  - Lymphocytes: 27%
  - Monocytes: 5%
- Urinalysis:
  - Urine sediment demonstrates the presence of the following organism:

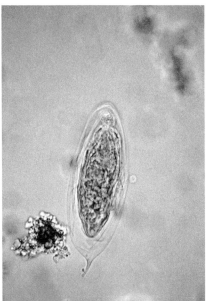

18. What is the most likely etiological agent of this infection?

A. *Ascaris lumbricoides*

B. *Coxiella burnetii*

C. *Francisella tularensis*

D. *Plasmodium falciparum*

E. *Schistosoma haematobium*

19. Which of the following is the most appropriate management for this patient?

A. Administration albendazole

B. Administration of chloroquine

C. Administration of praziquantel

D. Administration of streptomycin

E. No antibiotic therapy should be administered

20. The most likely mechanism of transmission of this infection is:

A. Bite of a mosquito

B. Bite of a tick

C. Contact with an infected animal

D. Ingestion of ova

E. Skin penetration by larvae

21. A 63-year-old woman returns from a vacation to the Virgin Islands in the Caribbean. During her last 2 days there she started feeling ill with a fever and just felt "bad." Three days after she returns from her trip she visits her primary care physician. She mentions she has had fever up to 39°C (102.3°F), joint and muscle pain, and just yesterday she noticed a rash on her stomach. She also notifies the clinician that she received numerous mosquito bites while on vacation. At the time of her visit, her temperature is 38.7°C (101.7°F). A blanching maculopapular rash is observed on her trunk, back, and arms. The rest of her physical examination is normal. Serological testing demonstrates the presence of IgM antibody for a specific alphavirus, which confirms the diagnosis. Which of the following is the most likely agent of this infection?

A. Chikungunya virus

B. Dengue virus

C. Ebola virus

D. Hantavirus

E. Zika virus

Source: Harriott M. Microbiology in Your Pocket.
New York, NY: Thieme; 2017

22. A 35-year-old man who lives in a rural area of Connecticut experiences joint pain and swelling of his right knee. He self-medicates with an over-the-counter analgesic for several days and continues life as usual. While shaving one morning, the man becomes rather alarmed when he notices the left side of his face is drooping. He lives alone so he asks a neighbor to drive him to the emergency department of the nearest hospital. As part of the history, on admission, the attending physician learns that the man spends a considerable amount of time outdoors. Which of the following cutaneous findings is most likely to be in this man's recent history?

A.

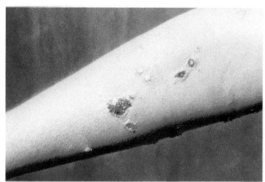

Source: CDC

B.

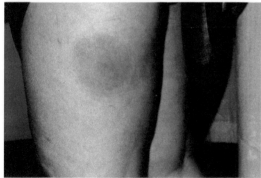

Source: CDC

C.

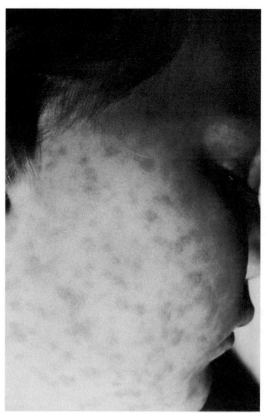

Source: CDC

D.

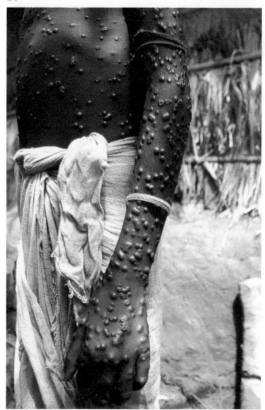

Source: CDC/Jean Roy

E.

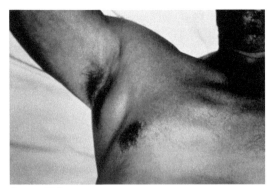

Source: CDC

23. A 23-year-old woman presents to her physician with a lesion on her right thumb. She states she recently took in a stray cat. Physical examination is notable for several scratches on her right hand and enlarged axillary lymph nodes. Which of the following is the most likely causative agent of this infection?

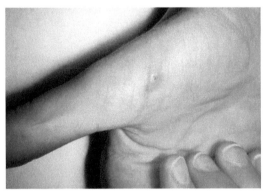

Source: CDC/Dr. Thomas F. Sellers, Emory University

A. Bartonella henselae

B. Borrelia burgdorferi

C. Pasteurella multocida

D. Rickettsia rickettsii

E. Staphylococcus aureus

24. The most accurate predictor of HIV-infected CD4+ lymphocytes in a patient with AIDS is:

A. Age of AIDS patient

B. Coinfection with Streptococcus pneumoniae

C. Gender of AIDS patient

D. Level of HIV RNA in plasma

E. Premature aging (senescence) of the immune system

25. A nurse returning from a medical relief trip to Guinea in West Africa develops a fever during the flight home. He identifies his concern to immigration officials in New York and is transferred and housed in isolation for the next 3 weeks. Blood, urine, and respiratory secretions should be screened for which of the following virus families?

A. Bunyaviridae

B. Filoviridae

C. Flaviviridae

D. Orthomyxoviridae

E. Togaviridae

26. A 12-year-old girl is carried in to the emergency department by her frightened parents after she had collapsed in their home. She had been experiencing a fever for the past 24 hours and a diffuse rash over her torso. The morning of hospital admission, the girl began vomiting and was complaining of muscle aches. On examination, her temperature `is 38.9°C (102.2°F) and her systolic blood pressure is 50 mm Hg. The physician notices significant vaginal erythema on removal of a tampon. Laboratory tests show that her phosphokinase creatinine levels are 2.5 times normal levels. Soon after her arrival she goes into cardiac arrest and attempts to resuscitate are unsuccessful. What is the most likely mechanism that caused the girl's death?

A. Adenylate cyclase activation

B. Antigenic cross-reactivity

C. Cross-linking T cell receptor and MHC II

D. Endotoxic shock

E. Type III secretion system

27. A 42-year-old man returns to his home in Los Angeles following a 2-week trip to Kenya. He had participated in a low-cost safari that involved sleeping in tents for several nights in the Masai Mara national park without mosquito protection. The man experienced symptoms that mimicked influenza including fever and chills, headache, and generalized body aches. Because he was experiencing these symptoms in July he went to an urgent care clinic. On examination, the urgent care physician notices symptoms of jaundice and suspected that the man's travel history was related to his illness. Immunization with which of the following would have most likely prevented the patient's travel-related illness?

A. Adjuvant

B. Attenuated virus vaccine

C. Conjugate vaccine

D. Subcellular vaccine

E. Toxoid

28. A 24-year-old man presents to the emergency department with a 2-day history of fever, headache, retro-orbital eye pain, and severe muscle and joint pain. Patient history is significant for returning from Argentina 1 week ago, where he was doing his second medical mission through his university. He had also become sick with a similar sickness and high fever after his first visit to Argentina. Vital signs are a temperature of 40°C (104°F) and blood pressure is 80/60 mm Hg. Physical examination reveals a maculopapular rash on his face. Laboratory results reveal elevated hematocrit, leukopenia, thrombocytopenia, and elevated AST levels. Which of the following receptors can increase the level of infection with the etiologic agent causing disease in this patient?

A. CD4

B. Complement receptor 2 (CR2)

C. DC-SIGN

D. Endothelial protein C (EPC) receptor

E. Fc receptor

29. A 16-year-old girl presents to the emergency department complaining of a bright red rash, joint pain, fever, headache, and eye pain for the past 5 days. Patient history is significant for returning from Puerto Rico on spring break 6 days ago. Vital signs are a temperature of 40.3°C (104.5°F) and blood pressure is 90/60 mm Hg. Physical examination reveals the presence of spontaneous petechiae. Based on the travel history, a tourniquet test is performed, which is positive. Which of the following laboratory findings is most likely be observed in this patient?

A. Decreased hematocrit

B. Decreased prothrombin time

C. Hyperproteinemia

D. Leukopenia

E. Normal AST levels

30. A 32-year-old woman is brought to the emergency department with severe abdominal pain, persistent vomiting with blood, restlessness, and a bloody nose. Patient history is significant for 5 days of high fever with headache, joint pain, rash, and retro-orbital eye pain after returning from a trip to Thailand. Physical examination reveals a temperature of 36.4°C (97.5°F), a respiratory rate of 36 breaths per minute, and is cold and clammy to the touch. Laboratory values demonstrate a 20% rise in hematocrit levels, elevated AST levels, severe thrombocytopenia, leukopenia, and a positive tourniquet test. Which of the following is the most likely etiologic agent causing this disease?

A. Chikungunya virus

B. Dengue virus

C. West Nile virus

D. Yellow fever virus

E. Zika virus

31. A 15-year-old girl is brought to her pediatrician by her mother with a chief complaint that her daughter has had "flu-like" symptoms for the past 3 days, including severe headache, high fever, joint and muscle pain, and severe pain behind her eye. Patient history is significant for a trip to Brazil 1 week ago. Physical examination reveals a temperature of 39.9°C (103.8°F) and a bright petechial rash that began today according to the mother. Laboratory results indicate leukopenia, thrombocytopenia, and elevated AST levels. Which of the following cell types is targeted for infection by the etiologic agent that is causing this disease?

A. Alveolar macrophages

B. Keratinocytes

C. Monocytes

D. Platelets

E. Red blood cells

15.2 Answers and Explanations

Easy	Medium	Hard

1. **Correct: Catalase positive, coagulase positive (B)**

(B) Overall, the most common pathogen of infective endocarditis is *Staphylococcus aureus*, a gram-positive coccus that is catalase positive and coagulase positive (answer choice B). In patients with a history of intravenous drug use (IVDU), *S. aureus* remains the most frequent agent implicated in endocarditis. Most often in endocarditis, the mitral and aortic valves are infected. However, in IVDU, the tricuspid valve is often infected because of the introduction of pathogens from the venous circulation to the right side of the heart. The modified Duke criteria are used for the diagnosis of infective endocarditis and include several facets including clinical presentation, laboratory testing, and cardiac studies. Nonspecific clinical findings of infective endocarditis include Osler's nodes (painful lesions of the extremities), Janeway lesions (erythematous lesions on the palms and soles), and Roth spots (retinal lesions). Osler's nodes and Roth spots are mediated by immune complexes whereas Janeway lesions are due to septic emboli. **(A)** All staphylococci species are catalase positive; however, only *S. aureus* is coagulase positive. Answer choice A describes the general category termed coagulase-negative staphylococci. One of the main clinically isolated species of coagulase-negative staphylococci is *S. epidermidis*. Coagulase-negative staphylococci are more commonly associated with prosthetic valve endocarditis rather than native valve endocarditis. There is no evidence in this case that the woman has a prosthetic valve and overall *S. aureus* is the most common agent of infective endocarditis; hence, answer choice A is incorrect. **(C)** *Streptococcus* species, especially viridans streptococci, are also common agents of infective endocarditis. Viridans streptococci are catalase negative and α-hemolytic. Like staphylococci, streptococci are gram-positive cocci. Viridans streptococci are most often associated with endocarditis, especially in individuals with poor dentition or a history of recent dental work. While it is possible that α-hemolytic streptococci may be involved in IVDU-associated endocarditis, it is more likely that *S. aureus* is involved. **(D, E)** Gram-negative pathogens, especially those of the HACEK group, are also common agents of endocarditis. However, enteric pathogens, such as *Escherichia coli*, which are lactose-positive (fermenters), oxidase negative **(D)**, and *Pseudomonas aeruginosa*, which are lactose negative (non-fermenters), oxidase positive **(E)**, are not typical agents of infective endocarditis. Of the answer choices provided, the most likely agent of this infection is *S. aureus*.

2. Correct: Heart murmur (B)

(B) This is a case of bacterial endocarditis most likely caused by the viridans streptococci group. In addition to the findings described in this case, a heart murmur is most likely to be observed. Several of the organisms classified in this group colonize the teeth and may be introduced into the bloodstream during dental procedures. The presentation of Osler's nodes, Janeway lesions (nodular lesions on the finger and toe pads, palms, and soles of the feet), splinter hemorrhages in the nail beds, and Roth spots (retinal lesions) are clinical presentations of endocarditis. Infective endocarditis with viridans streptococci may be indolent (slowly progressing) due to the low virulence of these organisms. **(A)** Headache and stiff neck would most likely indicate bacterial meningitis and this patient most likely has infectious endocarditis. *Streptococcus pneumoniae* may be implicated in rare cases of infective endocarditis and there is a possibility of developing secondary meningitis. However, in this case, a heart murmur is the best answer choice. **(C)** Myocardial abscess can be caused by *Staphylococcus aureus*. There is no evidence to suggest that a myocardia abscess is present in this case. The case presentation and etiology do not match *S. aureus* endocarditis, which has a fulminant course. **(D)** Antistreptolysin O titers indicate infection with *Streptococcus pyogenes*. *S. pyogenes* can cause pharyngitis and acute rheumatic fever is a sequela. Streptolysin O is a circulating virulence factor produced by *S. pyogenes*. **(E)** A positive tuberculin test indicates exposure to *Mycobacterium tuberculosis*. There is no evidence to suggest that this man has a high risk for exposure to *M. tuberculosis*.

3. Correct: Have fastidious growth requirements (B)

(B) Bacteria that constitute the HACEK group (*Haemophilus species*, *Aggregatibacter actinomycetemcomitans*, *Cardiobacterium hominis*, *Eikenella*

corrodens, *Kingella kingae*) have fastidious growth requirements. Bacteria in the HACEK group are all gram-negative rods or coccobacilli. These organisms can be cultured but may require additional nutrients and need CO_2 to grow. As a result of the fastidious growth requirements, these organisms may fail to grow on routine laboratory media. Hence infections with the HACEK group are often referred to as culture-negative endocarditis. *E. corrodens* tends to be easier to identify as this organism causes corrosion or pitting of the agar surface and has a bleach-like odor. **(A)** Strict (also called obligate) anaerobes include bacteria such as *Clostridium* or *Bacteroides* that use electron acceptors other than oxygen. Depending on their production of superoxide dismutase and catalase, the oxygen sensitivity of obligate anaerobes may vary from 0.5 to 8%. **(C)** *Mycoplasma pneumoniae*, a causative agent of walking pneumonia, and *Chlamydia trachomatis*, a causative agent of sexually transmitted infections, are examples of bacteria that lack a cell wall. The HACEK organisms all have a cell wall. **(D)** Bordet–Gengou agar is a selective media used for the cultivation of *Bordetella pertussis*, a gram-negative bacterium that causes whooping cough. **(E)** Thayer–Martin is a selective media used to culture pathogenic *Neisseria* species, particularly *N. meningitidis* and *N. gonorrhoeae*. See Appendix F for a list of high-yield bacteriology media.

4. Correct: Peripheral blood, Giemsa stain (A)

(A) The differential diagnosis in this case could include several infections and causative agents. However, the agent of this infection can be narrowed down to tick-borne infections that are common to the South Central United States. These infections include Rocky Mountain spotted fever (RMSF), Lyme disease, tularemia, human granulocytic anaplasmosis (HGA), and human monocytic ehrlichiosis (HME). Of these, the only pathogens represented in the answer choice are *Anaplasma* and *Ehrlichia*, which infect granulocytic cells (answer choice A shows a granulocytic cell). Classic laboratory findings in *Anaplasma* and *Ehrlichia* infections include thrombocytopenia, leukopenia, and elevated aminotransferases. A characteristic feature of infections with *Anaplasma* and *Ehrlichia* is the presence of inclusion bodies termed morulae in the cytoplasm of the infected cell as seen in answer choice A. The main species of *Ehrlichia* that infect humans are *E. chaffeensis* and *E. ewingii*. While *E. ewingii* infects granulocytes (like *Anaplasma*), *E. chaffeensis* infects monocytes; hence infections with this species are termed HME. It is not possible to microscopically distinguish *Anaplasma* from *E. ewingii* based on microscopy alone. Molecular testing, such as PCR can aid in a definite identification. RMSF and Lyme disease are best diagnosed with serology. The agent of tularemia, *Francisella tularensis*, is a gram-negative coccobacillus that will grow in blood culture bottles. Furthermore, tularemia tends to be much more serious and therefore patients are often more acutely ill compared to other tick-borne infections. None of the images supports these pathogens; hence, *Anaplasma* is the best answer. See Appendix L for a list of common vector-borne infections and corresponding vectors. **(B)** This is an image of *Leishmania* amastigotes. *Leishmania* is a protozoan parasite that infects macrophages. This case is unlikely to be due to *Leishmania* since the woman has not travelled to an endemic area. *Leishmania* is transmitted by the bite of a sandfly. **(C)** This image depicts a gametocyte of *Plasmodium falciparum*, an agent of malaria. This woman does not have a history of travel to a malaria endemic country; hence, this answer is incorrect. *Plasmodium* is protozoan parasites that infect red blood cells. The most common manifestations of malaria are cyclic fever and chills. **(D)** This image shows a trypomastigote of *Trypanosoma*, a flagellated protozoon parasite. This is unlikely to be the agent of this infection since infections are mainly seen in tropical countries outside of the United States. Since this woman's travel history is not significant for travel outside of the United States, infection with this pathogen is unlikely. Clinically significant species of *Trypanosoma* include *T. cruzi*, which is transmitted by reduviid bugs (i.e., kissing bugs, triatomine) and *T. brucei gambiense* and *T. brucei rhodesiense*, which are transmitted by tsetse flies. **(E)** Answer choice E shows an image of spirochetes in a blood smear. Spirochetes that may be seen in peripheral blood smears include *Leptospira* and *Borrelia*. *Leptospira* is unlikely to be the agent of this infection because it is not tick-borne and the infection in this case is most likely due to a tick bite. There are many species of *Borrelia* that are clinically significant, including *B. burgdorferi*, *B. recurrentis*, and *B. hermsii*. *B. burgdorferi* and *B. hermsii* are tick-borne while *B. recurrentis* is louse-borne. Clinical manifestations of this infection do not match infection with either *Leptospira* or *B. hermsii*. *Leptospira* causes a biphasic illness and classic findings of the acute phase include fever and conjunctival suffusion. Liver and renal dysfunction may be seen (Weil's disease) during the immune phase of the infection. *B. recurrentis* and *B. hermsii* both cause relapsing fever with repetitive cycles of abrupt fever followed by an afebrile phase. *B. burgdorferi* is the agent of Lyme disease and is not typically seen in blood smears.

5. Correct: *Francisella tularensis* (D)

(D) This man most likely has ulceroglandular tularemia caused by *Francisella tularensis*. The ulcer on his finger is an eschar, which most often forms at the site of inoculation. Because of this man's exposure to rabbits, the lymphadenopathy and the Gram stain findings of gram-negative coccobacilli, the most likely causative agent is *F. tularensis*. *F. tularensis* is

a zoonotic intracellular gram-negative coccobacillus. Commonly associated animals include small rodents and rabbits. This pathogen can also be transmitted by the bite of a tick, ingestion, and inhalation. Depending on the mechanism of transmission, different clinical manifestations may be observed. The most common form is ulceroglandular tularemia as described in this case, which occurs following a tick bite or contact with an infected animal. Another term for this infection is lymphocutaneous or lymphangitis in which cutaneous infections develop into draining sinus tracts that travel along the lymphatic channel. *F. tularensis*, if cultured in the laboratory, can pose harm to the laboratory staff. Additionally, patient specimens containing *F. tularensis*, if handled incorrectly, can also result in laboratory-acquired infections. Hence, if tularemia is suspected, clinicians should notify the clinical microbiology laboratory. Alternatively, serology may also aid in diagnosis. **(A)** *Bacillus anthracis* is a gram-positive rod and not a gram-negative coccobacillus as described in this case. Cutaneous anthrax is the most common manifestation of anthrax. Infections are characterized by lesions that begin as small, painless, erythematous pruritic papules that develop a central vesicle or bulla and eventually become painless necrotic ulcers with black depressed eschars. Edema of surrounding tissue may be present due to the production of an exotoxin. *B. anthracis* is a normal inhabitant of the soil and may infect various herbivores. Humans may be infected following contact with contaminated soil or handling of hides from infected animals, such as goats. **(B)** *Corynebacterium* are gram-positive rods; hence, this answer is incorrect. Most often *C. diphtheriae* causes respiratory infections; however, this pathogen may also be an agent of skin infections. Skin infections are more common in tropical countries. Infections are transmitted by direct contact with skin lesions from infected individuals. Lesions begin as papules that evolve into shallow ulcers with demarcated edges which may be covered with a grey–white membrane. **(C)** Like *F. tularensis*, *Coxiella burnetii* is a gram-negative coccobacillus. However, infections with *C. burnetii* do not typically result in skin manifestations or eschars, as seen in this case. Infections (i.e., Q fever) usually manifest as a febrile flu-like illness or atypical pneumonia. Primary infections may progress to the liver, resulting in hepatitis or the heart resulting in endocarditis. Transmission usually occurs following inhalation of aerosols from infected animals, especially goats and sheep. **(E)** Infections with *Orientia*, a *Rickettsia*-like organism, may result in eschar formation; however, this pathogen does not Gram stain. *Orientia tsutsugamushi* is the agent of scrub typhus that is transmitted by larval mites (chiggers) and infections are mainly seen in East Asia. This man has not travelled to an endemic area. Furthermore, his history of a hunting hobby indicates that tularemia is more likely to be the causative infection.

6. Correct: *Brucella abortus* (C)

(C) All the answer choices are zoonotic pathogens. However, because of this woman's occupation, clinical and laboratory findings, the most likely causative agent is *Brucella abortus. Brucella* species are small, gram-negative rods or coccobacilli. *Brucella* species are zoonotic pathogens and are associated with a variety of animals including goats and sheep (*B. melitensis*), cattle (*B. abortus*), and pigs/wild boar (*B. suis*). Meat packers, veterinarians, farmers, and other individuals in contact with these animals are at risk for infections. Infections are transmitted by ingestion of unpasteurized milk or other dairy products, inhalation of contaminated dust or aerosols or direct contact with contaminated animals or their sections. Infections are often nonspecific and indolent. Brucellosis is also referred to as undulant fever because the fever may peak during the day and defervesce during the night. Pain of the bones and joints may occur, which often affects the sacroiliac joint and large joints of the lower limbs. Like *Francisella*, *Brucella* can pose a risk to laboratory personnel, so the clinical laboratory should be notified of potential *Brucella* cases. In addition to culture, serology may also aid in the diagnosis of *Brucella*. **(A)** Based on this woman's occupation as a meat packer, this woman is certainly at risk for anthrax. However, her symptoms are more indolent and are not characteristic of anthrax. *Bacillus anthracis*, a gram-positive rod, is the agent of anthrax and is a zoonotic pathogen that is commonly associated with herbivores such as goats and sheep. Cutaneous infections occur following contact with contaminated animals or hides, respiratory infections occur following inhalation of spores, and gastrointestinal anthrax occurs following ingestion of spores from contaminated meat. Osteoarticular infections are not commonly associated with anthrax. **(B)** *Bartonella henselae*, a tiny gram-negative rod, is also a zoonotic pathogen and is transmitted by the scratch of a cat or bite from a cat or infected flea. However, infections usually manifest as a febrile illness with regional lymphadenopathy referred to as cat scratch fever. It is possible this infection could be due to *B. henselae*; however, based on clinical manifestations and her occupation, cat scratch fever is less likely. **(D)** *Pasteurella multocida*, a gram-negative coccobacillus, is normal oral microbiota of cats and dogs and infections are transmitted following a bite or scratch from an infected animal. Infections usually manifest as skin or soft tissue infections. There is the possibility that an infection with *P. multocida* may progress to septic arthritis or osteomyelitis and symptoms may then include fever and osteoarticular pain as described in the question stem. However, there is no indication of an antecedent wound. Furthermore, *P. multocida* is usually transmitted by smaller animals (dogs and cats) rather than larger animals that would likely be present in a meat packing plant. **(E)** *Streptobacillus moniliformis* is a gram-negative rod that is the agent of rat bite fever, which is most often transmitted from the scratch or bite of an infected rodent. Infections are usually less indolent than *Brucella* and clinical manifestations include fever, headache, joint pain, and rash. Based on the Gram stain, patient's occupation as a meat packer and indolent nature of this infection, this is more likely to be a case of brucellosis than rat bite fever.

7. Correct: Warthin–Starry stain (D)

(D) This infection is most likely caused by the spirochete *Leptospira interrogans* as indicated by the positive microscopic agglutination test (MAT). Like all spirochetes, *Leptospira* does not Gram stain well. The Warthin–Starry stain (answer choice D) is a silver stain and is useful for the identification of bacteria that do not stain well or at all with common stains such as Gram or Giemsa stains. With the Warthin–Starry stain, bacteria stain dark brown or black and the background is yellow (see image at the end of this answer). *Leptospira* is a zoonotic infection and the typical reservoir is rodents, but cattle, horses, pigs, and dogs may also harbor this pathogen. The organism is shed in the urine of infected animals and humans become infected following exposure to contaminated soil, water, urine, or other body fluid from these animals. High-risk activities include contact with contaminated water, such as in this case. Leptospirosis is a mild self-limiting infection or can manifest as an acute febrile disease. Conjunctival suffusion is often seen in infections. The pathogen may disseminate and subsequently result in meningitis, pulmonary hemorrhage, and renal and hepatic dysfunction (Weil's disease). The MAT is the standard test used for the diagnosis of leptospirosis, however; it is not readily available. The MAT test utilizes live *Leptospira* antigens to detect antibodies, if present, from the patient's serum. Therefore, serology and molecular assays are most often used for the diagnosis of leptospirosis. **(A)** The Gram stain is the most commonly used stain in the clinical microbiology laboratory but is not useful in visualizing spirochetes or other pathogens such as *Rickettsia*, *Chlamydia*, and *Mycoplasma*. The Gram stain differentially stains organisms pink or purple based on cell wall properties. Although spirochetes have a gram-negative cell wall, most spirochetes do not stain with the Gram stain. **(B)** Periodic-acid Schiff (PAS) stain is used for the visualization of carbohydrates in cell walls of fungi and human cells. This is stain in not typically used for the identification of spirochetes; hence, this answer is incorrect. **(C)** The trichrome stain is typically used to identify protozoan parasites, not spirochetes, which are bacteria. **(E)** The Kinyoun stain is an acid-fast stain used mainly for the identification of *Mycobacteria*. However, some bacteria, notably *Nocardia*, also stain with a modified version of acid-fast stains. Spirochetes are not acid-fast.

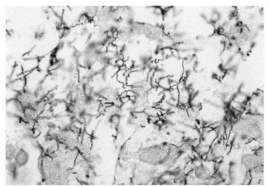

Source: CDC/Dr. Edwin P. Ewing, Jr.

8. Correct: Murine typhus (B)

(B) This man most likely has bubonic plague caused by *Yersinia pestis*, which is transmitted by the bite of a flea. Murine typhus (answer choice B) is also transmitted by the bite of a flea. In bubonic plague, swollen and inflamed lymph nodes or buboes are present and are most often seen in the groin and axillae. The ends of *Yersina* stain more readily than the center, giving the organism a bipolar appearance with Giemsa stain, which is often described as safety-pin–like (see image at the end of this answer). Other mechanisms of *Y. pestis* transmission include contact with contaminated animal fluid or tissue, which may result in bubonic or septicemic plague. While many animals are potential reservoirs of *Y. pestis*, small rodents such as mice, prairie dogs, and squirrels are commonly implicated in transmission. Domestic cats or dogs have also been known to be reservoirs (due to the carriage of rodent fleas) and humans may become infected following a scratch or bite from an infected cat or dog. Person-to-person transmission may also occur following exposure to respiratory droplets from an infected human. In the United States cases of plague have been noted in the Southwest, especially in New Mexico, Arizona, Utah, and Colorado as well as in California. The causative agent of murine (or endemic) typhus is *Rickettsia typhi*. In murine typhus constitutional symptoms are followed by a maculopapular rash that starts on the trunk and moves to the extremities, usually sparing the palms and soles. See Appendix L for a list of common vector-borne infections and corresponding vectors. **(A)** Babesiosis is caused by the protozoan parasite *Babesia* and is transmitted by the bite of a tick, not a flea. Babesiosis is characterized by fever and chills without periodicity. Buboes are not characteristic of babesiosis. **(C)** Rickettsialpox is caused by *Rickettsia akari* and is transmitted

by a mite and not a flea. In rickettsialpox a papule develops at the mite bite site. This papule eventually develops into a vesicle and then an eschar that encrusts. This organism does not infect the lymph nodes. **(D)** Trench fever is transmitted by lice, which makes this answer incorrect. The causative agent of trench fever is *Bartonella quintana*. *B. quintana* (and *B. henselae)* is also an agent of bacillary angiomatosis. Infections are characterized by flu-like symptoms, bone pain, and a macular rash, usually on the trunk. Another species of *Bartonella, B. henselae* may infect lymph nodes and is transmitted by a cat bite, cat scratch or infected flea resulting in cat scratch fever/disease. **(E)** Yellow fever is caused by a virus, the yellow fever virus, and is transmitted by mosquitoes, not fleas. Yellow fever is a febrile illness with conjunctival injection that may progress to hepatitis or hemorrhagic fever. This organism is mainly limited to tropical areas and would not typically be associated with Eastern California.

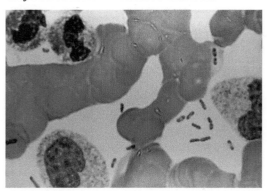

Source: CDC

9. Correct: *Wuchereria bancrofti* (E)

(E) Severe lymphedema or elephantiasis is a classic finding observed in infections with the filarial nematodes, *Wuchereria bancrofti* (answer choice E) and *Brugia malayi*. Infections may be asymptomatic, acute, or chronic. Chronic infections may result in severe lymphedema (see image [i] at the end of this answer), as described in this case. Adult worms reside in the lymphatics but produce microfilariae that migrate to the blood and lymph. Infections may be diagnosed by the identification of microfilariae in Giemsa stained blood smears, as shown in the question stem. The microfilariae are nocturnal; hence, blood specimens obtained at night are more likely to contain the parasite. Both *Wuchereria* and *Brugia* are transmitted by the bite of a mosquito. *B. malayi* is mainly seen in Southeast Asia whereas *W. bancrofti* is mainly seen in the Indian subcontinent and sub-Saharan Africa. **(A)** *Dracunculus medinensis* is a nematode that causes guinea worm disease. This worm is not typically seen in peripheral blood smears. Furthermore, clinical manifestations of guinea worm

343

disease differ from the symptoms described in this case. Therefore, this answer is incorrect. Humans become infected with *D. medinensis* following ingestion of water containing copepods, which contain *D. medinensis* larvae. Infections occur approximately 12 months after transmission and are characterized by constitutional symptoms followed by a skin papule, usually located on the lower extremities. As the papule becomes larger, it becomes more painful and the worm eventually emerges from the papule (see image [ii] at the end of this answer). This infection is most common in Africa, India, and the Middle East. **(B)** Similar to *Wuchereria*, *Loa loa* is a filarial nematode. The microfilariae of *L. loa* look very similar to *Wuchereria* microfilariae microscopically (see image [iii] at the end of this answer). However, the clinical findings seen in this case differ from infections with *L. loa*, so answer choice B is incorrect. There are two characteristic features of infections with *L. loa*: calabar swelling and eye worm. Calabar swellings are localized areas of transient subcutaneous swelling/angioedema, especially of the extremities and around the face. The area around the swelling may be itchy. In eye worm, the adult worm may cross the surface of the eye and even the bridge of the nose. *L. loa* is transmitted by the bite of a deerfly, also called mango fly. Infections are mainly seen in Central Africa. **(C)** *Strongyloides stercoralis* is a nematode and the diagnostic form of the pathogen is the rhabditiform larvae (see image [iv] at the end of this answer), which may be seen in the stool or respiratory specimens. Infections are mainly asymptomatic but if symptomatic, clinical manifestations differ from infections with *Wuchereria* and *Brugia*. Gastroenteritis, pneumonitis, and urticaria are the most common findings of strongyloidiasis. Severe lymphadenitis as described in this case is not typically observed. Infections are transmitted following skin penetration by the infective filariform larvae. Infections occur worldwide but are endemic in tropical countries, including African nations. **(D)** *Onchocerca volvulus* (see image [v] at the end of this answer) is another filarial parasite that looks very similar to *Wuchereria* and *Brugia*. *O. volvulus* most often causes eye infections, including lesions, keratitis, and uveitis. Infections are often referred to as "river blindness" and are transmitted by the bite of a black fly. *O. volvulus* may also cause a pruritic

rash and nodules in subcutaneous tissue. In rare cases, this pathogen may also cause severe edema. However, the most common causative agents of lymphatic filariasis are *Wuchereria* and *Brugia*; hence, answer choice D is incorrect.

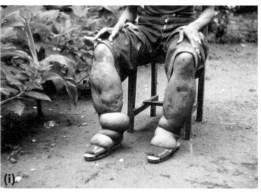

(i)

Source: CDC

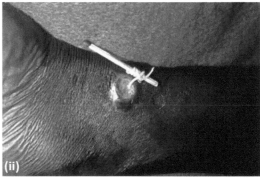

(ii)

Source: CDC

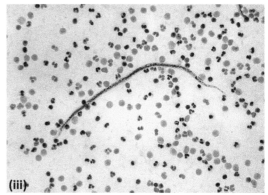

(iii)

Source: CDC/Dr. Lee Moore

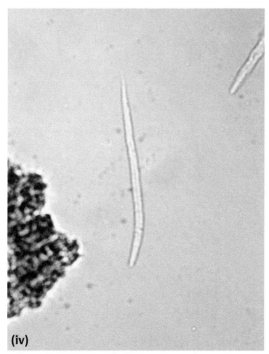

(iv)

Source: Harriott M. Microbiology in Your Pocket. New York, NY: Thieme; 2017

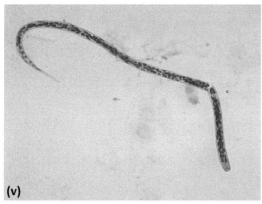

(v)

Source: CDC/Dr. Lee Moore

10. Correct: Atovaquone plus azithromycin (B)

(B) This infection is due to *Babesia*, a protozoon parasite that infects red blood cells. Infections can be treated with atovaquone plus azithromycin. Atovaquone is mainly used in the treatment of *Babesia* and *Pneumocystis*. This agent interferes with the electron transport chain of the pathogen. Azithromycin is a macrolide that inhibits bacterial protein synthesis. In the United States, *B. microti* is a commonly isolated *Babesia* species and the merozoites of *B. microti* may resemble a Maltese cross or rosette (see image at the end of this answer). Note that *Babesia* is transmitted via the bite of the tick. The same species of tick also transmits *B. burgdorferi* (Lyme disease) *Anaplasma* (anaplasmosis), and Powassan virus. In the United States, *B. microti* and Lyme disease are found primarily in the Northeast. **(A)** Albendazole is an antihelminthic agent that destroys

the cytoskeleton of parasites. It is effective against some protozoa but not *Babesia*; hence, answer choice A is incorrect. Albendazole is mainly used to treat nematodes (roundworms) and some cestodes (mainly *Taenia solium*; neurocysticercosis) and some trematodes. **(C)** Doxycycline is an antibacterial agent that inhibits protein synthesis and is used for many infections, including bacterial tick-borne infections, such as rickettsial diseases, ehrlichiosis, and anaplasmosis. Doxycycline is not effective against *Babesia*, which is a tick-borne parasitic infection. **(D)** Nifurtimox is used in the treatment of infections caused by the protozoan parasite, *Trypanosoma*. Nifurtimox is not typically used in the management of *Babesia*. The mechanism of action of this agent is not completely understood but it is thought to induce the formation of toxic free radicals leading to DNA damage. **(E)** Miltefosine induces cell death by interfering with lipids and cytochrome c oxidase. This agent is used in the treatment of leishmaniasis, caused by the protozoa *Leishmania*. Miltefosine is not used in the management of babesiosis.

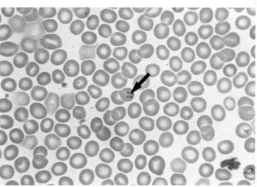

Source: CDC/Dr. Mae Melvin

11. Correct: Antigen variation (A)

(A) This man has relapsing fever caused by *Borrelia* species. *Borrelia* species can vary the antigens on the cell surface leading to the inability of the immune system to recognize the pathogen (i.e., antigenic variation, answer choice A). This leads to subsequent episodes of fever and other symptoms. Two common species of *Borrelia* include *B. recurrentis* and *B. hermsii*. *B. recurrentis* is seen worldwide but is endemic in parts of Africa and is transmitted by lice. *B. hermsii* is also seen worldwide but is transmitted by ticks. In relapsing fever there is an abrupt onset of fever, chills and other constitutional symptoms, which last a few days. During the afebrile period, the patient may feel well; however, after a few days (typically within 2 weeks), the fever and symptoms occur again. Other common findings of relapsing fever include hypotension, petechiae, and myocarditis. **(B)** Endotoxin is synonymous with lipopolysaccharide (LPS). *Borrelia* has gram-negative cell walls that contain LPS, which may contribute to the development of the fever. But it is the

345

ability of the organism to escape the host immune system by varying the antigens on the cell surface that mainly contributes to the pathogenesis of recurrent fever. Therefore, answer choice B is incorrect. **(C)** This answer is incorrect because *B. recurrentis* and *B. hermsii* are found in the bloodstream but do not invade into RBCs. Pathogens that do infect RBCs include *Plasmodium, Babesia, Bartonella quintana*, and parvovirus B19. **(D)** This answer is incorrect because *B. recurrentis* and *hermsii* do not produce secreted toxins (i.e., exotoxins). **(E)** This answer is incorrect because there is no evidence to suggest that *B. recurrentis* and *hermsii* undergo molecular mimicry. Molecular mimicry occurs when a foreign antigen resembles a self-antigen resulting in a nonspecific immune response against the self-antigen. An example of molecular mimicry is the development of rheumatic fever following *Streptococcus pyogenes* infections.

12. Correct: Hypnozoite (B)

(B) This girl most likely has malaria as indicated by the fever, chills, and image (presented in the question stem) depicting the ring form of *Plasmodium* species in her blood smear. In this case the infecting species is most likely to be *P. vivax* or *P. ovale* due to the recurrence of infection. Relapses with these two species occur due to hypnozoites (answer choice B), which are dormant forms that reside in the liver and may be reactivated after initial infection. Malaria is widely seen in tropical countries and is transmitted by the bite of the female *Anopheles* mosquito. The protozoan parasite lives in RBCs, which can lead to RBC destruction and hemolytic anemia. The fever and chills occur at regular intervals or paroxysms (species dependent; every 48 or 72 hours) because all of the parasites within the host RBCs are at approximately the same stage of development. Fever is induced when RBCs rupture and merozoites are released. This may be followed by a period of intense sweating and chills. **(A, C, D, E)** The gametocyte, merozoite, schizont, and trophozoite are all morphological forms of *Plasmodium* but are not responsible for the recurrence of infection. *Plasmodium* species possess over two dozen morphological forms. The trophozoite or ring form is the earliest form. The immature schizont is the beginning stage of the developed asexual sporozoa trophozoite. This form will then mature and fully develop, which is characterized by the presence of mature merozoites. The gametocytes can be categorized into two forms: microgametocyte or male sex cell and macrogametocyte or female sex cell. See following image for an overview of the *Plasmodium* life cycle.

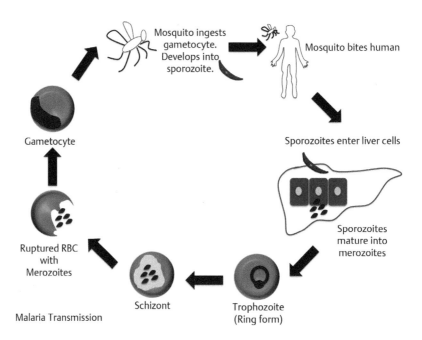

13. Correct: Antigenic variation (B)

(B) This is a case of malaria that was acquired by the traveler while on a trip to Ghana where the disease is endemic. Prophylaxis can prevent acquiring malaria and the fact that the student failed to maintain her dosage or was prescribed ineffective medication due to resistance of the endemic *Plasmodium* strains (chloroquine resistance is widespread) contributed to the appearance of disease upon her return to the United States. Antigenic variation is responsible for the expression of different proteins on the surface of *Plasmodium* species confounding the host immune response to parasitemia. Different species of the malaria pathogen exhibit synchronized life cycles in the bloodstream with *P. vivax*, *P. ovale*, and *P. falciparum* following a tertian cycle. (A) ADP-ribosylation is the enzymatic mechanism of some bacterial cytotoxins such as cholera toxin and pertussis toxin. (C) Molecular mimicry refers to the convergent evolution that results in the surface proteins of a pathogen sharing sequence homology with host protein. One example is the M protein of *Streptococcus pyogenes* that induces cross-reactive antibodies to human myosin protein. (D) Signal transduction is a process used by prokaryotic and eukaryotic cells to respond to environmental signals. (E) Type III secretion is responsible for the direct injection of effector proteins into mammalian cells by bacterial pathogens such as *Yersinia pestis*. Type III secretion requires direct cell-to-cell contact.

14. Correct: Thick and thin blood films (E)

(E) The periorbital edema (Romaña's sign; see image [i] at the end of this answer) is a classic finding in Chagas disease, caused by *Trypanosoma cruzi*, a flagellated protozoan parasite. Chagas disease is mainly seen in Central and South America and is transmitted via a reduviid bug (also called triatomine or kissing bug). The bug defecates in the bite site and when the infected individual scratches the site, the parasite enters the host and migrates to tissue. These tissue forms or amastigotes mature into flagellated trypomastigotes (see image [ii] at the end of this answer) in the peripheral blood and are the diagnostic form of the pathogen. Trypomastigotes are best seen with thick and thin blood films. (A) Culture on blood agar, a nonselective medium, is a good method of diagnosing common bacterial infections, such as those caused by urinary tract or respiratory pathogens. *T. cruzi*, the causative agent of this infection, does not grow on blood agar. (B) Lowenstein–Jensen agar is a selective

and differential agar for *Mycobacterium* species. *T. cruzi*, the causative agent of this infection, does not grow on Lowenstein–Jensen agar. (C) KOH preparations are used in the diagnosis of fungal infections. KOH can aid in dissolving keratin and other cellular material from clinical specimens, allowing for better visualization of yeast and hyphal elements. *Trypanosoma cruzi*, the causative agent of this infection, would be better visualized with thick and thin blood films, which are usually Giemsa stained. (D) The stool ova and parasite examination is the classic diagnostic test to determine if an enteric parasite is present in the stool. Stool specimens are usually stained with trichrome stains and evaluated microscopically for parasites. *Trypanosoma* would not be seen in the stool or stain with trichrome stain; hence, answer choice E is the best answer.

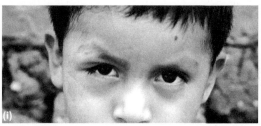

Source: CDC/Dr. Mae Melvin

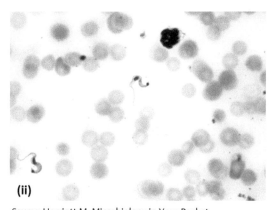

(ii)

Source: Harriott M. Microbiology in Your Pocket. New York, NY: Thieme; 2017

15. Correct: Doxycycline (B)

(B) This man's occupation as a farmer, his exposure to farm animals, his clinical findings, and his laboratory tests indicate that the most likely infecting agent is *Coxiella burnetii*, a small gram-negative coccobacillus. Acute infections with this pathogen are referred to as Q fever and the drug of choice is doxycycline, a tetracycline that inhibits protein synthesis. See

Appendix I for a list of major antibiotic classes and mechanisms of action. Other effective agents include fluoroquinolones and macrolides. Note that patients may also be asymptomatic and treatment may not be indicated in these cases. Laboratory diagnosis of infection is usually confirmed by serological analysis (of phase I and phase II antibodies) or molecular testing. For serological analysis, serum is drawn early during the infection and then again approximately 3 to 4 weeks later (paired serum). A fourfold or greater increase in the titer (of phase II antibodies) is consistent with acute infection. Human transmission of *Coxiella* most often occurs following inhalation of the pathogen. Infections are frequently associated with contaminated placenta and other fluids from pregnant animals. Other mechanisms of infection include ingestion of unpasteurized dairy products. (Note: *Coxiella* antibodies are divided into phase I and phase II antibodies. Diagnosis of acute infections is dependent on at least a fourfold rise in titer of phase II antibodies. In contrast, during chronic infections phase I titers will be increased over time and greater than phase II titers. See the Centers for Disease Control and Prevention [CDC] website on Q fever for more information on phase I and phase II antibodies.) **(A)** Ceftriaxone is used in several infections including infections with the gram-negative pathogens *Neisseria* and *Haemophilus* but not for *Coxiella*. **(C)** Nafcillin, a β-lactam antibiotic is mainly used in the treatment of methicillin-sensitive staphylococcal infections. **(D)** Nitrofurantoin is a broad-spectrum antimicrobial used for the treatment of uncomplicated cystitis. This agent interferes with bacterial carbohydrate metabolism. **(E)** Penicillin is a β-lactam agent that inhibits cell wall synthesis and is used in a number of infections but is not indicated for Q fever.

16. Correct: Endocarditis (B)

(B) The most common finding of chronic Q fever is infective endocarditis. *Coxiella* may also affect the bones and joints resulting in pain. **(A, C, D)** Cellulitis, megacolon, and meningitis are not typical findings of acute or chronic infections with *C. burnetii*. **(E)** Pneumonia, most often atypical pneumonia, is a finding of acute, not chronic, Q fever. Another classic finding of acute Q fever is hepatitis.

17. Correct: *Ehrlichia chaffeensis* (D)

(D) This boy most likely has ehrlichiosis or human monocytic ehrlichiosis (HME) as it is often referred to. This pathogen is transmitted by a tick bite and camping puts this child at risk for infection. See Appendix L for a list of common vector-borne diseases and corresponding vectors. This bacterial pathogen is an obligate intracellular organism that infects monocytes and inclusion bodies termed morulae may be seen within infected cells. Common clinical manifestations of HME include fever, conjunctival injection, and a rash. Note that the rash most often does not affect the palms and soles and most often the rash is seen in children but not adults. **(A)** *Anaplasma* and *Ehrlichia* are closely related bacterial pathogens. Both are obligate intracellular pathogens that are transmitted by ticks and clinical manifestations are often indistinguishable. Furthermore, infected cells with either pathogen may contain morulae. However, *Anaplasma* infects granulocytic cells and not monocytes; hence, this answer choice is incorrect. **(B)** *Babesia microti* is a protozoan parasite that is also transmitted by a tick. However, this pathogen infects red blood cells, not monocytes. **(C)** *Borrelia burgdorferi* is the agent of Lyme disease, a tick-borne infection. This spirochete-shaped bacterium is mainly extracellular; hence, it would most likely not be visualized within monocytes. **(E)** *Rickettsia rickettsii* is an obligate intracellular bacterium and is tick-borne. This pathogen causes Rocky Mountain spotted fever (RMSF). Symptoms are very similar to *Ehrlichia* and *Anaplasma* infections. However, the rash of RMSF is frequently noted on the palms and soles as well as on the body. Furthermore, *R. rickettsii* most often infects endothelial cells and not monocytes; hence, answer choice D (*Ehrlichia*) is more likely the causative agent in this case.

18. Correct: *Schistosoma haematobium* (E)

(E) The image presented in the question stem shows an ovum of *Schistosoma haematobium* and the patient is exhibiting signs of acute schistosomiasis. This trematode or fluke is mainly seen in Africa and the Middle East. Typical manifestations of schistosomiasis include urticaria, angioedema, arthralgias, fever, chills, and headache. Schistosomiasis is a type IV hypersensitivity reaction and can be caused by other schistosomes as well including *S. mansoni* and *S. japonicum*. Adult *S. haematobium* worms live in the venous plexus of the bladder and the eggs are then released in the urine. Elevated eosinophil counts are often present in these infections. The terminal spine, as seen in the image in the question stem, is the key to identifying *S. haematobium* ova. *S. mansoni* has a large lateral spine while *S. japonicum* has a small lateral spine which aids in the differentiation of these pathogens. **(A)** *Ascaris lumbricoides* is a nematode worm that may cause gastrointestinal symptoms when the pathogen is in the gastrointestinal tract or pulmonary symptoms as larvae migrate through the lungs. The manifestations described in this case do not resemble an *Ascaris* infection. However, similar to schistosomiasis, eosinophilia may be present in infections caused by other helminthes, including *Ascaris*. **(B)** *Coxiella burnetii*, a gram-negative coccobacillus and obligate intracellular pathogen, is the causative agent of Q fever. Q fever may manifest with an acute onset of fever, headache, and myalgia.

Q fever may also present acutely as a pneumonia or hepatitis. *C. burnetti* infections are associated with sheep, cows and goats and infections are transmitted by inhalation. Farmers and veterinarians are at increased risk for infection. This man's travel history and finding of the ova in the urine indicate that *S. haematobium* is the agent of this infection. **(C)** *Francisella tularensis* is a gram-negative rod or coccobacillus. There are several forms of disease and all start with an acute onset of chills, fever, and malaise. The most common form of infection is ulceroglandular tularemia in which a painful papule develops at the site of inoculation. The papule eventually becomes necrotic and leaves an ulcer with an eschar. Tularemia is transmitted via the bite of a tick or handling of infected animals, especially rabbits. The clinical findings and travel history indicate that *S. haematobium* is more likely the agent of this infection. **(D)** *Plasmodium* species are protozoan parasites and are the causative agents of malaria. Malaria is mainly seen in tropical countries and the characteristic features of malaria are paroxysms of fever and chills. *Plasmodium* infects red blood cells, and the thick and thin blood films aid in diagnosis. Based on this man's travel history, malaria is certainly a plausible agent of infection. However, his exposure to water and the finding of the ova in the urine sediment indicate that *S. haematobium* is the most likely agent of this infection.

19. Correct: Administration of praziquantel (C)

(C) The image presented in the question stem shows a *Schistosoma haematobium* ovum and the patient is exhibiting signs of acute schistosomiasis. Praziquantel is an antihelminthic agent that can be used in the treatment of flukes including schistosomiasis and *Clonorchis sinensis*, the human liver fluke. The exact mechanism of action is unknown, but praziquantel increases the permeability of the parasite cell membrane. **(A)** Albendazole is a broad-spectrum antihelmintic agent that is used to treat roundworm (*Ascaris lumbricoides*) and hookworm (*Ancylostoma duodenale* and *Necator americanus*) infections, neurocysticercosis (*Taenia solium*), and hydatid disease (*Echinococcus granulosus*). Albendazole inhibits tubulin polymerization that ultimately results in destruction of the cytoplasmic microtubules. **(B)** Chloroquine is used in the treatment of malaria, which is caused by *Plasmodium* parasites. It is important to note that there is increasing resistance of *Plasmodium* to this agent so alternative agents may have to be used. The exact mechanism of action is unknown, but chloroquine is thought to interact with the *Plasmodium* DNA. **(D)** Streptomycin, an aminoglycoside that inhibits protein synthesis, may be used in the management of the febrile illness, tularemia, caused by *Francisella tularensis*. **(E)** Some febrile illnesses including mild cases of Q

fever caused by *Coxiella burnetii* are self-limiting and antimicrobial therapy is not warranted.

20. Correct: Skin penetration by larvae (E)

(E) The image presented in the question stem shows a *Schistosoma haematobium* ovum and the patient is exhibiting signs of acute schistosomiasis. *Schistosoma* ova are deposited in fresh water and develop into larvae. Miracidia, larval forms, enter fresh water snails and continue development. Cercaria, another morphological form of the organism, is then released from the snails and can penetrate human skin (answer choice E). This man's exposure to fresh water put him at risk for this organism. **(A)** *Plasmodium* parasites and many other pathogens are transmitted via a bite of a mosquito. See Appendix L for a list of common infections transmitted by mosquitos. **(B)** Many pathogens are transmitted via ticks including *Borrelia burgdorferi*, the causative agent of Lyme disease. Tularemia may also be transmitted via the bite of a tick. **(C)** Many zoonotic pathogens cause febrile illness including *Francisella* and *Coxiella*. *Francisella* is associated with voles, muskrats, beavers, and rabbits and is found mainly in the Northern Hemisphere. Infections may occur via direct contact with an infected animal, animal products, or inhalation. *Coxiella* is associated with goats, sheep, and cattle. **(D)** *Ascaris lumbricoides* and many other parasites are transmitted via ingestion of ova or eggs. *Schistosoma* is transmitted by cercariae that penetrate human skin.

21. Correct: Chikungunya virus (A)

(A) Based on this woman's travel history and that she was bitten by mosquitos, arthropod-borne infections such as dengue, Zika, and chikungunya are most likely. All three, present with similar clinical findings, are transmitted by mosquitos. Classic findings in these three infections include muscle or joint pain, headache, retro-orbital pain, rash, and conjunctivitis. In this case, the serological analysis confirmed the identity of the causative agent, an alphavirus. Alphaviruses are part of the togavirus family and the only pathogen in the answer choice that is in this category is chikungunya virus (answer choice A). Other togaviruses of clinical interest include rubella, eastern equine encephalitis (EEE), western equine encephalitis (WEE), and Venezuelan equine encephalitis (VEE). See Appendix N for a list of clinically significant viruses and their corresponding characteristics. **(B, E)** Infections with dengue and Zika virus present in a very similar manner and may be found in similar tropical regions. However, both of these viruses are part of the flavivirus family and not the alphavirus group or togavirus family. **(C)** Ebola infections may present as febrile illness with a rash or present with hemorrhagic fever. Infections with Ebola virus, a filovirus, are mainly seen in West Africa. This woman's travel history and clinical manifestations are not consistent with Ebola. Furthermore, Ebola is a filovirus and not a togavirus. **(D)** Hantavirus is a bunyavirus that presents as a febrile illness with shock and pulmonary edema or hemorrhagic fever. Infections are transmitted from aerosols from rodent excreta. Hantavirus may be seen worldwide in select regions. The clinical manifestations in this case do not resemble infection with Hantavirus. Moreover, serological testing demonstrates that the agent of this infection is an alphavirus/togavirus and not bunyavirus.

22. Correct: (B)

(B) The causative agent of Lyme disease is *Borrelia burgdorferi*, a spirochete that is transmitted to humans by ticks. Answer B shows a bullseye or target-shaped rash of Lyme disease. The white-tailed deer is an animal reservoir and incidence of disease is greatest in the northeastern United States and parts of the Midwest. The initial sign of infection (within 1 week) is a bullseye-shaped rash accompanied by fever and other nonspecific symptoms. Approximately 1 month after infection, the patient may experience severe headache, neck stiffness, facial or Bell's palsy (droop on one or both sides of the face), arthritis, heart palpitations, dizziness, memory loss, and neuralgia (nerve pain). **(A)** This is an image of impetigo, which is caused by *Streptococcus pyogenes* or *Staphylococcus aureus*. Infection with *S. pyogenes* may lead to sequelae such as acute glomerulonephritis but not the neurologic symptoms seen in this patient. **(C)** This is an image of the rash of Rocky Mountain spotted fever (RMSF), which is also transmitted to humans by the bite of a tick. The causative agent of this infection is *Rickettsia rickettsii*. The Rickettsiae are intracellular parasites with RMSF predominating in the southeastern United States. The petechiae (rash) for this disease are characteristic, appearing on the palms and soles of the feet. **(D)** This image depicts the classic findings of smallpox caused by Variola virus. This infection was eradicated in 1977, but may be found in rare cases in rural Afghanistan and Pakistan. Any significant appearance of the disease would be through an act of bioterrorism. The differential diagnosis is with chickenpox with the distinction that the smallpox vesicles are all at the same stage of development. With chickenpox the vesicles are at different stages of development. **(E)** This image shows the swollen lymph nodes seen in bubonic plague. Rare cases of bubonic plague occur each year in the United States (average seven per year); typically, sylvatic plague transmitted by the bite of a flea carrying the causative agent *Yersinia pestis*. Wild rodents serve as a reservoir of the bacterial pathogen. The organism has a tropism for the lymphatics causing the grossly swollen lymph nodes (buboes). Dissemination of the organism and disseminated intravascular coagulation cause tissue death

and necrosis leading to gangrenous acral regions of the body hence the term "black death."

23. Correct: *Bartonella henselae* (A)

(A) Because of the cutaneous manifestations and the lymphadenopathy this infection is most likely due to *Bartonella henselae*, the agent of cat scratch fever. An inhabitant of the oral cavity of cats, *B. henselae* may be transferred to their claws and be the source of regional lymphadenopathy near a scratch. While the bacterium may cause chronic lymphadenopathy in children through repeated injury it is a self-limiting infection in otherwise healthy individuals. Immunocompromised injured patients may develop bacillary angiomatosis (vascular infection) and hepatic or splenic peliosis (hemorrhagic lesions). **(B)** *Borrelia burgdorferi* is the causative agent of Lyme disease transmitted to humans through the bite of a tick. Early stages of infection are characterized by a bull's-eye–shaped rash surrounding the inoculation site (see image at the end of this answer). **(C)** *Pasteurella multocida* causes cellulitis following a dog or cat bite. It will not usually cause the lymph node involvement seen with *B. henselae*. **(D)** Rocky Mountain spotted fever (RMSF) also transmitted to humans by the bite of a tick with *Rickettsia rickettsii* as the causative agent of infection. The Rickettsiae are intracellular parasites with RMSF predominating in the southeastern United States. The petechiae (rash) for this disease are characteristic, appearing on the palms and soles of the feet. **(E)** *Staphylococcus aureus* would most likely occur through autologous transmission and would most likely cause a pruritic skin lesion at the site of injury.

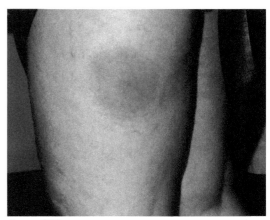

Source: CDC

24. Correct: Level of HIV RNA in plasma (D)

(D) There is direct correlation between the level of HIV RNA in the plasma and the number of infected CD4+ lymphocytes in AIDS patients. **(A)** Age can contribute to the immunocompetence of a patient but it does not directly correlate with the number of HIV-infected CD4+ lymphocytes. **(B)** AIDS patients may suffer from bacterial pneumonias due to their immunocompromised status. However, the super-infection would not contribute to a decline in CD4+ lymphocytes. **(C)** Women have a greater biological and social susceptibility to HIV infection but gender does not directly correlate with the number of HIV-infected CD4+ lymphocytes. **(E)** Premature aging (senescence) of the immune system contributing to CD4+ T lymphocyte decline is an evolving paradigm of HIV infection. Immune activation induced by HIV infection or other factors may contribute to immune response dysregulation.

25. Correct: Filoviridae (B)

(B) Ebola is in the Filoviridae family and is an agent of viral hemorrhagic fever. Suspicion of infection in this case is based on travel history to West Africa and nurse's role as a medical relief worker while in Guinea. The Filoviridae can cause severe hemorrhagic fever in humans and nonhuman primates and include the Marburgvirus and Ebolavirus families. There is a zoonotic lifecycle with bats serving as a reservoir for human infection. See Appendix N for a list of clinically significant viruses and key characteristics. **(A)** Bunyaviridae are found in and transmitted by arthropods (e.g., mosquitoes, ticks, and sandflies) and, in the case of hantavirus, rodents, and can occasionally infect humans. Examples are the tick-borne Crimean–Congo hemorrhagic fever and the sin nombre virus, which was discovered to cause a cluster of cases of hantavirus pulmonary syndrome in the southwestern United States. **(C)** Flaviviridae are found in arthropod vectors (ticks and mosquitoes) and can infect humans. Mosquito-transmitted Flaviviridae include yellow fever, dengue fever, Japanese encephalitis, West Nile viruses, and Zika virus. Flaviviruses are transmitted by ticks and are responsible of encephalitis and hemorrhagic diseases: tick-borne encephalitis, Kyasanur Forest disease, Alkhurma disease, and Omsk hemorrhagic fever. **(D)** Orthomyxoviridae is a family of viruses that includes influenza A, which causes pandemics in humans. Orthomyxoviridae cause zoonotic infections. **(E)** Togaviridae is a family of viruses with humans, mammals, birds, and mosquitoes as natural hosts. This family includes the mosquito-borne alphaviruses (chikungunya virus, eastern equine encephalitis [EEE], western equine encephalitis [WEE], and others), which cause arthritis and encephalitis, and the respiratory Rubiviruses, which are also in this family including the rubella virus that is the agent of rubella.

26. Correct: Cross-linking T cell receptor and MHC II (C)

(C) Cross-linking T cell receptor and MHC II are descriptions of a superantigen. In this case, the causative agent is most likely *Staphylococcus aureus*. The girl was most likely vaginally colonized by toxic

shock syndrome toxin (TSST)-producing strains of *S. aureus*. The presence of a tampon exacerbated bacterial growth and TSST production. Although cases of TSS have declined precipitously with greater public awareness, there remains a risk particularly with girls entering menstrual period. **(A)** ADP-ribosylating exotoxins such as cholera toxin and pertussis toxin activate adenylate cyclase resulting in a net increase in intracellular cyclic AMP levels. **(B)** M protein produced by *Streptococcus pyogenes* induces the production of cross-reactive antibodies that react with heart muscle protein. This is the mechanism of post-streptococcal sequelae and rheumatic heart disease. **(D)** Endotoxin is a component of the gram negative outer membrane. Although the girl presented with the signs and symptoms of shock a more likely etiology was the gram-positive bacterium *S. aureus* colonizing her vagina. **(E)** Bacterial pathogens such as *Yersinia pestis* use type III secretion to inject effector proteins into mammalian cells. Type III secretion requires bacterial cell and mammalian cell contact.

27. Correct: Attenuated virus vaccine (B)

(B) This is a case of yellow fever that was contracted by a traveler returning from an area where the disease is epidemic. This infection may be prevented by immunization with an attenuated virus vaccine. Yellow fever is caused by a virus of the Flaviviridae family, a positive-sense RNA virus. The vaccine is composed of live virus that has been attenuated by multiple passages in tissue cell culture. **(A)** Adjuvants are used to potentiate the immune response to vaccines. **(C)** Conjugate vaccines are developed for immunization against encapsulated bacterial pathogens such as *Streptococcus pneumoniae* and *Haemophilus influenzae*. Because polysaccharide capsule is a poor immunogen, a conjugate comprising capsule and proteins such as diphtheria toxoid is used as a vaccine. This serves the purpose of boosting a memory response. **(D)** Subcellular vaccines include toxoids, conjugated capsular vaccines, and recombinant surface antigens of hepatitis B. **(E)** Toxoids are inactivated protein toxins that serve as vaccines. Examples include diphtheria and tetanus toxoids.

28. Correct: Fc receptor (E)

(E) This patient has dengue fever, as suggested by his recent travel to a dengue-endemic area, a high fever, corresponding laboratory values, and severe eye, joint, and muscle pain. In individuals who have been exposed to dengue virus before, the preexisting antibodies specific for dengue can lead to "antibody-dependent enhancement" of infection. In antibody-dependent enhancement, the antibodies induced by the first infection bind to the current dengue virus and bind to Fc receptors on monocytes and macrophages. These antibody-bound viruses are more readily phagocytosed after binding to the Fc receptors and initiate replication in these phagocytes, resulting in an increased number of infected cells, amount of virus produced, and the severity of disease. **(A)** This answer is incorrect because CD4 is a receptor for HIV. It is unlikely based on the information given that this individual was exposed to HIV. While there can be a leukopenia and elevated AST levels during acute HIV infection, elevated hematocrit would not be expected. Finally, the presence of retro-orbital eye pain is not consistent with HIV presentation. **(B)** This answer is incorrect because the complement receptor 2 (CR2) binds to Epstein–Barr virus and is one of the receptors required for EBV entry. While EBV can result in elevated temperature and liver enzymes, the triad of classical symptoms of infectious mononucleosis (pharyngitis, fever, and lymphadenopathy) are not demonstrated in this patient. **(C)** This answer is incorrect because DC-SIGN enhances HIV infection by binding HIV and "presenting" it to CD4+ T cells. DC-SIGN is found on dendritic cells at mucosal sites, where HIV can enter. HIV bound to DC-SIGN is shuttled back to the lymph nodes as dendritic cells migrate from the site of infection to the draining lymph nodes to present antigen. Therefore, HIV binding to DC-SIGN increases the likelihood of infection through dendritic cells interacting with CD4+ T cells. As described further, it is unlikely that this individual is HIV-positive. **(D)** This answer is incorrect because EPC-receptor is critical in the process of *Plasmodium falciparum* infection. *P. falciparum* is not endemic in Argentina and this individual does not show typical signs of a cycle of high fever with defervescence that is seen in malaria.

29.   Correct: Leukopenia (D)

(D) This individual is infected with dengue virus and demonstrating symptoms of dengue hemorrhagic fever (DHF). Major laboratory findings in these individuals are leukopenia, thrombocytopenia, increased hematocrit (due to plasma leakage), hypoproteinemia, elevated AST levels, and increased prothrombin time. **(A)** This answer is incorrect because the levels of hematocrit can increase by 20% over baseline during DHF due to plasma leakage. **(B)** This answer is incorrect because individuals with DHF typically demonstrate an increased prothrombin time. **(C)** This answer is incorrect because individuals with DHF typically exhibit hypoproteinemia, also mainly due to plasma leakage. **(E)** This answer is incorrect because during DHF, the AST levels can typically be increased 2 to 5 times the normal range.

30.   Correct: Dengue virus (B)

(B) This patient is infected with dengue virus and is transitioning from DHF to dengue shock syndrome (DSS). Not all patients that have dengue hemorrhagic fever (DHF) will progress to DSS, but advanced warning signs include severe abdominal pain, protracted vomiting, marked change in temperature, and/or change in mental status. Early signs of DSS include restlessness, cold clammy skin, rapid weak pulse, and/or hypotension. The tourniquet test can be used to screen for dengue virus infections and is an indication of capillary fragility and thrombocytopenia. For this test a patient's blood pressure is measured and recorded. The blood pressure cuff is then inflated to half way between the systole and diastolic pressure for 5 minutes. A positive test is one in which there are more than 10 petechiae/square inch. **(A)** This answer is incorrect because chikungunya virus infection does not lead to shock. Both dengue and chikungunya should be considered in patients with acute onset of fever and polyarthralgias, especially if they have recently traveled to a location that is affected by these two viruses. However, chikungunya virus is more likely to manifest with high fever, severe arthralgia, rash, lymphopenia, and arthritis, while dengue infection is more likely to present with neutropenia, thrombocytopenia, hemorrhage, shock, and death. **(C)** This answer is incorrect because while West Nile virus is transmitted via mosquito and can present with fever, headache, body aches, and rash (as is seen in this patient), West Nile virus does not present with hemorrhagic fevers. **(D)** This answer is incorrect for a few reasons. First and foremost, yellow fever is not a risk in Thailand. According to the CDC, yellow fever is a risk when traveling to South America and sub-Saharan Africa. Second, while there can be many similarities between yellow fever and dengue fever, individuals with severe yellow fever infection (or the "period of intoxication") will demonstrate icteric hepatitis (hence the name "yellow fever"). **(E)** This answer is incorrect because Zika virus infection does not typically present with a high fever and does not induce a thrombocytopenia and leukocytopenia. Furthermore, Zika virus infection does not induce a hemorrhagic fever. Zika virus infection can induce a mild headache, rash, some joint and muscle pain, but can also present with a conjunctivitis, which is not typically seen in dengue infections.

31.   Correct: Monocytes (C)

(C) This girl has been infected with dengue virus which infects monocytes. There is some evidence that dengue can also infect lymphocytes (with most of the evidence pointing to B lymphocytes as the target), but this still is somewhat controversial. Infections of Fc-bearing monocytes are also thought to contribute to the antibody-dependent enhancement of infection during a secondary infection with dengue. In this situation, the antibody from a previous response increases the infection of monocytes with antibody-bound dengue virus using Fc receptors on monocytes to increase the level of infection. **(A)** This answer is incorrect because the patient is infected with dengue virus, which is not an inhaled pathogen, like influenza. Dengue exposure occurs through the bite from an infected *Aedes aegypti* mosquito. While dengue virus can infect monocytes, it typically does not target alveolar macrophages. **(B)** This answer is incorrect because dengue is not currently known to infect keratinocytes. After a bite from a dengue virus-infected *Aedes aegypti* mosquito, the virus either goes into the blood of the capillary found in the dermis or may be found deposited in the surrounding dermis and/or epidermis. However, to date, there is no evidence that keratinocytes of the epidermis are targeted by dengue virus. **(D)** This answer is incorrect because even though individuals with dengue exhibit thrombocytopenia, this is not due to dengue infection and direct destruction of platelets. The thrombocytopenia associated with dengue infection is thought to be due to dengue virus-induced bone marrow hypoplasia, platelet destruction by complement involving antiplatelet antibodies, and increased platelet consumption due to disseminated intravascular coagulation. **(E)** This answer is incorrect because red blood cells are not infected by dengue viruses. In the differential for dengue virus infection is *Plasmodium* sp. (the cause of malaria), which can infect red blood cells and lead to high fevers. However, this patient does not show typical signs of the cycle of high fever with defervescence that is typically seen in malaria.

Appendices

Appendix A: Overview of Immune System

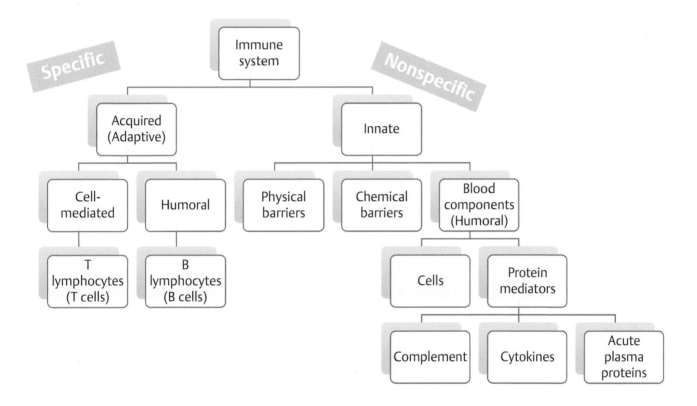

Appendix B: Key Cellular Markers

Cellular Marker	Function
Macrophages and dendritic cells	
CD1d	Presents lipid antigens to NKT cells
CD14 and TLR-4 (CD284)	LPS receptors, complex of proteins that binds to LPS on Gram negative bacteria
CR3 (or CD11b, Mac-1α)	Complement C3b receptor, opsonization, and phagocytosis
FcγRIII (CD16)	IgG Fcγ receptor, opsonization, and phagocytosis → antibody-dependent cellular cytotoxicity (ADCC)
MHC class I molecules	Antigen presentation to CD8+ cytotoxic T cells, expressed on nucleated cells
MHC class II molecules	Antigen presentation to CD4+ helper T cells, expressed on antigen-presenting cells (APC)
CD40	Binds with CD40L ligand (CD154) on T cells → co-activation of antigen-presenting cells (APCs) and cytokine expression
B7-1 (CD80, CD28L)	Binds with CD28 receptor on T cells → T cell co-stimulation
B7-2 (CD86, CD28L)	Binds with CD28 receptor on T cells → T cell co-stimulation
T cells	
CD3	Component of the TCR complex → signal transduction pathway → T cell activation
CD4	Present on TH1, TH2, TH17, and Treg T cell subsets; binds to MHC class II molecules
CD8	Present on cytotoxic T cell lymphocytes, binds to MHC class I molecules
CD28	T cell co-receptor, binds to B7 ligands on APCs → T cell co-stimulation
CTLA-4 (CD152)	Binds to B7 ligands on APCs after T cell activation → delivers inhibitory signals to the T cell
CD25	α chain of T cell IL-2R, IL-2 ligand binding → stimulation of T cells; expressed on T regulatory cells
CD40L (CD154)	Ligand, binds to CD40 receptor on APCs → co-stimulation of APCs
B cells	
CD19	Present on circulating B cells; negative regulator of BCR signaling
CD20	Present on circulating B cells
CD21	Present on circulating B cells, receptor for Epstein–Barr virus (EBV)
FcγRII (CD32)	IgG Fcγ receptor, mediates feedback inhibition of B cell antibody production
CD40	Binds with CD40L ligand on T cells → co-activation of APCs and cytokine expression
NK cells	
FcγRIII (CD16)	IgG Fcγ receptor, opsonization and phagocytosis → ADDC
CD56	Present on NK cells, cell adhesion molecule
Others	
CD45RA	Marker for nAïve T cells
CD45RO	Marker for memOry T cells
CD69	Nonspecific marker of immune cell activation, present on activated macrophages, B cells, T cells, and NK cells
Fas (CD95)	Death receptor, mediates signal transduction pathway → activation of caspases → apoptosis
FasL (CD178)	Ligand for the death receptor, mediates signal transduction pathway → activation of caspases → apoptosis

Green = Macrophages and dendritic cells

Red = T cells

Blue = B cells

Orange = NK Cells

Purple = Others

Appendix C: Complement–An Overview

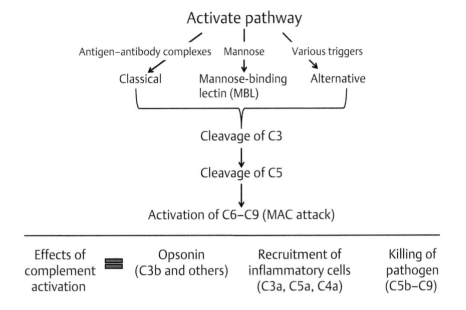

Appendix D: Cytokines

Cytokine	Major Cell Source(s)	Biological Function(s)
Interferons		
IFN-α, IFN-β (type I IFNs)	• Any virus-infected cell • Various leukocytes	• Upregulation of cellular antiviral defenses • Upregulation of MHC-I molecules expression • Activation of NK cells • Differentiation of CTLs
IFN-γ (type II IFN)	• CD4+ TH1 subset of T cells • NK cells • Activated cytotoxic CD8+ T cells	• Activation of macrophages • Inhibition of CD4+ TH2 subset of T cells • Promotion of isotype switch to IgG3 production
Tumor necrosis factors		
TNF-α (or cachectin)	• Dendritic cells, macrophages, NK cells • Endothelial and epithelial cells • Fibroblasts	• Activation of macrophages and T cells (pro-inflammatory) • Activation of endothelial cells through upregulation of cell adhesion molecules • Promotion of tumor cell killing • Promotion of weight loss, wasting (cachexia)
Lymphotoxin-α	• T cells, B cells	• Promotion of tumor cell killing through apoptosis, endothelial cell activation
Interleukins		
IL-1	• Dendritic cells, macrophages • Endothelial and epithelial cells • Fibroblasts	• Promotion of acute phase response • Activation of macrophages and T cells (pro-inflammatory) • Induction of fever at hypothalamus • Activation of endothelial cells through upregulation of cell adhesion molecules
IL-6	• T cells • Dendritic cells, macrophages • Endothelial and epithelial cells • Fibroblasts	• Promotion of acute phase response • Activation of macrophages and T cells (pro-inflammatory) • Induction of fever at hypothalamus • Activation of endothelial cells through upregulation of cell adhesion molecules • Differentiation of B and T cell subsets • Promotion of TH17 differentiation with TGF-β
IL-2	• CD4+ TH1 cells • Activated naïve CD4+ T cells	• Activation of B and T cell proliferation • Activation of NK cells
IL-8 (or CXCL-8)	• Macrophages • Endothelial and epithelial cells	• Promotion of neutrophil chemotaxis
IL-12	• Dendritic cells, macrophages	• Differentiation of TH1 cells • Activation of NK cells
IL-17	• CD4+ TH17 cells	• Activation of neutrophils • Stimulation of epithelia to produce pro-inflammatory cytokines • Important in fighting certain fungal infections
IL-4	• CD4+ TH2 cells • Mast cells	• Promotion of B cell growth • Promotion of TH2 cell differentiation • Promotion of isotype switch to IgE, IgG1, IgG2, and IgG4 production • Inhibition of TH1 cells
IL-5	• CD4+ TH2 cells • Mast cells	• Promotion of eosinophilia
IL-9	• CD4+ TH2 cells	• Stimulation of mast cells

(Continued)

Cytokine	Major Cell Source(s)	Biological Function(s)
IL-13	• CD4+ TH2 cells • Mast cells	• Promotion of B cell growth • Promotion of allergic airway inflammation
BAFF	• Follicular dendritic cells, macrophages	• Promotion of B cell growth and survival
IL-10	• CD4+ Treg subset of T cells • CD4+ TH2 cells • Macrophages	• Immunoregulation (anti-inflammatory) • Inhibition of TH1 T cells and macrophages • Promotion of B cell growth and survival
TGF-β	• CD4+ Treg cells • Various leukocytes	• Immunoregulation (anti-inflammatory) • Inhibition of macrophages, T cells, B cells, and NK cells • Promotion of isotype switch to IgA production
IL-3	• T cells, thymic epithelial cells, stromal cells	• Differentiation of hematopoietic stem cells
IL-7	• Stromal cells of bone marrow and thymus	• Promotion of progenitor B and T cell development
Other molecules		
GM-CSF	• Stromal cells • T cells	• Differentiation and growth of myeloid stem cells

Color Key Based on Major Functions of Cytokines:

Pro-inflammatory

Anti-inflammatory

Cytotoxic

Allergies and eosinophilia

B cell growth

Stem cell development

Appendix E: Hypersensitivity Reactions

Name	Type I Immediate Hypersensitivity	Type II Antibody-Mediated Cytolysis	Type III Immune Complex Hypersensitivity	Type IV Delayed-Type or Cell-Mediated Hypersensitivity
Timing	Immediate	Variable	Variable	Delayed
Antigen	Soluble	Cell surface	Soluble	Soluble
Antibody	IgE	IgG IgM	IgG IgM	None
Cellular and chemical effectors	Mast cells/basophils	Complement	Complement Neutrophils	TH1 cells Macrophages Cytotoxic T cells
Mechanism	Antigen binds to IgE which is on surface of mast cells. This results in mast cell degranulation and release of vasoactive mediators such as histamine.	Antibody binds to antigen which is on target cell surface. This results in complement activation or antibody-dependent cell-mediated cytotoxicity (ADCC).	Immune complexes (i.e., antigen–antibody) deposit on tissue, which results in complement activation and neutrophil infiltration.	Antigen binds to T cell which results in lymphokine production and activation of macrophages. Activated macrophages produce pro-inflammatory cytokines.

Examples	• Bee sting
	• Atopic diseases, such as:
	  • Allergic rhinitis
	  • Asthma
	  • Eczema
	  • Anaphylaxis
		• Anti-glomerular basement membrane antibody disease
		• Autoimmune hemolytic anemia
		• Graves' disease
		• Myasthenia gravis
		• Rh-factor reactions
		• Transfusion reaction
			• Serum sickness
			• Systemic lupus erythematosus (SLE)
			• Post-infectious glomerulonephritis
			• Membranous nephropathy
				• Contact dermatitis
				• Tuberculin reaction

Appendix F: Media

Media	Purpose	Comments
Blood	Enriched, nonselective media that supports the growth of a wide variety of bacteria and some fungi	Enriched with red blood cells, some bacteria may hemolyze red blood cells leading to hemolysis Alpha hemolysis – partial hemolysis; beta hemolysis – complete hemolysis; gamma hemolysis – no hemolysis
Chocolate	Enriched, nonselective media that supports growth of a wide variety of bacteria and some fungi; supports the growth of *Haemophilus* and *Neisseria*	Enriched with X (hemin) and V (NAD) factors
Eosin methylene blue (EMB)	Selective for enteric gram-negative bacilli Differential for lactose reactions	*E. coli* produces a green metallic sheen
Hektoen	Selective for enteric gram-negative bacilli Differential for lactose reactions and hydrogen sulfide (H_2S)	Lactose positive = orange/yellow; lactose negative = clear/colorless H_2S positive = black colonies; H_2S negative = green colonies

(Continued)

Media	Purpose	Comments
MacConkey **Lactose positive** **Lactose negative**	Selective for enteric gram-negative bacilli Differential for lactose reactions	Contains bile salts and crystal violet to prevent the growth of gram-positive organisms Lactose positive = pink/red; lactose negative = clear/colorless
MacConkey with Sorbitol **Sorbitol positive** **Sorbitol negative**	Selective for enteric gram-negative bacilli Differential for enterohemorrhagic *E. coli* (EHEC or *E. coli* O157:H7)	Lactose positive = pink/red; lactose negative = clear/colorless Sorbitol positive = pink/red; sorbitol negative = clear/colorless
Thiosulfate citrate bile salts sucrose (TCBS) **Sucrose positive** **Sucrose negative** *Vibrio parahaemolyticus* on TCBS agar	Selective for Vibrio Differential for sucrose reactions	Sucrose positive = yellow; sucrose negative = green
Thayer–Martin	Selective for pathogenic *Neisseria*	
Regan–Lowe	Selective for *Bordetella pertussis*	
Bordet–Gengou	Selective for *Bordetella pertussis*	
Buffered charcoal yeast extract (BCYE)	Selective for *Legionella*	
Cystine tellurite	Selective for *Corynebacterium diphtheriae*	
Loefflers	Selective for *Corynebacterium diphtheriae*	
Lowenstein–Jensen	Selective for *Mycobacterium*	

Appendix G: Gram Stain Reactions for Select Clinically Significant Bacteria

Gram-positive cocci	Gram-positive bacilli	Gram-negative cocci	Gram-negative bacilli	Gram-negative coccobacilli	Organisms that Gram stain poorly
Chains: Enterococcus Streptococcus **Chains and pairs:** Streptococcus pneumoniae **Clusters:** Staphylococcus	Bacillus Clostridium Erysipelothrix Gardnerella Lactobacillus Listeria monocytogenes Propionibacterium acnes **Branching:** Actinomyces Nocardia (also modified acid fast) **Palisading, pleomorphic:** Corynebacterium diphtheriae	Moraxella **Pairs:** Neisseria	**Curved:** Campylobacter Helicobacter Vibrio **Aerobes:** Bartonella Citrobacter Enterobacter Escherichia coli Legionella Klebsiella Proteus Pseudomonas Salmonella Serratia Shigella Yersinia **Anaerobes:** Bacteroides Fusobacterium	Bordetella pertussis Brucella Coxiella Francisella Haemophilus Pasteurella	**Spirochetes:** Borrelia Leptospira Treponema **Other:** Chlamydia / Chlamydophila Mycobacterium Mycoplasma Anaplasma Ehrlichia Rickettsia Ureaplasma

Color Key Based on Gram Stain Reaction:

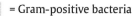

= Gram-positive bacteria

= Gram-negative bacteria

Appendix H: Gram Stain Reactions and Morphologies

Gram-positive cocci

Clusters   Chains   Pairs (diplococci)

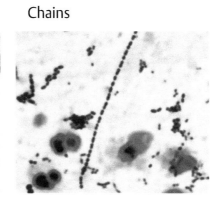 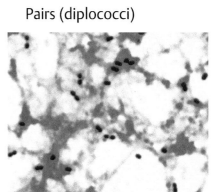

Gram-positive rods (bacilli)

Pleomorphic   With spores

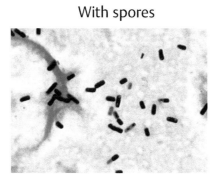 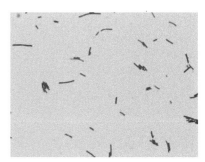

Gram-negative cocci

Pairs (diplococci)

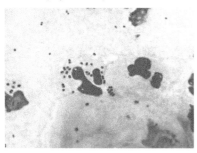

Gram-negative rods (bacilli)

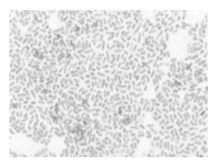 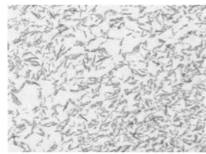 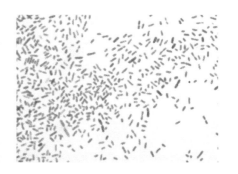

Appendix I: Antibiotics

Group	Example	Mechanism of Action	Spectrum of Activity (Examples)
Glycopeptides	Vancomycin		Narrow spectrum • Mainly Gram-positive
Polypeptide	Bacitracin		Moderate spectrum • Mainly Gram-positive
β-lactam Penicillins	Penicillin G (IV) Penicillin V (Oral)		Moderate spectrum • Mainly Gram-positive and some Gram-negative
β-lactam Antistaphylococcal penicillins (penicillin-ase-resistant penicillins)	Oxacillin Nafcillin Methicillin		Narrow spectrum • Mainly Gram-positive
β-lactam Amino-penicillins	Ampicillin (IV) Amoxicillin (Oral)		Moderate spectrum • Mainly Gram-positive and some Gram-negative
β-lactam Carboxy-penicillins + β-lactamase inhibitor	Ticarcillin + Clavu-lanic acid		Broad spectrum • Gram-positive and some Gram-negative including *P. aeruginosa*
β-lactam Ureido-peniclllins + β-lactamase inhibitor	Piperacillin + Tazobactam		Broad spectrum • Gram-positive and some Gram-negative including *P. aeruginosa*
β-lactam Cephalosporin – 1st generation	Cefazolin Cephalexin	Inhibition of cell wall synthesis	Moderate spectrum • Mainly Gram-positive and some Gram-negative
β-lactam Cephalosporin – 2nd generation	Cefuroxime Cefoxitin Cefotetan Cefaclor Cefprozil Cefpodoxime		Moderate spectrum • Mainly Gram-positive and some Gram-negative
β-lactam Cephalosporin – 3rd generation	Cefotaxime Ceftriaxone Ceftazidime Cefixime		Moderate spectrum • Mainly Gram-positive and some Gram-negative including *P. aeruginosa* (Ceftazidime only)
β-lactam Cephalosporin – 4th generation	Cefipime		Broad spectrum • Gram-positive and Gram-negative including *P. aeruginosa*
β-lactam Cephalosporin – 5th generation	Ceftaroline		Moderate spectrum (only approved for Gram-positive but has broader activity including vs. methicillin-resistant *Staphylococcus aureus*)
β-lactam Monobactam	Aztreonam		Narrow spectrum • Mainly Gram-negative

(Continued)

Group	Example	Mechanism of Action	Spectrum of Activity (Examples)
β-lactam Carbapenems	Doripenem Ertapenem Imipenem Meropenem		Broad spectrum
Sulfonamides (most often used in conjunction with Trimethoprim)	Sulfamethoxazole		Broad spectrum
Trimethoprim (most often used in conjunction with Sulfonamides)	Trimethoprim	Inhibition of folate synthesis	Broad spectrum
Trimethoprim-Sulfamethoxazole (TMP-SMX)	Trimethoprim-Sulfamethoxazole		Broad spectrum
Quinolones/Fluoroquinolones	Nalidixic acid Ciprofloxacin Levofloxacin Moxifloxacin Norfloxacin Ofloxacin	Inhibition of DNA replication and transcription	Broad spectrum
Rifampin	Rifampin		Broad spectrum
Aminoglycosides	Amikacin Gentamicin Kanamycin Neomycin Streptomycin Tobramycin	Inhibition of protein synthesis Target: 30S ribosome subunit	Broad spectrum • Very active against Gram-negative
Glycylcyclines	Tigecycline		Broad spectrum
Tetracyclines	Doxycycline Minocycline Tetracycline		Broad spectrum
Chloramphenicol	Chloramphenicol		Broad spectrum
Lincosamides	Clindamycin		Narrow spectrum Mainly Gram-positive
Macrolides	Azithromycin Clarithromycin	Inhibition of protein synthesis Target: 50S ribosome subunit	Broad spectrum
	Erythromycin		Narrow spectrum
Oxazolidinones	Linezolid		Narrow spectrum Mainly Gram-positive
Streptogramins	Dalfopristin/quinupristin		Narrow spectrum Mainly Gram-positive
Polymyxins (cyclic peptides)	Colistin Polymyxin B	Disruption of bacterial cell membranes	Broad spectrum

Appendix J: Bacterial Virulence Factors A–Z

Virulence Factor	Organism	Mechanism of Action	Role in Pathogenesis
ActA	*Listeria monocytogenes*	Actin-nucleating protein	Promotes intracellular and cell-to-cell motility and spread
Alginate	*Pseudomonas aeruginosa*	Acetylated polysaccharide; mucoid colony morphology	Lung colonization; defense response; contributes to biofilm formation
α-toxin	*Clostridium perfringens*	Phospholipase, hydrolyzes membrane-associated lecithin	Tissue necrosis and gas gangrene; kills phagocytes
α-toxin	*Staphylococcus aureus*	Pore-forming cytolysin; complement-like mechanism	Tissue necrosis; dissemination
Anthrax toxin	*Bacillus anthracis*	Three component toxin: **Edema toxin (ET):** Soluble adenylate cyclase enzyme; increases cAMP and disrupts host cell function **Lethal toxin (LT):** Metalloprotease that cleaves MAPK kinase; disrupts host cell signal transduction **Protective antigen (PA):** Receptor-binding subunit for edema toxin and lethal toxin to enter host cells; anti-PA antibody confers protective immunity	ET induces edema seen in cutaneous anthrax LT kills macrophages; induces lethal shock of systemic anthrax
Botulinum toxin (7 serotypes A–G)	*Clostridium botulinum*	Proteolytic cleavage of synaptobrevins involved in vesicular contents release; blocks presynaptic release of acetylcholine neurotransmitter in peripheral nervous system	Flaccid descending paralysis
Capsule	*Escherichia coli* Group A streptococci Group B streptococci *Haemophilus influenzae* *Neisseria meningitidis* *Staphylococcus aureus* *Streptococcus pneumoniae* *Yersinia* spp.	Prevents opsonization of microbe; interferes with complement function	Resistance to phagocytosis; contributes to invasive infections: septicemia, meningitis

(Continued)

Virulence Factor	Organism	Mechanism of Action	Role in Pathogenesis
Cell wall components	*Streptococcus pneumoniae*	Teichoic acid and peptidoglycan induce cytokine production; promote inflammatory response	Pneumonia: Fever and lung damage, bloody sputum Meningitis: Exudation across blood–brain barrier
Cholera toxin	*Vibrio cholerae*	A/B5 cytotoxin: **A subunit:** Catalyzes ADP-ribosylation of G proteins; increases cAMP levels; alters cell physiology **B subunits:** Bind ganglioside receptor on intestinal enterocytes	Contributes to fluid loss and profuse "rice–water" diarrhea
Colonization factor antigens (CFAI–IV)	Enterotoxigenic *Escherichia coli* (ETEC)	Adherence to intestinal epithelium receptors	Colonization of small intestine to allow watery diarrhea
Defect in organelle trafficking (Dot) proteins	*Legionella pneumophila*	Type IV secretion system; injects proteins into host cell	Intracellular survival in macrophage
Diphtheria toxin	*Corynebacterium diphtheriae*	A/B cytotoxin: A subunit ADP-riboxylates eukaryotic elongation factor 2; blocks protein synthesis	Systemic toxinosis; pseudomembrane formation in pharynx
Elastases (LasA, LasB)	*Pseudomonas aeruginosa*	Elastin degradation	**Cystic fibrosis:** Contributes to lung damage **Keratitis:** Contributes to corneal perforation
Elementary body	*Chlamydia spp:* *Chlamydia trachomatis* *Chlamydia pneumoniae*	Infectious life cycle stage	Receptor-mediated entry into mammalian epithelial cells
Exfoliative toxins (ETA, ETB)	*Staphylococcus aureus*	Proteolytic cleavage of desmoglein "glue" that holds desmosomal junctions together; separation between stratum spinosum and stratum granulosum	Desquamation associated with staphylococcal scalded skin syndrome (SSSS)
Exotoxin A	*Pseudomonas aeruginosa*	A/B cytotoxin: A subunit ADP-riboxylates eukaryotic elongation factor 2; blocks protein synthesis	Tissue damage; inhibition of phagocyte function
Exoenzyme S (ExoS) Exoenzyme U (ExoU)	*Pseudomonas aeruginosa*	Enters host cells by type III secretion system; ADP-ribosylate G proteins; disrupts signal transduction	Tissue damage; inhibition of phagocyte function

(Continued)

Virulence Factor	Organism	Mechanism of Action	Role in Pathogenesis
Filamentous hemagglutinin (Fha)	*Bordetella pertussis*	Binds to sulfated glycolipids of ciliated respiratory epithelium	Colonization of respiratory tract
Heat labile toxin (LT)	Enterotoxigenic *E. coli* (ETEC)	A/B5 cytotoxin: **A subunit:** Catalyzes ADP-ribosylation of G proteins; increases cAMP levels; alters cell physiology **B subunits:** Bind ganglioside receptor on host cells	Contributes to fluid loss and watery diarrhea
Heat stable toxin (ST)	Enterotoxigenic *E. coli* (ETEC)	Hormone-like activity; increases cGMP levels; alters cell physiology	Contributes to fluid loss and watery diarrhea
Hyaluronidase	*Staphylococcus aureus*	Hydrolyzes connective tissue	Exoprotein for spreading through tissue planes
Internalins	*Listeria monocytogenes*	Adherence and invasion	Invasion of intestinal epithelium
Intimin	Enterohemorrhagic *E. coli* (EHEC) Enteropathogenic *E. coli* (EPEC)	Induces actin rearrangement	Contributes to attaching/effacing lesions, hemorrhagic colitis
Intracellular multiplication (Icm) proteins	*Legionella pneumophila*	Type IV secretion system; proteins injected into host cell	Intracellular survival in macrophage
Invasins	*Salmonella spp:* *S. enteritidis* *S. typhi* *Yersinia spp:* *Y. pestis* *Y. enterocolitica* *Y. pseudotuberculosis*	Actin cytoskeletal rearrangement in epithelial cells; membrane ruffling (*Salmonella spp*)	Facilitates uptake of bacteria into nonprofessional phagocytes
Invasion plasmid antigens	Shigella species: *S. dysenteriae* (Group A) *S. flexneri* (Group B) *S. boydii* (Group C) *S. sonnei* (Group D)	Actin cytoskeletal rearrangement in intestinal M cells	Uptake into M cells; cell-to-cell spread in the intestinal epithelium

(Continued)

Virulence Factor	Organism	Mechanism of Action	Role in Pathogenesis
Invasive adenylate cyclase	Bordetella pertussis	Enzyme injected into ciliated respiratory epithelial cells; stimulates cAMP production and increases cAMP levels; alters cell physiology	Fluid loss; alteration of monocyte migration
Leukocidin (PVL)	Staphylococcus aureus	Catalytically disrupts phospholipid metabolism	Leukocyte membrane damage and killing; immune response evasion
Lipoarabinomannan	Mycobacterium tuberculosis	Cell wall glycolipid	Suppresses T cell proliferation; prevents macrophage activation
Lipooligosaccharide (LOS)	Neisseria spp: N. gonorrhoeae N. meningitidis	Neisseria LPS associated with outer membrane; antigenically variable	Confers serum resistance; induces inflammatory response; blood vessel thrombosis; disseminated intravascular coagulation (DIC)
Listeriolysin O (LLO)	Listeria monocytogenes	Pore-forming cytolysin	Facilitates escape of the pathogen from intracellular vacuoles
Low calcium response (LcrV)	Yersinia spp. Y. pestis Y. enterocolitica Y. pseudotuberculosis	Released by type III secretion system; regulates translocation of Yops proteins into host cells	Controls injection of toxic proteins into host cells
M protein	Streptococcus pyogenes	Surface-associated fibrils; subject to antigenic variation	Anti-phagocytic; cross-reactive antibodies and molecular mimicry contribute to immunologic phenomena: rheumatic heart disease, acute glomerulonephritis
Macrophage infectivity promoter (Mip)	Legionella pneumophila	Peptidyl prolyl isomerase enzyme	Intracellular survival in macrophage
Mucinase	Helicobacter pylori Vibrio cholerae	Degrades mucus	Facilitates colonization of the GI mucosal epithelium
Mycolic acid (cord factor)	Mycobacterium tuberculosis	Cell wall glycolipid	Resistance to killing by non-activated macrophages; contributes to granuloma formation
Opacity proteins (Opa)	Neisseria gonorrhoeae	Antigenically variable outer membrane proteins	Confound humoral immune response
Outer surface proteins (Osps, Erps, Vls, VMP)	Borrelia spp: B. burgdorferi B. hermsii B. recurrentis	Immunoprotective antigens; antigenically variable outer membrane proteins	Contribute to inflammatory arthritis syndrome; contribute to recurring disease relapses

(Continued)

Virulence Factor	Organism	Mechanism of Action	Role in Pathogenesis
Pertussis toxin	*Bordetella pertussis*	A/B5 cytotoxin secreted by type IV secretion system **A subunit:** Catalyzes ADP-ribosylation of Gi protein; Increases cAMP levels in host cells; alters cell physiology **B subunits:** Receptor-binding	Fluid loss; alteration of monocyte migration
Phospholipase	*Legionella pneumophila* *Listeria monocytogenes* *Rickettsia* spp: *Rickettsia rickettsii* *Rickettsia prowazekii*	Hydrolyzes phospholipids	Escape from endocytotic vacuoles; survival inside phagocytes; cell-to-cell spread
Pili associated with pyelone-phritis (PAP)	Uropathogenic *E. coli*	Bind P group antigens (globobiose) on uroepithelium	Colonization of the urethra, bladder, and kidneys
Pilin (Pil)	*Neisseria gonorrhoeae*	Antigenically variable adhesin	Confounds humoral immune response
Plasminogen activator	*Yersinia pestis*	Activates conversion of plasminogen to active plasmin enzyme	Dissolves fibrin clots; prevents chemotaxis of PMNs
Pneumolysin	*Streptococcus pneumoniae*	Pore-forming cytolysin	Kills ciliated respiratory epithelial cells; impairs PMN function; lung inflammation
Protein A	*Staphylococcus aureus*	Binds to the Fc portion of IgG	Evasion of immune response
Protein G	*Streptococcus pyogenes*	Binds to the Fc portion of IgG	Evasion of immune response
Rck protein	*Salmonella enteritidis*	Outer membrane adhesin; serum resistance	Evasion of opsonization and complement killing
Reticulate body	*Chlamydia* spp: *Chlamydia trachomatis* *Chlamydia pneumoniae*	Intracellular replicative life cycle stage	Persistent infections
Salmonella pathogenicity islands I and II (SPI, SPII)	*Salmonella enteritidis*	Type III secretion system; membrane ruffling and invasion	Phagolysosomal survival; contribute to systemic infection
Shiga toxin Shiga-like toxin	*Shigella dysenteriae* 1 Enterohemorrhagic *E. coli* (EHEC)	A/B5 cytotoxin: **A subunit:** Catalytically inactivates eukaryotic ribosomes **B subunits:** Bind receptor	Tissue necrosis in kidneys; hemolytic uremic syndrome (HUS)

(Continued)

(Continued)

Virulence Factor	Organism	Mechanism of Action	Role in Pathogenesis
Staphylococcal enterotoxins (7 serotypes SAE [A–D])	*Staphylococcus aureus*	Superantigens that induce cytokine release	Emesis associated with food poisoning
Staphylokinase	*Staphylococcus aureus*	Activates conversion of plasminogen to active plasmin enzyme	Dissolves fibrin clots
Streptococcal pyrogenic exotoxin	*Streptococcus pyogenes*	Superantigen that induces massive cytokine storm	Fever, rash, shock; T-cell hyper-stimulation, endotoxin sensitivity
Streptokinase	*Streptococcus pyogenes*	Activates conversion of plasminogen to active plasmin enzyme	Dissolves fibrin clots
Streptolysin O (SLO) Streptolysin S (SLS)	*Streptococcus pyogenes*	Pore-forming cytolysins	Evasion of immune response; heart tissue damage
Tetanus toxin (tetanospasmin)	*Clostridium tetani*	Proteolytic cleavage of synaptobrevins involved in vesicular contents release; blocks presynaptic release of inhibitory neurotransmitters Gly and GABA in central nervous system	Spastic paralysis
Toxic shock syndrome toxin (TSST-1)	*Staphylococcus aureus*	Superantigen that induces massive cytokine storm	Fever, rash, shock; T cell hyper-stimulation, endotoxin sensitivity
Toxic oxygen radicals	*Mycoplasma pneumoniae*	Secreted peroxide and superoxide radicals	Ciliated respiratory epithelium damage
Toxin A and B	*Clostridium difficile*	Glucosylation of G proteins; alters cell physiology; disrupts actin cytoskeletal polymerization	Intestinal mucosa damage; pseudomembrane formation, colitis
Transferrin binding protein	*Neisseria gonorrhoeae*	Scavenges iron from transferrin	Iron acquisition

Virulence Factor	Organism	Mechanism of Action	Role in Pathogenesis

Urease	**Gastric infections:**
	Helicobacter pylori
	
	Urinary tract infections:
	Klebsiella pneumoniae
	Proteus spp:
	  P. mirabilis
	  P. vulgaris
	Staphylococcus saprophyticus
		Converts urea to ammonia and carbon dioxide	Neutralizes stomach acid; protects *H. pylori* from gstric acidic damage
			
			Contributes to struvite (ammonium–magnesium–phosphate or AMP) stone formation by urinary tract pathogens

VacA cytotoxin	*Helicobacter pylori*	Induces vacuole formation	Death of gastric mucosal epithelial cells
Vi antigen	*Salmonella typhi*	Capsular polysaccharide	Increased virulence, invasion

Yersinia outer membrane proteins (Yops)	*Yersinia spp.*
	  Yersinia pestis
	  Yersinia enterocolitica
	  Y. pseudotuberculosis
		Components of type III secretion system; effector Yops are kinase and phosphatase enzymes injected into cells; disrupt actin cytoskeletal polymerization	Disrupt macrophage and PMN functions

Appendix K: Pathogens by Organ System

System/Anatomic Site	Common Clinically Significant Pathogens			
	Bacteria	**Viruses**	**Fungi**	**Parasites**
Nervous system	*Escherichia coli K1* *Haemophilus influenzae* *Neisseria meningitidis* *Clostridium botulinum* *Clostridium tetani* *Listeria monocytogenes* *Streptococcus agalactiae* (Group B Strep) *Streptococcus pneumoniae* Viridans Group Streptococci	Arboviruses (e.g., West Nile virus) Coxsackie viruses Herpes simplex virus (1 & 2) Poliovirus Rabies virus Varicella zoster virus	*Cryptococcus neoformans* Zygomycetes (e.g., *Rhizopus, Mucor*)	*Naegleria fowleri* *Plasmodium falciparum* *Taenia solium* *Toxoplasma gondii*
Eye	*Chlamydia trachomatis* *Haemophilus influenzae* *Moraxella* species *Neisseria gonorrhoeae* *Pseudomonas aeruginosa* *Staphylococcus aureus* *Streptococcus pneumoniae*	Adenovirus Cytomegalovirus (CMV) Epstein–Barr virus (EBV) Herpes simplex virus (1 & 2) Varicella zoster virus	Zygomycetes	*Loa loa* *Onchocerca volvulus* *Toxoplasma* *Toxocara*
Ear	*Haemophilus influenzae* *Moraxella* species *Pseudomonas aeruginosa* *Staphylococcus aureus* *Streptococcus pneumoniae* *Streptococcus pyogenes* (Group A Strep)			
Respiratory system	*Chlamydophilia pneumoniae & psittaci* *Mycobacterium tuberculosis* (MTB) *Mycoplasma pneumoniae* *Bordetella pertussis* *Haemophilus influenzae* *Klebsiella pneumoniae* *Legionella pneumophilia* *Pseudomonas aeruginosa* *Yersinia pestis* *Bacillus anthracis (aerosolized)* *Corynebacterium diphtheriae* *Staphylococcus aureus* *Streptococcus pneumoniae* *Streptococcus pyogenes* (Group A Strep) *Streptococcus agalactiae* (Group B Strep)	Adenovirus Coronavirus, including SARS virus Coxsackie viruses Cytomegalovirus (CMV) Epstein–Barr virus (EBV) Influenza virus Measles virus Mumps virus Parainfluenza virus Respiratory syncytial virus (RSV) Rhinovirus Rubella virus	*Aspergillus* species *Blastomyces dermatitidis* *Candida* species *Coccidioides immitis* *Cryptococcus neoformans* *Histoplasma capsulatum* *Paracoccidioides brasiliensis* *Pneumocystis jirovecii* *Sporothrix schenckii* Zygomycetes	*Ascaris lumbricoides* *Strongyloides stercoralis*

(Continued)

System/ Anatomic Site	Common Clinically Significant Pathogens			
	Bacteria	Viruses	Fungi	Parasites
Cardiovascular system	*Borrelia burgdorferi*	Coxsackie virus	*Candida* species	*Trypanosoma* species
	Pseudomonas aeruginosa			
	Corynebacterium diphtheriae			
	Enterococcus species			
	Staphylococcus aureus			
	Staphylococcus epidermidis			
	Viridans Group Streptococci			
Gastrointestinal system and associated organs	*Bacteroides* species	Adenovirus	Microsporidia	*Ancylostoma duodenale*
	Campylobacter species	Hepatitis A virus		*Ascaris lumbricoides*
	Enteraggregative *Escherichia coli* (EAEC)	Hepatitis B virus		*Cryptosporidium parvum*
	Enterohemorrhagic *Escherichia coli* (EHEC)	Hepatitis C virus		*Cyclospora*
	Enteroinvasive *Escherichia coli* (EIEC)	Hepatitis D virus		*Echinococcus granulosus*
	Enteropathogenic *Escherichia coli* (EPEC)	Hepatitis E virus		*Diphyllobothrium latum*
	Enterotoxogenic *Escherichia coli* (ETEC)	Norovirus		*Entamoeba histolytica*
	Helicobacter pylori	Rotavirus		*Enterobius vermicularis*
	Salmonella species			*Giardia lamblia*
	Shigella species			*Isospora belli*
	Vibrio cholerae			*Necator americanus*
	Yersinia entercolitica			*Strongyloides stercoralis*
	Bacillus cereus			*Taenia saginata*
	Clostridioides difficile			*Taenia solium*
	Clostridium perfringens			*Trichuris trichiura*
	Listeria monocytogenes			
	Staphylococcus aureus			
Genital tract	*Chlamydia trachomatis*	Herpes simplex virus (1 & 2)	*Candida* species	*Trichomonas vaginalis*
	Mycoplasma hominis	Human papillomavirus (HPV)		
	Treponema pallidum			
	Ureaplasma urealyticum			
	Haemophilus ducreyi			
	Klebsiella granulomatis			
	Neisseria gonorrhoeae			
	Gardnerella vaginalis (gram variable)			

(Continued)

System/ Anatomic Site	Common Clinically Significant Pathogens			
	Bacteria	**Viruses**	**Fungi**	**Parasites**
Urinary tract	*Mycoplasma hominis* *Ureaplasma urealyticum*		*Candida* species	*Schistosoma haematobium*
	Escherichia coli *Klebsiella pneumoniae* *Proteus mirabilis* *Pseudomonas aeruginosa*			
	Corynebacterium urealyticum *Enterococcus* species *Staphylococcus aureus* *Staphylococcus saprophyticus* *Streptococcus agalactiae* (Group B Strep)			
Systemic/blood/ lymph	*Borrelia burgdorferi* *Leptospira* *Rickettsia* species	Cytomegalovirus (CMV) Epstein–Barr virus (EBV) Human immunodeficiency virus (HIV) Human T cell lymphotropic virus Parvovirus B19	*Aspergillus* species *Candida* species *Sporothrix schenckii*	*Babesia* species *Brugia malayi* *Leishmania* species *Loa loa* *Onchocerca volvulus* *Plasmodium* species *Schistosoma japonicum* *Schistosoma mansoni* *Trypanosoma* species *Wuchereria bancrofti*
	Bacteroides species *Bartonella* species *Brucella* *Coxiella burnetti* *Francisella tularensis* *Neisseria meningitidis* *Pasteurella multocida* *Salmonella typhi* *Yersinia pestis*			
Skin and musculoskeletal system	*Borrelia burgdorferi* *Mycobacterium leprae* *Rickettsia* species *Treponema pallidum*	Coxsackie viruses Herpes simplex virus (1 & 2) Human herpesviruses (HHV-6, HHV-7, HHV-8) Human papillomavirus (HPV) Measles virus Poxvirus Parvovirus B19 Rubella virus Varicella zoster virus	*Blastomyces dermatitidis* *Coccidioides immitis* *Cryptococcus neoformans* Dermatophytes (Trichophyton, Epidermophyton, Microsporum) *Sporothrix schenckii*	Ectoparasites *Leishmania* species *Onchocerca volvulus* *Trichinella spiralis* *Trypanosoma* species
	Neisseria gonorrhoeae *Yersinia pestis* *Actinomyces israelii* *Bacillus anthracis* *Clostridium perfringens* *Nocardia* species *Staphylococcus aureus* *Streptococcus pyogenes* (Group A Strep)			

Color Key:

    = Gram-positive bacteria

    = Purple = Gram-negative bacteria

    = Bacteria that do not Gram stain

    = Viruses

    = Fungi

    = Parasites

Appendix L: Vector-Borne Infections

	Mosquito	Tick	Flea	Mite (Chigger)	Lice	Sandfly
Bacteria		• Tularemia (*Francisella tularensis*) • Recurrent fever (*Borrelia hermsii* and other non *B. recurrentis* species) • Human granulocytic anaplasmosis (HGA) (*Anaplasma*) • Human monocytic ehrlichiosis (HME) (*Ehrlichia*) • Lyme disease (*Borrelia burgdorferi*) • Rocky Mountain spotted fever (*Rickettsia rickettsii*; RMSF)	• Cat-scratch fever (*Bartonella henselae*) • Plague (*Yersinia pestis*) • Murine (endemic) typhus (*Rickettsia typhi*)	• Rickettsialpox (*Rickettsia akari*) • Scrub typhus (*Orientia tsutsugamushi*)	• Trench fever and bacillary angiomatosis (*Bartonella quintana*) • Relapsing fever (*Borrelia recurrentis*) • Epidemic typhus (*Rickettsia prowazekii*)	• Oroya fever; also called Carrion's disease (*Bartonella bacilliformis*)
Virus	• Chikungunya • Dengue • Eastern, Western and Venezuelan equine encephalitis • Japanese encephalitis • St. Louis encephalitis • West Nile • Yellow fever • Zika	• Colorado tick virus				
Parasite	• Lymphadenitis (*Wuchereria bancrofti* and *Brugia malayi*) • Malaria (*Plasmodium*)	• Babesiosis (*Babesia*)				• Leishmaniasis (*Leishmania*)

Other:

- Black fly
  - River blindness (*Onchocerca volvulus*)
- Deer fly (also called mango fly)
  - *Loa loa*
- Reduviid bug also called triatome and kissing bug
  - Chagas disease (*Trypanosoma cruzi*)
- Tsetse fly
  - African sleeping sickness *(Trypanosoma brucei* subsp. *gambiense* and *rhodensiense)*

Color Key:

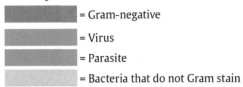

= Gram-negative

= Virus

= Parasite

= Bacteria that do not Gram stain

Appendix M: Characteristic AIDS-Defining Infectious Diseases

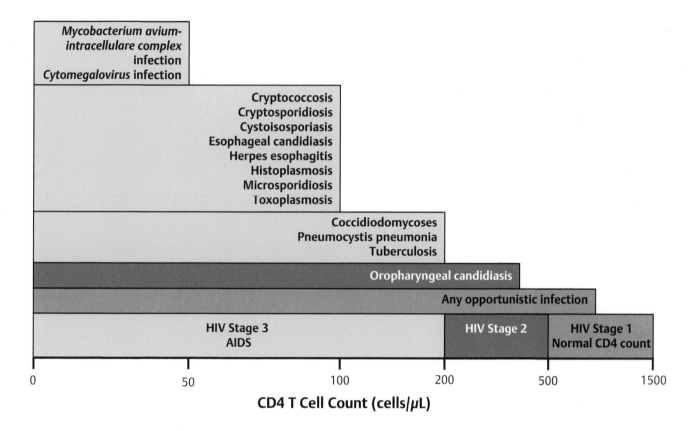

CD4 T Cell Count (cells/µL)

Appendix N: Viruses

Virus	Family	Genome	Envelope	Disease/Clinical Signs
Herpes simplex virus-1 (HSV-1) (HHV-1)	Herpesvirus	ds-DNA	Yes	• Vesicular orolabial and genital lesions • Meningoencephalitis • Keratitis (classically with dendritic ulcers)
Herpes simplex virus-2 (HSV-2) (HHV-2)	Herpesvirus	ds-DNA	Yes	• Vesicular genital lesions • Meningoencephalitis, including neonates after vaginal delivery
Varicella zoster virus (HHV-3)	Herpesvirus	ds-DNA	Yes	• Varicella or "chickenpox" • Herpes zoster of "shingles"; may be complicated by post-herpetic neuralgia

Epstein–Barr virus (HHV-4)	Herpesvirus	ds-DNA	Yes	• Infectious mononucleosis
				• EBV-associated lymphoproliferative diseases:
				  o Burkitt lymphoma
				  o Nasopharyngeal cancer
				  o Post-transplant lymphoproliferative disorder

Cytomegalovirus (HHV-5)	Herpesvirus	ds-DNA	Yes	• Infectious mononucleosis • Retinitis • Pneumonitis • Esophagitis • Hepatitis • Gastroenteritis • Congenital CMV syndrome
Human herpes virus-6 (HHV-6)	Herpesvirus	ds-DNA	Yes	• Roseola infantum or "Sixth disease"
Human herpes virus-8 (HHV-8)	Herpesvirus	ds-DNA	Yes	• Kaposi sarcoma (classically in AIDS)
Adenovirus	Adenovirus	ds-DNA	No	• Conjunctivitis • Gastroenteritis • Genitourinary infection • Respiratory infection
BK virus JC virus	Polyomavirus	ds-DNA	No	• BK: Polyomavirus nephropathy • JC: Progressive multifocal leukoencephalopathy
Human papillomavirus (HPV)	Papillomavirus	ds-DNA	No	• Condylomata acuminate or "genital warts" (low-risk HPV: 6, 11) • Cervical cancer (high-risk HPV: 16, 18, 31, 33) • Head and neck papilloma and squamous cell cancer
Molluscum contagiosum virus	Poxvirus	ds-DNA	Yes	• Molluscum contagiosum (pink/white papules with characteristic central umbilication)
Variola (smallpox) virus	Poxvirus	ds-DNA	Yes	• Smallpox; officially eradicated in 1980
Parvovirus B19	Parvovirus	ss-DNA	No	• Erythema infectiosum or "Fifth disease" • Hydrops fetalis if *in utero* infection • Aplastic crisis in sickle cell disease
Hepatitis A virus (HAV)	Picornavirus	(+) ss-RNA	No	• Self-limited acute hepatitis • Fecal-oral transmission

(Continued)

Virus	Family	Genome	Envelope	Disease/Clinical Signs
Hepatitis B virus (HBV)	Hepadnavirus	Partial ds-DNA, circular genome	Yes	• Acute, fulminant, and/or chronic hepatitis • May cause cirrhosis and hepatocellular cancer • Parenteral transmission
Hepatitis C virus (HCV)	Flavivirus	(+) ss-RNA	Yes	• Chronic hepatitis • May cause cirrhosis and hepatocellular cancer • Parenteral transmission
Hepatitis D virus (HDV)	Deltavirus	(−) ss-RNA	Yes	• Requires HBV for infection • Super-infection has worse prognosis than co-infection • Parenteral transmission
Hepatitis E virus (HEV)	Hepevirus	(+) ss-RNA	No	• Self-limited acute hepatitis • Fecal-oral transmission • 20% mortality rate in pregnant women
Coxsackie virus (a non-polio enterovirus)	Picornavirus	(+) ss-RNA	No	• Hand, foot, and mouth disease and herpangina • Myocarditis, pericarditis • Aseptic meningitis
Echovirus (a non-polio enterovirus)	Picornavirus	(+) ss-RNA	No	• Carditis • Aseptic meningitis
Polio virus (an enterovirus)	Picornavirus	(+) ss-RNA	No	• Poliomyelitis
Rhinovirus	Picornavirus	(+) ss-RNA	No	• Upper respiratory tract infection of the "common cold"
Norovirus	Calicivirus	(+) ss-RNA	No	• Gastroenteritis
Human immunodeficiency virus (HIV)	Retrovirus	(+) ss-RNA	Yes	• Acquired immunodeficiency syndrome (AIDS)
Human T cell lymphotropic virus (HTLV)	Retrovirus	(+) ss-RNA	Yes	• T cell leukemia and lymphoma
Human coronavirus	Coronavirus	(+) ss-RNA	Yes	• Respiratory infection: common cold
Severe Acute Respiratory Syndrome coronavirus (SARS-CoV)	Coronavirus	(+) ss-RNA	Yes	• Respiratory infection: SARS
Middle East Respiratory Syndrome coronavirus (MERS-CoV)	Picornavirus	(+) ss-RNA	Yes	• Respiratory infection: MERS
Influenza viruses A, B, C	Orthomyxovirus	(−) ss-RNA Segmented genome	Yes	• Respiratory infection: influenza • May be complicated by secondary *Staphylococcus aureus* bacterial pneumonia
Measles virus	Paramyxovirus	(−) ss-RNA	Yes	• Measles
Mumps virus	Paramyxovirus	(−) ss-RNA	Yes	• Mumps: may cause parotitis, orchitis, pancreatitis
Parainfluenza virus	Paramyxovirus	(−) ss-RNA	Yes	• Laryngotracheobronchitis or "croup" in young children
Respiratory syncytial virus (RSV)	Paramyxovirus	(−) ss-RNA	Yes	• Respiratory infection: bronchiolitis is babies
Rubella virus	Togavirus	(+) ss-RNA	Yes	• Rubella in kids/adults • Congenital rubella syndrome
Alphavirus Chikungunya	Togavirus	(+) ss-RNA	Yes	• Febrile illness

Virus	Family	Genome	Envelope	Disease/Clinical Signs

Alphavirus
  Eastern equine encephalitis
  Western equine encephalitis
  Venezuelan equine encephalitis
	Togavirus	(+) ss-RNA	Yes	• Encephalitis

Dengue virus	Flavivirus	(+) ss-RNA	Yes	• Hemorrhagic and "break-bone" fever
West Nile virus	Flavivirus	(+) ss-RNA	Yes	• Flu-like syndrome • Meningoencephalitis
Yellow fever virus	Flavivirus	(+) ss-RNA	Yes	• Hemorrhagic fever
Zika virus	Flavivirus	(+) ss-RNA	Yes	• Zika fever
Ebola virus Marburg virus	Filovirus	(−) ss-RNA	Yes	• Hemorrhagic fever
Hantavirus	Bunyavirus	(−) ss-RNA	Yes	• Hemorrhagic fever
California encephalitis virus Lacrosse virus	Bunyavirus	(−) ss-RNA	Yes	• Encephalitis
Rabies virus	Rhabdovirus	(−) ss-RNA	Yes	• Rabies
Rotavirus	Reovirus	ds-RNA	No	• Gastroenteritis
Colorado tick virus	Reovirus	ds-RNA	No	• Febrile illness
Lassa virus	Arenavirus	Ambisense RNA	Yes	• Febrile illness; possible hemorrhagic fever

Color Key:

Red = DNA virus

Blue = RNA virus

Appendix O: Hepatitis

	Hepatitis A virus (HAV)	Hepatitis B virus (HBV)	Hepatitis C virus (HCV)	Hepatitis D virus (HDV)	Hepatitis E virus (HEV)
Alternative name	Infectious	Serum	Non-A, non-B Posttransfusion	Delta agent	Enteric Non-A, non-B
Virus properties	Picornavirus SS +RNA	Hepadnavirus DS DNA	Flavivirus SS +RNA	Incomplete virion RNA	Hepevirus SS +RNA
Transmission	Fecal-oral	Body fluids: blood, semen, other fluids Vertical	Primary: contaminated blood Other: sexual, vertical	Needs HBV to replicate; see HBV	Fecal-oral
Average incubation (days)	28	120	45	See HBV	40
Chronicity	No	Yes	Yes	Yes	No
Long-term sequelae of chronic infections	None; no chronic form	Cirrhosis, liver failure, hepatocellular carcinoma	Cirrhosis, hepatocellular carcinoma	See HBV	None; no chronic form
Serology	Acute: IgM anti-HAV Convalescent: IgG anti-HAV Past infection/immunity: total anti-HAV	IgM anti-HBc: acute HBsAg: acute; chronic (> 6 months) Total anti-HBc: acute, chronic, resolved Anti-HBs: recovery/immunity	Cannot distinguish acute from chronic Anti-HCV HCV RNA	Anti-HDV: present in co-infections and superinfections	Acute: IgM anti-HEV Late acute and convalescent: IgG anti-HEV
Vaccination	Inactivated	Recombinant	None	None	None
Antimicrobial	None	Pegylated interferon alpha 2a, entecavir, tenofovir	Interferon Protease (NS3/4A) inhibitors NS5A inhibitors Polymerase (NS5B) inhibitors	See HBV	None

Abbreviations: DS, double stranded; HBc, hepatitis B core; HBsAg, hepatitis B surface antigen; Ig, immunoglobulin; SS, single stranded.

Appendix P: Parasite

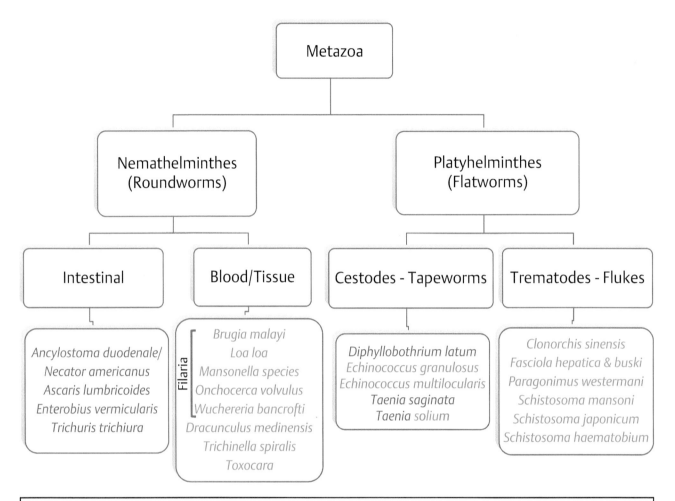

Color Key:
Intestinal pathogens are listed in red.
Blood and tissue parasites are in green.
Some parasites may affect both the gastrointestinal system and the blood and tissue. Those parasites are listed in both red and green.

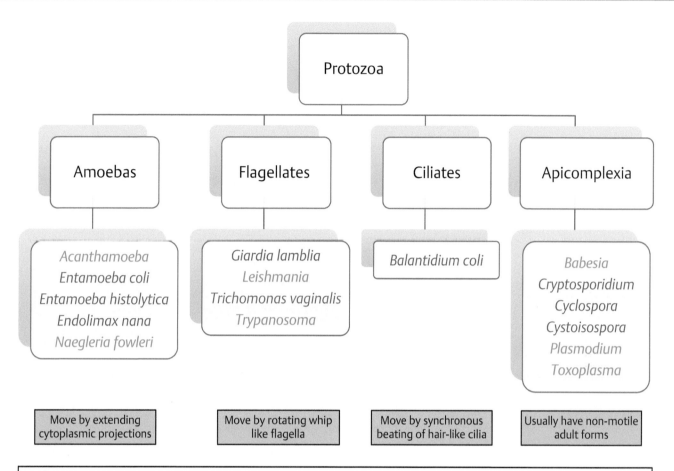

Protozoa

| Amoebas | Flagellates | Ciliates | Apicomplexia |

Amoebas
Acanthamoeba
Entamoeba coli
Entamoeba histolytica
Endolimax nana
Naegleria fowleri

Flagellates
Giardia lamblia
Leishmania
Trichomonas vaginalis
Trypanosoma

Ciliates
Balantidium coli

Apicomplexia
Babesia
Cryptosporidium
Cyclospora
Cystoisospora
Plasmodium
Toxoplasma

| Move by extending cytoplasmic projections | Move by rotating whip like flagella | Move by synchronous beating of hair-like cilia | Usually have non-motile adult forms |

Color Key:
Intestinal pathogens are listed in red.
Urogenital pathogens in blue.
Blood and tissue parasites are in green.
Some parasites may affect both the gastrointestinal system and the blood and tissue. Those parasites are listed in both red and green.

Index